Nur...
Diag...

i

Handbook of
Nursing
Diagnosis

14TH EDITION

Lynda Juall Carpenito, RN, MSN, CRNP
Family Nurse Practitioner
ChesPenn Health Services
Chester, Pennsylvania
Nursing Consultant
Mullica Hill, New Jersey

 Wolters Kluwer | Lippincott Williams & Wilkins
Health

Philadelphia · Baltimore · New York · London
Buenos Aires · Hong Kong · Sydney · Tokyo

Acquisitions Editor: Patrick Barbera   *Illustration Coordinator:* Brett MacNaughton
Supervising Product Manager: Betsy Gentzler   *Manufacturing Coordinator:* Karin Duffield
Editorial Assistant: Jacalyn Clay   *Prepress Vendor:* S4Carlisle, Inc.
Design Coordinator: Joan Wendt

14th Edition

9 8 7 6 5 4 3 2 1

Printed in China.

Library of Congress Cataloging-in-Publication Data
Carpenito, Lynda Juall.
  Handbook of nursing diagnosis / Lynda Juall Carpenito. — 14th ed.
    p. cm.
  Summary: "This handbook is the ideal quick reference to nursing diagnoses and collaborative problems authored by the foremost authority on NANDA International diagnoses. The practical, easy-access format helps you reach accurate nursing diagnoses with speed and confidence. Sections cover nursing diagnoses, health promotion and wellness diagnoses, collaborative problems, and diagnostic clusters"— Provided by publisher.
  Includes bibliographical references and index.
  ISBN 978-1-60831-110-1 (pbk.)
  1. Nursing diagnosis—Handbooks, manuals, etc. I. Title.
  RT48.6.C385 2013
  616.07′5—dc23

                        2012015988

Care has been taken to confirm the accuracy of the information presented and to describe generally accepted practices. However, the author, editors, and publisher are not responsible for errors or omissions or for any consequences from application of the information in this book and make no warranty, expressed or implied, with respect to the currency, completeness, or accuracy of the contents of the publication. Application of this information in a particular situation remains the professional responsibility of the practitioner; the clinical treatments described and recommended may not be considered absolute and universal recommendations.

The author, editors, and publisher have exerted every effort to ensure that drug selection and dosage set forth in this text are in accordance with the current recommendations and practice at the time of publication. However, in view of ongoing research, changes in government regulations, and the constant flow of information relating to drug therapy and drug reactions, the reader is urged to check the package insert for each drug for any change in indications and dosage and for added warnings and precautions. This is particularly important when the recommended agent is a new or infrequently employed drug.

Some drugs and medical devices presented in this publication have Food and Drug Administration (FDA) clearance for limited use in restricted research settings. It is the responsibility of the health care provider to ascertain the FDA status of each drug or device planned for use in his or her clinical practice.

To Olen, my son

for your wisdom and commitment to justice

for our quiet moments and embraces

for Olen Jr. and Aiden

for your presence in my life

. . . I am grateful

for you are my daily reminder of what is

really important . . .

love, health, and human trust

Preface

Many nurses, and even some faculty, question the usefulness of nursing diagnosis. Unfortunately, nursing diagnosis is still joined at the hip with traditional care planning. It is time to separate these conjoined twins so that both can function separately. Nursing diagnosis defines the science and art of nursing. It is as imperative to nurses and the nursing profession as medical diagnoses are to physicians. It serves to organize nursing's knowledge in the literature, in research, and in the clinician's mind. Do not underestimate the importance of this classification. A clinician with expertise in nursing diagnoses can hypothesize several explanations for a client's anger, such as fear, anxiety, grieving, powerlessness, or spiritual distress. Without this knowledge, the client is simply angry.

Care planning as it is taught in schools of nursing is an academic exercise. This is not wrong, but as the student progresses into the senior year, this academic care plan must be transformed into a clinically useful product. Students will progress to utilizing a standardized care plan *rather* than creating them. Copying from books, such as this one, does not enhance one's knowledge of nursing diagnosis and critical analysis. Students should start with a standardized document (electronic or pre-printed) and then revise it according to the specific data they have acquired while caring for their client. For example, each student would have a standardized care plan for an individual experiencing abdominal surgery. If the person also has diabetes mellitus, then the collaborative problem *Risk for Complications of Hypoglycemia/Hyperglycemia* would be added with monitoring interventions. If another client, post emergency abdominal surgery from motor vehicle trauma, lost his wife in the accident, then *Grieving* would be added.

Faculty, nurse managers, administrators, and clinicians need to do their part. Change is imperative. Nursing must defend its right to determine its documentation requirements, just as medicine has. If nursing continues to do business as usual, nursing as we want it—nursing as clients need it—will cease to exist. Nursing will continue to be defined by what we do and write and not by what we know.

From goals to specific interventions, *Handbook of Nursing Diagnosis* focuses on nursing. It provides a condensed, organized outline of clinical nursing practice designed to communicate creative clinical nursing. It is not meant to replace nursing textbooks, but rather to provide nurses who work in a variety of settings with the information they need without requiring a time-consuming review of the literature. It will assist students in transferring their theoretical knowledge to clinical practice; it can also be used by experienced nurses to recall past learning and to intervene in those clinical situations that previously went ignored or unrecognized.

The 14th edition is organized in three sections, with additional content available online. Section 1, Nursing Diagnoses, provides an alphabetical reference to nursing diagnoses, including Author's Notes and interventions for nursing care. Section 2 focuses on Health Promotion/Wellness Nursing Diagnoses. Section 3, Diagnostic Clusters, presents medical conditions with associated collaborative problems and nursing diagnoses, designed for easy reference in the clinical setting. Additional content for selected collaborative problems and sample generic care plans are available online at *http://thePoint.lww.com/CarpenitoHB14e*, using the access code printed in the front of this text.

Lynda Juall Carpenito, RN, MSN, CRNP

Contents

Introduction   1

Section 2

Health Promotion/Wellness Nursing Diagnoses ... 693

Section 3

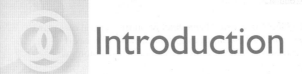

Introduction

Creating a Care Plan for Your Client

Step 1: Complete the Assessment From Your Course or the Agency

Ask your instructor which format to use.

Step 2: Refer to Section 3 Diagnostic Clusters in This Book for the Primary Medical Diagnosis of Your Client

Diagnoses such as:

- Diabetes mellitus
- Pneumonia
- Heart failure

OR

the surgical procedure the client has had such as:

- Abdominal surgery
- Hysterectomy
- Total joint replacement

Note: If a diagnostic cluster is not relevant to your assigned client, proceed to Step 3.

Step 3: Refer to http://thePoint.lww.com/ CarpenitoHB14e for Sample General Care Plans

For a general care plan with goals, interventions, and rationales for all hospitalized persons or a general care plan for all persons having surgery, collect a care plan from thePoint. These plans focus on the usual nursing diagnoses and collaborative problems present for persons admitted for medical problems or surgical procedures. Save the care plan to your computer so you can do the following:

- Add risk factors to the general care plan from your assessment data of your client.
- Delete or revise goals/interventions not useful for your client.

- Add additional priority diagnoses not on the general care plan, such as *Risk for Complications of Unstable Blood Glucose Level* if the person has diabetes mellitus and has had abdominal surgery.
- You can start your care plan with one of these plans. Now you will review the assessment data on your assigned client in Step 4.

 Carp's Cues

> You can find general medical and surgical care plans on thePoint. Consult you instructor on how you can use these general care plans.

Step 4: Identify the Client's Risk

Factors

Risk factors are situations, personal characteristics, disabilities, or medical conditions that can hinder the person's ability to heal, cope with stressors, and progress to his or her original health prior to hospitalization, illness, or surgery.

Before hospitalization:

- Did the client have an effective support system?
- Could the client perform self-care? Bathing? Feeding self?
- Did the client need assistance (e.g., ADLs, housekeeping, transportation)?
- Could the client walk unassisted?
- Did the client have memory problems?
- Did the client have hearing problems?
- Did the client smoke cigarettes?
- Did the client abuse alcohol or drugs?

What conditions or diseases does the client have that make him or her more vulnerable to:

- Falling
- Infection
- Nutrition/fluid imbalance
- Pressure ulcers
- High anxiety
- Physiologic instability (e.g., electrolytes, blood glucose, blood pressure, respiratory function, healing problems)

When you meet the assigned client, determine if any of the risk factors are present:

- Obesity
- Communication problems
- Movement difficulties
- Inadequate nutritional status
- Recent or ongoing stress (e.g., financial, death in family)

Write significant data on index card:

- Hearing problems
- No or ineffective support system
- Unhealthy lifestyle (e.g., little regular exercise, smokes, poor nutritional habits)
- Learning difficulties
- Ineffective coping skills (e.g., angry, depressed, unmotivated, denial)
- Obesity
- Fatigue
- Financial problems
- Negative self-efficacy
- Self-care difficulties

 Carp's Cues

Risk factors can be used as additional related factors for a nursing diagnosis on the general plan such as:

- *Anxiety* related to loss of job and hospital costs
- *Risk for Infection* related to compromised healing secondary to excess adipose tissue (obesity)

OR

An additional nursing diagnosis not on the general plan as:

- *Ineffective Self-Health Management* related to insufficient knowledge of risks and strategies to quit smoking
- *Impaired Verbal Communication* related to unavailable interpreter and compromised hearing
- *Ineffective Denial* related to continued smoking despite recent deep vein thrombosis
- *Fatigue* (refer to Related Factors under *Fatigue*)
- *Impaired Memory* (refer to Related Factors under *Impaired Memory*)

Step 5: Identify Strengths

Strengths are qualities or factors that will help the person to recover, cope with stressors, and progress to his or her original health (or as close as possible) prior to hospitalization, illness, or surgery. Examples of strengths are as follows:

- Positive spiritual framework
- Positive support system
- Ability to perform self-care
- No eating difficulties
- Effective sleep habits

- Alertness and good memory
- Financial stability
- Ability to relax most of the time
- Motivation, resiliency
- Positive self-esteem
- Internal locus of control
- Self-responsibility
- Positive belief that they will improve (self-efficacy)

Write a list on a card of the strengths of your assigned client and of their support systems.

The strengths of the client and of their support systems can be used to motivate them to cope with some difficult activities. Strengths are not nursing diagnoses, risks, or related factors. They are to be considered in planning care. For example, a person with a strong religious affiliation and a new cancer diagnosis may benefit from a dialogue session with their religious leader.

Step 6: Create Your Initial Care Plan

Print the general care plan (medical, surgical) for your assigned client. These general care plans reflect the usual, predicted care a client needs. Ask your instructor how you can use them to prevent excessive writing.

 Carp's Cues

In the remaining steps, collaborative problems are discussed. If you do not know about them, please refer to the section that follows care planning on the Bifocal Clinical Practice Model.

Step 7: Review the Collaborative Problems on the General Plan

Review the collaborative problems listed. These are the physiologic complications that you need to monitor. Do not delete any because they all relate to the condition or procedure that your client has had. You will need to add how often you should take vital signs, record intake and output, change dressings, etc. Ask the nurse to whom you are assigned for the frequency of monitoring.

Review each intervention for collaborative problems. Are any interventions unsafe or contraindicated for your client? For example, if your client has edema and renal problems, the fluid requirements may be too high for him or her. Ask a nurse or instructor for help here.

Review the collaborative problems on the general plan. Also review all additional collaborative problems that you found that are related to any medical or treatment problems. For example, if your client has diabetes mellitus, you need to add *Risk for Complications of Unstable Blood Glucose Level.*

Step 8: Review the Nursing Diagnoses on the General Plan

Review each nursing diagnosis on the plan.

- Does it apply to your assigned client?
- Does your client have any risk factors (see your index card) that could make this diagnosis worse?

An example on the General Medical Care Plan is *Risk for Injury related to unfamiliar environment and physical or mental limitations secondary to condition, medication, therapies, or diagnostic tests.*

Now look at your list of risk factors for your assigned client. Can any factors listed contribute to the client sustaining an injury? For example, is he or she having problems walking or seeing? Is he or she experiencing dizziness?

If your client has an unstable gait related to peripheral vascular disease (PVD), you would add the following diagnosis: *Risk for Injury related to unfamiliar environment and unstable gait secondary to peripheral vascular disease.*

Review each intervention for each nursing diagnosis:

- Are they relevant for your client?
- Will you have time to provide them?
- Are any interventions not appropriate or contraindicated for your assigned client?
- Can you add any specific interventions?
- Do you need to modify any interventions because of risk factors (see index card)?

Review the goals listed for the nursing diagnosis:

- Are they pertinent to your client?
- Can the client demonstrate achievement of the goal on the day you provide care?
- Do you need more time?
- Do you need to make the goal more specific for your client?

Delete goals that are inappropriate for your client. If your client will need more time to meet the goal, add "by discharge." If the client can accomplish the goal this day, write "by (insert date)" after the goal.

Using the same diagnosis *Risk for Injury related to unfamiliar environment and physical and mental limitations secondary to the condition, therapies, and diagnostic tests,* consider this goal:

- The client will request assistance with ADLs.

Indicators

- Identify factors that increase risk of injury.
- Describe appropriate safety measures.

If it is realistic for your client to achieve all the goals on the day of your care, you should add the date to all of them. If your client is confused, you can add the date to the main goal, but you would delete all the indicators because the person is confused. Or you could modify the goal by writing:

- Family member will identify factors that increase the client's risk of injury.

Remember that you cannot individualize a care plan for a client until you spend time with him or her, but you can add or delete interventions based on your preclinical knowledge of the client (e.g., medical diagnosis, coexisting medical conditions).

Step 9: Prepare the Care Plan (Written or Printed)

You can prepare the care plan by:

- Saving the online general care plan onto your computer, then deleting or adding specifics for your client (use another color or a different type font for additions/deletions), and printing it.
- Writing the care plan.

Ask your faculty person what options are acceptable. Using different colors or fonts allows your instructor to clearly see your analysis. Be prepared to provide rationales for why you added or deleted items.

Step 10: Initial Care Plan Completed

Now that you have a care plan of the collaborative problems and nursing diagnoses, which ones are associated with the primary condition for which your client was admitted? If your assigned client is a healthy adult undergoing surgery or was admitted for an acute medical problem and you have not assessed any significant factors in Step 1, you have completed the initial care plan. Go to Step 12.

Step 11: Additional Risk Factors

If your client has risk factors (on the index card) that you identified in Steps 1 and 2, evaluate if these risk factors make your assigned client more vulnerable to develop a problem. The following questions can help to determine if the client or family has additional diagnoses that need nursing interventions:

- Are additional collaborative problems associated with coexisting medical conditions that require monitoring? For example, if the client has diabetes mellitus, add *Risk for Complications of Unstable Blood Glucose Level.*
- Are there additional nursing diagnoses that, if not managed or prevented now, will deter recovery or affect the client's functional status? For example, a client who has recently experienced a death of a significant person needs *Grieving* added to the plan.

You can address nursing diagnoses not on the priority list by referring the client for assistance after discharge (e.g., counseling, weight loss program).

Step 12: Evaluate the Status of Your Client (After You Provide Care)

Collaborative Problems
Review the nursing goals for the collaborative problems:

- Assess the client's status.
- Compare the data to established norms (indicators).
- Judge if the data fall within acceptable ranges.
- Conclude if the client is stable, improved, unimproved, or worse.

Is your client stable or improved?

- If yes, continue to monitor the client and provide interventions indicated.
- If not, has there been a dramatic change (e.g., elevated blood pressure and decreased urinary output)? Have you notified the physician or advanced practice nurse? Have you increased your monitoring of the client? Communicate your evaluations of the status of collaborative problems to your clinical faculty and to the nurse assigned to your client.

Nursing Diagnosis
Review the goals or outcome criteria for each nursing diagnosis. Did the client demonstrate or state the activity defined in the goal? If yes, then document the achievement on your plan. If not and the client needs more time, change the target date. If time is not the issue, evaluate why the client did not achieve the goal. Was the goal:

- Not realistic because of other priorities?
- Not acceptable to the client?

Step 13: Document the Care You Provided and the Client's Responses on the Agency's Forms, Flow Records, and Progress Notes

Nursing Diagnoses Versus Collaborative Problems*

In 1983, Carpenito published the Bifocal Clinical Practice Model. In this model, nurses are accountable to treat two types of clinical judgments or diagnoses: nursing diagnoses and collaborative problems.

Nursing diagnoses are clinical judgments about individual, family, or community responses to actual or potential health problems/life processes. Nursing diagnoses provide the basis for selection of nursing interventions to achieve outcomes for which the nurse has accountability (NANDA, 1998; NANDA-I, 2012).

Collaborative problems are certain physiologic complications that nurses monitor to detect onset or changes in status. Nurses manage collaborative problems using physician-prescribed and nurse-prescribed interventions to minimize the complications of the events (Carpenito, 2013).

Nursing interventions are classified as nurse-prescribed or physician-prescribed. Nurse-prescribed interventions are those that the nurse can legally order for nursing staff to implement. Nurse-prescribed interventions treat, prevent, and monitor nursing diagnoses. Nurse-prescribed interventions manage and monitor collaborative problems. Physician-prescribed interventions represent treatments for collaborative problems that the nurse initiates and manages. Collaborative problems require both nursing-prescribed and physician-prescribed interventions. Box 1 represents these relationships.

The following illustrates the types of interventions associated with the collaborative problem *Risk for Complications of Hypoxemia:*

NP   1. Monitor for signs of acid-base imbalance.
NP/PP   2. Administer low flow oxygen as needed.
NP   3. Ensure adequate hydration.
NP   4. Evaluate the effects of positioning on oxygenation.
NP/PP   5. Administer medications as needed.
(NP: Nurse-prescribed; PP: Physician/Nurse-Practitioner-prescribed)

---

* The terminology for collaborative problems has been changed to Risk for Complications of (specify) from Potential Complications: (specify).

Box I RELATIONSHIP BETWEEN NURSING-PRESCRIBED INTERVENTIONS AND PHYSICIAN-PRESCRIBED INTERVENTIONS

Nursing-Prescribed Interventions

- Reposition q2h
- Lightly massage vulnerable areas
- Teach how to reduce pressure when sitting

Nursing Diagnoses

Risk for Impaired Skin Integrity related to immobility secondary to fatigue

Physician-Prescribed Interventions

Usually not needed

Nursing-Prescribed Interventions

- Maintain NPO state
- Monitor:
  Hydration
  Vital signs
  Intake/output
  Specific gravity
- Monitor electrolytes
- Maintain IV at prescribed rate
- Provide/encourage mouth care

Collaborative Problems

Risk for Complications of Fluid and Electrolyte Imbalances

Physician-Prescribed Interventions

- IV (type, amount)
- Laboratory studies

Selection of Collaborative Problems

As mentioned earlier, collaborative problems are different from nursing diagnoses. The nurse makes independent decisions regarding both collaborative problems and nursing diagnoses. The decisions differ in that, for nursing diagnoses, the nurse prescribes the definitive treatment for the situation and is responsible for outcome achievement; for collaborative problems, the nurse monitors the client's condition to detect onset or status of physiologic complications and manages the events with nursing- and physician-prescribed interventions. Collaborative problems are as follows:

Risk for Complications of Bleeding
Risk for Complications of Kidney Failure

The physiologic complications that nurses monitor usually are related to disease, trauma, treatments, and diagnostic studies. The following examples illustrate some collaborative problems:

Situation	Collaborative Problem
Anticoagulant therapy	*Risk for Complications of Bleeding*
Pneumonia	*Risk for Complications of Hypoxemia*

Outcome criteria or client goals are used to measure the effectiveness of nursing care. When a client is not progressing to goal achievement or has worsened, the nurse must reevaluate the situation. Box 2 represents the questions to be considered. If none of these options is appropriate, the situation may not be a nursing diagnosis.

Collaborative problems have nursing goals that represent the accountability of the nurse—to detect early changes and to co-manage with physicians. Nursing diagnoses have client goals that represent the accountability of the nurse—to achieve or maintain a favorable status after nursing care. Box 3 includes frequently used collaborative problems.

Box 2   EVALUATION QUESTIONS

Is the diagnosis correct?
Has the goal been mutually set?
Is more time needed for the plan to work?
Does the goal need to be revised?
Do the interventions need to be revised?

Box 3   CONDITIONS THAT NECESSITATE NURSING CARE

Nursing Diagnoses*

1. Health Perception—Health Management
    Contamination
        Contamination, Risk for
    Energy Field, Disturbed
    Growth and Development, Delayed
        Development, Risk for Delayed
        Failure to Thrive, Adult
        Growth, Risk for Disproportionate
    Health, Deficient Community
    Health Behavior, Risk-Prone
    Health Maintenance, Ineffective
    Immunization Status, Readiness for Enhanced
    Injury, Risk for
        Aspiration, Risk for
        Falls, Risk for
        Perioperative Positioning Injury, Risk for
        Poisoning, Risk for
        Suffocation, Risk for
        Thermal Injury, Risk for
        Trauma, Risk for
    Noncompliance
    Self-Health Management, Ineffective
    †Self-Health Management, Ineffective Community
    †Self-Health Management, Ineffective Family
    Self-Health Management, Readiness for Enhanced
    Surgical Recovery, Delayed

2. Nutritional—Metabolic
    Adverse Reaction to Iodinated Contrast Media, Risk for
    Allergy Response, Risk for
    Blood Glucose Level, Risk for Unstable
    Body Temperature, Risk for Imbalanced
        Hyperthermia
        Hypothermia
        Thermoregulation, Ineffective

(continued on page 12)

Box 3 CONDITIONS THAT NECESSITATE NURSING CARE (continued)

Breastfeeding, Ineffective
Breastfeeding, Interrupted
Breastfeeding, Readiness for Enhanced
Breast Milk, Insufficient
Electrolyte Imbalances, Risk for
Fluid Balance, Readiness for Enhanced
Fluid Volume, Deficient
    Fluid Volume, Risk for Deficient
Fluid Volume, Excess
Fluid Volume, Risk for Imbalanced
Infection, Risk for
†Infection Transmission, Risk for
Jaundice, Neonatal
    Jaundice, Risk for Neonatal
Latex Allergy Response
    Latex Allergy Response, Risk for
Nutrition, Imbalanced: Less Than Body Requirements
    Dentition, Impaired
    Infant Feeding Pattern, Ineffective
    Swallowing, Impaired
Nutrition, Imbalanced: More Than Body Requirements
    Nutrition, Imbalanced: More Than Body Requirements, Risk for
Nutrition, Readiness for Enhanced
Protection, Ineffective
    Dry Eye, Risk for
    Oral Mucous Membrane, Impaired
    Skin Integrity, Impaired
    Skin Integrity, Risk for Impaired
    Tissue Integrity, Impaired

3. Elimination
Bowel Incontinence
Constipation
    Constipation, Perceived
Diarrhea
Gastrointestinal Motility, Dysfunctional
    Gastrointestinal Motility, Risk for Dysfunctional
Urinary Elimination, Impaired
    †Continuous Urinary Incontinence

Box 3   CONDITIONS THAT NECESSITATE NURSING CARE (continued)

Functional Urinary Incontinence
Maturational Enuresis
Overflow Urinary Incontinence
Reflex Urinary Incontinence
Stress Urinary Incontinence
Urge Urinary Incontinence
Urge Urinary Incontinence, Risk for
Urinary Elimination, Readiness for Enhanced

4. Activity—Exercise
Activity Intolerance
Activity Planning, Ineffective
Activity Planning, Risk for Ineffective
Bleeding, Risk for
Cardiac Output, Decreased
Disuse Syndrome, Risk for
Diversional Activity, Deficient
Home Maintenance, Impaired
Infant Behavior, Disorganized
Infant Behavior, Risk for Disorganized
Infant Behavior, Readiness for Enhanced Organized
Intracranial Adaptive Capacity, Decreased
Lifestyle, Sedentary
Liver Function, Risk for Impaired
Mobility, Impaired Physical
Bed Mobility, Impaired
Transfer Ability, Impaired
Walking, Impaired
Wheelchair Mobility, Impaired
†Respiratory Function, Risk for Ineffective
Airway Clearance, Ineffective
Breathing Pattern, Ineffective
Gas Exchange, Impaired
Spontaneous Ventilation, Impaired
Ventilatory Weaning Response, Dysfunctional
†Ventilatory Weaning Response, Risk for Dysfunctional
Self-Care, Readiness for Enhanced
†Self-Care Deficit Syndrome
Feeding Self-Care Deficit

(continued on page 14)

Box 3 CONDITIONS THAT NECESSITATE NURSING CARE (continued)

    Bathing Self-Care Deficit
    Dressing Self-Care Deficit
    †Instrumental Self-Care Deficit
    Toileting Self-Care Deficit
Shock, Risk for
Sudden Infant Death Syndrome, Risk for
Tissue Perfusion, Ineffective
    Cardiac Tissue Perfusion, Risk for Decreased
    Cerebral Tissue Perfusion, Risk for Ineffective
    Gastrointestinal Tissue Perfusion, Risk for Ineffective
    Peripheral Neurovascular Dysfunction, Risk for
    Peripheral Tissue Perfusion, Ineffective
    Peripheral Tissue Perfusion, Risk for Ineffective
    Renal Perfusion, Risk for Ineffective
Vascular Trauma, Risk for
Wandering

5. Sleep—Rest
Sleep, Readiness for Enhanced
Sleep Pattern, Disturbed
    Insomnia
    Sleep Deprivation

6. Cognitive—Perceptual
Aspiration, Risk for
Comfort, Impaired
    Nausea
    Pain, Acute
    Pain, Chronic
Comfort, Readiness for Enhanced
Confusion, Acute
    Confusion, Risk for Acute
Confusion, Chronic
Decisional Conflict
Decision Making, Readiness for Enhanced
Dysreflexia, Autonomic
    Dysreflexia, Risk for Autonomic
Environmental Interpretation Syndrome, Impaired
Knowledge, Deficient
Knowledge (Specify), Readiness for Enhanced

Box 3 CONDITIONS THAT NECESSITATE NURSING CARE (continued)

Memory, Impaired
Neglect, Unilateral

7. Self-Perception
Anxiety
  Anxiety, Death
Fatigue
Fear
Hope, Readiness for Enhanced
Hopelessness
Human Dignity, Risk for Compromised
Neglect, Self
Power, Readiness for Enhanced
Powerlessness
  Powerlessness, Risk for
†Self-Concept, Distrubed
  Body Image, Disturbed
  Personal Identity, Disturbed
  Personal Identity, Risk for Disturbed
  Self-Esteem, Chronic Low
  Self-Esteem, Risk for Chronic Low
  †Self-Esteem, Disturbed
  Self-Esteem, Situational Low
  Self-Esteem, Risk for Situational Low
Self-Concept, Readiness for Enhanced

8. Role—Relationship
Childbearing Process, Ineffective
  Childbearing Process, Risk for Ineffective
†Communication, Impaired
  Communication, Impaired Verbal
Communication, Readiness for Enhanced
Family Processes, Dysfunctional
Family Processes, Interrupted
Family Processes, Readiness for Enhanced
Grieving
  †Grieving, Anticipatory
  Grieving, Complicated
  Grieving, Risk for Complicated

(continued on page 16)

Box 3   CONDITIONS THAT NECESSITATE NURSING CARE (continued)

Loneliness, Risk for
Parental Role Conflict
Parenting, Impaired
    Attachment, Risk for Impaired
Parenting, Readiness for Enhanced
Relationship, Ineffective
    Relationship, Risk for Ineffective
Relationship, Readiness for Enhanced
Role Performance, Ineffective
Social Interaction, Impaired
Social Isolation
Sorrow, Chronic

9. Sexuality—Reproductive

Childbearing Process, Readiness for Enhanced
Maternal/Fetal Dyad, Risk for Disturbed
Sexuality Patterns, Ineffective
    Sexual Dysfunction

10. Coping—Stress Tolerance

Caregiver Role Strain
    Caregiver Role Strain, Risk for
Coping, Compromised Family
Coping, Disabled Family
Coping, Ineffective
    Coping, Defensive
    Denial, Ineffective
    Impulse Control, Ineffective
Coping, Ineffective Community
Coping, Readiness for Enhanced
Coping, Readiness for Enhanced Community
Coping, Readiness for Enhanced Family
Post-Trauma Syndrome
    Post-Trauma Syndrome, Risk for
    Rape-Trauma Syndrome
Relocation Stress [Syndrome]
    Relocation Stress [Syndrome], Risk for
Resilience, Impaired Individual
Resilience, Readiness for Enhanced

Box 3   CONDITIONS THAT NECESSITATE NURSING CARE (continued)

Resilience, Risk for Compromised
†Self-Harm, Risk for
    Self-Mutilation
    Self-Mutilation, Risk for
    Suicide, Risk for
Stress Overload
Violence, Risk for Other-Directed
Violence, Risk for Self-Directed

11. Value—Belief
Moral Distress
    †Moral Distress, Risk for
Religiosity, Readiness for Enhanced
Spiritual Distress
    Religiosity, Impaired
    Religiosity, Risk for Impaired
    Spiritual Distress, Risk for
Spiritual Well-Being, Readiness for Enhanced

‡Collaborative Problems

Risk for Complications of Cardiac/Vascular Dysfunction
RC of Decreased Cardiac Output
RC of Dysrhythmias
RC of Pulmonary Edema
RC of Cardiogenic Shock
RC of Thromboembolic/Deep Vein Thrombosis
RC of Hypovolemia
RC of Peripheral Vascular Insufficiency
RC of Hypertension
RC of Congenital Heart Disease
RC of Angina
RC of Endocarditis
RC of Pulmonary Embolism
RC of Spinal Shock
RC of Ischemic Ulcers

Risk for Complications of Respiratory Dysfunction
RC of Hypoxemia

(continued on page 18)

Box 3 CONDITIONS THAT NECESSITATE NURSING CARE (continued)

RC of Atelectasis/Pneumonia
RC of Tracheobronchial Constriction
RC of Pleural Effusion
RC of Tracheal Necrosis
RC of Ventilator Dependency
RC of Pneumothorax
RC of Laryngeal Edema

Risk for Complications of Renal/Urinary Dysfunction
RC of Acute Urinary Retention
RC of Renal Failure
RC of Bladder Perforation
RC of Renal Calculi

Risk for Complications of Gastrointestinal/Hepatic/Biliary Dysfunction
RC of Paralytic Ileus/Small Bowel Obstruction
RC of Hepatic Failure
RC of Hyperbilirubinemia
RC of Evisceration
RC of Hepatosplenomegaly
RC of Curling's Ulcer
RC of Ascites
RC of Gastrointestinal Bleeding

Risk for Complications of Metabolic/Immune/Hematopoietic Dysfunction
RC of Hypoglycemia/Hyperglycemia
RC of Negative Nitrogen Balance
RC of Electrolyte Imbalances
RC of Thyroid Dysfunction
RC of Hypothermia (Severe)
RC of Hyperthermia (Severe)
RC of Sepsis
RC of Acidosis (Metabolic, Respiratory)
RC of Alkalosis (Metabolic, Respiratory)
RC of Hypo/Hyperthyroidism
RC of Allergic Reaction
RC of Donor Tissue Rejection
RC of Adrenal Insufficiency

Box 3   CONDITIONS THAT NECESSITATE NURSING CARE (continued)

RC of Anemia
RC of Thrombocytopenia
RC of Opportunistic Infection
RC of Polycythemia
RC of Sickling Crisis
RC of Disseminated Intravascular Coagulation

Risk for Complications of Neurological/Sensory Dysfunction

RC of Increased Intracranial Pressure
RC of Stroke
RC of Seizures
RC of Spinal Cord Compression
RC of Meningitis
RC of Cranial Nerve Impairment (Specify)
RC of Paralysis
RC of Peripheral Nerve Impairment
RC of Increased Intraocular Pressure
RC of Corneal Ulceration
RC of Neuropathies

Risk for Complications of Muscular/Skeletal Dysfunction

RC of Osteoporosis
RC of Joint Dislocation
RC of Compartment Syndrome
RC of Pathologic Fractures

Risk for Complications of Reproductive Dysfunction

RC of Fetal Distress
RC of Postpartum Bleeding
RC of Gestational Hypertension
RC of Hypermenorrhea
RC of Polymenorrhea
RC of Syphilis
RC of Prenatal Bleeding
RC of Preterm Labor

Risk for Complications of Medication Therapy Adverse Effects

RC of Adrenocorticosteroid Therapy Adverse Effects
RC of Antianxiety Therapy Adverse Effects

(continued on page 20)

> ## Box 3   CONDITIONS THAT NECESSITATE
> ##   NURSING CARE (continued)
>
> RC of Antiarrhythmic Therapy Adverse Effects
> RC of Anticoagulant Therapy Adverse Effects
> RC of Anticonvulsant Therapy Adverse Effects
> RC of Antidepressant Therapy Adverse Effects
> RC of Antihypertensive Therapy Adverse Effects
> RC of Beta-Adrenergic Blocker Therapy Adverse Effects
> RC of Calcium-Channel Blocker Therapy Adverse Effects
> RC of Angiotensin-Converting Enzyme Therapy Adverse Effects
> RC of Antineoplastic Therapy Adverse Effects
> RC of Antipsychotic Therapy Adverse Effects
> RC of Diuretic Therapy Adverse Effects

*The Functional Health Patterns were identified in Gordon, M. (1994).
   Nursing diagnosis: Process and application. New York: McGraw-Hill, with minor
   changes by the author.
†These diagnoses are not currently on the NANDA-I list but have been included for
   clarity and usefulness.
‡Frequently used collaborative problems are represented on this list. Other situations not
   listed here could qualify as collaborative problems.

Some physiologic complications, such as pressure ulcers and infection from invasive lines, are problems that nurses can prevent. Prevention is different from detection. Nurses do not prevent paralytic ileus but, instead, detect its presence early to prevent greater severity or even death. Physicians cannot treat collaborative problems without nursing knowledge, vigilance, and judgment.

Formulate Nursing Diagnoses Correctly

Types of Nursing Diagnoses

A nursing diagnosis can be actual, risk, or a wellness or syndrome type.

- *Actual:* An actual nursing diagnosis describes a clinical judgment that the nurse has validated because of the presence of major defining characteristics.
- *Risk:* A risk nursing diagnosis describes a clinical judgment that an individual/group is more vulnerable to develop the problem

than others in the same or a similar situation because of risk factors.

- *Wellness:* A wellness nursing diagnosis is a clinical judgment about an individual, family, or community in transition from a specific level of wellness to a higher level of wellness (NANDA-I, 2012).
- *Syndrome:* A syndrome diagnosis comprises a cluster of actual or risk nursing diagnoses that are predicted to present because of a certain situation or event.
- Possible nursing diagnosis is not a type of diagnosis as are actual, risk, and syndrome. Possible nursing diagnoses are a diagnostician's option to indicate that some data are present to confirm a diagnosis but are insufficient at this time.

Diagnostic Statements

The diagnostic statement describes the health status of an individual or group and the factors that have contributed to the status.

One-Part Statements
Wellness nursing diagnoses will be written as one-part statements: *Readiness for Enhanced* _____ (e.g., *Readiness for Enhanced Parenting*). Related factors are not present for wellness nursing diagnoses because they would all be the same: motivated to achieve a higher level of wellness. Syndrome diagnoses, such as *Rape-Trauma Syndrome*, have no "related to" designations.

Two-Part Statements
Risk and possible nursing diagnoses have two parts. The validation for a risk nursing diagnosis is the presence of risk factors. The risk factors are the second part, as in:

Risk Nursing Diagnosis Related to Risk Factors
Possible nursing diagnoses are suspected because of the presence of certain factors.

Two-Part Statement Examples
Risk for Impaired Skin Integrity related to immobility secondary to fractured hip
Possible Self-Care Deficit related to impaired ability to use left hand secondary to IV

Designating a diagnosis as possible provides the nurse with a method to communicate to other nurses that a diagnosis may be present. Additional data collection is indicated to rule out or confirm the tentative diagnosis.

Three-Part Statements

An actual nursing diagnosis consists of three parts.

Diagnostic label + contributing factors + signs and symptoms

The presence of major signs and symptoms (defining characteristics) validates that an actual diagnosis is present. This is the third part. It is not possible to have a third part for risk or possible diagnoses because signs and symptoms do not exist.

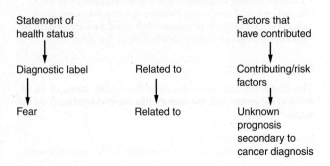

Three-Part Statement Examples

Anxiety related to unpredictable nature of asthmatic episodes as evident by statements of "I'm afraid I won't be able to breathe"

Urge Incontinence related to diminished bladder capacity secondary to habitual frequent voiding as evident by inability to hold off urination after desire to void and report of voiding out of habit, not need

The presence of a nursing diagnosis is determined by assessing the individual's health status and ability to function. Functional health patterns and the corresponding nursing diagnoses are listed in Box 3. If significant data are collected in a particular functional pattern, the next step is to check the related nursing diagnoses to see whether any of them are substantiated by the data that are collected.

Client Validation

The process of validating a nursing diagnosis should not be done in isolation from the client or family. Individuals are the experts on themselves. During assessments and interactions, nurses are provided a small glimpse of their clients. Diagnostic hunches or inferences about data should be discussed with clients for their input. Clients are given opportunities to select what they want assistance with, which problems are important to them, and which ones are not.

Clinical Example

After the screening assessment has been completed, the nurse applies each of the following questions to each functional or need area:

• Is there a possible problem in a specific area?
• Is the person at risk (or high risk) for a problem?
• Does the person desire to improve his/her health?

For example, after assessing a client's elimination pattern, the nurse would then analyze the data. Does this person have a possible problem with constipation or diarrhea? If yes, the nurse would then ask the person more focused questions to confirm

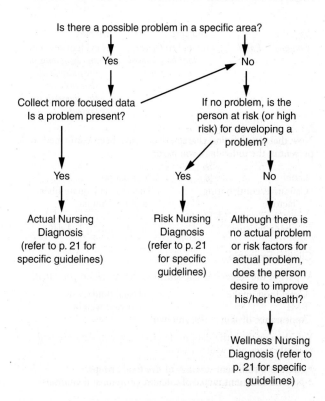

the presence of the defining characteristics of constipation or diarrhea. If these defining characteristics are not present, then there is no actual diagnosis of *Constipation or Diarrhea*. Is there a risk diagnosis? To determine this, the nurse will assess for risk factors of *Constipation or Diarrhea* (listed under related/risk factors). If none of these are present, there is no risk for *Constipation or Diarrhea*.

Lastly, if there is no actual or at risk elimination nursing diagnosis, the nurse can ask whether the individual would like to improve his or her elimination patterns. If the answer is yes, the wellness diagnosis *Potential for Enhanced Elimination* is the appropriate choice.

Actual Nursing Diagnoses

Actual nursing diagnoses are written in two- or three-part statements:

1st part	2nd part	3rd part
Diagnostic Label	related to *factors that have caused or contributed*	as evident by *signs and symptoms in the individual that indicate the diagnosis is present*

Now that the defining characteristics have been confirmed to be present in the individual, you have:

Label	Constipation
Causative/contributing factors:	related to inadequate fiber and fluid intake
Signs/symptoms: (defining characteristics)	as evident by reports of dry, hard stools, q 3–4 days

Clinical Example

As part of the screening assessment under nutrition you elicit:

Usual food intake	Usual fluid intake
BMI	Current weight
Appearance of skin, nails, and hair	

You then analyze the data to determine which data are within a normal range, and which are not:

• Are there sufficient servings of five food groups?
• Is there sufficient intake of calcium, protein, and vitamins?

- Is the fat intake <30% of total caloric intake?
- Does the person drink at least 6 to 8 cups of water besides coffee or soft drinks?
- Does the appearance of skin, hair, and nails reflect a healthy nutrition pattern?
- Is the person's weight within normal limits for height?

For example, in a specific person, Mr. Jewel, you find there is:

- Appropriate weight for height
- Insufficient fluid intake (four 8-oz. glasses of water/juice)
- Insufficient vegetable intake (two servings)
- Excess intake of bread, cereal, rice, and pasta (eight servings)
- Dry skin and hair

From your assessment, you have confirmed that a nursing diagnosis is present because the person has signs or reports symptoms that represent those listed as defining characteristics under that specific diagnosis. These are usually the person's complaints.

At this point, you have two parts of the diagnostic statement—the first and third, but not the second:

Imbalanced Nutrition: less than body requirement related to _____, as evident from dry skin and hair, dietary intake (low in fiber, vegetables, fluids, and high in CHO)

Now you want to determine what has caused or contributed to Mr. Jewel's imbalanced nutrition. Look at the list of related factors or risk factors under *Imbalanced Nutrition*. Do any relate to Mr. Jewel's situation? Does Mr. Jewel think his diet is inadequate? If he says no, "lack of knowledge" would be the third part of your diagnostic statement. If he says yes, but it is not important to him to change his habits at his age, you will need to talk with him. Perhaps he has a problem with constipation or energy. Maybe a change of diet could help. When you are assured that Mr. Jewel understands the reasons for a balanced diet, but see that he has decided to continue his present diet, record his decision and your attempts to influence that decision.

Select Priority Diagnoses

Priority Criteria

Nurses cannot treat all the nursing diagnoses and collaborative problems that an individual client, family, or community has. Attempts to do this will result in frustration for the nurse and the client. By identifying a priority set—a group of nursing diagnoses and collaborative problems that take precedence over other nursing diagnoses or collaborative problems—the nurse can best

direct resources toward goal achievement. It is useful to differentiate priority diagnoses from those that are important, but not
priority.

Priority diagnoses are those nursing diagnoses or collaborative problems that, if not managed now, will deter progress to
achieve outcomes or will negatively affect the client's functional
status.

Nonpriority diagnoses are those nursing diagnoses or collaborative problems for which treatment can be delayed to a later time
without compromising present functional status. How does the
nurse identify a priority set? In an acute-care setting, the client
enters the hospital for a specific purpose, such as surgery or other
treatments for acute illness.

- What are the nursing diagnoses or collaborative problems
  associated with the primary condition or treatments (e.g.,
  surgery)?
- Are there additional collaborative problems associated with
  coexisting medical conditions that require monitoring (e.g.,
  hypoglycemia)?
- Are there additional nursing diagnoses that, if not managed
  now, will deter recovery or affect the client's functional status
  (e.g., *High Risk for Constipation*)?
- What problems do the client perceive as priority?

Use of Consultants/Referrals

How are other diagnoses not on the diagnostic cluster selected for
a client's problem list? Limited nursing resources and increasingly
reduced client care time mandate that nurses identify important
nursing diagnoses that can be addressed later and do not need to
be included on the client's problem list. For example, for a client
hospitalized after myocardial infarction who is 50 pounds overweight, the nurse would want to explain the effects of obesity on
cardiac function and refer the client to community resources for
a weight-reduction program after discharge. The discharge summary record would reflect the teaching and the referral; a nursing
diagnosis related to weight reduction would not need to appear on
the client's problem list.

Summary

Making accurate nursing diagnoses takes knowledge and practice. If the nurse uses a systematic approach to nursing diagnosis
validation, then accuracy will increase. The process of making
nursing diagnoses is difficult because nurses are attempting to

diagnose human responses. Humans are unique, complex, and ever-changing; thus, attempts to classify these responses have been difficult.

References

Carpenito, L. J. (2013). *Nursing diagnosis: Application to clinical practice* (14th ed.). Philadelphia: Lippincott Williams & Wilkins.

North American Nursing Diagnosis Association. (2008). National conference, Miami, FL.

NANDA International. (2012). *Nursing diagnoses: Definitions and classification 2012–2014*. Ames, IA: Wiley-Blackwell.

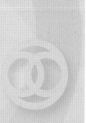

Section I

Nursing Diagnoses

ACTIVITY INTOLERANCE

NANDA-I Definition

Insufficient physiologic or psychological energy to endure or complete required or desired daily activities

Defining Characteristics

Major (Must Be Present)

An altered physiologic response to activity

Respiratory
Exertional dyspnea*   Shortness of breath
Excessively increased rate   Decreased rate

Pulse
Weak   Failure to return to preactivity
Excessively increased   level after 3 minutes
Rhythm change   EKG changes reflecting
Decreased   arrhythmias or ischemia*

Blood Pressure
Abnormal blood pressure response to activity
Failure to increase with activity
Increased diastolic pressure greater than 15 mm Hg

Minor (May Be Present)

Verbal report of weakness*   Verbal report of fatigue*
Pallor or cyanosis   Confusion
Verbal reports of vertigo

Related Factors

Any factors that compromise oxygen transport, physical conditioning, or create excessive energy demands that outstrip the client's physical and psychological abilities can cause activity intolerance. Some common factors follow.

Pathophysiologic

Related to imbalance between oxygen supply/demand

Related to compromised oxygen transport system secondary to:

Cardiac
Cardiomyopathies   Congestive heart failure
Dysrhythmias   Angina
Myocardial infarction (MI)   Valvular disease
Congenital heart disease

Respiratory
Chronic obstructive pulmonary disease (COPD)
Bronchopulmonary dysplasia
Atelectasis

Circulatory
Anemia   Peripheral arterial disease
Hypovolemia

Related to increased metabolic demands secondary to:

Acute or Chronic Infections
Viral infection   Mononucleosis
Endocrine or metabolic   Hepatitis
  disorders

Chronic Diseases
Renal   Hepatic
Inflammatory   Musculoskeletal
Neurologic

Related to inadequate energy sources secondary to:
Obesity   Inadequate diet
Malnourishment

Treatment Related

Related to increased metabolic demands secondary to:
Malignancies   Surgery
Diagnostic studies   Treatment schedule/frequency

Related to compromised oxygen transport secondary to:
Hypovolemia   Bed rest*   Immobility*

Situational (Personal, Environmental)

Related to inactivity secondary to:
Depression   Sedentary lifestyle*
Inadequate social support   Insufficient knowledge

Related to increased metabolic demands secondary to:
Assistive equipment (walkers, crutches, braces)
Extreme stress
Pain
Environmental barriers (e.g., stairs)

Climate extremes (especially hot, humid climates)
Air pollution (e.g., smog)
Atmospheric pressure (e.g., recent relocation to high-altitude
    living)

Related to inadequate motivation secondary to:

Fear of falling	Pain
Depression	Dyspnea
Obesity	Generalized weakness*

Maturational

Older adults may have decreased muscle strength and flexibility,
as well as sensory deficits. These factors can undermine body
confidence and may contribute directly or indirectly to activity
intolerance.

 Author's Note

Activity Intolerance is a diagnostic judgment that describes a client with
compromised physical conditioning. This client can engage in therapies
to increase strength and endurance. *Activity Intolerance* is different
than *Fatigue*; *Fatigue* is a pervasive, subjective draining feeling. Rest
does treat *Fatigue*, but it can also cause tiredness. Moreover, in *Activity
Intolerance*, the goal is to increase tolerance to activity; in *Fatigue*,
the goal is to assist the client to adapt to the fatigue, not to increase
endurance.

NOC

Activity Intolerance

Goal

The client will progress activity to (specify level of activity desired),
evidenced by these indicators:

- Identify factors that aggravate activity intolerance.
- Identify methods to reduce activity intolerance.
- Maintain blood pressure within normal limits 3 minutes after
  activity.

NIC

Activity Tolerance, Energy Management, Exercise Promotion, Sleep Enhancement,
Mutual Goal Setting

Interventions

Elicit From the Client Their Personal Goals to Improve
Their Health

Monitor the Client's Response to Activity and Record Response

- Take resting pulse, blood pressure, and respirations.
- Consider rate, rhythm, and quality (if signs are abnormal—
  e.g., pulse above 100—consult with physician about advisability of increasing activity).
- If signs are normal or if physician approves, have the client
  perform the activity.
- Take vital signs immediately after activity.
- Have the client rest for 3 minutes; take vital signs again.
- Discontinue the activity if the client responds with:
  - Complaints of chest pain, vertigo, or confusion
  - Decreased pulse rate
  - Failure of systolic blood pressure to increase
  - Decreased systolic blood pressure
  - Increased diastolic blood pressure by 15 mm Hg
  - Decreased respiratory response
- Reduce the intensity or duration of the activity if:
  - The pulse takes longer than 3 to 4 minutes to return to
    within 6 beats of the resting pulse.
  - The respiratory rate increase is excessive after the activity.

Increase the Activity Gradually

- Increase tolerance for activity by having the client perform the
  activity more slowly, for a shorter time, with more rest pauses,
  or with more assistance.
- Minimize the deconditioning effects of prolonged bed rest and
  imposed immobility:
  - Begin active range of motion (ROM) at least twice a day. For
    the client who is unable, the nurse should perform passive
    ROM.
  - Encourage isometric exercise.
  - Encourage the client to turn and lift self actively unless
    contraindicated.
  - Promote optimal sitting balance and tolerance by increasing
    muscle strength.
  - Gradual increase tolerance by starting with 15 minutes the
    first time out of bed.
  - Have the client get out of bed three times a day, increasing
    the time out of bed by 15 minutes each day.

- Practice transfers. Have the client do as much active movement as possible during transfers.
- Promote ambulation with or without assistive devices.
- Provide support when the client begins to stand.
- If the client cannot stand without buckling the knees, he or she is not ready for ambulation; help the client to practice standing in place with assistance.
- Choose a safe gait. (If the gait appears awkward but stable, continue; stay close by and give clear coaching messages, e.g., "Look straight ahead, not down.")
- Allow the client to gauge the rate of ambulation.
- Provide sufficient support to ensure safety and prevent falling.
- Encourage the client to wear comfortable walking shoes (slippers do not support the feet properly).

Discuss Effects of Condition on Role Responsibilities, Occupation, and Finances

Determine Adequacy of Sleep (See Disturbed Sleep Pattern for More Information)

- Plan rest periods according to the client's daily schedule. (They should occur throughout the day and between activities.)
- Encourage the client to rest during the first hour after meals. (Rest can take many forms: napping, watching TV, or sitting with legs elevated.)

Promote a Sincere "Can-Do" Attitude

- Identify factors that undermine the client's confidence, such as fear of falling, perceived weakness, and visual impairment.
- Explore possible incentives with the client and the family; consider what the client values (e.g., playing with grandchildren, returning to work, going fishing, performing a task or craft).
- Allow the client to set the activity schedule and functional activity goals. If the goal is too low, negotiate (e.g., "Walking 25 feet seems low. Let's increase it to 50 feet. I'll walk with you.").
- Plan a purpose for the activity, such as sitting up in a chair to eat lunch, walking to a window to see the view, or walking to the kitchen to get some juice.
- Help the client to identify progress. Do not underestimate the value of praise and encouragement as effective motivational techniques. In selected cases, assisting the client to keep a written record of activities may help to demonstrate progress.

Interventions for Clients With Chronic Pulmonary Insufficiency

- Encourage conscious controlled-breathing techniques during increased activity and times of emotional and physical stress (techniques include pursed-lip and diaphragmatic breathing).
- Teach pursed-lip breathing. The person should breathe in through the nose, then breathe out slowly through partially closed lips while counting to seven and making a "pu" sound. (Often, people with progressive lung disease learn this naturally.)
- Teach diaphragmatic breathing:
  - Place your hands on the client's abdomen below the base of the ribs and keep them there while he or she inhales.
  - To inhale, the client relaxes the shoulders, breathes in through the nose, and pushes the stomach outward against your hands. The client holds the breath for 1 to 2 seconds to keep the alveoli open, then exhales.
  - To exhale, the client breathes out slowly through the mouth while you apply slight pressure at the base of the ribs.
  - Have the client practice this breathing technique several times with you; then, the client should place his or her own hands at the base of the ribs to practice alone.
  - Once the technique has been learned, have the client practice it a few times each hour.
  - Encourage gradual increase in daily activity to prevent "pulmonary crippling."
  - Encourage the client to use adaptive breathing techniques to decrease the work of breathing.
- Discuss physical barriers at home and at work (e.g., number of stairs) and ways of alternating expenditure of energy with rest pauses (place a chair in bathroom near sink to rest during daily hygiene).
- Explain the importance of supporting arm weight to reduce the work of respiratory muscles (Breslin, 1992).
- Teach how to increase unsupported arm endurance with lower extremity exercises performed during exhalation (Breslin, 1992).
- While in the hospital, discuss the effects of smoking on the cardiovascular, respiratory, circulatory, and musculoskeletal systems with a focus on the specific health problems of the individual.
- Determine readiness for quitting.

INEFFECTIVE ACTIVITY PLANNING

Ineffective Activity Planning
Risk for Ineffective Activity Planning

NANDA-I Definition

Inability to prepare for a set of actions fixed in time and under certain conditions

Defining Characteristics*

Verbalization of fear toward a task to be undertaken
Verbalization of worries toward a task to be undertaken
Excessive anxieties toward a task to be undertaken
Failure pattern of behavior
Lack of plan
Lack of resources
Lack of sequential organization
Procrastination
Unmet goals for chosen activity

Related Factors*

Compromised ability to process information
Defensive flight behavior when faced with proposed solution
Hedonism
Lack of family support
Lack of friend support
Unrealistic perception of events
Unrealistic perception of personal competence

 Author's Note

This newly accepted NANDA-I nursing diagnosis can represent a problematic response that relates to many existing nursing diagnoses such as *Chronic Confusion, Self-Care Deficit, Anxiety, Ineffective Denial, Ineffective Coping,* and *Ineffective Self-Health Management.* This author recommends that *Ineffective Activity Planning* should be seen as a sign or symptom. The questions are:

• What activities are not being planned effectively? Self-care? Self-health management?
• What is preventing effective activity planning? Confusion? Anxiety? Fear? Denial? Stress overload?

Examples are:

- *Stress Overload* related to unrealistic perception of events as evidence by impaired ability to plan... (specify activity)
- *Ineffective Self-Health Management* related to lack of plan, lack of resources, lack of social support as evidence by impaired ability to plan... (specify activity)
- *Anxiety* related to compromised ability to process information and unrealistic perception of personal competence as evident by impaired ability to plan... (specify activity)

Risk For Ineffective Activity Planning

NANDA-I Definition

At risk for an inability to prepare for a set of actions fixed in time and under certain conditions

Risk Factors*

Compromised ability to process information
Defensive flight behavior when faced with proposed solution
Hedonism
History of procrastination
Ineffective support system
Insufficient support system
Unrealistic perception of events
Unrealistic perception of personal competence

 Author's Note

Refer to *Ineffective Activity Planning*.

RISK FOR ADVERSE REACTION TO IODINATED CONTRAST MEDIA

NANDA-I Definition

At risk for any noxious or unintended reaction associated with the use of iodinated contrast media that can occur within seven (7) days after contrast agent injection

Risk Factors

Pathophysiologic

Underlying disease (e.g., heart disease, pulmonary disease, blood dyscrasias, endocrine disease, renal disease, pheochromocytoma, autoimmune disease)*
Collagen vascular disease
Sickle cell disease
Myeloma
Polycythemia
Paraproteinemia syndrome/disease (e.g., multiple myeloma)
Diabetes mellitus treated with insulin or oral medications
History of a kidney transplant, renal tumor, renal surgery, or single kidney
History of end-stage liver disease
History of severe congestive heart failure
Dehydration*
Elevated creatinine levels
Recent history (1 month) of: (Robbins & Pozniak, 2010)
    Major infection (e.g., pneumonia, sepsis, osteomyelitis)
    Vascular ischemia of extremities (e.g., amputation, arterial thrombosis)
    Venous or arterial thrombosis
    Major surgery or vascular procedure (e.g., amputation, transplantation, CABG)
    Multiorgan system failure

Treatment Related

>20 mg iodine
Chemotherapy or amino glycoside within past month
Concurrent use of medications (e.g., beta-blockers, interleukin-2, metformin, nephrotoxic medications* NSAIDs)

Fragile veins (e.g., prior or actual chemotherapy treatment or radiation in the limb to be injected, multiple attempts, to obtain intravenous access, indwelling intravenous lines in place for more than 24 hours, previous axillary lymph node dissection in the limb to be injected, distal intravenous access sites: hand, wrist, foot, ankle)*

Physical and chemical properties of the contrast media (e.g., iodine concentration, viscosity, high osmolality, ion toxicity, unconsciousness)*

Situational (Personal, Environmental)

Females > Males
Anxiety*
Generalized debilitation*
History of allergies*(food, medications, hay fever)
History of previous adverse effect from iodinated contrast media*

Maturational

Older than 60 years   Extremes of age*

 Author's Note

This new NANDA-I nursing diagnosis represents a clinical situation in which iodinated contrast media is infused for radiographic diagnostic tests. Reactions can be mild and self-limiting (e.g., scattered uticaria, nausea) to severe and life-threatening (e.g., cardiac arrhythmias, seizures). Nurses caring for individuals scheduled for these tests must be aware of individuals who are at higher risk for adverse events. Nurses in radiology departments are responsible for assessing for high risk individuals, reviewing renal function status of individual prior to the procedure, monitoring for early signs or reactions, and using protocols when indicated.

This clinical situation can be described with this nursing diagnosis. In contrast, *Risk for Complications of Contrast Media* is more appropriate as a collaborative problem, since interventions required are nurse and physician prescribed with protocols for treatment of adverse events. The interventions included with this diagnosis can be used with *Risk for Adverse Reaction to Iodinated Contrast Media* or *Risk for Complications of Contrast Media*.

NOC

Vital Signs, Coping, Medication Response, Peripheral Vascular Access, Peripheral Tissue Perfusion

Goal

The client will report risk factors for adverse reaction and any symptoms experienced during infusion, evidenced by the following indicators:

- State risk factors for adverse reactions.
- Report any sensations that are felt during and after infusion.
- Describe delayed reactions and the need to report.

NIC

Teaching: individual, Vital Sign Monitoring Venous Access Device, Maintenance, Anxiety Reduction, Circulatory Precautions

Peripheral Sensation Management, Preparatory Sensory Information: Procedure

Interventions

Assess for Factors That Increase Risk for Contrast Medium Adverse Reactions

- Refer to risk factors.
- Review with the client/significant others previous experiences with contrast media infusions.
- Consult with radiologist if indicated.

Prepare the Client for the Procedure

On Unit

- Explain the procedure (e.g., administration, sensations that may be felt such as mild, warm flushing at site of injection, which may spread over body and may be more intense in perineum, metallic taste).
- Evaluate level of anxiety. Consult with prescribing physician, and/or NP if anxiety is high.
- Ensure that the client is well hydrated prior to procedure. Consult with physician and/or NP for hydration ordered if indicated (Maddox, 2002).
- For clients who can drink: administer 500 mL prior to procedure and 2500 mL over 24 hours after the procedure.
- Intravenous: 0.95 OR 0, 45% saline, 100 mL per hour beginning 4 hours prior to procedure and continuing for 24 hours after the procedure UNLESS contraindicated.
- Assure serum creatinine/clearance results are documented. Consult with radiologist if abnormal.
- Assess if the client has received metformin or other oral hyperglycemic agents before. Withhold metformin for 48 hours after the procedure.

- Determine when the last contrast media was infused.
- Consult with radiologist/physician/NP if needed.

In Radiology Department

- Ensure that emergency equipment and medications are available:
  - EKG machine
  - Respiratory equipment (oxygen, bag-valve mask, airways)
  - Emergency medications
  - Crash cart
  - IV fluids
- Ensure that the client is well hydrated prior to procedure.
- Explain the procedure (e.g., administration, sensations that may be felt such as mild, warm flushing at site of injection, which may spread over body, may be more intense in perineum, metallic taste).
- Evaluate level of anxiety. Consult with prescribing physician or NP if anxiety is high.
- Encourage continuous conversation and feedback from the client during the procedure (Singh & Daftary, 2008).
- Anxiety, apprehension, and fear may contribute to reactions (Singh & Daftary, 2008).
- Follow protocol for administration of contrast media (e.g., site preparation, rate of infusion, warming of ICM).
- Monitor the client's emotional and physiologic response continuously during infusion.
- Refer to Table II.1 for signs/symptoms of adverse reactions.
- Monitor for extravasation of contrast by assessing for swelling, erythema, pain that usually abates with no residual problems.
- If extravasation is suspected (Robbins & Pozniak, 2010):
  - Discontinue injection/infusion.
  - Notify responsible physician.
  - Elevate the affected extremity above the heart.
  - Provide brief compression for no more than 1 minute.
  - Follow agency protocol for documentation and reporting.
  - Consult with plastic surgeon if swelling or pain progresses, decreased capillary refill is present, sensation alters, and/or skin ulcers or blisters.

Explain Delayed Contrast Reactions

- Advise the client/family that a delayed contrast reaction can occur anytime between 3 hours to 7 days following the administration of contrast.
- Explain that delayed reaction can be cutaneous exanthem, pruritus without urticaria, nausea, vomiting, drowsiness, and headache.

- Advise them to report signs/symptoms to responsible physician/NP.
- Advise to go to ER if symptoms increase or difficulty swallowing or breathing occurs (Siddiqi, 2011).

Table II.1	CONTRAST MEDIUM REACTIONS	
Idiosyncratic		
Mild Reactions		
Scattered urticaria	Pruritus	Rhinorrhea
Nausea	Brief belching	Vomiting
Diaphoresis	Coughing	Dizziness
Moderate Reactions		
Persistent vomiting	Diffuse urticaria	Headache
Facial edema	Tachycardia	Hypertension
Palpitations	Mild bronchospasm or dyspnea	Abdominal cramps
Severe Reactions		
Life-threatening arrhythmias	Laryngeal edema	Overt bronchospasm
Pulmonary edema	Seizures	Syncope
Death		
Nonidiosyncratic		
Bradycardia	Hypotension	Vasovagal reactions
Neuropathy	Cardiovascular reactions	Extravasation
Delayed reactions mouth Nausea/vomiting	Sensations of warmth	Metallic taste in mouth

Siddiqi, N. (2011). Contrast medium reactions. *Medscape.* Retrieved from http://emedicine.medscape.com/article/422855-overview

RISK FOR ALLERGY RESPONSE

NANDA-I Definition

Risk of an exaggerated immune response or reaction to substances

Risk Factors

Treatment Related

Pharmaceutical agents (e.g., penicillin*, sulfa)
Adhesive tape
Latex

Situational (Personal, Environmental)

Chemical products (e.g., bleach*, solvents, paint, glue)
Animals (e.g., dander)
Environmental substances* (e.g., mold, dust mites, hay)
Food (e.g., peanuts, shellfish, mushrooms*, citrus fruits, sulfites)
Insect stings*
Repeated exposure to environmental substances*
Down pillows, quilts
Cosmetics*, lotions, creams, perfumes
Nickel
Plants (e.g., tomato, poison ivy)

Maturational

Genetic predisposition to atopic disease

 Author's Note

This new NANDA-I diagnosis can represent a diagnosis with the nursing assessments and educational interventions that can assist individuals and families with the prevention of allergic responses. The collaborative problem *Risk for Complications of Allergic Reaction* that can be found on http://thePoint.lww.com/CarpenitoHB14 is indicated when nursing and medical interventions are needed for an allergic reaction.

NOC

Immune Hypersensitivity Control

Goal

The client will report less or no allergy symptoms as evidenced by the following indicators:

• Describe strategies to avoid exposure.
• Describe methods to reduce environmental exposure.
• Describe pharmaceutical management of a reaction.

NIC

Allergy Management

Environmental Risk Protection

Interventions

Refer the Client to Allergy Specialist for Testing and Treatment if the Client Has Food Allergies

Instruct the Client on How to Reduce Allergens in Home (Asthma and Allergy Foundation of America, 2011; Mayo Clinic Staff, 2011)

Develop Weekly/Monthly Cleaning Routine

- Damp-mop wood or linoleum flooring and vacuum carpeting. Use a vacuum cleaner with a small-particle or a high-efficiency particulate air (HEPA) filter.
- Use a damp cloth to clean other surfaces, including the tops of doors, windowsills, and window frames.
- Vacuum weekly with a vacuum cleaner that has a small-particle or HEPA filter. Wash area rugs and floor mats weekly. Shampoo wall-to-wall carpets periodically.
- If you have allergies, either wear a dust mask while cleaning or ask someone who does not have allergies to do the cleaning.
- Change or clean heating and cooling system filters once a month.
- Use HEPA filters in your whole-house central-air system, or in room air-cleaning devices. Replace filters regularly.

Bedroom

- Encase pillows, mattresses, and box springs in dust-mite-proof covers.
- Wash sheets once a week in 130-degree hot water to kill mites and their eggs.
- Replace mattresses every 10 years.
- Replace pillows every 5 years.
- Remove, wash, or cover comforters. Choose bedding made of synthetic materials, not down.

Kitchen

- Install and use a vented exhaust fan. Most stovetop hoods simply filter cooking particulates without venting outside.
- Wash dishes daily. Scrub the sink and faucets as well.
- Wipe excessive moisture. Discard moldy or out-of-date food.
- Regularly empty and clean dripping pan and clean or replace moldy rubber seals around doors.

- Place garbage in a can with an insect-proof lid and empty trash daily. Keep the kitchen free of food crumbs.
- Clean cabinets and countertops with detergent and water. Check under-sink cabinets for plumbing leaks. Store food, including pet food in sealed containers.
- Never leave food or garbage out to attract roaches.
- Store food in airtight containers in or out of the refrigerator.
- Wipe the stovetop right after cooking to remove food particles that attract insects, and remove crumbs and/or spilled items on countertops right away.
- Use poison baits, boric acid, and insect traps to kill cockroaches. People with asthma should avoid using liquid or spray pesticides.
- Wash dishes immediately after eating; avoid piling dishes in the sink.
- Use a covered/sealed trash can in the kitchen.
- Keep stovetop items covered. Use the kitchen fan when cooking to keep steam and moisture from condensing on kitchen surfaces.
- Use easy-to-clean kitchen flooring. Wash floor mats weekly to remove small food particles.

Bathroom
- Install and use an exhaust fan to reduce moisture while taking baths or showers.
- Towel-dry the tub and enclosure after use. Scrub mold from tub, shower, and faucets with bleach. Clean or replace moldy shower curtains and bathmats.
- Scrub mold from plumbing fixtures. Repair leaks.
- Remove wallpaper and install tile, or paint walls with mold-resistant enamel paint.
- Remove mold as soon as you see it anywhere in the bathroom.
- Fix leaky pipes under the sink, in the shower/tub, and behind the toilet.
- Use the fan/vent when showering to keep air circulating.
- Use washable floor mats, and wash them weekly.
- Use a mold/mildew spray to clean moldy areas, including shower curtains, tiles, etc.
- Wash the "show towels" and bath towels weekly.
- Wipe the sink and counter every day to remove puddles of water and moisture.

Windows/Doors
- Close windows and rely on air conditioning during pollen season. Clean mold and condensation from window frames and sills. Use double-paned windows if you live in a cold climate.

- Use washable curtains made of plain cotton or synthetic fabric. Replace horizontal blinds with washable roller-type shades.

Humidity
- Vent clothes dryer outside.
- Choose an air filter that has a small-particle or HEPA filter. Try adjusting your air filter so that it directs clean air toward your head when you sleep.
- Maintain temperature at 70° F (21° C) and keep relative humidity no higher than 50%. Clean or replace small-particle filters in central heating and cooling systems and in room air conditioners at least once a month.

Pets
- Never allow pets on the bed.
- Keep pet sleeping areas and/or bird cages out of bedrooms.
- Bath pets at least twice a week which may reduce the amount of allergen in the dander they shed.

Fireplaces
- Avoid use of wood-burning fireplaces or stoves.

Kid's Room
- Create a "healthy-room" for your child.
- Use special mite-proof mattress and pillow covers.
- Wash sheets once a week in 130° F hot water to kill dust mites and their eggs with bleach to kill mold.
- Wash stuffed toys every week in 130° F hot water to kill dust mites and their eggs with bleach to kill mold.
- Place nonwashable stuffed toys in the freezer once a week for 24-hours to kill dust mites, then rinse them in cold water to remove dead mites.
- Keep kids' toys away from pets and storing them in a covered, dry place where pets cannot get them.
- Don't allow your kids to sleep with stuffed toys (mites from the bed will get onto the toys, and vice versa).
- Make sure all clothes are fully dry before putting them in drawers and closets.
- Tell kids to wipe their feet and shake out their coats before coming inside, to keep any outside pollen from coming in on their clothes.
- Tell kids to put their clothes in the laundry immediately after coming in from the outdoors, rather than on the floor or back in drawers, to minimize pollen exposure.

Living Room
- Vacuum furniture and curtains/drapes once a week.
- Use washable slip covers and cushions. Wash them in 130° F hot water once a week.

- Keep pets off of the furniture.
- Use easy-to-clean flooring, and avoid carpeting where moisture can get trapped.
- Use blinds and other easy-to-clean window treatments, or wash and dry curtains once a month.
- Never eat on the floor or on furniture.

Basement
- Find and fix all leaks, seams, and cracks in the foundation that let moisture seep in.
- Fix leaks and drips in pipes in and around the water heater and central HVAC system.
- Remove and clean mold wherever it appears. Apply mold prevention paint sealer.

Flooring
- Be vigilant about keeping flooring surfaces clean. Every type of flooring is a potential breeding ground for allergens, whether it's carpet, tile, or hardwood.
- Do not install wall-to-wall carpeting if you do not have to. It is harder to remove moisture, mold, and other allergens that are hidden in it.
- Vacuum all flooring weekly.

Instruct on Treatments at Home if Symptoms Occur

- Instruct to consult with allergist, primary care provider (physician, NP) regarding medical management of symptoms at home (e.g., Benadryl).
- Insure that the client has an Epi-pen, knows when and how to use it, and has transportation to the ER.
- Advise of the need to check expiration dates.

Do Not Allow Smoking Anywhere Inside Your House

Seek Immediate Emergency Care If:

- Facial edema occurs.
- Change in voice.
- Difficulty breathing or swallowing.

Call 911, Do Not Drive to the ER

Wear an Allergy ID Bracelet, Carry a List of Allergies, and/or Store a List of Allergies in Cell Phone in Designated Site

Refer to Allergy Specialist for Skin Testing and Treatment

ANXIETY

Anxiety

Death Anxiety

NANDA-I Definition

Vague uneasy feeling of discomfort or dread accompanied by an autonomic response (the source often unspecific or unknown to the individual); a feeling of apprehension caused by anticipation of danger. It is an alerting signal that warns of impending danger and enables the individual to take measures to deal with threat.

Defining Characteristics

Major (Must Be Present)

Manifested by symptoms from each category—physiologic, emotional, and cognitive; symptoms vary according to level of anxiety (Whitley, 1994).

Physiologic

Increased pulse*

Increased respiration*

Diaphoresis*

Voice quivering*

Palpitations

Urinary frequency, hesitancy, urgency*

Insomnia*

Facial flushing* or pallor

Body aches and pains (especially chest, back, neck)

Paresthesias

Increased blood pressure*

Pupil dilation*

Trembling, twitching*

Nausea*

Diarrhea*

Fatigue*

Dry mouth*

Restlessness*

Faintness*/dizziness

Anorexia*

Emotional

Client states feeling:

Apprehensive*

Jittery*

Loss of control

Persistent increased helplessness*

Vigilance*

Tension or being "keyed up"

Anticipation of misfortune

Client exhibits:

Irritability*/impatience
Crying
Startle reaction
Withdrawal
Self-deprecation

Angry outbursts
Tendency to blame others*
Criticism of self and others
Lack of initiative
Poor eye contact*

Cognitive

Impaired attention*; difficulty
    concentrating*
Forgetfulness*
Orientation to past
Hyperattentiveness
Diminished ability to learn*
Lack of awareness of
    surroundings

Rumination*
Blocking of thoughts (inability
    to remember)
Preoccupation*
Confusion*

Related Factors

Pathophysiologic

Any factor that interferes with physiologic stability.

Related to respiratory distress secondary to:
Chest pain
Mind-altering drugs

Cancer diagnosis

Treatment Related

Related to (examples):
Impending surgery
Effects of chemotherapy

Invasive procedure

Situational (Personal, Environmental)

Related to threat to self-concept secondary to:
Change in or threat to role
    status/function* and
    prestige
Failure (or success)
Ethical dilemma (Varcarolis,
    2011)
Exposure to phobic object or
    situation
Intrusive, unwanted thoughts

Flashbacks
Lack of recognition from
    others
Loss of valued possessions
Fear of panic attack
Unmet needs
Cessation of ritualistic
    behavior

Related to loss of significant others secondary to:

Threat of death*   Divorce
Cultural pressures   Moving
Temporary or permanent   Death
  separation

Related to threat to biologic integrity secondary to:

Dying   Assault
Invasive procedures   Disease (specify)

Related to change in environment secondary to:

Hospitalization   Natural disasters
Retirement   Refugee issues
Environmental pollutants   Military or political
Moving   deployment
Safety hazards   Airline travel
Incarceration

Related to change in socioeconomic status secondary to:

Unemployment   New job
Promotion   Displacement

Related to idealistic expectations of self and unrealistic goals (specify)

Maturational

Infant/Child

Related to separation

Related to unfamiliar environment, people

Related to changes in peer relationships

Related to death of (specify) with unfamiliar rituals and grieving adults

Adolescent

Related to death of (specify)

Related to threat to self-concept secondary to:

Sexual development   Peer relationship changes
Academic failure

Adult

Related to threat to self-concept secondary to:

Pregnancy   Parenting
Career changes   Effects of aging

Related to previous pregnancy complications, miscarriage, or fetal death

Related to lack of knowledge of changes associated with pregnancy

Related to lack of knowledge about labor experience

Older Adult

Related to threat to self-concept secondary to:

Sensory losers	Motor losses
Financial problems	Retirement changes

 Author's Note

Several researchers have examined the nursing diagnoses of *Anxiety* and *Fear* (Jones & Jakob, 1984; Taylor-Loughran, O'Brien, LaChapelle, & Rangel, 1989; Whitley, 1994; Yokom, 1984). Differentiation of these diagnoses focuses on whether the threat can be identified. If so, the diagnosis is *Fear*; if not, it is *Anxiety* (NANDA, 2012). This differentiation, however, has not proved useful for clinicians (Taylor-Loughran et al., 1989).

Anxiety is a vague feeling of apprehension and uneasiness in response to a threat to one's value system or security pattern (May, 1977). The client may be able to identify the situation (e.g., surgery, cancer), but actually the threat to self relates to the enmeshed uneasiness and apprehension. In other words, the situation is the source of, but is not itself, the threat. In contrast, fear is feelings of apprehension related to a specific threat or danger to which one's security patterns respond (e.g., flying, heights, snakes). When the threat is removed, fear dissipates (May, 1977). Anxiety is distinguished from fear, which is feeling afraid or threatened by a clearly identifiable external stimulus that represents danger to the person. Anxiety is unavoidable in life and can serve many positive functions by motivating the person to take action to solve a problem or to resolve a crisis (Varcarolis, Carson, & Shoemaker, 2010).

Anxiety and fear produce a similar sympathetic response: cardiovascular excitation, pupillary dilation, sweating, tremors, and dry mouth. Anxiety also involves a parasympathetic response of increased gastrointestinal (GI) activity; in contrast, fear is associated with decreased GI activity. Behaviorally, the fearful person exhibits increased alertness and concentration, with avoidance, attack, or decreasing the risk of threat. Conversely, the anxious person experiences increased tension, general restlessness, insomnia, worry, and helplessness and vagueness concerning a situation that cannot be easily avoided or attacked.

Clinically, both anxiety and fear may coexist in a response to a situation. For example, a client facing surgery may be fearful of pain and anxious about possible cancer. According to Yokom (1984), "Fear can be allayed by withdrawal from the situation, removal of the offending object, or by reassurance. Anxiety is reduced by admitting its presence and by being convinced that the values to be gained by moving ahead are greater than those to be gained by escape."

Anxiety Level, Coping, Impulse Self-Control

Goal

The client will relate increased psychological and physiologic comfort, evidenced by the following indicators:

• Describe own anxiety and coping patterns.
• Identifies two strategies to reduce anxiety.

Anxiety Reduction, Impulse Control Training, Anticipatory Guidance

Interventions

Nursing interventions for *Anxiety* can apply to any client with anxiety regardless of etiologic and contributing factors.

Assist the Client to Reduce Present Level of Anxiety

• Assess level of anxiety: mild, moderate, severe, or panic.
  • Provide reassurance and comfort.
  • Stay with the client.
  • Do not make demands or ask the client to make decisions.
  • Support present coping mechanisms (e.g., allow the client to talk, cry); do not confront or argue with defenses or rationalizations.
  • Speak slowly and calmly.
  • Be aware of your own concern and avoid reciprocal anxiety.
  • Convey empathic understanding (e.g., quiet presence, touch, allowing crying, talking).
  • Provide reassurance that a solution can be found.
  • Remind the client that feelings are not harmful.
  • Respect personal space.
• If anxiety is at severe or panic level:
  • Provide a quiet, nonstimulating environment with soft lighting.
  • Remain calm in your approach.
  • Use short, simple sentences; speak slowly.
  • Give concise directions.
  • Focus on the present.
  • Remove excess stimulation (e.g., take the client to a quieter room); limit contact with others who are also anxious (e.g., other clients, family).

- Provide physical measures that will aid in relaxation such as warm baths, back massage, aromatherapy, and music.
- Consult a physician for possible pharmacologic therapy, if indicated.
- Provide an opportunity to exercise (e.g., walk fast).
- If the client is hyperventilating or experiencing dyspnea:
  - Demonstrate breathing techniques; ask the client to practice the technique with you.
  - Acknowledge the client's fear and give positive reinforcement for efforts.
  - Acknowledge feelings of helplessness.
  - Avoid suggesting that the client "relax." Do not leave the client alone.
  - Provide assistance with all tasks during acute episodes of dyspnea.
  - During an acute episode, do not discuss preventive measures.
  - During nonacute episodes, teach relaxation techniques (e.g., tapes, guided imagery).

When Anxiety Diminishes, Assist the Client in Recognizing Anxiety and Causes

- Help the client to see that mild anxiety can be a positive catalyst for change and does not need to be avoided.
- Request validation of your assessment of anxiety (e.g., "Are you uncomfortable now?").
- If the client says yes, continue with the learning process; if the client cannot acknowledge anxiety, continue supportive measures until he or she can.
- When the client can learn, determine usual coping mechanisms: "What do you usually do when you get upset?" (e.g., read, discuss problems, distance, use substances, seek social support).
- Assess for unmet needs or expectations; encourage recall and description of what client experienced immediately before feeling anxious.
- Assist in reevaluation of perceived threat by discussing the following:
  - Were expectations realistic? Too idealistic?
  - Was it possible to meet expectations?
  - Where in the sequence of events was change possible?
- "Keep focused on manageable problems; define them simply and concretely" (Varcarolis, 2011).
- Teach anxiety interrupters to use when the client cannot avoid stressful situations:
  - Look up. Lower shoulders.
  - Control breathing.

- Slow thoughts. Alter voice.
- Give self-directions (out loud, if possible).
- Exercise.
- "Scruff your face"—changes facial expression.
- Change perspective: imagine watching a situation from a distance (Grainger, 1990).

Reduce or Eliminate Problematic Coping Mechanisms

- Depression, withdrawal (see *Ineffective Coping*)
- Violent behavior (see *Risk for Other-Directed Violence*)
- Denial
  - Develop an atmosphere of empathic understanding.
  - Assist in lowering the level of anxiety.
  - Focus on the present situation.
  - Give feedback about current reality; identify positive achievements.
  - Have the client describe events in detail; focus on specifics of who, what, when, and where.
- Numerous physical complaints with no known organic base (Maynard, 2004)
  - Encourage expression of feelings.
  - Give positive feedback when the client is symptom free.
  - Acknowledge that symptoms must be burdensome.
  - Encourage interest in the external environment (e.g., volunteering, helping others).
  - Listen to complaints.
  - Evaluate secondary gains the client receives and attempt to interrupt the cycle; see the client regularly, not simply in response to somatic complaints.
  - Engage in discussions not related to symptoms.
- Anger (e.g., demanding behavior, manipulation; with adults, see *Ineffective Coping*)
- Unrealistic expectations of self (Lyon, 2002)
  - Help to set realistic goals with short-term daily or weekly goals.
  - Allow for setbacks.
  - Use positive self-talk.
  - Practice "thought stopping" with toxic thinking.
- Toxic thoughts (Lyon, 2002)
  - Avoid assigning negative meaning to an event.
  - Avoid "reading someone else's mind."
  - Avoid all-or-nothing, black-or-white thinking.
  - Avoid making the worst of a situation.
  - Attempt to fix the problem; avoid assigning blame.
- Teach to recognize that certain autonomic thinking can trigger anxiety (e.g., should, never, always).
- Role-play alternative thinking (Varcarolis, 2011).

Promote Resiliency

- Avoid minimizing positive experiences.
- Gently encourage humor.
- Encourage optimism.
- Encourage discussion with significant others.
- Encourage the client to seek spiritual comfort through religion, nature, prayer, meditation, or other methods.

Initiate Health Teaching and Referrals as Indicated

- Refer people identified as having chronic anxiety and maladaptive coping mechanisms for ongoing mental health counseling and treatment.
- Instruct in nontechnical, understandable terms regarding illness and associated treatments.
- Instruct (or refer) the client for assertiveness training.
- Instruct the client to increase exercise and reduce TV watching (refer to *Risk-Prone Health Behavior* for specific interventions).
- Instruct in use of relaxation techniques (e.g., aromatherapy [orange, lavender] hydrotherapy, music therapy, massage).
- Explain the benefits of foot massage and reflexology (Grealish, Lomasney, & Whiteman, 2000; Stephenson, Weinrich, & Tavakoli, 2000).
- Provide telephone numbers for emergency intervention: hotlines, psychiatric emergency room, and on-call staff if available.

Pediatric Interventions

- Explain events that are sources of anxiety using simple, age-appropriate terms and illustrations, such as puppets, dolls, and sample equipment.
- Allow child to wear underwear and have familiar toys or objects.
- Assist the child to cope with anxiety (Hockenberry & Wilson, 2009):
  - Establish a trusting relationship.
  - Minimize separation from parents.
  - Encourage expression of feelings.
  - Involve the child in play.
  - Prepare the child for new experiences (e.g., procedures, surgery).
  - Provide comfort measures.
  - Allow for regression.
  - Encourage parental involvement in care.
  - Allay parental apprehension and provide them information.
- Assist a child with anger.
  - Encourage the child to share anger (e.g., "How did you feel when you had your injection?").

- Tell the child that being angry is okay (e.g., "I sometimes get angry when I can't have what I want.").
- Encourage and allow the child to express anger in acceptable ways (e.g., loud talking, running outside around the house).

Maternal Interventions

- Discuss expectations and concerns regarding pregnancy and parenthood with the woman alone, her partner alone, and then together as indicated.
- Acknowledge anxieties and their normality (Lugina, Christensson, Massawe, Nystrom, & Lindmark, 2001):
  - *1 week postpartum:* worried about self (e.g., feeling tired and nervous about breasts, perineum, and infection)
  - *1 week postpartum:* worried about baby's health (e.g., baby's eyes, respirations, temperature, safety, and crying)
  - *6 weeks postpartum:* worried about partner's reaction to her and baby

Geriatric Interventions

- Explore the client's worries (e.g., financial, security, health, living arrangements, crime, violence).

Death Anxiety

NANDA-I Definition

Vague uneasy feeling of discomfort or dread generated by perceptions of a real or imagined threat to one's existence

Defining Characteristics*

Client reports:

Worry about the impact of one's own death on significant others

Feeling powerless over dying

Fear of loss of mental abilities when dying

Fear of pain related to dying

Fear of suffering related to dying

Deep sadness

Fear of the process of dying

Concerns of overworking the caregiver

Negative thoughts related to death and dying

Fear of prolonged dying

Fear of premature death

Fear of developing a terminal illness

Related Factors

A diagnosis of a potentially terminal condition or impending death can cause this diagnosis. Additional factors can contribute to death anxiety.

Situational (Personal, Environmental)

*Related to discussions on topic of death**

*Related to near death experience**

*Related to perceived proximity of death**

*Related to uncertainty of prognosis**

*Related to anticipating suffering**

*Related to confronting reality of terminal disease**

*Related to observations related to death**

*Related to anticipating pain**

*Related to nonacceptance of own mortality**

*Related to uncertainty about life after death**

*Related to uncertainty about an encounter with a higher power**

*Related to uncertainty about the existence of a higher power**

*Related to experiencing the dying process**

*Related to anticipating impact of death on others**

*Related to anticipating adverse consequences of general anesthesia**

Related to personal conflict with palliative versus curative care

Related to conflict with family regarding palliative versus curative care

Related to fear of being a burden

Related to fear of unmanageable pain

Related to fear of abandonment

Related to unresolved conflict (family, friends)

Related to fear that one's life lacked meaning

Related to social disengagement

Related to powerlessness and vulnerability

Author's Note

The inclusion of *Death Anxiety* in the NANDA-I classification creates a diagnostic category with the etiology in the label. This opens the NANDA-I list to many diagnostic labels with etiology (e.g., separation anxiety, failure anxiety, and travel anxiety). Many diagnostic labels can take this same path: fear as claustrophobic fear, diarrhea as traveler's diarrhea, decisional conflict as end-of-life decisional conflict.

Specifically, end-of-life situations create multiple responses in clients and significant others. Some of these are shared and expected of those involved. These responses could be described with a syndrome diagnosis as End-of-Life Syndrome. This author recommends its development by nurses engaged in palliative and hospice care.

NOC

Dignified Life Closure, Fear, Self-Control, Client Satisfaction, Decision-Making, Family Coping

Goal

The client will report diminished anxiety or fear, as evidenced by the following indicators:

- Share feelings regarding dying.
- Identify specific requests that will increase psychological comfort.

NIC

Limit Setting, Patient Rights Protection, Family Support, Dying Care, Coping Enhancement, Active Listening, Emotional Support, Spiritual Support

Interventions

For a Client With New or Early Diagnosis of a Potentially Terminal Condition

- Allow the client and family separate opportunities to discuss their understanding of the condition. Correct misinformation.
- Access valid information regarding condition, treatment options, and stage of condition from primary provider (physician, nurse practitioner).
- Ensure a discussion of the prognosis if known.

For the Client Experiencing a Progression of a Terminal Illness

- Explore with the client his or her understanding of the situation and feelings.

- Ensure that the primary physician or nurse practitioner initiate a discussion regarding the situation and options desired by the client.
- Discuss with family and client palliative care and strategies that can be used for dyspnea, pain, and other discomforts (Yarbro, Wujcik, & Gobel, 2011).
- Elicit from the client and client's family specific requests for end-of-life care.
- Provide family with explanation of changes in their loved one that may occur as death nears (e.g. death rattle, anorexia, nausea, weakness, withdrawal, decreased perfusion in extremities) (Yarbro, Wujcik, & Gobel, 2011).
- Avoid giving a specific time for the expected time of death. "It is helpful to give a range of time, such as 'hours to days,' 'days to weeks,' or 'weeks to months'" (Yarbro, Wujcik, & Gobel, 2011).
- Provide opportunities for the person to discuss end-of-life decisions. Be direct and empathetic.
- Encourage the client to reconstruct his or her world view:
  - Allow the client to verbalize feelings about the meaning of death.
  - Advise the client that there are no right or wrong feelings.
  - Advise the client that responses are his or her choice.
  - Acknowledge struggles.
  - Encourage dialogue with a spiritual mentor or close friend.
- Allow significant others opportunities to share their perceptions and concerns. Advise them that sadness is expected and normal.
- Discuss the value of truthful conversations (e.g., sorrow, mistakes, disagreements).
- To foster psychospiritual growth, open dialogue with the client specifically (Yakimo, 2006):
  - If your time is indeed shortened, what do you need to get done?
  - Are there people whom you need to contact in order to resolve feelings or unfinished business?
  - What do you want to do with the time you have left?
- If appropriate, offer to help the client contact others to resolve conflicts (old or new) verbally or in writing. Validate that forgiveness is not a seeking reconciliation, "but a letting go of a hurt" (Yakimo, 2006).
- The nurse through listening can help the client with personal growth.
- Explain preparatory depression and associate behaviors to significant others (Yakimo, 2006).
- Realization of impending death.
- Reviewing what their life has meant.

- Reflections on life review and sorrow of impeding losses.
- Encourage significant others to allow for life review and sorrow and not to try and cheer him or her up.
- Respect the dying client's wishes (e.g., few or no visitors, modifications in care, no heroic measures, food or liquid preferences).
- Encourage the client to:
  - Tell life stories and reminisce.
  - Discuss leaving a legacy: donation, personal articles, or taped messages.
- Encourage reflective activities, such as personal prayer, meditation, and journal writing.
- Return to a previously pleasurable activity. Examples include painting, music, woodworking, and quilting.
- Return of the gift of love to others by listening, praying for others, sharing personal wisdom gained from illness, and creating legacy gifts.
- Aggressively manage unrelieved symptoms (e.g., nausea, pruritus, pain, vomiting, fatigue).
- Initiate referrals and health teaching as indicated to explain palliative care (Miller, 2009):
  - Ensure the primary focus is on comfort, psychosocial, and spiritual well-being rather than improving physical function.
  - Manage distressing symptoms (e.g., pain, thirst, nausea, dyspnea, constipation, dry mouth).
  - Educate and support family and significant others.
  - Consult, educate, and support professional caregivers.
- Initiate referrals and health teaching as indicated to explain hospice care:
  - Hospice has designated caregivers, nurses, social service, physicians, and nurse practitioners in the program.
  - Hospice provides palliative care in homes and health care settings.
  - Refer to educational resources (e.g., National Hospice and Palliative Care Organization, www.nhpco.org).

RISK FOR BLEEDING

See also *Risk for Complications of Bleeding* on http://thePoint.lww.com/CarpenitoHB14.

NANDA-I Definition

At risk for a decrease in blood volume that may compromise health

Risk Factors*

Aneurysm

Circumcision

Deficient knowledge

Disseminated intravascular coagulopathy

History of falls

Gastrointestinal disorders (e.g., gastric ulcer disease, polyps, varices)

Impaired liver function (e.g., cirrhosis, hepatitis)

Inherent coagulopathies (e.g., thrombocytopenia)

Postpartum complications (e.g., uterine atony, retained placenta)

Pregnancy-related complications (e.g., placenta previa, molar pregnancy, placenta abruptio [placental abruption])

Trauma

Treatment-related side effects (e.g., surgery, medications, administration of platelet-deficient blood products, chemotherapy)

 Author's Note

This NANDA-I diagnosis represents several collaborative problems.

Goals/Interventions

Refer to http://thePoint.lww.com/CarpenitoHB14 for the specific collaborative problems such as *Risk for Complications of Hypovolemia, Risk for Complications of Bleeding, Risk for Complications of GI Bleeding, Risk for Complications of Prenatal Bleeding, Risk for Complications of Postpartum Hemorrhage,* or *Risk for Complications of Anticoagulant Therapy Adverse Effects.*

RISK FOR UNSTABLE BLOOD GLUCOSE LEVEL

See also *Risk for Complications of Hypo/Hyperglycemia* on http://thePoint.lww.com/CarpenitoHB14.

NANDA-I Definition

At risk for variation of blood glucose/sugar levels from the normal range that may compromise health

Risk Factors*

Deficient knowledge of diabetes management (e.g., action plan)
Developmental level
Dietary intake
Inadequate blood glucose monitoring
Lack of acceptance of diagnosis
Lack of adherence to diabetes management (e.g., adhering to action plan)

Lack of diabetes management (e.g., action plan)
Medication management
Physical activity level
Physical health status
Pregnancy
Rapid growth periods
Stress
Weight gain
Weight loss

 Author's Note

This nursing diagnosis represents a situation that requires collaborative intervention with medicine. This author recommends that the collaborative problem *Risk for Complications of Hypo/Hyperglycemia* be used instead. Students should consult with their faculty for advice about whether to use *Risk for Unstable Blood Glucose Level* or *Risk for Complications of Hypo/Hyperglycemia*. Refer to http://thePoint.lww.com/CarpenitoHB14 for interventions for these specific diagnoses. In addition, the nursing diagnosis of *Ineffective Self-Health Management* relates to insufficient knowledge of blood glucose monitoring, dietary requirements of diabetes mellitus, need for exercise and prevention of complications, and risk of infection. Refer to Section 1 under *Ineffective Self-Health Management* for more information.

RISK FOR IMBALANCED BODY TEMPERATURE

Risk for Imbalanced Body Temperature

Hyperthermia

Hypothermia

Ineffective Thermoregulation

NANDA-I Definition

At risk for failure to maintain body temperature within normal range

Risk Factors

Treatment Related

Related to cooling effects of:

Parenteral fluid infusion/blood transfusion

Cooling blanket

Dialysis

Operating suite

Situational (Personal, Environmental)

Related to:

Consumption of alcohol

Exposure to extremes of environmental temperature*

Inappropriate clothing for environmental temperature*

Inability to pay for shelter, heat, or air conditioning

Extremes of weight*

Dehydration*/malnutrition

Newborn birth environment exposure

Maturational

Related to ineffective temperature regulation secondary to extremes of age (e.g., newborn, older adult)*

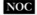 Author's Note

Risk for Imbalanced Body Temperature includes those at risk for *Hyperthermia*, *Hypothermia*, *Ineffective Thermoregulation*, or all of these. If the client is at risk for only one (e.g., *Hypothermia* but not *Hyperthermia*), then it is more useful to label the problem with the specific diagnosis (*Risk for Hypothermia*). If the client is at risk for two or more, then *Risk for Imbalanced Body Temperature* is more appropriate. The focus of nursing care is preventing abnormal body temperatures by identifying and treating those with normal temperature who demonstrate risk factors that nurse-prescribed interventions (e.g., removing blankets, adjusting environmental temperature) can control. If the imbalance is related to a pathophysiologic complication that requires nursing and medical interventions, then the problem should be labeled as a collaborative problem (e.g., *RC of Severe Hypothermia related to hypothalamus injury*). The focus of concern then becomes monitoring to detect and report significant temperature fluctuations and implementing collaborative interventions (e.g., a warming or cooling blanket) as ordered. See also Author's Note for *Hyperthermia* and *Hypothermia*.

NOC

Thermoregulation

Goal

The client will demonstrate a temperature within normal limits for age evidenced by the following indicators:

- Report measures to prevent temperature fluctuations.
- Report episodes of chills, diaphoresis, shivering, cool skin.

NIC

Temperature Regulation, Temperature Regulation: Intraoperative, Environmental Management

Interventions

- Monitor temperature as needed (1 to 4 hours). Use continuous temperature monitoring for vulnerable individuals (e.g., critically ill adults, neonates, infants).
- Use oral thermometers if possible.
- Maintain consistent room temperature of 72° F (22.2° C). Avoid drafts.
- During bathing, expose only small sections of the body. After washing, cover the area with absorbent blanket.
- Ensure that optimal nutrition and hydration is achieved.
- Refer to *Ineffective Thermoregulation* for interventions for newborns.
- Refer to *Hypothermia* or *Hyperthermia* for interventions to prevent body temperature disruptions.

Hyperthermia

NANDA-I Definition

Body temperature elevated above normal range

Defining Characteristics

Major (Must Be Present)

Temperature higher than 100° F (37.8° C) orally or 101° F (38.8° C) rectally

Minor (May Be Present)

Flushed skin*
Tachycardia*
Tachypnea*
Shivering/goose pimples
Warm to touch*

Malaise/fatigue/weakness
Loss of appetite
Specific or generalized aches
    and pains (e.g., headache)

Related Factors

Treatment Related

Related to decreased ability to perspire* secondary to (specify)

Situational (Personal, Environmental)

Related to:
Exposure to hot environment*
Inappropriate clothing* for
    climate

No access to air conditioning
Newborn hospital environment
    warming equipment

Related to decreased circulation secondary to:
Extremes of weight   Dehydration*

Related to insufficient hydration for vigorous activity*

Maturational

Related to ineffective temperature regulation secondary to age (refer to
Ineffective *Thermoregulation)**

 Author's Note

The nursing diagnoses *Hypothermia* and *Hyperthermia* represent people
with temperature below and above normal, respectively. Some of these
states are treatable by nursing interventions, such as correcting external causes (e.g., inappropriate clothing, exposure to elements [heat or
cold], and dehydration). Nursing care centers on preventing or treating
mild hypothermia and hyperthermia. As life-threatening situations that
require medical and nursing interventions, severe hypothermia and hyperthermia represent collaborative problems and should be labeled *RC
of Hypothermia* or *RC of Hyperthermia*.

Temperature elevation from infections, other disorders (e.g., hypo-
thalamic), or treatments (e.g., hypothermia units) require collaborative
treatment. If desired, the nurse could use the nursing diagnosis *Impaired
Comfort* and the collaborative problem *RC of Hypothermia* or *RC of
Hyperthermia*.

NOC

Thermoregulation

Goal

The client will maintain body temperature as evidenced by the following indicators:

- Identify risk factors for hyperthermia.
- Reduce risk factors for hyperthermia.

NIC

Fever Treatment, Temperature Regulation, Environmental Management, Fluid Management

Interventions

Remove or Reduce Contributing Risk Factors

Dehydration
- Monitor intake and output and provide favorite beverage. Teach the importance of maintaining adequate fluid intake (at least 2,000 mL a day of cool liquids unless contraindicated by heart or kidney disease). Explain the importance of not relying on thirst sensation as an indication of the need for fluid.
- Recommended fluid replacement for moderate activities in hot weather (DeFabio, 2000) is as follows:
  - 78° to 84.9° F (25.6° to 29.4° C)   16 oz/hour
  - 85° to 89.9° F (29.4° to 32.2° C)   24 oz/hour
  - Greater than 90° F (32.2° C)   32 oz/hour
- See also *Deficient Fluid Volume*.
- Avoid caffeine and alcohol.

Environmental Warmth/Exercise
- Assess whether clothing or bedcovers are too warm for the environment or planned activity.
- Remove excess clothing or blankets (remove hat, gloves, or socks, as appropriate) to promote heat loss. Encourage wearing loose cotton clothing.
- Provide air conditioning, dehumidifiers, fans, or cool baths or compresses as appropriate.
- Teach the importance of increasing fluid intake during warm weather and exercise. Advise against exercising in hot weather.

Initiate Health Teaching as Indicated

- Explain that children and older adults are more at risk for hyperthermia.
- Teach the early signs of hyperthermia or heat stroke:
  - Flushed skin
  - Fatigue
  - Headache/confusion
  - Loss of appetite
  - Nausea/vomiting
  - Muscle cramps
- Teach the client to take cool baths several times a day in hot temperatures, avoiding soap to prevent skin drying.
- Teach the client to apply ice packs or cool, wet towels to the body, from toes to thighs and fingertips to axillae (Nicoll, 2002).
- Explain the need to avoid alcohol, caffeine, and large, heavy meals during hot weather.
- Stress the need to report persistent elevated temperature.
- Teach the need to wear a hat or use an umbrella during sun exposure.

Pediatric Interventions

- Determine if fever is drug-related (e.g., anticholinergics, amphetamines, epinephrine, acetaminophen [large doses], antihistamines [large doses], phenothiazines).
- Explain to parents that fever is a protective measure and not harmful unless high (e.g., 100° F [> 41.1° C]).
- Caution not to sponge, which causes extreme chilling.
- Explain appropriate clothing for infants and children in warm weather.

Geriatric Interventions

Refer to *Ineffective Thermoregulation*, Geriatric Interventions.

Hypothermia

NANDA-I Definition

Body temperature below normal range

Defining Characteristics†

Body temperature below normal range*
Cool skin*
Hypertension*
Pallor*

Piloerection*
Shivering*
Slow capillary refill*
Tachycardia*

Related Factors

Situational (Personal, Environmental)

Related to:

Exposure to cool environment* (e.g., surgical suite)
Evaporation from skin in cool environment* (e.g., during bathing, surgery)

Inappropriate clothing*
Inability to pay for shelter or heat
Malnutrition*

Related to decreased circulation secondary to:
Extremes of weight
Consumption of alcohol*

Dehydration
Inactivity*

Maturational

Related to ineffective temperature regulation secondary to age (e.g., neonate, older adult)

Author's Note

Because more serious hypothermia (temperatures below 95° F or 35° C rectally) can cause severe pathophysiologic consequences, such as decreased myocardial and respiratory function, the nurse must report these low readings to the physician. This is a collaborative problem: *of Hypothermia*. Nurses most often initiate nurse-prescribed interventions for mild hypothermia (temperatures between 95° F [35° C] and 97° F [36° C] rectally) to prevent more serious hypothermia. Nurses are commonly responsible for identifying and preventing *Risk for Hypothermia*. See also *Risk for Imbalanced Body Temperature*.

NOC

Thermoregulation

---

† Adapted from Carroll, S. M. (1989). Nursing diagnosis: Hypothermia. In R. M. Carroll-Johnson (Ed.), *Classification of nursing diagnosis: Proceedings of the eighth conference*. Philadelphia, PA: J. B. Lippincott.

Goal

The client will maintain body temperature within normal limits evidenced by the following indicators:

- Identify risk factors for hypothermia.
- Reduce risk factors for hypothermia.

NIC

Hypothermia Treatment, Temperature Regulation, Temperature Regulation: Intraoperative, Environmental Management

Interventions

Assess for Risk Factors

Refer to Related Factors.

Monitor Body and Environmental Temperatures

Reduce or Eliminate Causative or Contributing Factors, If Possible

Prolonged Exposure to Cold Environment
- Assess room temperatures at home.
- Teach the client to keep room temperatures at 70° to 75° F (21.1° to 23.9° C) or to layer clothing.
- Explain the importance of wearing a hat, gloves, warm socks, and shoes to prevent heat loss.
- Discourage going outside when temperatures are very cold.
- Acquire an electric blanket, warm blankets, or down comforter and flannel sheets for the bed.
- Provide a hot bath before the client becomes cold.
- Teach the client to wear close-knit undergarments to prevent heat loss.
- Explain that more clothes may be needed in the morning, when body metabolism is lowest.
- Consult with social services to identify sources of financial assistance, warm clothing, blankets, shelter.
- Teach the importance of preventing heat loss before body temperature is actually lowered.
- Acquire warm socks, sweaters, gloves, and hats.

Neurovascular/Peripheral Vascular Disease
- Keep room temperature at 70° to 74° F (21.1° to 23.3° C).
- Assess for adequate circulation to the extremities (i.e., satisfactory peripheral pulses).
- Instruct the client to wear warm gloves and socks to reduce heat loss.

- Teach the client to take a warm bath if he or she cannot get warm.

Initiate Health Teaching If Indicated

- Explain the relationship of age as a risk for hypothermia.
- Teach the early signs of hypothermia: cool skin, pallor, blanching, redness, slurred speech, and confusion (Nicoll, 2002).
- Explain the need to drink 8 to 10 glasses of water daily and to consume frequent, small meals with warm liquids.
- Explain the need to avoid alcohol during periods of very cold weather.

Reduce Heat Loss During Surgery

- Warmed blankets or, when possible, circulating water blankets
- Limit exposed areas
- Warmed fluids (intravenous, irrigating)
- Heating and humidifying inhaled gases
- The greatest reduction in temperature is during the first hour of surgery.

Pediatric and Geriatric Interventions

For Extremes of Age (Newborns, Older Adults)

- Maintain room temperature at 70° to 74° F (21.1° to 23.3° C).
- Instruct the adult client to wear hat, gloves, and socks if necessary to prevent heat loss.
- Explain to family members that newborns, infants, and older adults are more susceptible to heat loss (see also *Ineffective Thermoregulation*).

During Intraoperative Experience

- For children and older adults, unless hypothermia is desired to reduce blood loss, consider the following interventions (Puterbough, 1991):
  - Increase ambient temperature of the operating room (OR) before the case.
  - Use a portable radiant heating lamp to provide additional heat during surgery.
  - Cover with warm blankets when arriving in the OR.
  - When possible, use warming blankets.
  - When prepping for surgery and during surgery, keep as much of the client's body surface covered as possible.
  - Warm prep set, blood, fluids, anesthesia, and irrigants.
  - Replace wet gowns and drapes with dry ones.
  - Keep head well covered.

- Continue heat-conserving interventions postoperatively.
- Children and older adults can become hypothermic in a moderately cold OR environment (Miller, 2009; Hockenberry & Wilson, 2009).

Ineffective Thermoregulation

NANDA-I Definition

Temperature fluctuation between hypothermia and hyperthermia

Defining Characteristics

Refer to Defining Characteristics for *Hypothermia* and *Hyperthermia*

Related Factors

Situational (Personal, Environmental)

Related to:

Fluctuating environmental
  temperatures
Cold or wet articles (clothes,
  cribs, equipment)
Inadequate housing

Wet body surface
Inadequate clothing for
  weather (excessive,
  insufficient)

Maturational

Related to limited metabolic compensatory regulation secondary to age (e.g., neonate, older adult)

 Author's Note

Ineffective Thermoregulation is a useful diagnosis for people with difficulty maintaining a stable core body temperature over a span of environmental temperatures. This diagnosis most commonly applies to older adults and newborns. Thermoregulation involves balancing heat production and heat loss. Nursing care focuses on manipulating external factors (e.g., clothing and environmental conditions) to maintain body temperature within normal limits and on teaching prevention strategies.

NOC

Thermoregulation

Goals

- The infant will have a temperature 97.5° to 98.6° F (36.4° to 37° C).
- The parent will explain techniques to avoid heat loss at home.
  - List situations that increase heat loss.
  - Demonstrate how to conserve heat during bathing.
  - Demonstrate how to take infant's temperature.
  - State appropriate attire for outdoor/indoor climates.

NIC

Temperature Regulation, Environmental Management, Newborn Monitoring, Vital Sign Monitoring

Interventions

Pediatric Interventions

Reduce or Eliminate the Sources of Heat Loss in Infants

Evaporation
- After delivery, quickly dry skin and hair with a heated towel and place infant in a prewarmed, heated environment.
- When bathing, provide a warm environment or bathe under a heat source.
- Wash and dry in sections to reduce evaporation.
- Limit time in contact with wet clothing or blankets.

Convection
- Avoid drafts (e.g., air conditioning, fans, windows, open port-holes on isolette).
- Place sides of radiant warmer bed up at all times.
- Use only portholes for infant access in isolette whenever possible.

Conduction
- Warm all articles for care (e.g., stethoscopes, scales, hands of caregivers, clothes, bed linens).
- Place infant close to mother to conserve heat and promote bonding.
- Warm or cover any equipment that may come in contact with the infant's skin.

Radiation

- Limit objects in the room that absorb heat (e.g., metal).
- Place crib or bed as far away from walls (outside) or windows as possible.

Monitor Temperature of Infants

- If temperature is below normal:
  - Wrap in two blankets.
  - Put on head cap.
  - Assess for environmental sources of heat loss.
  - If hypothermia persists for > 1 hour, notify physician.
  - Assess for complications of cold stress such as hypoxia, respiratory acidosis, hypoglycemia, fluid and electrolyte imbalances, weight loss.
- If temperature is above normal:
  - Loosen blanket.
  - Remove cap, if on.
  - Assess environment for thermal gain.
  - If hyperthermia persists for > 1 hour, notify physician.

Assess for Signs of Sepsis (Respiratory Function, Skin, Poor Feeding, Irritability, Signs of Localized Infections [Skin, Umbilicus, Circumcision, Eyes]).

Teach Caregiver Why Infant Is Vulnerable to Temperature Fluctuations (Cold and Heat).

Demonstrate How to Conserve Heat During Bathing

Instruct That It Is Not Necessary to Check Temperature Routinely at Home

Teach to Check Temperature If Infant Is Hot, Sick, or Irritable

Geriatric Interventions

- Explain age-related changes that interfere with thermoregulation (Miller, 2009):
  - Cold (e.g., inefficient vasoconstriction, decreased cardiac output, decreased subcutaneous tissue, delayed and diminished shivering)
  - Heat (e.g., delayed sweating response, diminished sweating response)
- Explain that these changes will distort perception of environmental temperatures.
- Investigate even a slight elevation of temperature. Use tympanic route for temperatures, not oral or axillary.
- Teach how to prevent hypothermia and hyperthermia (refer to *Hypothermia, Hyperthermia*).

BOWEL INCONTINENCE

NANDA-I Definition

Change in normal bowel habits characterized by involuntary passage of stool

Defining Characteristics*

Constant dribbling of soft stool
Fecal odor
Fecal staining of bedding
Fecal staining of clothing
Inability to delay defecation
Urgency
Inability to recognize urge to defecate

Inattention to urge to defecate
Recognizes rectal fullness but reports inability to expel formed stool
Red perianal skin
Self-report of inability to recognize rectal fullness

Related Factors

Pathophysiologic

Related to rectal sphincter abnormality secondary to:
Anal or rectal surgery
Anal or rectal injury

Obstetric injuries
Peripheral neuropathy

Related to overdistention of rectum secondary to chronic constipation

Related to loss of rectal sphincter control* secondary to:
Progressive neuromuscular disorder
Spinal cord compression

Cerebral vascular accident
Spinal cord injury
Multiple sclerosis

Related to impaired reservoir capacity* secondary to:
Inflammatory bowel disease
Chronic rectal ischemia

Treatment Related

Related to impaired reservoir capacity* secondary to:
Colectomy
Radiation proctitis

Situational (Personal, Environmental)

Related to inability to recognize, interpret, or respond to rectal cues secondary to:
Depression
Impaired cognition*

Author's Note

This diagnosis represents a situation in which nurses have multiple responsibilities. Clients experiencing bowel incontinence have various responses that disrupt functioning, such as embarrassment and skin problems related to the irritative nature of feces on skin.

For some spinal cord-injured clients, *Bowel Incontinence* related to lack of voluntary control over rectal sphincter would be descriptive.

NOC

Bowel Continence, Tissue Integrity

Goal

The client will evacuate a soft, formed stool every other day or every third day:

- Relate bowel elimination techniques.
- Describe fluid and dietary requirements.

NIC

Bowel Incontinence Care, Bowel Training, Bowel Management, and Skin Surveillance

Interventions

Assess Contributing Factors

Refer to Related Factors.

Assess the Client's Ability to Participate in Bowel Continence

- Ability to reach toilet
- Control of rectal sphincter
- Intact anorectal sensation
- Orientation, motivation

Plan a Consistent, Appropriate Time for Elimination

- Institute a daily bowel program for 5 days or until a pattern develops, then move to an alternate-day program (morning or evening).
- Provide privacy and a nonstressful environment.
- Offer reassurance and protect from embarrassment while establishing the bowel program.
- Implement prompted voiding program.

Teach Effective Bowel Elimination Techniques

- Position a functionally able client upright or sitting. If he or she is not functionally able (e.g., quadriplegic), place the client in left side-lying position.
- For a functionally able client, use assistive devices (e.g., dil stick, digital stimulator, raised commode seat, lubricant, gloves) as appropriate.
- For a client with impaired upper extremity mobility and decreased abdominal muscle function, teach bowel elimination facilitation techniques as appropriate:
  - Abdominal massage
  - Forward bends
  - Pelvic floor exercises
  - Sitting push-ups
  - Valsalva maneuver
- Maintain an elimination record or a flow sheet of the bowel schedule that includes time, stool characteristics, assistive methods used, and number of involuntary stools, if any.

Explain Fluid and Dietary Requirements for Good Bowel Movements

- Ensure client drinks 8 to 10 glasses of water daily.
- Design a diet high in bulk and fiber. Refer to *Constipation* for specific dietary instructions.
- Teach the client about caffeine and explain why it should be avoided.

Explain Effects of Activity on Peristalsis

- Assist in determining the appropriate exercises for the client's functional ability.

Initiate Health Teaching, as Indicated

- Explain the hazards of using stool softeners, laxatives, suppositories, and enemas.
- Explain the signs and symptoms of fecal impaction and constipation. Refer to *Dysreflexia* for additional information.
- Initiate teaching of a bowel program before discharge. If the client is functionally able, encourage independence with the bowel program; if not, incorporate assistive devices or attendant care, as needed.
- Explain the effects of stool on the skin and ways to protect the skin. Refer to *Diarrhea* for interventions.

INEFFECTIVE BREASTFEEDING

NANDA-I Definition

Dissatisfaction or difficulty a mother, infant, or child experiences with the breastfeeding process

Defining Characteristics

Unsatisfactory breastfeeding process*
Perceived inadequate milk supply*
Infant inability to latch on to maternal breast correctly*
Observable signs of inadequate infant intake*; poor weight gain, voids, or stools
No observable signs of oxytocin release*
Nonsustained or insufficient opportunity for suckling at the breast*
Persistence of sore nipples beyond the first week of breastfeeding
Infant exhibiting fussiness and/or crying of infant within the first hour after breastfeeding*, unresponsive to other comfort measures*
Infant arching or crying at the breast, resisting latching on*

Related Factors

Physiologic

Related to difficulty of neonate to attach or suck secondary to:*

Infant or maternal breast anomaly* (i.e., cleft lip/palate on infant)
Poor infant sucking reflex*
Prematurity*, late preterm

Previous breast surgery*
Inverted nipples, inadequate let-down reflex
Failure to thrive

Situational (Personal, Environmental)

Related to maternal fatigue

*Related to maternal anxiety**

*Related to maternal ambivalence**

Related to multiple birth

Related to inadequate nutrition intake

Related to inadequate fluid intake

*Related to previous history of unsuccessful breastfeeding**

*Related to nonsupportive partner/family**

*Related to knowledge deficit**

Related to interruption in breastfeeding secondary to ill mother, ill infant*

Related to work schedule and/or barriers in the work environment

*Related to infant receiving supplemental feedings with artificial nipple**

Related to medications (Hale, 2010)

 Author's Note

In managing breastfeeding, nurses strive to reduce or eliminate factors that contribute to *Ineffective Breastfeeding* or factors that can increase vulnerability for a problem using the diagnosis *Risk for Ineffective Breastfeeding*.

In the acute setting after delivery, little time will have elapsed for the nurse to conclude that there is no problem in breastfeeding, unless the mother is experienced. For many mother–infant dyads, *Risk for Ineffective Breastfeeding related to inexperience with the breastfeeding process* would represent a nursing focus on preventing problems in breastfeeding. *Risk* would not be indicated for all mothers.

NOC

Breastfeeding Establishment: Infant, Breastfeeding Establishment: Maternal, Breastfeeding Management, Knowledge: Breastfeeding

Goals

Mother

The mother will report confidence in establishing satisfying, effective breastfeeding.
The mother will demonstrate effective breastfeeding independently.

Indicators
• Identify factors that deter breastfeeding.
• Identify factors that promote breastfeeding.
• Demonstrate effective positioning.

Infant

Infant will show signs of adequate intake, evidenced by these indicators: wet diapers, weight gain, relaxed, feeding.

NIC
Breastfeeding Assistance, Lactation Counseling

Interventions

Assess for Causative or Contributing Factors

- Lack of knowledge
- Lack of role model or support (partner, physician, family)
- Discomfort
- Leaking or loss of control of bodily fluid
- Engorgement
- Nipple soreness
- Embarrassment
- Attitudes and misconceptions of mother
- Social pressure against breastfeeding
- Change in body image
- Change in sexuality
- Feelings of being tied down
- Stress
- Lack of conviction regarding decision to breastfeed
- Sleepy, unresponsive infant
- Infant with hyperbilirubinemia
- Fatigue
- Separation from infant (premature or sick infant, sick mother)
- Barriers in workplace

Promote Open Dialogue

- Assess knowledge
  - Has the woman taken a class in breastfeeding?
  - Has the woman attended a breastfeeding support group prior to delivery?
  - Has she read anything on the subject?
  - Does she have friends who are breastfeeding their babies?
  - Did her mother breastfeed?
- Explain myths and misconceptions. Ask the mother to list anticipated difficulties. Common myths include the following:
  - My breasts are too small.
  - My breasts are too large.
  - My mother couldn't breastfeed.
  - How do I know my milk is good?
  - How do I know the baby is getting enough?
  - The baby will know that I'm nervous.
  - I have to go back to work, so what's the point of breastfeeding for a short time?

- I'll never have any freedom.
- Breastfeeding will cause my breasts to sag.
- My nipples are inverted, so I can't breastfeed.
- My husband won't like my breasts anymore.
- I'll have to stay fat if I breastfeed.
- I can't breastfeed if I have a cesarean section.
- You cannot get pregnant when breastfeeding.
- Build on the mother's knowledge
  - Clarify misconceptions.
  - Explain process of breastfeeding.
  - Offer literature.
  - Show video.
  - Discuss advantages and disadvantages.
  - Bring breastfeeding mothers together to talk about breastfeeding and their concerns.
  - Discuss contraindications to breastfeeding.
- Support mother's decision to breastfeed or bottle-feed.

Assist Mother During First Feedings

- Promote relaxation
  - Position comfortably, using pillows (especially cesarean-section mothers). The use of breastfeeding support pillows will also promote comfort in bringing the infant up to her to feed.
  - Use a footstool or phone book to bring knees up while sitting.
  - Use relaxation breathing techniques. Encourage relaxing and opening/pulling shoulders back to promote oxygenation and blood flow to the breast tissue (physical therapy).
- Demonstrate different positions and rooting reflex
  - Sitting
  - Lying
  - Football hold
  - Skin-to-skin
- Instruct the mother to place a supporting hand on the baby's bottom and turn the body toward her (promotes security in infant).
- Show the mother how she can help the infant latch on. Tell her to look at where the infant's nose and chin are on her breast and to compress her breast with her thumb and middle finger behind these contact points.
- Skin-to-skin
  - Use of skin-to-skin contact for a minimum of 1 hour per day has been shown to bring the mother's milk in an average of 18 hours faster.
  - Skin-to-skin allows infant vital signs to be regulated.

- Allows for infant to be colonized by beneficial bacteria from the mother.
- Infants will cry less; breasts will warm or cool depending on the needs of baby's body temperature.
- The more skin-to-skin contact in the first few days will help extend the breastfeeding experience (Newman & Pittman, 2006).
- Show the mother how to grasp her breast with her fingers under the breast and her thumbs on the top; this way she can roll the nipple toward the roof of the baby's mouth (avoid scissors hold, which constricts milk flow). This will aid in a deeper latch.
- Make sure the baby grasps a good portion of the areola, not just the nipple.
- Observe gliding action of the jaw, which indicates proper latch-on and suck.
- The infant should not be chewing or simply sucking with the lips.
- Listen for swallowing or observe the chin as it drops slightly during a swallow.
- Observe for bruising, creasing, or beveling of nipple tip after feeding.

Promote Successful Breastfeeding

- Advise the mother to increase feeding times gradually
  - Allow infant to finish the first breast before moving to the second.
  - Allow the infant unrestricted, unlimited access to the breast.
  - Average feeding time may be 5 to 45 minutes on each side (Walker, 2006).
- Instruct the mother to offer both breasts at each feeding
  - Alternate the beginning side each time.
  - Demonstrate how to support the infant's head at the nape of the neck to allow the chin to contact the underside of the areola, and allow the infant to latch with nose touching breast (explain that nose may touch breast). This will change the position of the nipple in the infant's mouth.
  - Demonstrate how the mother can place her finger in the infant's mouth to break the seal before removing from the breast.
  - Demonstrate ways to awaken the infant, which may be necessary before offering the second breast (e.g., change diaper, massage infant). Do not use a cold, wet wash cloth to wipe over the infant.
- Discuss burping
  - Inform the mother that burping may be unnecessary with breastfed infants but to always attempt.
  - If the infant grunts and seems full between breasts, the mother should attempt to burp the infant, and then continue feeding.

Provide Follow-Up Support During Hospital Stay

- During the hospital stay, develop a care plan so other health team members are aware of any problems or needs. Tell the mother to be flexible as the plan of care may change throughout the day and over the next few days and weeks as the infant's feeding behaviors change.
- Allow for flexibility of feeding schedule; avoid scheduling feedings. Strive for 10 to 12 feedings every 24 hours according to the infant's size and need (frequent feedings help prevent or reduce breast engorgement). Feeding on demand will aid in milk supply increasing. Allow the infant unlimited, unrestricted access to the breasts.
- Try not to use artificial nipples and pacifiers during the first 4 weeks.
- Ensure that the mother has resources for breastfeeding assistance when leaving the hospital.
- Encourage exclusive breastfeeding and do not encourage the use of artificial baby milk unless medically indicated.
- Encourage latching the baby during the first hour after birth.
- Promote rooming-in (AzDHS, 2010).
- Allow for privacy during feedings.
- Be available for questions.
- Be positive even if the experience is difficult.
- Reassure the mother that this is a learning time for her and the infant. They will develop together as the days pass.
- Heat and massage prior to each feeding throughout the engorgement phase will help to reduce painful engorgement (AzDHS, 2010).

Teach Ways to Control Specific Nursing Problems (May Need Assistance of Lactation Consultant).

- Engorgement
  - Wear correct-fitting support brassiere day and night.
  - Apply warm compresses with firm massage for 5 to 10 minutes before breastfeeding.
  - Nurse frequently (on demand).
  - Use hand expression, hand pump, or electric pump to tap off some of the tension before putting the infant to the breast.
  - Massage breasts and apply a warm washcloth before expression.
  - Encourage rooming-in and feeding on demand.
- Sore nipples
  - Apply a warm, moist compress for 5 to 10 minutes after breastfeeding.
  - Keep nipples warm and dry.

- If nipple pain is too great, pumping breast milk for 24 to 36 hours instead of the infant breastfeeding may be needed in order to allow healing. Suggest alternate positions to rotate the infant's grasps. Allow the breasts to dry after each feeding.
- Keep nursing pads dry.
- Coat the nipples with breast milk (which has healing properties) and allow to air dry.
- A lactation consultant should be seen prior to using nipple shields as improper use may result in a decrease in milk supply.
- Explain that nipple soreness usually resolves within 7 to 10 days as long as the latch has been corrected.
- Stasis, mastitis
  - If one area of the breast is sore or tender, apply moist heat before each breastfeeding session.
  - Gently massage the breast from the base toward the nipple before beginning to breastfeed and during feeding.
  - Breastfeed frequently and change the infant's position during feeding.
  - Rest frequently.
  - Monitor for signs and symptoms of mastitis: chills, body aches, fatigue, and fever above 100.4° F.
  - Consult primary care provider if painful area accompanied by signs and symptoms of mastitis do not resolve within 24 to 48 hours. Observe for signs of abscess.
- Difficulty with baby grasping nipple. Consult with a lactation specialist if indicated.
  - Cup the breast with the fingers underneath.
  - Position the baby for the mother's and infant's comfort (turn the baby's abdomen toward the mother's body).
  - Stroke the infant's lips gently with the nipple tip.
  - Hand-express some milk into the infant's mouth.
  - Roll nipples to bring them out before feeding. Use a nipple shell between feedings to help extend inverted nipples. Remove shield after let-down.
  - Assess the infant's suck—the baby may need assistance in the development of suck. Suck training may be needed (Palmer, 2006).

Encourage Verbal Expression of Feelings Regarding Changes in Body

- Many women dislike leaking and lack of control. Explain that this is temporary.
- Demonstrate the use of a nursing pad. To prevent irritation from the use of a disposable pad, the client should not use the

waterproof backing; cotton (washable) pads seem to reduce irritation. Must keep nipples clean, cool, and dry.
- Breasts change from "sexual objects" to implements of nutrition, which can affect the sexual relationship. Sexual partners will get milk if they suck on the woman's nipples, and orgasm releases milk. Infant suckling is "sensual" and may cause guilt or confusion in the woman. Encourage discussion with other mothers. Include the partner in at least one discussion to assess his or her feelings and how they affect the breastfeeding experience.
- Explore the woman's feelings about self-consciousness during feedings.
  - Where?
  - Around whom?
  - What is the partner's reaction to when and where she breastfeeds?
  - Demonstrate the use of a shawl for modesty, allowing breastfeeding in public.
  - Remind the mother that what she is doing is normal and natural.

Assist the Family With the Following:

- Sibling reaction
  - Explore feelings and anticipation of problems. An older child may be jealous of contact with the baby. Mother can use this time to read to the older child.
  - The older child may want to breastfeed. Allow him or her to try; usually, the child will not like it.
  - Stress the older child's attributes: freedom, movement, and choices.
- Fatigue and stress
  - Explore the situation.
  - Encourage the mother to make herself and the infant a priority.
  - Encourage her to limit visitors for the first 2 weeks to allow optimum bonding and learning to breastfeed for mother and baby.
  - Emphasize that the mother will need support and assistance during the first 4 weeks. Encourage the support person to help as much as possible.
  - Encourage the mother not to try to be "superwoman," but to ask directly for help from friends or relatives or to hire someone.
- Feelings of being enslaved
  - Allow the mother to express feelings.
  - Encourage her to seek assistance and to pump milk to allow others to feed the baby at 3 to 4 weeks of age.

- Advise her that she can store harvested breast milk for 8 hours at room temperature, 3 days in the refrigerator, and 6 months in the freezer. (*Note:* Tell the woman never to microwave frozen breast milk, as doing so destroys its immune properties and may cause uneven heating which may burn the infant's mouth.)
- Remember that time between feedings will get longer (every 2 hours for 4 weeks, then every 3 to 4 hours for 3 months), but this is not definite. Feeding patterns will change as infant ages and goes through growth spurts.

Initiate Referrals, as Indicated

- Refer to lactation consultant if indicated by:
  - Lack of confidence
  - Ambivalence
  - Problems with infant suck and latch-on
  - Infant weight drop or lack of urination
  - Barriers in the workplace
  - Prolonged soreness
  - Hot, tender spots on the breast
- Refer to La Leche League.
- Refer to childbirth educator and childbirth class members.
- Refer to other breastfeeding mothers.

INTERRUPTED BREASTFEEDING

NANDA-I Definition

Break in the continuity of the breastfeeding process as a result of inability or inadvisability to put baby to breast for feeding

Defining Characteristics*

Infant receives no nourishment at the breast for some or all feedings

Maternal desire to eventually provide breast milk for child's nutritional needs

Maternal desire to maintain breastfeeding for child's nutritional needs

Related Factors*

Maternal or infant illness
Prematurity
Maternal employment

Contraindications (e.g., drugs,
    true breast milk, jaundice)
Need to wean infant abruptly

 Author's Note

This diagnosis represents a situation, not a response. Nursing interventions do not treat the interruption but, instead, its effects. The situation is interrupted breastfeeding; the responses can vary. For example, if continued breastfeeding or use of a breast pump is contraindicated, the nurse focuses on the loss of this breastfeeding experience using the nursing diagnosis *Grieving*.

If breastfeeding continues with expression and storage of breast milk, teaching, and support, the diagnosis will be *Risk for Ineffective Breastfeeding related to continuity problems secondary to (specify)* (e.g., maternal employment). If difficulty is experienced, the diagnosis would be *Ineffective Breastfeeding related to interruption secondary to (specify) and lack of knowledge*.

INSUFFICIENT BREAST MILK

NANDA-I Definition

Low production of maternal breast milk

Defining Characteristics*

Infant
Constipation
Does not seemed satisfied after
    sucking
Frequent crying
Voids small amounts of con-
    centrated urine (less than
    4–6 times a day)

Long breastfeeding time
Wants to suck very frequently
Refuses to suck
Weight gain is lower than
    500 gm in a month (compar-
    ing two measures)

Related Factors

Infant
Ineffective latching on
Rejection of breast
Ineffective sucking

Short sucking time
Insufficient opportunity to
    suckle

Mother
Alcohol intake
Medication side effects (e.g.,
    contraceptives, diuretics)
Malnutrition

Tobacco smoking/use
Pregnancy
Fluid volume depletion (e.g.,
    dehydration, hemorrhage)

 Author's Note

In managing breastfeeding, nurses strive to reduce or eliminate factors that contribute to *Ineffective Breastfeeding* or factors that can increase vulnerability for a problem using the diagnosis *Risk for Ineffective Breastfeeding*.

In the acute setting after delivery, too little time will have lapsed for the nurse to conclude that there is no problem in breastfeeding, unless the mother is experienced. For many mother–infant dyads, *Risk for Ineffective Breastfeeding related to inexperience with the breastfeeding process* would represent a nursing focus on preventing problems in breastfeeding. Risk would not be indicated for all inexperienced mothers.

Insufficient Breast Milk is a new NANDA-I accepted diagnosis that represents a more specific diagnosis under *Ineffective Breastfeeding*. When this specific etiology can be identified with *Ineffective Breastfeeding*, the nurse can use either one.

Goals/Interventions

Refer to *Ineffective Breastfeeding*

DECREASED CARDIAC OUTPUT

See also *Risk for Complications of Decreased Cardiac Output* on http://thePoint.lww.com/CarpenitoHB14.

NANDA-I Definition

Inadequate blood pumped by the heart to meet metabolic demands of the body

Defining Characteristics*

Altered heart rate/rhythm (e.g., arrhythmias, bradycardia, EKG changes, palpitations, tachycardia)
Altered preload (e.g., edema, decreased central venous pressure, decreased pulmonary artery wedge pressure [PAWP])
Altered contractility
Altered afterload
Behavioral/Emotional (anxiety, restlessness)

Related Factors*

Altered heart rate   Altered afterload
Altered rhythm   Altered contractility
Altered stroke volume   Altered preload

 Author's Note

This nursing diagnosis represents a situation in which nurses have multiple responsibilities. People experiencing decreased cardiac output may display various responses that disrupt functioning (e.g., activity intolerance, disturbed sleep–rest, anxiety, fear). Or they may be at risk for developing such physiologic complications as dysrhythmias, cardiogenic shock, and congestive heart failure.

When *Decreased Cardiac Output* is used clinically, associated goals usually are written:

• Systolic blood pressure is greater than 100
• Urine output is greater than 30 mL/h
• Cardiac output is greater than 5
• Cardiac rate and rhythm are within normal limits

These goals do not represent parameters for evaluating nursing care, but for evaluating the client's status. Because they are monitoring criteria that the nurse uses to guide implementation of nurse-prescribed and physician-prescribed interventions, students consult with faculty to determine which diagnosis to use: *Decreased Cardiac Output* or *Risk for Complications of Decreased Cardiac Output*. Refer to *Activity Intolerance related to insufficient knowledge of adaptive techniques needed secondary to impaired cardiac function* and *RC of Cardiac/Vascular Dysfunction* on http://thePoint.lww.com/CarpenitoHB14 for specific interventions.

CAREGIVER ROLE STRAIN

Caregiver Role Strain
Risk for Caregiver Role Strain

Definition

Difficulty in performing family/significant other caregiver role (NANDA)

**A state in which a person is experiencing physical, emotional, social, and/or financial burden(s) in the process of giving care to a significant other.

Defining Characteristics

Expressed or Observed
Insufficient time or physical energy
Difficulty performing required caregiving activities
Conflicts between caregiving responsibilities and other important roles (e.g., work, relationships)
Apprehension about the future for the care receiver's health and ability to provide care
Apprehension about the care receiver's care when caregiver is ill or deceased
Feelings of depression or anger
Feelings of exhaustion and resentment

Related Factors

Pathophysiologic

Related to unrelenting or complex care requirements secondary to:

Addiction*	Disability
Chronic mental illness	Progressive dementia
Cognitive problems*	Unpredictability of illness
Debilitating conditions (acute, progressive)	course*

**This definition has been added by Lynda Juall Carpenito, the author, for clarity and usefulness.

Treatment Related

*Related to 24-hour care responsibilities**

Related to time-consuming activities (e.g., dialysis, transportation)

*Related to complexity of activities**

*Related to increasing care needs**

Situational (Personal, Environmental)

*Related to years of caregiving**

*Related to unpredictability of care situation or illness course**

*Related to inadequate informal support**

*Related to unrealistic expectations of caregiver by care receiver, self, or others**

*Related to pattern of impaired individual coping (e.g., abuse, violence, addiction)**

*Related to compromised physical or mental health of caregiver**

Related to history of poor relationship or family dysfunction**

*Related to history of marginal family coping**

Related to duration of caregiving required

Related to isolation

Related to insufficient respite

*Related to insufficient finances**

*Related to inadequate community resources**

Related to no or unavailable support

Related to insufficient resources

*Related to inexperience with caregiving**

*Related to deficient knowledge about community resources**

Maturational

Infant, Child, and Adolescent

Related to unrelenting care requirements secondary to:
Developmental delay   Physical disabilities (specify)
Mental disabilities (specify)

Author's Note

"Health care policies that rely on caregiver sacrifice can be made to appear cost-effective only if the emotional, social, physical, and financial costs incurred by the caregiver are ignored" (Winslow & Carter, 1999, p. 285). Worldwide, family caregivers provide the most care for dependent persons of all ages whether living in developing countries or developed countries (AARP, 2009). The care receivers have physical and/or mental disabilities, which can be temporary or permanent. Some disabilities are permanent but stable (e.g., blindness); others signal progressive deterioration (e.g., Alzheimer's disease).

Caring and caregiving are intrinsic to all close relationships. They are "found in the context of established roles such as wife–husband, child–parent" (Pearlin, Mullan, Semple, & Skaff, 1990, p. 583). Under some circumstances, caregiving is "transformed from the ordinary exchange of assistance among people standing in close relationship to one another to an extraordinary and unequally distributed burden" (Pearlin et al., 1990, p. 583). It becomes a dominant, overriding component occupying the entire situation (Pearlin et al.).

Caregiver Role Strain represents the burden of caregiving on the physical and emotional health of the caregiver and its effects on the family and social system of the caregiver and care receiver. *Risk for Caregiver Role Strain* can be a very significant nursing diagnosis because nurses can identify those at high risk and assist them to prevent this grave situation.

Chronic sorrow has been associated with caregivers of people with mental illness and children with chronic illness. See *Chronic Sorrow* for more information.

NOC

Caregiver Well-Being, Caregiver Lifestyle Disruption, Caregiver Emotional Health, Caregiver Role Endurance Potential, Family Coping, Family Integrity

Goals

The caregiver will report a plan to decrease the caregiver's burden:

- Share frustrations regarding caregiving responsibilities.
- Identify one source of support.
- Identify two changes that would improve daily life if implemented.

The family will establish a plan for weekly support or help:

- Relate two strategies to increase support.
- Convey empathy to caregiver regarding daily responsibilities.

NIC

Caregiver Support, Respite Care, Coping Enhancement, Family Mobilization, Mutual Goal Setting, Support System Enhancement, Anticipatory Guidance

Interventions

Assess for Causative or Contributing Factors

Refer to Related Factors

Provide Empathy and Promote a Sense of Competency

- Allow caregiver to share feelings.
- Emphasize the difficulties of the caregiving responsibilities.
- Convey admiration of the caregiver's competency.
- Evaluate effects of caregiving periodically (depression, burnout).

Promote Realistic Appraisal of the Situation

- Determine how long the caregiving has taken place (Winslow & Carter, 1999).
- Ask the caregiver to describe future life in 3 months, 6 months, and 1 year.
- Discuss the effects of present schedule and responsibilities on physical health, emotional status, and relationships.
- Discuss positive outcomes of caregiving responsibilities (for self, care receiver, family).
- Evaluate if behavior is getting worse.

Promote Insight Into the Situation

- Ask the caregiver to describe "a typical day":
  - Caregiving and household tasks
  - Work outside the home
  - Role responsibilities
- Ask the caregiver to describe:
  - At-home leisure activities (daily, weekly)
  - Outside-the-home social activities (weekly)
- Engage other family members in discussion, as appropriate
- Caution the caregiver about the danger of viewing helpers as less competent or less essential
- Explain that dementia causes memory loss, which results in the following (Young, 2001):
  - Repetitive questions
  - Denial of memory loss
  - Forgetting
  - Fluctuations in memory

Assist Caregiver to Identify Activities for Which He or She Desires Assistance

- Care receiver's needs (hygiene, food, treatments, mobility; refer to *Self-Care Deficits*)
  - Laundry
  - House cleaning
  - Meals
  - Shopping, errands
  - Transportation
  - Appointments (doctor, hairdresser)
  - Yard work
  - House repairs
  - Respite (hours per week)
  - Money management

Stress Importance of Health Promotion

- Rest–exercise balance
- Effective stress management (e.g., yoga, relaxation training, creative arts)
- Low-fat, high–complex-carbohydrate diet
- Supportive social networks
- Appropriate screening practices for age
- Maintain a good sense of humor; associate with others who laugh
- Advise caregivers to initiate phone contacts or visits with friends or relatives rather than waiting for others to do it.

Engage Family to Appraise Situation (Apart from Caregiver) (Shields, 1992).

- Allow the family to share frustrations.
- Share the need for the caregiver to feel appreciated.
- Discuss the importance of regularly acknowledging the burden of the situation for the caregiver.
- Discuss the benefits of listening without giving advice.
- Differentiate the types of social support (emotional, appraisal, informational, instrumental).
- Emphasize the importance of emotional and appraisal support, and identify sources of this support.
- Regular phone calls
- Cards, letters
- Visits
- Stress "that in many situations, there are no problems to be solved, only pain to be shared" (Shields, 1992).
- Discuss the need to give the caregiver "permission" to enjoy self (e.g., vacations, day trips).
- Allow caregiver opportunities to respond to "How can I help you?"

Assist with Accessing Informational and Instrumental Support

- Provide information that is needed with problem-solving strategies.
- Provide information that is needed for skill-building.

Role Play How to Ask for Help With Activities

- For example: "I have three appointments this week, could you drive me to one?" "I could watch your children once or twice a week in exchange for you watching my husband."
- Identify all possible sources of volunteer help: family (siblings, cousins), friends, neighbors, church, and community groups.
- Discuss how most people feel good when they provide a "little help."

Advise Caregivers About Sources of More Information

- National Center for Women's Health Information (www.womenshealth.gov)
- National Health Statistics (www.cdc.gov/ncbddd/disabilityand-health/family.html)
- If appropriate, discuss if and when an alternative source of care (e.g., nursing home) may be indicated.
- Evaluate factors that reduce the stress of deciding on nursing home placement (Hagen, 2001):
  - Low level of guilt
  - Independence in the relationship
  - Availability of support from others
  - Low fear of loneliness
  - Positive or neutral nursing home attitudes
  - Positive sense of life without care burden

Initiate Health Teaching and Referrals, if Indicated

- Explain the benefits of sharing with other caregivers.
  - Support group
  - Individual and group counseling
  - Telephone buddy system with another caregiver
- Identify community resources available (e.g., counseling, social service, day care).
- Arrange a home visit by a professional nurse or a physical therapist to provide strategies to improve communication, time management, and caregiving.
- Engage others to work actively to increase state, federal, and private agencies' financial support for resources to enhance caregiving in the home.

🌱 Pediatric Interventions

* Determine parents' understanding of and concerns about child's illness, course, prognosis, and related care needs.
* Elicit the effects of caregiving responsibility on:
  * Personal life (work, rest, leisure)
  * Marriage (time alone, communication, decisions, attention)
* Assist parents to meet the well siblings' needs for:
  * Knowledge of sibling's illness and relationship to own health
  * Sharing feelings of anger, unfairness, embarrassment
  * Discussions of future of ill sibling and self (e.g., family planning, care responsibilities)
* Discuss strategies to help siblings adapt.
  * Include in family decisions when appropriate.
  * Keep informed about ill child's condition.
  * Maintain routines (e.g., meals, vacations).
  * Prepare for changes in home life.
  * Promote activities with peers.
  * Avoid making the ill child the center of the family.
  * Determine what daily assistance in caregiving is realistic.
  * Plan for time alone.
* Advise teachers of home situation.
* Address developmental needs. See *Delayed Growth and Development*.
* Advise that caregiving activities produce fatigue that can increase over time (Williams, 2000).
* Discuss strategies to reduce caregiver fatigue (Williams, 2000).
  * Partner support
  * Household help
  * Child care for siblings
  * Provisions to ensure adequacy of caregiver's sleep

Risk for Caregiver Role Strain

NANDA-I Definition

At risk for caregiver vulnerability for felt difficulty in performing the family caregiver role

Risk Factors

Primary caregiver responsibilities for a recipient who requires regular assistance with self-care or supervision because of physical or mental disabilities in addition to one or more of the Related Factors for *Caregiver Role Strain*.

Author's Note

Refer to *Caregiver Role Strain*.

NOC

Refer to *Caregiver Role Strain*.

Goal

The client will relate a plan for how to continue social activities despite caregiving responsibilities.

• Identify activities that are important for self.
• Relate intent to enlist the help of at least two people weekly.

NIC

Refer to *Caregiver Role Strain*.

Interventions

Explain Causes of Caregiver Role Strain

Refer to Related Factors for *Caregiver Role Strain*.

Teach Caregiver and Significant Others to Be Alert for Danger Signals (Murray, Zentner, & Yakimo, 2009)

• No matter what you do, it is never enough.
• You believe you are the only client in the world doing this.
• You have no time or place to be alone for a brief respite.
• Family relationships are breaking down because of the caregiving pressures.
• Your caregiving duties are interfering with your work and social life.
• You are in a "no-win situation" and will not admit difficulty.
• You are alone because you have alienated everyone who could help.
• You are overeating, under eating, abusing drugs or alcohol, or being harsh and abusive with others.
• There are no more happy times. Love and care have given way to exhaustion and resentment. You no longer feel good about yourself or take pride in what you are doing.

Explain the Four Types of Social Support to All Involved

• Emotional (e.g., concern, trust)
• Appraisal (e.g., affirms self-worth)

- Informational (e.g., useful advice, information for problem solving)
- Instrumental assistance (e.g., caregiving) or tangible assistance (e.g., money, help with chores)

Discuss the Implications of Daily Responsibilities with the Primary Caregiver

- Encourage caregiver to set realistic goals for self and care recipient.
- Discuss the need for respite and short-term relief.
- Encourage caregiver to accept offers of help.
- Practice asking for help; avoid "they should know I need help" thinking and martyrdom behavior.
- Caution on viewing others as not "competent enough."
- Discuss that past conflicts will not disappear. Try to work on resolution and emphasize today.

Stress Importance of Daily Health Promotion

- Rest–exercise balance
- Effective stress management
- Low-fat, high-complex-carbohydrate diet
- Supportive social networks
- Appropriate screening practices for age
- Maintain a good sense of humor; associate with others who laugh.
- Advise caregivers to initiate phone contacts or visits with friends or relatives rather than waiting for others to do it.

Assist Those Involved to Appraise the Situation

- What is at stake? What are the choices?
- Provide accurate information and answers to encourage a realistic perspective.
- Initiate discussions concerning stressors of home care (e.g., physical, emotional, environmental, financial).
- Emphasize the importance of respites to prevent isolating behaviors that foster depression.
- Discuss with nonprimary caregivers their responsibilities in caring for the primary caregiver.
- Where is there help? Direct the family to community agencies, home health care organizations, and sources of financial assistance as needed. (Refer to *Impaired Home Maintenance*.)

Discuss With All Household Members the Implications of Caring for an Ill Family Member

- Available resources (e.g., finances, environmental)
- 24-hour responsibility

- Effects on other household members
- Likelihood of progressive deterioration
- Sharing of responsibilities with other household members, siblings, and neighbors
- Likelihood of exacerbation of long-standing conflicts
- Effects on lifestyle
- Alternative or assistive options (e.g., community-based providers, group living, nursing home)

Assist Caregiver to Identify Activities for Which He or She Desires Assistance

Refer to *Caregiver Role Strain*.

Assist with Accessing Informational and Instrumental Support

Refer to *Caregiver Role Strain*.

Initiate Health Teaching and Referrals, if Indicated

Refer to *Caregiver Role Strain*.

INEFFECTIVE CHILDBEARING PROCESS

Ineffective Childbearing Process

Risk for Ineffective Childbearing Process

NANDA-I Definition

Pregnancy and childbirth process and care of the newborn that does not match the environmental context, norms, and expectations

Defining Characteristics*

During Pregnancy
Does not access support systems appropriately
Does report appropriate physical preparations
Does not report appropriate prenatal lifestyle (e.g., nutrition, elimination, sleep, bodily movement, exercise, personal hygiene)

Does not report availability of support systems
Does not report managing unpleasant symptoms in pregnancy
Does not report realistic birth plan
Does not seek necessary knowledge (e.g., labor and delivery, newborn care)
Failure to prepare necessary newborn care items
Inconsistent prenatal health visits
Lack of prenatal visits
Lack of respect for unborn baby

During Labor and Delivery

Does not access support systems appropriately
Does not report lifestyle (e.g., diet, elimination, sleep, bodily movement, personal hygiene) that is appropriate for the stage of labor
Does not report availability of support systems
Does not demonstrate attachment behavior to the newborn
Does not respond appropriately to the onset of labor
Lacks proactivity during labor and delivery

After Birth

Does not access support systems appropriately
Does not demonstrate appropriate baby feeding techniques
Does not demonstrate appropriate breast care
Does not demonstrate attachment behavior to the newborn
Does not demonstrate basic baby care techniques
Does not provide safe environment for the baby
Does not report appropriate postpartum lifestyle (e.g., diet, elimination, sleep, bodily movement, exercise, personal hygiene)
Does not report availability of support systems

Related Factors

Deficient knowledge (e.g., of labor and delivery, newborn care)
Domestic violence
Inconsistent prenatal health visits
Lack of appropriate role models for parenthood
Lack of cognitive readiness for parenthood
Lack of maternal confidence
Lack of a realistic birth plan
Lack of sufficient support systems
Maternal powerlessness
Suboptimal maternal nutrition
Substance abuse
Unplanned pregnancy
Unsafe environment

Author's Note

This new NANDA-I diagnosis represents numerous situations and factors that can compromise the well-being of a mother and her relationship with her infant during labor and delivery and after birth. It can be used to organize a standard of care for all pregnant women during the process of labor and delivery and after birth.

Imbedded in this broad diagnosis is a multitude of specific actual or risk problematic responses; some examples are as follows:

Risk for Dysfunctional Family Processes
Interrupted Family Processes
Altered Nutrition
Risk-Prone Health Behavior
Ineffective Coping
Powerlessness
Ineffective Self-Health Management

Risk for Ineffective Childbearing Process would be the standard of care on the appropriate units.

If *Ineffective Childbearing Process* is validated, it may be more clinically useful to use a more specific nursing diagnosis. However, if there are multiple related factors complicating the childbearing process, this diagnosis would be useful.

Due to the extensive art and science of nursing that is related to this specialty diagnosis, the author refers the reader to Maternal-Child Nursing literature for goals and interventions.

Risk for Ineffective Childbearing Process

NANDA-I Definition

Risk for a pregnancy and childbirth process and care of the newborn that does not match the environmental context, norms, and expectations

Risk Factors*

Deficient knowledge (e.g., of labor and delivery, newborn care)
Domestic violence
Inconsistent prenatal health visits
Lack of appropriate role models for parenthood
Lack of cognitive readiness for parenthood
Lack of maternal confidence
Lack of prenatal health visits
Lack of a realistic birth plan
Lack of sufficient support systems
Maternal powerlessness

Maternal psychologic distress   Unsafe environment
Suboptimal maternal; nutrition   Unplanned pregnancy
Substance abuse

 Author's Note

Refer to Author's Note under *Ineffective Childbearing Process*.

IMPAIRED COMFORT**

Impaired Comfort
Acute Pain

Chronic Pain

Nausea

NANDA-I Definition

Perceived lack of ease, relief, and transcendence in physical, psychospiritual, environmental, cultural, and social dimensions

Defining Characteristics

The client reports or demonstrates discomfort.

Autonomic response in acute pain
  Increased blood pressure
  Increased pulse
  Increased respirations
  Diaphoresis
  Dilated pupils
Guarded position
Facial mask of pain
Crying, moaning
Inability to relax*
Irritability*

Reports*
  Abdominal heaviness
  Anxiety
  Being cold or hot
  Being uncomfortable
  Lack of privacy
  Malaise
  Nausea
  Pruritus
  Treatment related side effects
    (medications, radiation)
  Disturbed sleep pattern
  Itching
  Vomiting

**This diagnosis was developed by Lynda Juall Carpenito.

Related Factors

Any factor can contribute to impaired comfort. The most common are listed below.

Biopathophysiologic

Related to uterine contractions during labor

Related to trauma to perineum during labor and delivery

Related to involution of uterus and engorged breasts

Related to tissue trauma and reflex muscle spasms secondary to:

Musculoskeletal Disorders
Fractures	Arthritis
Contractures	Spinal cord disorders
Spasms	Fibromyalgia

Visceral Disorders
Cardiac	Intestinal
Renal	Pulmonary
Hepatic	

Cancer

Vascular Disorders
Vasospasm	Phlebitis
Occlusion	Vasodilation (headache)

Related to inflammation of, or injury
Nerve	Joint
Tendon	Muscle
Bursa	Juxta-articular structures

Related to fatigue, malaise, or pruritus secondary to contagious diseases:
Rubella	Chicken pox
Hepatitis	Mononucleosis
Pancreatitis	

Related to effects of cancer on (specify)

Related to abdominal cramps, diarrhea, and vomiting secondary to:
Gastroenteritis	Influenza
Gastric ulcers	

Related to inflammation and smooth muscle spasms secondary to:
Gastrointestinal infections	Renal calculi

Treatment Related

Related to tissue trauma and reflex muscle spasms secondary to:
Accidents
Burns
Diagnostic tests (venipuncture, invasive scanning, biopsy)
Surgery

Related to nausea and vomiting secondary to:
Anesthesia   Side effects of (specify)
Chemotherapy

Situational (Personal, Environmental)

Related to fever

Related to immobility/improper positioning

Related to overactivity

Related to pressure points (tight cast, elastic bandages)

Related to allergic response

Related to chemical irritants

Related to unmet dependency needs

Related to severe repressed anxiety

Maturational

Related to tissue trauma and reflex muscle spasms secondary to:
Infancy: Colic
Infancy and early childhood: Teething, ear pain
Middle childhood: Recurrent abdominal pain, growing pains
Adolescence: Headaches, chest pain, dysmenorrhea

 Author's Note

There is an ethical duty to relieve pain (Johnson, 2005). Deandrea et al. reported that 40% of individuals with cancer pain are under-treated (2010). Nurses should be as aggressive in advocating for effective pain relief for their clients as they would be if the client was their child, mother, partner, or best friend. Those most in need for effective pain relief may be the poor, uneducated, substance abuser and others who are voiceless in the health care system.

A diagnosis not on the current NANDA-I list, *Impaired Comfort* can represent various uncomfortable sensations (e.g., pruritus, immobility, NPO status). For a client experiencing nausea and vomiting, the nurse should assess whether *Impaired Comfort, Risk for Impaired Comfort or*

Risk for Imbalanced Nutrition: Less Than Body Requirements is appropriate. Short-lived episodes of nausea, vomiting, or both (e.g., postoperatively) is best described with *Impaired Comfort* related to effects of anesthesia or analgesics. When nausea/vomiting may compromise nutritional intake, the appropriate diagnosis may be *Risk for Imbalanced Nutrition: Less Than Body Requirements related to nausea and vomiting secondary to (specify). Impaired Comfort* also can be used to describe a cluster of discomforts related to a condition or treatment, such as radiation therapy.

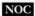

Symptom Control; Comfort Status

Goal

The client will report acceptable control of symptoms as evidenced by the following indicators:

- Describe factors that increase symptoms.
- Describe measures to improve comfort.

Pruritus Management, Fever Treatment, Environmental Management: Comfort

Interventions
Assess for Sources of Discomfort

- Pruritus
- Prolonged bed rest
- Fever

Reduce Pruritus and Promote Comfort

Maintain Hygiene Without Producing Dry Skin
- Encourage frequent baths:
  - Use cool water when acceptable.
  - Use mild soap (Castile, lanolin) or soap substitute (Williams, 2009).
  - Blot skin dry; do not rub.
- Apply cornstarch lightly to skin folds by first sprinkling on hand (to avoid caking of powder); for fungal conditions, use antifungal or antiyeast powder preparations [Mycostatin (nystatin)] or miconazole cream.
- Massage pruritic scar tissue with cocoa butter daily (Field et al., 2000).

Prevent Excessive Dryness

- Lubricate skin with a moisturizer or emollients, unless contra-indicated; pat on with hand or gauze.
- Apply lubrication after bath, before skin is dry, to encourage moisture retention.
- Apply wet dressings continuously or intermittently. Provide 20- to 30-min tub soaks of 32° to 38° F; water can contain oatmeal powder, Aveeno, cornstarch, or baking soda.
- Avoid excessive warmth or dryness, perfumes, cosmetics, deodorants, rough fabrics, fatigue, stress, and monotony (lack of distractions) (Thorns & Edmonds, 2000; Yarbro, Wujcik, & Gobel, 2011).

Promote Comfort and Prevent Further Injury

- Advise against scratching; explain the scratch–itch–scratch cycle.
- Secure order for topical corticosteroid cream for local inflamed pruritic areas; apply sparingly and occlude area with plastic wrap at night to increase effectiveness of cream and prevent further scratching.
- Secure an antihistamine order if itching is unrelieved.
- Use mitts (or cotton socks), if necessary, on children and con-fused adults.
- Maintain trimmed nails to prevent injury; file after trimming.
- Remove particles from bed (food crumbs, caked powder).
- Use old, soft sheets and avoid wrinkles in bed; if bed protector pads are used, place draw sheet over them to eliminate direct contact with the skin.
- Avoid using perfumes and scented lotions.
- Avoid contact with chemical irritants/solutions.
- Wash clothes in a mild detergent and put through a second rinse cycle to reduce residue; avoid use of fabric softeners.
- Prevent excessive warmth by the use of cool room tempera-tures and low humidity, light covers with bed cradle; avoid overdressing.
- Apply ointments with gloved or bare hand, depending on type, to lightly cover skin; rub creams into the skin.
- Use frequent, thin applications of ointment, rather than one thick application.

Proceed With Health Teaching, When Indicated

- Explain causes of pruritus and possible prevention methods.
- Explain factors that increase symptoms (e.g., low humidity, heat).
- Explain interventions that relieve symptoms (e.g., fluid intake of 3,000 mL/day unless contraindicated).

- Teach about medications, such as diuretics, that decrease skin moisture (Williams, 2009).
- Advise about exposure to sun and heat and protective products.
- Teach the client to avoid fabrics that irritate skin (wool, coarse textures).
- Teach the client to wear protective clothing (rubber gloves, apron) when using chemical irritants.
- Refer for allergy testing, if indicated.
- Provide opportunity to discuss frustrations.
- For further interventions, refer to *Ineffective Coping* if pruritus is stress related.

For a Client on Bed Rest
- Vary position at least every 2 h unless other variables necessitate more frequent changes.
- Use small pillows or folded towels to support limbs.
- Vary positions with flexion and extension, abduction, or adduction.
- Use prone position if tolerable.

Pediatric Interventions

- Explain to children why they should not scratch.
- Dress child in long sleeves, long pants, or a one-piece outfit to prevent scratching.
- Avoid overdressing child, which will increase warmth.
- Give child a tepid bath before bedtime; add two cups of cornstarch to bath water.
- Apply Caladryl lotion to weeping pruritic lesions; apply with small paintbrush.
- Use cotton blankets or sheets next to skin.
- Remove furry toys that may increase lint and pruritus.
- Teach child to press or (if permitted) put a cool cloth on the area that itches, but not to scratch.

Maternal Interventions

- Teach the following to prevent strain on back muscles:
  - Avoid heavy lifting; use leg muscles, not back muscles.
  - Place one foot higher than the other when standing for prolonged periods.
  - Wear heels lower than one inch.
  - Wear maternity girdle and exercise daily (e.g., walk, stretch).
  - Apply heat or cold to back two or three times daily.
- If leg cramps occur and are not caused by thrombophlebitis, teach the client to flex or bend foot and not massage. Instruct the client to stretch calf muscles before going to bed.

Acute Pain

NANDA-I Definition

Unpleasant sensory and emotional experience arising from actual or potential tissue damage or described in terms of such damage (International Association for the Study of Pain); sudden or slow onset of any intensity from mild to severe with anticipated or predictable end and a duration of <6 months

Defining Characteristics

Self-Report of Pain Quality and Intensity

(Attempt to use with all clients)

For Clients Unable to Provide Self-Report (in Order of Preference)

Presence of pathologic condition or procedure known to cause pain
Physical responses such as diaphoresis, changes in blood pressure or pulse, pupil dilation, change in respiratory rate, guarding, grimacing, moaning, crying, or restlessness
Surrogate reporting (family members, caregivers)
Response to an analgesic trial

Related Factors

See *Impaired Comfort*.

Author's Note

Nursing management of pain presents specific challenges. Is acute pain a response that nurses treat as a nursing diagnosis or collaborative problem? Is acute pain the etiology of another response that better describes the condition that nurses treat? Does some cluster of nursing diagnoses represent a pain syndrome or chronic pain syndrome (e.g., *Fear, Risk for Ineffective Family Coping, Impaired Physical Mobility, Social Isolation, Ineffective Sexuality Patterns, Risk for Colonic Constipation, Fatigue*)? McCaffery and Beebe (1989) cite 18 nursing diagnoses that can apply to people experiencing pain. Viewing pain as a syndrome diagnosis can provide nurses with a comprehensive nursing diagnosis for people in pain to whom many related nursing diagnoses could apply.

NOC

Comfort Level, Pain Control

Goal

The client will experience a satisfactory relief measure as evidenced by (specify):

- Increased participation in activities of recovery
- Reduction in pain behaviors (specify)
- Improvement in mood, coping

NIC

Pain Management, Medication Management, Emotional Support, Teaching: Individual, Hot/Cold Application, Simple Massage

Interventions

Assess for Factors That Decrease Pain Tolerance

- Disbelief from others; uncertainty of prognosis
- Fatigue
- Fear (e.g., of addiction or loss of control)
- Monotony
- Financial and social stressors
- Lack of knowledge

Reduce or Eliminate Factors That Increase Pain

Disbelief from Others
- Establish a supportive accepting relationship:
  - Acknowledge the pain.
  - Listen attentively to the client's discussion of pain.
  - Convey that you are assessing pain because you want to understand it better (not determine if it really exists).
- Assess the family for any misconceptions about pain or its treatment:
  - Explain the concept of pain as an individual experience.
  - Discuss factors related to increased pain and options to manage.
  - Encourage family members to share their concerns privately (e.g., fear that the client will use pain for secondary gains if he or she receives too much attention).

Lack of Knowledge/Uncertainty
- Explain the cause of the pain, if known.
- Relate the severity of the pain and how long it will last, if known.
- Explain diagnostic tests and procedures in detail by relating the discomforts and sensations that the client will feel; approximate the duration.
- Support individual in addressing specific questions regarding diagnosis, risks, benefits of treatment, and prognosis. Consult with the specialist or primary care provider.

Fear
- Provide accurate information to reduce fear of addiction.
  - Explore reasons for the fear.
  - Explain the difference between drug tolerance and drug addiction.
- Assist in reducing fear of losing control.
  - Include the client in setting a realistic pain goal and in adopting strategies for pain control that are congruent with his/her beliefs and experiences.
  - Provide privacy for the client's pain experience.
  - Attempt to limit the number of health care providers who provide care.
  - Allow the client to share intensity of pain; express to the client how well he or she tolerated it.
  - Involve the social worker or case manager if social or financial concerns exist.
- Provide information to reduce fear that the medication will gradually lose its effectiveness.
  - Discuss drug tolerance.
  - Discuss interventions for drug tolerance with the physician (e.g., changing the medication, increasing the dose, decreasing the interval, adding adjunct therapy).
  - Discuss the effect of relaxation techniques on medication effects.

Fatigue
- Determine the cause of fatigue (sedatives, analgesics, sleep deprivation).
- Explain that pain contributes to stress, which increases fatigue.
- Assess present sleep pattern and the influence of pain on sleep.
- Provide opportunities to rest during the day and with periods of uninterrupted sleep at night (must rest when pain is decreased).
- Consult with physician for an increased dose of pain medication at bedtime.
- Refer to *Insomnia* for specific interventions to enhance sleep.

Monotony
- Discuss with the client and family the therapeutic uses of distraction, along with other methods of pain relief.
- Emphasize that the degree to which a client can be distracted from the pain is not at all related to the existence or intensity of the pain.
- Explain that distraction usually increases pain tolerance and decreases pain intensity; however, after the distraction ceases, the client may have an increased awareness of pain and fatigue.
- Vary the environment if possible.

If the client is on bed rest:
- Encourage family to decorate the client's room with flowers, plants, and pictures.
- Provide music, videos, and video games.
- Consult with a recreational therapist for appropriate tasks.

If the client is at home:
- Encourage the client to plan an activity for each day, preferably outside the home.
- Discuss the possibility of learning a new skill (e.g., a craft, a musical instrument).
- Teach a method of distraction during acute pain that is not a burden (e.g., count items in a picture, count silently to self, or play cards); breathe rhythmically; listen to music and increase the volume as pain increases.

Collaborate With the Client About Possible Methods to Reduce Pain Intensity

Consider the Following Before Selecting a Specific Pain-Relief Method:
- Client's willingness (motivation) and ability to participate
- Preference
- Support of significant others for method
- Contraindications (allergy, health problem)
- Method's cost, complexity, precautions, and convenience

Explain the Various Noninvasive Pain-Relief Methods to the Client and Family and Why They Are Effective:
- Discuss the use of heat applications,* their therapeutic effects, indications, and related precautions.
  - Hot water bottle
  - Warm tub
  - Hot summer sun
  - Electric heating pad
  - Moist heat pack
  - Thin plastic wrap over painful area to retain body heat (e.g., knee, elbow)

- Discuss the use of cold applications,* their therapeutic effects, indications, and related precautions.
  - Cold towels (wrung out)
  - Cold water immersion for small body parts
  - Ice bag
  - Cold gel pack
  - Ice massage
- Explain the therapeutic uses of menthol preparations, massage, and vibration.
- Teach the client to avoid negative thoughts about ability to cope with pain.
- Practice distraction (e.g., guided imagery, music).
- Practice relaxation techniques.

Provide Optimal Pain Relief With Prescribed Analgesics

- Use oral route when feasible, intravenous or rectal routes if needed with permission.
- Avoid intramuscular routes due to erratic absorption and unnecessary pain.
- Assess vital signs, especially respiratory rate, before administration.
- Consult with pharmacist for possible adverse interactions with other medications (e.g., muscle relaxants, tranquilizers).
- Understand pain therapies, including the peak and duration of selected routes of administration of opioid therapy (Dunwoody et al., 2008).
- Use a preventive approach:
  - Medicate before an activity (e.g., ambulation) to increase participation, but evaluate the hazard of sedation.
  - Instruct the client to request PRN pain medication before the pain is severe.
  - Collaborate with physician/nurse practitioner to order medications on a 24-hour schedule basis rather than PRN unless the client is sedated.
- Determine the type of pain from the individual's description. Consult with physician or advance practice nurse to determine appropriate analgesia. The types of pain include (McMenamin, 2011):
  - Somatic pain is described as aching, gnawing, or throbbing pain.
  - Visceral or soft tissue pain is typically described as dull, aching, cramping, and generally not localized. It is caused by compression, infiltration, or distention of viscera.
  - Visceral and somatic pain are responsive to opioids and nonsteroidal anti-inflammatory drugs (NSAIDs).

- Neuropathic pain is described as burning, stabbing, stinging, electric, pins and needles, shooting, or numbness.
- Opioids alone usually do not manage this type of pain. It is responsive to anticonvulsants (gabapentin), selective serotonin reuptake inhibitors (SSRIs), tricyclic antidepressants (TCAs), clonidine, Lidoderm patches®, and N-methyl-D-aspartate receptor antagonists (NMDAs) such as ketamine or methadone.
- Muscle spasm is described as cramping, spasm, or tightening and responds to muscle relaxants (e.g., Soma, Flexeril).

Assess the Client's Response to the Pain-Relief Medication

- After administration, return in 30 min to assess effectiveness.
- Ask the client to rate severity of pain before the medication and amount of relief received.
- Ask the client to indicate when the pain began to increase. How long it has been since the last pain medication? After a certain activity (e.g., ambulation, dressing change)?
- Advise the client to request pain medication earlier. Plan pain relief measures prior to activities.
- Consult with physician if a dosage or interval change is needed; the dose may be increased by 50% until effective (Agency for Health Care Policy and Research [AHCPR], 1992).
- Collaborate with the physician to multimodal analgesia.

Reduce or Eliminate Common Side Effects of Opioids

Sedation
- Assess whether the cause is the opioid, fatigue, sleep deprivation, or other drugs (e.g., sedatives, antiemetics).
- Assess for signs of respiratory depression (decreased level of consciousness, respiratory rate below 8, decreased oxygen saturation) and report to physician or nurse practitioner.
- Inform the client that drowsiness usually occurs the first 2 to 3 days, then subsides.
- Advise the client to ask for assistance to avoid injury (e.g., falls).
- If drowsiness is excessive, consult with physician to slightly reduce the dose and/or add non-sedating adjuvant pain medication.

Constipation (Refer to *Constipation*)

Nausea and Vomiting (Refer to *Nausea*)

Dry Mouth (Refer also to *Impaired Oral Mucous Membranes*)
- Explain that opioids decrease saliva production.
- Instruct the client to rinse mouth often, suck on sugarless sour

candies, eat pineapple chunks or watermelon (if permissible), and drink liquids often.
- Explain the necessity of good oral hygiene and dental care.

Assist Family to Respond Optimally to the Client's Pain Experience

- Assess the family's knowledge of pain and response to it.
- Give accurate information to correct misconceptions (e.g., addiction, doubt about pain).
- Provide each family member with opportunities to discuss fears, anger, and frustrations privately; acknowledge the difficulty of the situation.
- Incorporate family members in the pain-relief modality, if possible (e.g., stroking, massage).
- Praise their participation and concern.

Minimize Procedural and Diagnostic Pain

- Anticipate pain and pre-medicate the client prior to painful procedures (e.g., sedation).
- Consider the use of either intradermal 0.9% sodium chloride next to the vein or a topical anesthetic per protocol prior to intravenous starts.
- Encourage the use of relaxation or guided imagery during procedures.

Initiate Health Teaching, as Indicated

- Discuss with the client and family noninvasive pain-relief measures (e.g., relaxation, distraction, massage, music).
- Teach the techniques of choice to the client and family.
- Explain the expected course of the pain (resolution) if known (e.g., fractured arm, surgical incision).
- Provide the client with written guidelines for weaning from pain medications when the acute event is relieved.

Pediatric Interventions

Assess the Child's Pain Experience

- Determine the child's concept of the cause of pain, if feasible.
- Ask the child to point to the area that hurts.
- Determine the intensity of the pain at its worst and best. Use a pain assessment scale appropriate for the child's developmental age. Use the same scale the same way each time and encourage its use by parents and other health care professionals. Indicate on the care plan which scale to use and how (introduction of scale, language specific for child); attach copy if visual scale.

- Ask the child what makes the pain better and what makes it worse.
- Include the parents' rating of their child's pain in assessment. Parents and nurses can rate a child's pain differently. The parents' observation is often more accurate.
- Assess whether fear, loneliness, or anxiety is contributing to pain.
- Assess effect of pain on sleep and play. Note: A child who sleeps, plays, or both can still be in pain (sleep and play can serve as distractions) or adequately medicated for pain.
- With infants, assess crying, facial expressions, body postures, and movements. Infants exhibit distress from environmental stimuli (light, sound) as well as from touch and treatments.
- Use tactile and vocal stimuli to comfort infants, but assess the effect of comfort measures (does it increase or decrease distress?) and individualized intervention.
- Explain the pain source to the child using verbal and sensory (visual, tactile) explanations (e.g., perform treatment on doll, allow the child to handle equipment). Explicitly explain and reinforce to the child that he or she is not being punished.

Assess the Child and Family for Misconceptions About Pain or Its Treatment

- Explain to the parents the necessity of good explanations to promote trust.
- Explain to the parents that the child may cry more openly when they are present, but that their presence is important for promoting trust.
- Parents and older children may have misconceptions about analgesia and may fear narcotic use/abuse. Emphasize that narcotic use for moderate or severe pain does not lead to addiction. Discuss with parents and older children that "say no to drugs" does not apply to analgesia for pain prescribed by physicians and monitored by physicians and nurses.

Promote Security with Honest Explanations and Opportunities for Choice

Promote Open, Honest Communication
- Tell the truth; explain:
  - How much it will hurt
  - How long it will last
  - What will help the pain
- Do not threaten (e.g., do not tell the child, "If you don't hold still, you won't go home").
- Explain to the child that the procedure is necessary so he or she can get better and that holding still is important so it can be done quickly.

- Discuss with parents the importance of truth-telling. Instruct them to:
  - Tell the child when they are leaving and when they will return.
  - Relate to the child that they cannot take away pain, but that they will be with him or her (except in circumstances when parents are not permitted to remain).
- Allow parents opportunities to share their feelings about witnessing their child's pain and their helplessness.

Prepare the Child for a Painful Procedure

- Discuss the procedure with the parents; determine what they have told the child.
- Explain the procedure in words suited to the child's age and developmental level (see *Delayed Growth and Development* for age-related needs).
- Relate the likely discomforts (e.g., what the child will feel, taste, see, or smell). "You will get an injection that will hurt for a little while and then it will stop."
- Be sure to explain when an injection will cause two discomforts: the prick of the needle and the absorption of the drug.
- Encourage the child to ask questions before and during the procedure; ask the child to share what he or she thinks will happen and why.
- Share with the child older than 12 years that:
  - You expect the child to hold still and that it will please you if he or she can.
  - It is all right to cry or squeeze your hand if it hurts.
- Find something to praise after the procedure, even if the child could not hold still.
- Arrange to have the parents present for procedures (especially for children younger than 10 years); describe what to expect to the parents before the procedure, and give them a role during the procedure (e.g., hold the child's hand, talk to the child).

Reduce the Pain During Treatments When Possible

- If restraints must be used, have sufficient clientele available so that the procedure is not delayed.
- If injections are ordered, try to obtain an order for oral or IV analgesics instead. If injections must be used:
  - Expect the child (older than 2 or 3 years) to hold still.
  - Have the child participate by holding the Band-Aid for you.
  - Tell the child how pleased you are that he or she helped.
  - Pull the skin surface as taut as possible (for IM).
  - Comfort the child after the procedure.
- Tell child step-by-step what is going to happen right before it is done.

- Offer the child the option of learning distraction techniques for use during the procedure. (The use of distraction without the child's knowledge of the impending discomfort is not advocated because the child will learn to mistrust.):
  - Tell a story with a puppet.
  - Blow a party noisemaker.
  - Ask the child to name or count objects in a picture.
  - Ask the child to look at the picture and to locate certain objects ("Where is the dog?").
  - Ask child to tell you about his or her pet.
  - Ask child to count your blinks.
- Avoid rectal thermometers in preschoolers; if possible, use electronic oral or ear probes.
- Provide the child with privacy during the painful procedure; use a treatment room rather than the child's bed.
- The child's bed should be a "safe" place.
- No procedures should be done in the playroom or schoolroom.

Provide the Child Optimal Pain Relief with Prescribed Analgesics

- Medicate child before painful procedure or activity (e.g., dressing change, ambulation).
- Consult with physician for a change of the IM route to the IV route.
- Assess appropriateness of medication, dose, and schedule for cause of pain, child's weight, and child's response, not age.
- Along with using pain assessment scales, observe for behavioral signs of pain (because the child may deny pain); if possible, identify specific behaviors that indicate pain in an individual child.
- Assess the potential for use of patient-controlled analgesia (PCA), which provides intermittent controlled doses of IV analgesia (with/without continuous infusion) as determined by the child's need. Children as young as 5 years can use PCA. Parents of children physically unable can administer it to them. PCA has been found safe and to provide superior pain relief compared with conventional-demand analgesia.
- Consult with physician about the use of epidural infusion of morphine for the treatment of postoperative pain. Epidural morphine infusion has been used safely in both adults and children in nonintensive care settings.

Reduce or Eliminate the Common Side Effects of Opioids

Sedation
- Assess whether the cause is the opioid, fatigue, sleep deprivation, or other drugs (sedatives, antiemetics).

- If drowsiness is excessive, consult with physician to slightly reduce the dose.

Constipation
- Explain to older children why pain medications cause constipation.
- Increase roughage in diet (e.g., fruits; 1 teaspoon of bran on cereal).
- Encourage child to drink 8 to 10 glasses of liquid each day.
- Teach child how to do abdominal isometric exercises if activity is restricted (e.g., "Pull in your tummy; now relax your tummy; do this ten times each hour during the day").
- Instruct child to keep a record of exercises (e.g., make a chart with a star sticker placed on it whenever the exercises are done).
- Refer to *Constipation* for additional interventions.

Dry Mouth
- Explain to older children that narcotics decrease saliva production.
- Instruct child to rinse mouth often, suck on sugarless sour candies, eat pineapple chunks and watermelon, and drink liquids often.
- Explain the necessity of brushing teeth after every meal.

Assist Child with the Aftermath of Pain

- Tell the child when the painful procedure is over. Pick up the small child to indicate it is over.
- Encourage child to discuss pain experience (draw or act out with dolls).
- Encourage child to perform the painful procedure using the same equipment on a doll under supervision.
- Praise the child for his or her endurance and convey that he or she handled the pain well regardless of actual behavior (unless the child was violent to others).
- Give the child a souvenir of the pain (Band-Aid, badge for bravery).
- Teach child to keep a record of painful experiences and to plan a reward each time he or she achieves a behavioral goal, such as a gold star (reward) for each time the child holds still (goal) during an injection. Encourage achievable goals; holding still during an injection may not be possible for every child, but counting or blowing may be.

Collaborate With Child to Initiate Appropriate Noninvasive Pain-Relief Modalities

- Encourage mobility as much as indicated, especially when pain is lowest.

- Discuss with child and parents activities that they like and incorporate them in daily schedule (e.g., clay modeling, painting).
- Discuss with the child older than 7 years that thinking about something else can decrease the pain and demonstrate the effects.
  - Ask child to count to 100 (or count your eye blinks).
  - As child is counting, apply gentle pressure to Achilles tendon (pinch back of heel).
  - Gradually increase the pressure.
  - Ask child to stop counting but keep pressure on heel.
- Ask if the child can feel the discomfort in his or her heel now and if the child felt it during counting.
- Consider the use of transcutaneous electrical nerve stimulation (TENS) for procedural, acute, and chronic pain. TENS has been studied and used effectively in children with postoperative pain, headache, and procedural pain, without adverse effects.
- Refer to guidelines for noninvasive pain-relief measures.

Assist Family to Respond Optimally to Child's Pain Experience

- Assess family's knowledge of and response to pain (e.g., do parents support the child who has pain?).
- Assure parents that they can touch or hold their child, if feasible (e.g., demonstrate that touching is possible even with tubes and equipment).
- Give accurate information to correct misconceptions (e.g., the necessity of the treatment even though it causes pain).
- Provide parents opportunities to discuss privately their fears, anger, and frustrations.
- Acknowledge the difficulty of the situation.
- Incorporate parents in the pain-relief modality if possible (e.g., stroking, massage, distraction).
- Praise their participation and concern.
- Negotiate goals of pain management plan; reevaluate regularly (e.g., pain-free, decreased pain).

Initiate Health Teaching and Referrals, if Indicated

- Provide child and family with ongoing explanations.
- Use the care plan to promote continuity of care for hospitalized child.
- Use available mental health professionals, if needed, for assistance with guided imagery, progressive relaxation, and hypnosis.

- Use available pain service (pain team) at pediatric health care centers for an interdisciplinary and comprehensive approach to pain management in children.
- Refer parents to pertinent literature for themselves and children (see Bibliography).

Maternal Interventions

- Advise the woman that she will be assisted in managing her labor. Explore her wishes.
- Determine the role the expectant father chooses for the labor and birth experience: coach, teammate, or witness, or support the doula or coach.
- Explain all procedures before initiation.
- Provide comfort techniques as desired (e.g., walking, music, massage, acupressure, shower, baths, hot or cold applications, hypnosis, imagery) (Pillitteri, 2010).
- Instruct woman not to use breathing techniques too early.
- Engage the woman in pleasant dialogue and thoughts about specific subjects (e.g., other children, favorite friends, new baby, memorable vacation).
- As labor progresses to active stage:
  - Evaluate effectiveness of breathing techniques.
  - If pain or anxiety is not reduced, consult with midwife or physician for a new plan.
  - Evaluate fatigue level.
  - Assess how well the labor partner is anticipating the woman's needs.
  - Encourage ambulation and position changes every 20 to 30 min.
  - Position changes can prevent or correct malposition of the fetus, promote rotation and labor progress, and reduce lower back pain.
  - Approach the woman in an unhurried, gentle manner.

Chronic Pain

NANDA-I Definition

Unpleasant sensory and emotional experience arising from actual or potential tissue damage or described in terms of such damage (International Association for the Study of Pain); sudden or slow onset of any intensity from mild to severe with anticipated or predictable end and a duration of >6 months

Defining Characteristics

Major (Must Be Present)

The client reports that pain has existed for more than 6 months (may be the only assessment data present).

Minor (May Be Present)

Discomfort	Guarded movement
Anger, frustration, depression because of situation	Muscle spasms
	Redness, swelling, heat
Facial mask of pain	Color changes in the affected
Anorexia, weight loss	area
Insomnia	Reflex abnormalities

Related Factors

See *Impaired Comfort*.

 Author's Note

Chronic or persistent pain is common in 80% of older adults. One survey of 10,291 clients revealed prevalence of 10.1% for back pain, 7.1% for leg and foot pain, 4.1% for hand and arm pain, and 3.5% for headache (Hardt et al., 2008).

It is well known that chronic pain affects coping, sleep, sexual activity, socialization, family processes, nutrition, spirituality, and activity tolerance. Approximately 50% of clients with persistent pain also suffer from depression or anxiety disorder (Weisburg & Boatwright, 2007).

 NOC

Comfort Level, Pain: Disruptive Effects, Pain Control, Depression Control

Goals

The client will relate improvement of pain and increased daily activities as evidenced by the following indicators:

• Relate that others validate that their pain exists.
• Practice selected noninvasive pain-relief measures.

The child will demonstrate coping mechanism for pain, methods to control pain and the pain cause/disease, as evidenced by increased play and usual activities of childhood, and the following indicators:
• Communicate improvement in pain verbally, by pain assessment scale, or by behavior (specify).

- Maintain usual family role and relationships throughout pain experience, as evidenced by (specify).

NIC

Pain Management, Medication Management, Exercise Promotion, Mood Management, Coping Enhancement

Interventions

Assess the Client's Pain Experience

Assess for Factors that Decrease Pain Tolerance

See *Acute Pain*.

Reduce or Eliminate Factors that Increase Pain

See *Acute Pain*.

Determine with the Client and Family the Effects of Chronic Pain on the Client's

- Physical well-being (fatigue, strength, appetite, sleep, function, constipation, nausea)
- Psychologic well-being (anxiety, depression, coping, control, concentration, sense of usefulness, fear, enjoyment)
- Spiritual well-being (religiosity, uncertainty, positive changes, sense of purpose, hopefulness, suffering, meaning of pain, transcendence)
- Social well-being (family support, family distress, sexuality, affection, employment, isolation, financial burden, appearance, roles, relationships)

Assist the Client and Family to Cope With the Mood Effects of Persistent Pain

- Explain the relationship between chronic pain and mood disorders (e.g., anger, anxiety, depression).
- Encourage verbalization concerning difficult situations.
- Listen carefully.
- See *Ineffective Coping* for additional interventions.

Collaborate With the Client About Possible Methods to Reduce Pain Intensity

See *Acute Pain*.

Collaborate With the Client to Initiate Appropriate Nonpharmaceutical Pain-Relief Measures**

See *Acute Pain*.

**May require a primary care provider's order.

Provide Pain Relief with Prescribed Analgesics**

- Determine preferred route of administration: oral, IM, IV, or rectal.
- Assess the client's response to the medication. For those admitted to acute care settings:
  - After administration, return in 30 min to assess effectiveness.
  - Ask the client to rate severity of pain before the medication and amount of relief received.
  - Ask the client to indicate when the pain began to increase (e.g., activity, dressing change).
  - Consult with the physician/advanced practice nurse if a dosage or interval change is needed.
- For outpatients:
  - Ask the client to keep a record of when he or she takes medication and kind of relief received.
  - Instruct the client to consult physician with questions concerning medication dosage.
- Encourage the use of oral medications as soon as possible.
  - Consult with physician for a schedule to change from IM to IV or oral.
  - Explain to the client and family that oral medications can be as effective as IM.
- Explain how the transition will occur:
  - Begin oral medication at a larger dose than necessary (loading dose).
  - Continue PRN IV medication but use as a backup for pain unrelieved by oral medication.
  - Gradually reduce IM IV medication dose.
- Use the client's account of pain to regulate oral doses.
- Consult with physician about possibly adding aspirin or acetaminophen to medication regimen.

Discuss Fears (Individual, Family) of Addiction and Under Treatment of Pain

- Explain tolerance versus addiction.

Reduce or Eliminate Common Side Effects of Opioids

See *Acute Pain*.

Assist Family to Respond Optimally to the Client's Pain Experience

See *Acute Pain*.

- Encourage family to seek assistance if needed for specific problems, such as coping with chronic pain: family counselor; financial and service agencies (e.g., American Cancer Society).

**May require a primary care provider's order.

Promote Optimal Mobility

- Discuss the value of exercise (e.g., walking, yoga, or stretching).
- Plan daily activities when pain is at its lowest level.

Initiate Health Teaching and Referrals as Indicated

- Discuss with the client and family the various treatment modalities available:
  - Family therapy
  - Behavior modification
  - Hypnosis
  - Exercise program
  - Group therapy
  - Biofeedback
  - Acupuncture

🌿 Geriatric Interventions

- Assessment of chronic pain in older adults can be particularly challenging due to co morbidities, polypharmacy, and possible effects of increased sensitivities to pain medication (Dewar, 2006).
- Special attention must be paid to the beliefs of the individual and the past experiences that they have had with pain and pain treatments (Dewar, 2006).
- Exploration of chronic pain should include its impact on the functionality of the individual within the community including shopping, home chores, and socialization, as well as the ability to perform activities of daily living (ADLs) (Dewar, 2006).

⚕ Pediatric Interventions

- Assess pain experiences by using developmentally appropriate assessment scales and by assessing behavior. Incorporate child and family in ongoing assessment. Identify potential for secondary gain for reporting pain (e.g., companionship, attention, concern, caring, distraction); include strategies for meeting identified needs in plan of care.
- Set short-term and long-term goals for pain management with child and family and evaluate regularly (e.g., totally or partially relieve pain, control behavior, or anxiety associated with pain).
- Promote normal growth and development; involve family and available resources, such as occupational, physical, and child life therapists.

- Promote the "normal" aspects of the child's life: play, school, family relationships, physical activity.
- Promote a trusting environment for child and family.
- Believe the child's pain.
- Encourage child's perception that interventions are attempts to help.
- Provide continuity of care and pain management by health care providers (nurse, physician, pain team) and in different settings (inpatient, outpatient, emergency department, home).
- Use interdisciplinary team for pain management as necessary (e.g., nurse, physician, child life therapist, mental health therapist, occupational therapist, physical therapist, nutritionist).
- Identify myths and misconceptions about pediatric pain management (e.g., IM analgesia, narcotic use and dosing, assessment) in attitudes of health care professionals, child, and family; provide accurate information and opportunities for effective communication.
- Provide parents and siblings with opportunities to share their experiences and fears.

Nausea

NANDA-I Definition

A subjective phenomenon of an unpleasant feeling in the back of the throat and stomach that may or may not result in vomiting

Defining Characteristics*

Aversion toward food	Increased swallowing
Gagging sensation	Reports nausea
Increased salivation	Reports sour taste in mouth

Related Factors

Biopathophysiologic

Related to tissue trauma and reflex muscle spasms secondary to:

Acute gastroenteritis	Drug overdose
Peptic ulcer disease	Renal calculi
Irritable bowel syndrome	Uterine cramps associated
Pancreatitis	with menses
Infections (e.g., food poisoning)	Motion sickness

Treatment Related

Related to effects of chemotherapy, theophylline, digitalis, antibiotics, iron supplements

Related to effects of anesthesia

Situational (Personal, Environmental)*

Anxiety
Noxious odors, taste
Fear
Pain

Psychologic factors
Unpleasant visual stimulation

NOC

Comfort Level, Nutrition Status, Hydration

Goal

The client will report decreased nausea as experienced by the following indicators:

• Name foods or beverages that do not increase nausea.
• Describe factors that increase nausea.

NIC

Medication Management, Nausea Management, Fluid/Electrolyte Management, Nutrition Management

Interventions

Take Measures to Prevent Treatment-Related Nausea

• Aggressive management before, during, and after chemotherapy can prevent nausea (Yarbro, Wujcik, & Gobel, 2011).
• Aggressively prevent nausea and vomiting in those with risk factors (Pasero & McCaffery, 2011):
  • Female gender
  • Nonsmoker
  • History of motion sickness/postoperative nausea/vomiting
  • Use of volatile anesthetics within 0–2 hours, Nitrous oxide and or intraoperative and postoperative opioids.
  • Duration of surgery
  • Type of surgery (e.g., laparoscopic, ENT, neurosurgery, breast, plastic surgery)
• Consult with specialist to prevent postoperative nausea and vomiting intraoperatively and postoperatively (Pasero & McCaffery, 2011).

- Use multimodal analgesics to reduce the dose of opioids to lowest possible.
- Use multimodal antiemetics preinduction and at the end of surgery.

Promote Comfort During Nausea and Vomiting

- Protect those at risk for aspiration (immobile, children).
- Address the cleanliness of the client and environment.
- Provide an opportunity for oral care after each episode.
- Apply a cool, damp cloth to the client's forehead, neck, and wrists.

Reduce or Eliminate Noxious Stimuli

Pain
- Plan care to avoid unpleasant or painful procedures before meals.
- Medicate clients for pain 30 min before meals according to physician/NP's orders.
- Provide a pleasant, relaxed atmosphere for eating (no bedpans in sight, do not rush); try a "surprise" (e.g., flowers with meal).
- Arrange the plan of care to decrease or eliminate nauseating odors or procedures near mealtimes.

Fatigue
- Teach or assist the client to rest before meals.
- Teach the client to spend minimal energy preparing food (cook large quantities and freeze several meals at a time, request assistance from others).

Odor of Food
- Teach the client to avoid cooking odors—frying food, brewing coffee—if possible (take a walk; select foods that can be eaten cold).
- Suggest using foods that require little cooking during periods of nausea.
- Suggest trying sour foods.

Decrease Stimulation of the Vomiting Center

- Reduce unpleasant sights and odors. Restrict activity.
- Provide good mouth care after vomiting.
- Teach the client to practice deep breathing and voluntary swallowing to suppress the vomiting reflex.
- Instruct the client to sit down after eating, but not to lie down.
- Encourage the client to eat smaller meals and to eat slowly.
- Restrict liquids with meals to avoid overdistending the stomach; also, avoid fluids 1 hour before and after meals.

- Loosen clothing.
- Encourage the client to sit in fresh air or use a fan to circulate air.
- Advise the client to avoid lying flat for at least 2 hours after eating. (A client who must rest should sit or recline so that the head is at least 4 inches higher than the feet.)
- Advise the client to listen to music.
- Offer small amounts of clear fluids and foods and beverages with ginger.
- Offer muscle relaxation and distraction techniques to adult cancer patients.
- If qualified, use acupressure at pressure points post operatively.

Maternal Interventions

Teach That Various Interventions Have Been Reported to Help Control Nausea During Pregnancy

- Assure her that nausea is common during pregnancy (Pillitteri, 2010).
- Avoid fatigue and sudden movements.
- Avoid greasy, high-fat foods and strong odors.
- Eat high-protein meals and a snack before retiring.
- Chew gum or suck hard candies.
- Eat carbohydrates (e.g., crackers, toast, sour ball candy) on arising; Delay eating breakfast until nausea passes.
- Eat immediately when hungry.
- Do not go longer than 12 hours without eating.
- If nauseated, sip/consume carbonated beverages (e.g., Coke syrup, orange juice, ginger ale, and herbal teas such as ginger).
- Try deep breaths of fresh air
- Lie down to relieve symptoms.

Instruct the Pregnant Woman to Try One Food or Beverage Type at a Time (e.g., High-Protein Meals/Bedtime Snack)

- If nausea is not relieved, try another measure.
- Explain the use of acupressure and acupuncture. Refer to resources.

IMPAIRED COMMUNICATION**

Impaired Communication

Impaired Verbal Communication

**This diagnosis is not presently on the NANDA-I list but has been added for clarity and usefulness.

Definition

The state in which a person experiences, or is at risk to experience, difficulty exchanging thoughts, ideas, wants, or needs with others

Defining Characteristics

Major (Must Be Present)

Inappropriate or absent speech or response
Impaired ability to speak or hear

Minor (May Be Present)

Incongruence between verbal and nonverbal messages
Stuttering
Slurring
Word-finding problems
Weak or absent voice
Statements of being misunderstood or not understanding
Dysarthria
Aphasia
Language barrier

Related Factors

Pathophysiologic

Related to disordered, unrealistic thinking secondary to:
Schizophrenic disorder   Delusional disorder
Psychotic disorder   Paranoid disorder

Related to impaired motor function of muscles of speech secondary to:
Cerebrovascular accident ("Brain attack")
Oral or facial trauma
Brain damage (e.g., birth/head trauma)
Central nervous system (CNS) depression/increased intracranial
    pressure
Tumor (of the head, neck, or spinal cord)
Chronic hypoxia/decreased cerebral blood flow
Nervous system diseases (e.g., myasthenia gravis, multiple sclerosis, muscular dystrophy, Alzheimer's disease)
Vocal cord paralysis/quadriplegia

Related to impaired ability to produce speech secondary to:
Respiratory impairment (e.g., shortness of breath)
Laryngeal edema/infection
Oral deformities
Cleft lip or palate   Malocclusion or fractured jaw
Missing teeth   Dysarthria

Related to auditory impairment

Treatment Related

Related to impaired ability to produce speech secondary to:
Endotracheal intubation   Tracheostomy/tracheotomy/
Surgery of the head, face, neck,   laryngectomy
or mouth   Pain (especially of the mouth
CNS depressants   or throat)

Situational (Personal, Environmental)

Related to decreased attention secondary to fatigue, anger, anxiety, or pain

Related to no access to or malfunction of hearing aid

Related to psychologic barrier (e.g., fear, shyness)

Related to lack of privacy

Related to unavailable interpreter

Maturational

Infant/Child
Related to inadequate sensory stimulation

Older Adult (Auditory Losses)
Related to hearing impairment

Related to cognitive impairments secondary to (specify)

 Author's Note

Impaired Communication is clinically useful with individuals with commu-
nication-receptive deficits and language barriers.

Impaired Communication may not be useful to describe communication problems that are a manifestation of psychiatric illness or coping
problems. If nursing interventions focus on reducing hallucinations, fear,
or anxiety, *Confusion, Fear,* or *Anxiety* would be more appropriate.

NOC

Communication

Goal

The person will report improved satisfaction with ability to communicate as evidenced by the following indicators:

- Demonstrates increased ability to understand.
- Demonstrates improved ability to express self.
- Uses alternative methods of communication, as indicated.

NIC

Communication Enhancement: Speech, Communication Enhancement: Hearing Active Listening, Socialization Enhancement

Interventions

Identify a Method to Communicate Basic Needs

- Assess ability to comprehend, speak, read, and write
- Provide alternative methods of communication
  - Use a computer, pad and pencil, hand signals, eye blinks, head nods, and bell signals.
  - Make flash cards with pictures or words depicting frequently used phrases (e.g., "Wet my lips," "Move my foot," "I need a glass of water," or "I need a bedpan").
  - Encourage the person to point, use gestures, and pantomime.
- Using alternative forms of communication can help decrease anxiety, isolation, and alienation; promote a sense of control; and enhance safety (Iezzoni et al., 2004).

Identify Factors that Promote Communication

- Create atmosphere of acceptance and privacy
- Provide a non-rushed environment
- Use techniques to increase understanding
  - Face the client and establish eye contact if possible.
  - Use uncomplicated one-step commands and directives.
  - Have only one person talk (following a conversation among multiple parties can be difficult).
  - Encourage the use of gestures and pantomime.
  - Match words with actions; use pictures.
  - Terminate the conversation on a note of success (e.g., move back to an easier item).

- Validate that the client understands the message.
- Give information in writing to reinforce.

Initiate Health Teaching and Referrals, If Needed

- Seek consultation with a speech or audiology specialist.

Pediatric Interventions

- Use age-appropriate words and gestures (see *Delayed Growth and Development*, Table II.2).
- Initially talk to parent and allow the child to observe. Gradually include the child.
  - Approach the child slowly and speak in a quiet, unhurried, confident voice.
  - Assume an eye-level position.
  - Use simple words and short sentences.
  - Talk about something not related to the present situation (e.g., school, toy, hair, clothes).
- Offer choices as much as possible.
- Encourage the child to share concerns and fears.
- Allow the child an opportunity to touch and use articles (e.g., stethoscope, tongue blade).

Geriatric Interventions

- If the person can hear with a hearing aid, make sure that it is on and functioning.
- If the person can hear with one ear, speak slowly and clearly into the good ear. (It is more important to speak distinctly than to speak loudly.)
- If the person can read and write, provide pad and pencil at all times (even when going to another department).
- If the person can understand only sign language, have an interpreter with him or her as much as possible.
- Write and speak all important messages.
- Validate the person's understanding by asking questions that require more than "yes" or "no" answers. Avoid asking, "Do you understand?"
- Assess if cerumen impaction is impairing hearing.

Impaired Verbal Communication

NANDA-I Definition

Decreased, delayed, or absent ability to receive, process, transmit, and/or use a system of symbols

Defining Characteristics

Difficulty or inability to speak words but can understand others
Articulation or motor planning deficits

Related Factors

See *Impaired Communication*.

 NOC

Communication: Expressive Ability

Goal

The person will demonstrate improved ability to express self as
evidenced by the following indicators:

- Relate decreased frustration with communication.
- Use alternative methods as indicated.

 NIC

Active Listening, Communication Enhancement: Speech Deficit

Interventions

Identify a Method for Communicating Basic Needs

See *Impaired Communication for general interventions*.

Identify Factors That Promote Communication

For Clients with Dysarthria

- Reduce environmental noise (e.g., radio, TV) to increase the
  caregiver's ability to listen to words.
- Do not alter your speech or messages, because the client's
  comprehension is not affected; speak on an adult level.
- Encourage the client to make a conscious effort to slow down
  speech and to speak louder (e.g., "Take a deep breath between
  sentences.").
- Ask the client to repeat unclear words; observe for nonverbal
  cues to help understanding.
- If the client is tired, ask questions that require only short
  answers.
- If speech is unintelligible, teach use of gestures, written messages, and communication cards.

For Those Who Cannot Speak (e.g., Endotracheal Intubation, Tracheostomy)

- Reassure that speech will return, if it will. If not, explain available alternatives (e.g., esophageal speech, sign language).
- Do not alter your speech, tone, or type of message; speak on an adult level.
- Read lips for cues.

Promote Continuity of Care to Reduce Frustration

Observe for Signs of Frustration or Withdrawal

- Verbally address frustration over inability to communicate. Explain that both nurse and client must use patience.
- Maintain a calm, positive attitude (e.g., "I can understand you if we work at it.").
- Use reassurance (e.g., "I know it's difficult, but you'll get it.").
- Maintain a sense of humor.
- Allow tears (e.g., "It's OK. I know it's frustrating. Crying can let it all out.").
- For the client with limited speaking ability (e.g., can make simple requests, but not lengthy statements), encourage letter writing or keeping a diary to express feelings and share concerns.
- Anticipate needs and ask questions that need a simple yes or no answer.

Maintain a Specific Care Plan

- Write the method of communication that is used (e.g., "Uses word cards," "Points for bedpan" alphabet board, picture board writing materials).
- Record directions for specific measures (e.g., allow him to keep a urinal in bed).

Initiate Health Teaching and Referrals, as Indicated

- Teach communication techniques and repetitive approaches to significant others.
- Encourage the family to share feelings concerning communication problems.
- Seek consultation with a speech pathologist early in the treatment regimen.

🔹 Pediatric Interventions

- Establish a method of communication appropriate for age.
- If a young child is deprived of vocalization, teach basic language gestures (time, food, family relationships, emotions, animals, numbers, frequent requests).

- Consult with a speech pathologist for ongoing assistance.
- Discuss with parents or caregivers the importance of providing the child with a method of communication.

ACUTE CONFUSION

Acute Confusion

Risk for Acute Confusion

NANDA-I Definition

Abrupt onset of reversible disturbances of consciousness, attention, cognition, and perception that develop over a short period of time

Defining Characteristics

Major (Must be Present)

Abrupt onset of:
Fluctuation in cognition*   Fluctuation in level of consciousness*

Fluctuation in psychomotor activity
Increased agitation*   Incoherence
Reduced ability to focus   Fear
Disorientation   Anxiety
Increased restlessness*   Excitement
Hypervigilance

Symptoms are worse at night or when fatigued or in new situations.

Minor (May Be Present)

Illusions   Delusions
Hallucinations*   Misperceptions*

Related Factors

Related to abrupt onset of cerebral hypoxia or disturbance in cerebral metabolism secondary to (Miller, 2009):

Fluid and Electrolyte Disturbances
Dehydration   Hypokalemia
Acidosis/alkalosis   Hyponatremia/hypernatremia
Hypercalcemia/hypocalcemia   Hypoglycemia/hyperglycemia

Nutritional Deficiencies
Folate or vitamin B_{12} deficiency   Niacin deficiency
Anemia   Magnesium deficiency

Cardiovascular Disturbances
Myocardial infarction   Heart block
Congestive heart failure   Temporal arteritis
Dysrhythmias   Subdural hematoma

Respiratory Disorders
Chronic obstructive pulmonary disease: Tuberculosis and pneumonia
Pulmonary embolism

Infections
Sepsis   Urinary tract infection (especially
Meningitis, encephalitis   elderly)

Metabolic and Endocrine Disorders
Hypothyroidism/hyperthyroidism: Hypoadrenocorticism/
    hyperadrenocorticism
Hypopituitarism/hyperpituitarism: Postural hypotension,
    hypothermia/hyperthermia
Parathyroid disorders: Hepatic or renal failure

Central Nervous System (CNS) Disorders
Cerebral vascular accident   Head trauma
Multiple infarctions   Seizures and postconvulsive
Tumors   states
Normal-pressure hydrocephalus

Treatment Related

Related to a disturbance in cerebral metabolism secondary to:

Surgery
Therapeutic drug intoxication
    Neuroleptics: Opioids
    General anesthesia
Side effects of medication:
    Diuretics
    Digitalis
    Propranolol
    Atropine
    Oral hypoglycemics
    Anti-inflammatories
    Antianxiety agents
    Barbiturates
    Methyldopa

Disulfiram
Lithium
Phenytoin
Over-the-counter cold, cough, and sleeping preparations
Sulfa drugs
Ciprofloxacin
Metronidazole
Acyclovir
H2 receptor antagonists
Anticholinergics
Phenothiazines
Benzodiazepines

Situational (Personal, Environmental)

Related to disturbance in cerebral metabolism secondary to:
Withdrawal from alcohol, opioids, sedatives, hypnotics
Heavy metal or carbon monoxide intoxication

Related to:

Pain   Depression
Bowel impaction   Unfamiliar situations
Immobility

Related to chemical intoxications or medications (specify):

Alcohol   Methamphetamines
Cocaine   PCP
Methadone   Opioids, e.g., heroin

Author's Note

"Confusion" is a term nurses use frequently to describe an array of cognitive impairments. "Identifying a person as confused is just an initial step" (Rasin, 1990; Roberts, 2001). Confusion is a behavior that indicates a disturbance in cerebral metabolism. Reduced cerebral metabolism decreases neurotransmitter levels in the brain, especially acetylcholine and epinephrine. Acetylcholine is necessary for attention, learning, memory, and information processing (Rasin, 1990; Roberts, 2001).

The addition of *Acute Confusion* and *Chronic Confusion* to the NANDA-I list provides the nurse with more diagnostic clarity than *Confusion* or *Disturbed Thought Processes*. *Acute Confusion* has an abrupt onset with fluctuating symptoms; whereas *Chronic Confusion* describes long-standing or progressive degeneration. *Disturbed Thought Processes* is also a disruption of cognitive processes; however, the causes are related to coping problems or personality disorders.

NOC

Cognition, Cognitive Orientation, Distorted Thought Self-Control

Goal

The person will have diminished episodes of delirium as evidenced by the following indicators:

- Be less agitated.
- Participate in ADLs.
- Be less combative.

NIC

Delirium Management, Calming Technique, Reality Orientation, Environmental Management: Safety

Interventions

Assess for Causative and Contributing Factors

- Vision impairment
- Severe illness
- Dehydration (blood urea nitrogen/creatine over 18)
- Pre existing cognitive impairment

Environmental Factors

- Room changes
- Presence of medical or chemical restraint
- Absence of watch or clock
- Absence of support system
- Ensure that a thorough diagnostic workup has been completed.

Laboratory

- CBC and electrolytes
- TSH, T_4
- Vitamin B_{12} and folate, thiamine
- Serum thyroxine and serum-free thyroxine
- Rapid plasma reagin (RPR)
- Calcium and phosphate
- Na and K
- Creatinine, blood urea nitrogen
- AST, ALT, and bilirubin
- Serum glucose and fasting blood sugar
- Urinalysis

Diagnostic

- EEG
- CT scan
- Chest x-ray
- ECG

Psychiatric Evaluation
• Evaluate for depression.

Promote the Client's Sense of Integrity

• Examine knowledge and attitudes about confusion, especially in the aged.
• Educate family, significant others, and caregivers about the situation and coping methods (Young, 2001):
    • Explain the cause of the confusion.
    • Explain that the client does not realize the situation.
    • Explain the need to remain patient, flexible, and calm.
    • Stress the need to respond to the client as an adult.
    • Explain that the behavior is part of a disorder and is not voluntary.
• Maintain standards of empathic, respectful care.
    • Be an advocate when other caregivers are insensitive to the client's needs.
    • Function as a role model with coworkers.
    • Provide other caregivers with up-to-date information on confusion.
    • Expect empathic, respectful care and monitor its administration.
    • Attempt to obtain information for conversation (likes, dislikes; interests, hobbies; work history). Interview early in the day.
    • Encourage significant others and caregivers to speak slowly with a low voice pitch and at an average volume (unless hearing deficits are present), with eye contact, and as if expecting the client to understand.
• Provide respect and promote sharing.
    • Pay attention to what the client says.
    • Pick out meaningful comments and continue talking.
    • Call the client by name and introduce yourself each time you make contact; use touch if welcomed.
    • Use the name the client prefers; avoid "Pops" or "Mom," which can increase confusion and is unacceptable.
    • Convey to the client that you are concerned and friendly (through smiles, an unhurried pace, humor, and praise; do not argue).
    • Focus on the feeling behind the spoken word or action.

Provide Sufficient and Meaningful Sensory Input

• Reduce abrupt changes in schedule or relocation.
    • Keep the client oriented to time and place.
    • Refer to time of day and place each morning.
    • Provide the client with a clock and calendar large enough to see.

- Ensure corrective lenses are available and used.
- Use nightlights or dim lights at night.
- Use indirect lighting and turn on lights before dark.
- Provide the client with the opportunity to see daylight and dark through a window, or take the client outdoors.
- Single out holidays with cards or pins (e.g., wear a red heart for Valentine's Day).
- Reduce or eliminate:
  - Fatigue
  - Change in routine, environment, or caregiver
  - High-stimulus activity (e.g., crowds) or images (e.g., frightening pictures or movies)
  - Frustration from trying to function beyond capabilities or from being restrained
  - Pain, discomforts, illness, or side effects from medications
  - Competing or misleading stimuli (e.g., mirrors, television, costumes)
- Use adaptive devices to diminish sensory impediments (e.g., lighting, glasses, hearing aids).
- Encourage the family to bring in familiar objects from home (e.g., photographs with nonglare glass, afghan).
  - Ask the client to tell you about the picture.
  - Focus on familiar topics.
- In teaching a task or activity—such as eating—break it into small, brief steps by giving only one instruction at a time.
  - Remove covers from food plate and cups.
  - Locate the napkin and utensils.
  - Add sugar and milk to coffee.
  - Add condiments to food (sugar, salt, pepper).
  - Cut foods.
  - Offer simple explanations of tasks.
  - Allow the client to handle equipment related to each task.
  - Allow the client to participate in the task, such as washing his face.
  - Acknowledge that you are leaving and say when you will return.

Promote a Well Role

- Allow former habits (e.g., reading in the bathroom).
- Encourage the wearing of dentures.
- Ask the client/significant other about his usual grooming routine and encourage him to follow it.
- Provide privacy at all times; when it is necessary to expose a body surface, take precautions to cover all other areas (e.g., if washing a back, use towels or blankets to cover legs and front torso).

- Provide for personal hygiene according to the client's preferences (hair grooming, showers or bath, nail care, cosmetics, deodorants, fragrances).
- Discourage the use of nightclothes during the day; have the client wear shoes, not slippers.
- Promote mobility as much as possible.
- Have the client eat meals out of bed, unless contraindicated.
- Promote socialization during meals (e.g., set up lunch for four individuals in the lounge).
- Plan an activity each day to look forward to (e.g., bingo, ice cream sundae gathering).
- Encourage participation in decision-making (e.g., selecting what he wishes to wear).

Discuss Current Events, Seasonal Events (Snow, Water Activities); Share Your Interests (Travel, Crafts)

Do Not Endorse Confusion

- Do not argue with the client.
- Determine the best response to confused statements.
- Sometimes the confused client may be comforted by a response that reduces his or her fear; for example, "I want to see my mother," when his or her mother has been dead for 20 years. The nurse may respond with, "I know that your mother loved you."
- Direct the client back to reality; do not allow him or her to ramble.
- Adhere to the schedule; if changes are necessary, advise the client of them.
- Avoid talking to coworkers about other topics in the client's presence.
- Provide simple explanations that cannot be misinterpreted.
- Remember to acknowledge your entrance with a greeting and your exit with a closure ("I will be back in 10 minutes").
- Avoid open-ended questions.
- Replace five- or six-step tasks with two- or three-step tasks.

Prevent Injury to the Individual

- Follow institutional procedures for protecting confused persons (e.g., sitters).
- Explore other alternatives instead of restraints (Rateau, 2000). Put the client in a room with others who can help watch him.
- Enlist the aid of family or friends to watch the client during confused periods.
- If the client is pulling out tubes, use mitts instead of wrist restraints.

- Refer to *Risk for Injury* for strategies for assessing and manipulating the environment for hazards.
- Register with an emergency medical system, including the "wanderers' list" with the local police department.

Initiate Referrals, as Needed

- Refer caregivers to appropriate community resources.

Risk for Acute Confusion

NANDA-I Definition

At risk for reversible disturbances of consciousness, attention, cognition, and perception that develop over a short period of time

Risk Factors

Refer to Related Factors under *Acute Confusion*.

Refer to *Acute Confusion*.

Goal

The individual will demonstrate continued level of orientation, attention, and cognition.

Interventions

Refer to *Acute Confusion*.

CHRONIC CONFUSION

NANDA-I Definition

Irreversible, long-standing, and/or progressive deterioration of intellect and personality characterized by decreased ability to interpret environmental stimuli; decreased capacity for intellectual thought processes; and manifested by disturbances of memory, orientation, and behavior

Defining Characteristics

Major (Must Be Present)

Progressive or long-standing:

Cognitive or intellectual losses
  Loss of memory
  Inability to make choices, decisions
Loss of time sense
Inability to solve problems, reason
  Altered perceptions
  Poor judgment
Loss of language abilities
Affective or personality losses
  Loss of affect
  Diminished inhibition
  Loss of tact, control of temper
  Loss of recognition (others, environment, self)
  Increasing self-preoccupation

Psychotic features
  Antisocial behavior
  Loss of energy reserve
Cognitive or planning losses
Loss of general ability to plan
Progressively lowered stress threshold
Impaired ability to set goals, plan
  Purposeful wandering
  Violent, agitated, or anxious behavior
  Compulsive repetitive behavior
  Purposeless behavior
  Withdrawal or avoidance behavior

Related Factors

Pathophysiologic (Hall, 1991)

Related to progressive degeneration of the cerebral cortex secondary to:

Alzheimer's disease*   Combination
Multi-infarct dementia (MID)*

Related to disturbance in cerebral metabolism, structure, or integrity secondary to:

Pick's disease   Creutzfeldt–Jakob disease
Toxic substance injection   Degenerative neurologic disease
Brain tumors   Huntington's chorea
End-stage diseases   Psychiatric disorders
  (AIDS, cirrhosis, cancer, renal failure, cardiac failure, chronic obstructive pulmonary disease)

 Author's Note

Refer to *Acute Confusion.*

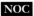

NOC

Cognitive Ability, Cognitive Orientation, Distorted Thought Self-Control, Surveillance: Safety, Emotional Support, Environmental Management, Fall Prevention, Calming Technique

Goal

The person will participate to the maximum level of independence in a therapeutic milieu as evidenced by the following indicators:

- Decreased frustration
- Diminished episodes of combativeness
- Increased hours of sleep at night
- Stabilized or increased weight

NIC

Dementia Management: Multisensory Therapy, Cognitive Stimulation, Calming Technique, Reality Orientation, Environmental Management: Safety

Interventions

Refer to Interventions Under Acute Confusion

Assess Who the Person Was Before the Onset of Confusion

- Educational level, career
- Hobbies, lifestyle
- Coping styles

Observe the Client to Determine Baseline Behaviors

- Best time of day
- Response time to a simple question
- Amount of distraction tolerated
- Judgment
- Insight into disability
- Signs/symptoms of depression
- Routine

Promote the Client's Sense of Integrity (Miller, 2009)

- Adapt communication to the client's level:
  - Avoid "baby talk" and a condescending tone of voice.
  - Use simple sentences and present one idea at a time.
  - If the client does not understand, repeat the sentence using the same words.
- Use positive statements; avoid "don'ts."
- Unless a safety issue is involved, do not argue.

- Avoid general questions, such as, "What would you like to do?" Instead, ask, "Do you want to go for a walk or work on your rug?"
- Be sensitive to the feelings the client is trying to express.
- Avoid questions you know the client cannot answer.
- If possible, demonstrate to reinforce verbal communication.
- Use touch to gain attention or show concern unless a negative response is elicited.
- Maintain good eye contact and pleasant facial expressions.
- Determine which sense dominates the client's perception of the world (auditory, kinesthetic, olfactory, or gustatory). Communicate through the preferred sense.

Promote the Client's Safety

- Ensure that the client carries identification.
- Adapt the environment so that the client can pace or walk if desired.
- Keep the environment uncluttered.
- Reevaluate whether treatment is needed. If needed, provide the following to promote safety.

Intravenous Therapy

- Camouflage tubing with loose gauze.
- Consider an intermittent access device instead of continuous IV therapy.
- If dehydration is a problem, institute a regular schedule for offering oral fluids.
- Use the least restrictive sites.

Urinary Catheters

- Evaluate causes of incontinence.
- Institute a specific treatment depending on type. Refer to *Impaired Urinary Elimination*.
- Place urinary collection bag at the end of the bed with catheter between rather than draped over legs. Velcro bands can hold the catheter against the leg.

Gastrointestinal Tubes

- Check frequently for pressure against nares.
- Camouflage gastrostomy tube with a loosely applied abdominal binder.
- If the client is pulling out tubes, use mitts instead of wrist restraints.
- Evaluate if restlessness is associated with pain. If analgesics are used, adjust dosage to reduce side effects.
- Put the client in a room with others who can help watch him or her.

- Enlist the aid of family or friends to watch the client during confused periods.
- Give the client something to hold (e.g., stuffed animal).

If Combative, Determine the Source of the Fear and Frustration

- Fatigue
- Misleading or inappropriate stimuli
- Change in routine, environment, caregiver
- Pressure to exceed functional capacity
- Physical stress, pain, infection, acute illness, discomfort

If a Dysfunctional Episode or Sudden Functional Loss Has Occurred

- Address the client by surname.
- Assume a dependent position to the client.
- Distract the client with cues that require automatic social behavior (e.g., "Mrs. Smith, would you like some juice now?").
- After the episode has passed, discuss the episode with the client.
- Document antecedents, behavior observed, and consequences.

Ensure Physical Comfort and Maintenance of Basic Health Needs

- Refer to *Self-Care Deficits*.

Select Modalities Involving the Five Senses (Hearing, Sight, Smell, Taste, and Touch) That Provide Favorable Stimuli for the Client

Music Therapy
- Determine the client's preferences. Play this music before the usual level of agitation for at least 30 min; assess response.
- Evaluate response, as some music can agitate individuals.
- Provide soft, soothing music during meals.
- Arrange group songfests with consideration to cultural/ethical orientation.
- Play music during other therapies (physical, occupational, and speech).
- Have the client exercise to music.
- Organize guest entertainment.
- Use client-developed songbooks (large print and decorative covers).

Recreation Therapy
- Encourage arts and crafts
- Suggest creative writing
- Provide puzzles
- Organize group games

Remotivation Therapy
• Organize group sessions into five steps (Dennis, 1984):

Step 1: Create a climate of acceptance (approx. 5 min).
  • Maintain a relaxed atmosphere; introduce leaders and participants.
  • Provide large-letter name tags and names on chairs.
  • Maintain assigned places for every session.

Step 2: Creating a bridge to reality (approx. 15 min).
  • Use a prop (visual, audio, song, picture, object, poem) to introduce the theme of the session.

Step 3: Share the world we live in (approx. 15 min).
  • Discuss the topic as a group.
  • Promote stimulation of senses.

Step 4: Appreciate the work of the world (approx. 20 min).
  • Discuss how the topic relates to their past experiences (work, leisure).

Step 5: Create a climate of appreciation (approx. 5 min).
  • Thank each member individually.
  • Announce the next session's topic and meeting date.
  • Use associations and analogies (e.g., "If ice is cold, then fire is. . . ?" "If day is light, then night is . . . ?").

• Choose topics for remotivation sessions based on suggestions from group leaders and group interests. Examples are pets, bodies of water, canning fruits and vegetables, transportation, and holidays.

Sensory Training
• Stimulate vision (with brightly colored items of different shape, pictures, colored decorations, kaleidoscopes).
• Stimulate smell (with flowers, soothing aromas from lavender or scented lotion).
• Stimulate hearing (play music with soothing sounds such as ocean or rain).
• Stimulate touch (massage, vibrating recliner, fuzzy objects, velvet, silk, stuffed animals).
• Stimulate taste (spices, salt, sugar, sour substances).

Reminiscence Therapy
• Consider instituting reminiscence therapy on a one-to-one or group basis. Discuss the purpose and Goals with the client care team. Prepare well before initiating.

Implement Techniques to Lower the Stress Threshold (Hall & Buckwalter, 1987; Miller, 2009)

Reduce Competing or Excessive Stimuli
• Keep the environment simple and uncluttered.

- Use simple written cues to clarify directions for use of radio and television.
- Eliminate or minimize unnecessary noise.

Plan and Maintain a Consistent Routine
- Attempt to assign the same caregivers.
- Elicit from family members specific methods that help or hinder care.
- Arrange personal care items in order of use (clothes, toothbrush, mouthwash, and so forth).
- Determine a daily routine with the client and family.
- Write down the sequence for all caregivers.
- Reduce the stress when change is anticipated:
  - Keep the change as simple as possible (e.g., minimal holiday decorations).
  - Ensure the client is well rested.
  - Institute change during the client's best time of day if possible.

Focus on the Client's Ability Level
- Do not request performance of function beyond ability.
- Express unconditional positive regard for the client.
- Modify environment to compensate for ability (e.g., use of Velcro fasteners, loose clothing, elastic waistbands).
- Use simple sentences; demonstrate activity.
- Do not ask questions that the client cannot answer.
- Avoid open-ended questions (e.g., "What do you want to eat?" "When do you want to take a bath?").
- Avoid using pronouns; name objects.
- Offer simple choices (e.g., "Do you want a cookie or crackers?").
- Use finger foods (e.g., sandwiches) to encourage self-feeding.

Minimize Fatigue (Hall, 1994)
- Provide rest periods twice daily.
- Choose a rest activity with the client, such as reading or listening to music.
- Encourage napping in recliner chairs, not in bed.
- Plan high-stress or fatiguing activities during the best time of day for the client.
- Allow the person to cease an activity at any time.
- Incorporate regular exercise in the daily plan.
- Be alert to expressions of fatigue and increased anxiety; immediately reduce stimuli.

Initiate Health Teaching and Referrals, as Needed
- Support groups
- Community-based programs (e.g., day care, respite care)
- Alzheimer's association (www.alz.org)
- Long-term care facilities

CONSTIPATION

Constipation

Perceived Constipation

NANDA-I Definition

Decrease in normal frequency of defecation accompanied by difficult or incomplete passage of stool and/or passage of excessively hard, dry stool

Defining Characteristics

Major (Must Be Present)

Hard, formed stool*
Defecation fewer than two
   times a week

Prolonged and difficult
   evacuation

Minor (May Be Present)

Distended abdomen*
Generalized fatigue*
Decreased bowel sounds

Straining with defecation*
Palpable rectal mass*

Related Factors

Pathophysiologic

Related to defective nerve stimulation, weak pelvic floor muscles, and immobility secondary to:
Spinal cord lesions
Spinal cord injury
Spina bifida
Cerebrovascular accident (CVA)/stroke
Neurologic diseases (multiple sclerosis, Parkinson's)
Dementia

Related to decreased metabolic rate secondary to:
Obesity
Pheochromocytoma
Hypothyroidism
Hyperparathyroidism

Uremia
Hypopituitarism
Diabetic neuropathy

Related to decreased response to urge to defecate secondary to:
Affective disorders

Related to pain (on defecation):
Hemorrhoids   Back injury

Related to decreased peristalsis secondary to hypoxia (cardiac, pulmonary)

Related to motility disturbances secondary to irritable bowel syndrome

Related to failure to relax anal sphincter or high resting pressure in the anal canal secondary to:
Multiple vaginal deliveries   Chronic straining

Treatment Related

Related to side effects of (specify):

Antidepressants	Calcium-channel blockers
Antacids (calcium, aluminum)	Calcium
Iron	Anticholinergics
Barium	Anesthetics
Aluminum	Narcotics (codeine, morphine)
Aspirin	Diuretics
Phenothiazines	Anti-Parkinson agents
Anticonvulsants	Chemotherapy

Related to effects of anesthesia and surgical manipulation on peristalsis

Related to habitual laxative use

Related to mucositis secondary to radiation

Situational (Personal, Environmental)

Related to decreased peristalsis secondary to:
Immobility   Stress
Pregnancy   Lack of exercise

Related to irregular evacuation patterns

Related to cultural/health beliefs

Related to lack of privacy

Related to inadequate diet (lack of roughage, fiber, thiamine) or fluid intake

Related to fear of rectal or cardiac pain

Related to faulty appraisal

Related to inability to perceive bowel cues

Author's Note

Constipation results from delayed passage of food residue in the bowel because of factors that the nurse can treat (e.g., dehydration, insufficient dietary roughage, immobility). *Perceived Constipation* refers to a faulty perception of constipation with self-prescribed overuse of laxatives, enemas, and/or suppositories.

NOC

Bowel Elimination, Hydration, Knowledge: Diet

Goal

The client will report bowel movements at least every 2 to 3 days as evidenced by the following indicators:

• Describe components for effective bowel movements.
• Explain rationale for lifestyle change(s).

NIC

Bowel Management, Fluid Management, Constipation/Impaction Management

Interventions

Assess Contributing Factors

Refer to Related Factors.

Promote Corrective Measures

Regular Time for Elimination
• Review daily routine.
• Advise the client to include time for defecation as part of his or her daily routine.
• Discuss a suitable time (based on responsibilities, availability of facilities, etc.).
• Provide a stimulus to defecation (e.g., coffee, prune juice).
• Advise the client to attempt to defecate about 1 hour or so after meals and that remaining in the bathroom for a suitable length of time may be necessary.

Adequate Exercise
• Review the current exercise pattern.
• Provide for frequent moderate physical exercise (if not contra-indicated).

- Provide frequent ambulation of the hospitalized client when tolerable.
- Perform range-of-motion exercises for the client who is bedridden.
- Teach exercises for increased abdominal muscle tone, unless contraindicated (Weeks, Hubbartt, & Michaels, 2000).
  - Contract abdominal muscles several times throughout the day.
  - Do sit-ups, keeping heels on floor with knees slightly flexed.
  - While supine, raise lower limbs, keeping knees straight.
- Turn and change positions in bed, lifting hips.
- Lift knees alternately to the chest, stretching arms out to side and up over the head.

Balanced Diet
- Review list of foods high in fiber:
  - Fresh fruits, fruit juices, and vegetables with skins
  - Beans (navy, kidney, lima), nuts, and seeds
  - Whole-grain breads, cereal, and bran
- Discuss dietary preferences.
- Consider any food intolerances or allergies.
- Include approximately 800 g of fruits and vegetables (about four pieces of fresh fruit and large salad) for normal daily bowel movement. Avoid cooked fruits.
- Suggest moderate use of bran at first (may irritate GI tract, produce flatulence, cause diarrhea or blockage).
- Gradually increase bran as tolerated (may add to cereals, baked goods, etc.). Explain the need for fluid intake with bran.
- Suggest 30 to 60 mL daily of a recipe of 2 cups of all-bran cereal, 2 cups of applesauce, and 1 cup of prune juice.
- Consider financial limitations (encourage the use of fruits and vegetables in season).

Adequate Fluid Intake
- Encourage intake of at least 2 L (8 to 10 glasses) unless contraindicated.
- Discuss fluid preferences.
- Set up regular schedule for fluid intake.
- Recommend drinking a glass of hot water 30 minutes before breakfast, which may stimulate bowel evacuation.
- Advise avoiding grapefruit juice, coffee, tea, cola, and chocolate drinks as daily fluid intake.

Optimal Position
- Provide privacy (close door, draw curtains around the bed, play the television or radio to mask sounds, have a room deodorizer available).

- Use the bathroom instead of a bedpan if possible. Allow suitable position (sitting and leaning forward, if not contraindicated).
- Elevate the legs on a footstool when on the toilet.
- Assist the client onto the bedpan if necessary; elevate the head of the bed to high Fowler's position or elevation permitted.

Conduct Health Teaching, as Indicated

- Explain the relationship of lifestyle changes to constipation.
- Instruct to advise health care professional if more than 3 days have passed without a bowel movement.
- Administer a mild laxative after oral administration of barium sulfate.**
- Assess elimination status while on antacid therapy (may be necessary to alternate magnesium-type antacid with other types).**
- Encourage increased intake of high-roughage foods and increased fluid intake as an adjunct to iron therapy (e.g., fresh fruits and vegetables with skins, bran, nuts, seeds, whole-wheat bread).
- Encourage early ambulation, with assistance if necessary, to counter effects of anesthetic agents.
- Assess elimination status while the client receives certain narcotic analgesics (morphine, codeine) and alert a physician if the client experiences difficulty with defecation.
- Advise the client about medications that cause constipation (e.g., antacids, bismuth, calcium channel blockers, clonidine, levodopa, iron, nonsteroidal anti-inflammatories, opiates, sucralfate [Shua-Haim, Sabo, & Ross, 1999]).
- Discuss laxative abuse (see *Perceived Constipation*).

Pediatric Considerations

- Discuss some causes of constipation in infants and children (e.g., underfeeding; high-protein, low-carbohydrate diet; lack of roughage; dehydration).
- If bowel movements are infrequent with hard stools:
  - With infants, add corn syrup to feeding or fruit to diet. Avoid apple juice or sauce.
  - With children, add bran cereal, prune juice, and fruits and vegetables high in bulk.
- Refer cases of persistent constipation for medical evaluation.
- Explain to adolescents the effects of fluids, fiber, and exercise on bowel function.

Maternal Considerations

- Explain the risks of constipation in pregnancy and postpartum:
  - Decreased gastric motility

** May require a primary care provider's order.

- Prolonged intestinal time
- Pressure of enlarging uterus
- Distended abdominal muscles (post)
- Relaxation of intestines (post)
- Iron supplements
- Explain aggravating factors for hemorrhoid development (straining at defecation, constipation, prolonged standing, wearing constrictive clothing).
- If woman has a history of constipation, discuss use of bulk-producing laxatives to soften bowels postdelivery.
- Assess abdomen (bowel sounds, distention, presence of flatus).
- Assess for hemorrhoids and perineal swelling.
- Provide relief of rectal or perineal pain.
- Instruct the client to take sitz baths and use cool, astringent compresses for hemorrhoids.
- Advise the importance of iron supplements for the fetus and not to discontinue due to constipation (Pillitteri, 2010).
- Refer to Interventions for preventing constipation.
- Iron supplements provide the iron stored for the fetus for growth and development (Pillitteri, 2010).

☘ Geriatric Interventions

- Discuss that individual bowel patterns vary (e.g., three times a day to three times a week).
- Discuss medications that can contribute to constipation (e.g., anticholinergics, narcotics, iron sulfate, psychotropic medications, aluminum and calcium antacids, tricyclic antidepressants, overuse of antidiarrheals).

Perceived Constipation

NANDA-I Definition

Self-diagnoses of constipation combined with abuse of laxatives, enemas, and/or suppositories to ensure a daily bowel movement

Defining Characteristics

Expectation of a daily bowel movement*
Overuse of laxatives, enemas, and/or suppositories*
Expectation of passage of stool at same time, every day*

Related Factors

Pathophysiologic

Related to faulty appraisal* secondary to:
Obsessive–compulsive disorders   Depression
Deterioration of the CNS   Impaired thought processes*

Situational (Personal, Environmental)
Related to inaccurate information secondary to:
Cultural health beliefs*   Family health beliefs*

 Author's Note

Refer to Author's Note under *Constipation*.

NOC

Bowel Elimination, Health Beliefs: Perceived Threat

Goal

The client will verbalize acceptance of a bowel movement every 1 to 3 days as evidenced by the following indicators:

- The client will not use laxatives regularly.
- The client will relate the causes of constipation.
- The client will describe the hazards of laxative use.
- The client will relate an intent to increase fiber, fluid, and exercise in daily life as instructed.

NIC

Bowel Management, Health Education, Behavior Modification, Fluid Management, Nutrition Management

Interventions

Assess Causative or Contributing Factors

- Cultural/familial belief
- Faulty appraisal

Explain That Bowel Movements Are Needed Every 2 to 3 Days, Not Daily

- Be sensitive to the client's beliefs.
- Be patient.

Explain the Hazards of Regular Laxative Use

- They provide only temporary relief and can promote constipation by interfering with peristalsis.
- They can interfere with absorption of vitamins A, D, E, and K.
- They can cause diarrhea.

If a Laxative Is Desired, Teach the Client How to Use Bulk-Forming Agents, Such as Psyllium Seed or Bran

- Start slowly with one-half the recommended dose.
- Increase the dose gradually over weeks.
- Refer to *Constipation* for interventions to promote optimal elimination.

INDIVIDUAL CONTAMINATION

Individual Contamination

Risk for Individual Contamination

NANDA-I Definition

Exposure to environmental contaminants in doses sufficient to cause adverse health effects

Defining Characteristics

Defining characteristics are dependent on the causative agent. Causative agents include pesticides*, chemicals*, biologics*, waste*, radiation*, and pollution*.

Pesticide Exposure Effects

Pulmonary
Anaphylactic reaction
Asthma
Irritation to nose and throat
Burning sensation in throat and chest
Pulmonary edema
Shortness of breath
Pneumonia
Upper airway irritation
Dyspnea
Bronchitis
Pulmonary fibrosis
COPD
Bronchiolitis
Airway hyperreactivity
Damage to the mucous membranes of the respiratory tract

Neurologic

Reye's-like syndrome	Peripheral neuropathy
Confusion	Pinpoint pupils
Anxiety	Blurred vision
Seizures	Headache
Decreased level	Dizziness
of consciousness	CNS excitation
Coma	Depression
Muscle fasciculation	Paresthesia
Skeletal muscle myotonia	

Gastrointestinal

Nausea, vomiting, diarrhea, and flu-like symptoms

Dermatologic

Chloracne

Cardiac

Cardiac dysrhythmia, tachycardia, bradycardia, conduction
block, and hypotension

Hepatic

Liver dysfunction

Chemical Exposure Effects

Pulmonary

Irritation of nose and throat, dyspnea, bronchitis, pulmonary
edema, and cough

Neurologic

Headache	Diplopia
Ataxia	Psychosis
Confusion	CNS depression
Seizures	Tremors
Lethargy	Weakness
Unconsciousness	Paralysis
Coma	Memory changes
Lacrimation	Encephalopathy
Ataxia	Hearing Loss
Vertigo	Parkinson's-like syndrome
Mood changes	Euphoria
Delirium	Narcosis
Hallucinations	Syncope
Nystagmus	Hyperthermia

Renal

Acetonuria and renal failure

Gastrointestinal

Nausea	Ulceration of the GI tract
Vomiting	Metabolic acidosis

Endocrine
Hyperglycemia, hypoglycemia

Dermatologic

Dermatitis	Conjunctivitis
Irritation of the skin and mucous membranes	Hyperpigmentation of skin and nails
Mucosal burns of eyes, nose, pharynx, and larynx	Dermal burns

Immunologic
Altered blood clotting and bone marrow depression

Reproductive
Shortening of menstrual cycle

Cardiac
Hypotension and chest pain

Ophthalmic
Pupil changes, blurred vision, severe eye pain, corneal irritation, temporary or permanent blindness

Hepatic

Jaundice	Hepatitis
Hepatomegaly	Pancreatitis

Biologic Exposure Effects

Bacteria
Anthrax (*Bacillus anthracis*): fever, chills, drenching sweats, profound fatigue, minimally productive cough, nausea and vomiting, and chest discomfort
Cholera (*Vibrio cholerae*): profuse watery diarrhea, vomiting, leg cramps, dehydration, and shock
Salmonella (*Salmonellosis*): fever, abdominal cramps, diarrhea (sometimes bloody), localized infection, and sepsis
E. coli (*Escherichia coli* 0157:H7): severe, bloody diarrhea and abdominal cramps; mild or no fever

Viruses
Smallpox (Variola virus): high fever, head and body aches, vomiting, and skin rash with bumps and raised pustules that crust, scab, and form a pitted scar

Ebola hemorrhagic fever (Ebola filovirus): headache, fever, joint and muscle aches, sore throat, and weaknesses followed by diarrhea, vomiting, stomachache, rash, red eyes, and skin rash

Lassa fever (Lassa virus): fever, retrosternal pain, sore throat, back pain, cough, abdominal pain, vomiting, diarrhea, conjunctivitis, facial swelling, proteinuria, and mucosal bleeding

Toxins

Ricin: respiratory distress, fever, cough, nausea, tightness in chest, heavy sweating, pulmonary edema, cyanosis, hypotension, respiratory failure, hallucinations, seizures, and blood in urine

Staphylococcal enterotoxin B: fever, headache, myalgia, malaise, diarrhea, sore throat, sinus congestion, rhinorrhea, hoarseness, and conjunctivitis

Radiation Exposure Effects

Oncologic

Skin cancer, thyroid cancer, and leukemia

Immunologic

Impaired response to immunizations, bone marrow suppression, autoimmune diseases

Genetic

DNA mutations, teratogenic effect including smaller head or brain size, poorly formed eyes, abnormally slow growth, and mental retardation

Neurologic

CNS damage, malfunctions of the peripheral nervous system, neuroautoimmune changes, and disturbances in neuroendocrine control

Dermatologic

Burns, skin irritation, dryness, inflammation, erythema, dry or moist desquamation, itching, blistering, and ulceration

Systemic radiation poisoning

Nausea, fatigue, weakness, hair loss, changes in blood chemistries, hemorrhage, diminished organ function, and death

Ophthalmic

Cataracts, degeneration of the macula

Cardiovascular

Changes in cardiovascular control, irregular heartbeat, changes in the electrocardiogram, development of atherosclerosis, hypertension, and ischemia

Pulmonary

Disturbances in respiratory volume, increase in the number of allergic illnesses, atypical cells in the bronchial mucosa

Gastrointestinal

Pathologic changes in the digestive system, inflammation of the duodenum, spontaneously hyperplasic mucous membranes

Waste Exposure Effects

Coliform bacteria: diarrhea and abdominal cramps

Giardia lamblia (protozoa): diarrhea, abdominal cramps, nausea, and weight loss

Cryptosporidium (protozoa): diarrhea, headache, abdominal cramps, nausea, vomiting, and low fever

Hepatitis A (enteric virus): lassitude, anorexia, weakness, nausea, fever, and jaundice

Helminths (parasitic worms): diarrhea, vomiting, gas, stomach pain, and loss of appetite

Fever

Pollution Exposure Effects

Pulmonary: coughing, wheezing, labored breathing, pulmonary and nasal congestion, exacerbated allergies, asthma exacerbation, pain when breathing, and lung cancer

Cardiac: chest pain

Neurologic: headaches, developmental delay

Reproductive: reduced fertility

Ophthalmic: eye irritation

Related Factors

Pathophysiologic

Presence of bacteria, viruses, and toxins

Nutritional factors (obesity, vitamin, and mineral deficiencies)

Pre-existing disease states

Gender (females have greater proportion of body fat, which increases the chance of accumulating more lipid-soluble toxins than men; pregnancy)

History of smoking

Treatment Related

Recent vaccinations

Insufficient or absent use of decontamination protocol

Inappropriate or no use of protective clothing

Situational (Personal, Environmental)

Flooding, earthquakes, or other natural disasters

Sewer-line leaks

Industrial plant emissions; intentional or accidental discharge of contaminants by industries or businesses

Physical factors: climactic conditions such as temperature, wind; geographic area

Social factors: crowding, sanitation, poverty, personal and household hygiene practices, and lack of access to health care
Biologic factors: presence of vectors (mosquitoes, ticks, rodents)
Bioterrorism
Occupation
Dietary practices

Environmental

Contamination of aquifers by septic tanks
Intentional/accidental contamination of food and water supply
Concomitant or previous exposures
Exposure to heavy metals or chemicals, atmospheric pollutants, radiation, bioterrorism, and disaster
Use of environmental contaminants in the home (pesticides, chemicals, radon, tobacco smoke)
Playing in outdoor areas where environmental contaminants are used
Type of flooring surface

Maturational

Developmental characteristics of children
Children younger than 5 years of age
Older adults
Gestational age during exposure

NOC

Anxiety Level, Fear Level, Grief Resolution, Health Beliefs: Perceived Threat, Immunization Behavior, Infection Control, Knowledge: Health Resources, Personal Safety Behavior, Community Risk Control, Safe Home Environment

Goal

Individual adverse health effects of contamination will be minimized.

NIC

Community Disaster Preparedness, Environmental Management, Anger Control Assistance, Anxiety Reduction, Grief Work Facilitation, Crisis Intervention, Counseling, Health Education, Health Screening, Immunization/Vaccination Management, Infection Control, Resiliency Promotion, Risk Identification

Interventions

General Interventions

Help Individuals Cope With Contamination Incident; Use Groups That Have Survived Terrorist Attacks as a Useful Resource for Victims

- Provide accurate information on risks involved, preventive measures, use of antibiotics, and vaccines.
- Assist victims in dealing with feelings of fear, vulnerability, and grief.
- Encourage victims to talk to others about their fears.
- Assist victims in thinking positively and moving to the future.

Specific Interventions

- Employ skin decontamination with dermal exposures.
- Clinical effects on body systems vary with exposure to specific agents. Monitor carefully and provide supportive care.
- Employ appropriate isolation precautions: universal, airborne, droplet, and contact isolation.

Monitor the Client for Therapeutic Effects, Side Effects, and Compliance With Postexposure Drug Therapy

Decontamination Procedure
- Primary decontamination of exposed personnel is agent specific.
  - Remove contaminated clothing.
  - Use copious amounts of water and soap or diluted (0.5%) sodium hypochlorite.
- For secondary decontamination from clothing or equipment of those exposed, use proper physical protection.

Risk for Individual Contamination

NANDA-I Definition

Accentuated risk of exposure to environmental contaminants in doses sufficient to cause adverse health effects

Risk Factors

See Related Factors under *Individual Contamination*.

NOC

Community Risk Control, Community Health Status, Health Beliefs: Perceived Threat, Knowledge: Health Resources, Knowledge: Health Behavior

Goal

The client will remain free of the adverse effects of contamination.

NIC

Community Disaster Preparedness Environmental Risk Protection, Environmental Management: Safety, Health Education, Health Screening, Immunization/Vaccination Management, Risk Identification, Surveillance: Safety

Interventions

General Interventions

Provide Accurate Information About Risks Involved and Preventive Measures

- Assist to deal with feelings of fear and vulnerability.
- Encourage them to talk to others about their fears.

Specific Interventions

Conduct Surveillance for Environmental Contamination

- Notify agencies authorized to protect the environment of contaminants in the area.
- Assist individuals in relocating to safer environment.
- Modify the environment to minimize risk.

FAMILY CONTAMINATION

Family Contamination

Risk for Family Contamination

NANDA-I Definition

Exposure to environmental contaminants in doses sufficient to cause adverse health effects

Defining Characteristics

Refer to Defining Characteristics for *Individual Contamination and Community Contamination*.

Related Factors

Refer to Related Factors for *Individual Contamination* and *Community Contamination*.

NOC

Refer to *Individual Contamination* and *Community Contamination* for possible NOC outcomes.

Goal

Family adverse health effects of contamination will be minimized.

NIC

Refer to *Individual Contamination and Community Contamination* for possible NOC outcomes. Also refer to appropriate NIC interventions based on family's defining characteristics.

Interventions

Refer to *Individual Contamination* and *Community Contamination* for possible interventions.

Risk for Family Contamination

NANDA-I Definition

At risk for exposure to environmental contaminants in doses sufficient to cause adverse health effects

Risk Factors

Refer to Related Factors under *Individual Contamination*.

Goal

Family will remain free of adverse effects of contamination.

Interventions

Refer to Interventions under *Risk for Individual Contamination*.

COMMUNITY CONTAMINATION

Community Contamination

Risk for Community Contamination

NANDA-I Definition

Exposure to environmental contaminants in doses sufficient to cause adverse health effects

Defining Characteristics

Clusters of clients seeking care for similar signs or symptoms
Signs and symptoms are dependent on the causative agent, which include pesticides, chemicals, biologics, waste, radiation, and pollution.*
Refer to *Individual Contamination* for specific contaminant-related health effects
Large numbers of clients with rapidly fatal illnesses
Sick, dying, or dead animals or fish; absence of insects
Measurement of contaminants exceeding acceptable levels

Related Factors

Pathophysiologic

Presence of bacteria, viruses, toxins

Treatment Related

Insufficient or absent use of decontamination protocol
Inappropriate or no use of protective clothing

Situational

Acts of bioterrorism
Flooding, earthquakes, natural disasters
Sewer line leaks
Industrial plant emissions; intentional or accidental discharge of
    contaminants by industries or businesses
Physical factors (climactic conditions such as temperature, wind;
    geographic area)
Social factors (crowding, sanitation, poverty, lack of access to
    health care)
Biologic factors (presence of vectors such as mosquitoes, ticks,
    rodents)

Environmental

Contamination of aquifers by septic tanks
Intentional/accidental contamination of food and water supply
Exposure to heavy metals or chemicals, atmospheric pollutants,
    radiation, bioterrorism, disaster; concomitant or previous
    exposure

Maturational

Community dynamics (participation, power and decision-making
    structure, collaborative efforts)

NOC

Community Competence, Community Disaster Readiness, Community Health Status,
Community Risk Control: Communicable Disease, Community Risk Control: Lead
Exposure, Grief Resolution, Community Risk Control: Violence, Infection Severity;
See *Individual Contamination* for Other Possible NOC Outcomes

Goals

- Community will use health surveillance data system to monitor for contamination incidents.
- Community will participate in mass casualty and disaster readiness drills.
- Community will utilize disaster plan to evacuate and triage affected members.
- Community exposure to contaminants will be minimized.
- Community health effects associated with contamination will be minimized.

NIC

Environmental Management, Environmental Risk Protection, Community Health Development, Bioterrorism Preparedness, Communicable Disease Management, Community Disaster Preparedness, Crisis Intervention, Health Education, Health Policy Monitoring, Infection Control, Surveillance: Community, Triage: Disaster, Triage: Emergency Center

Interventions

Monitor for Contamination Incidents Using Health Surveillance Data

Provide Accurate Information About Risks Involved, Preventive Measures, and Use of Antibiotics and Vaccines

- Encourage community members to talk to others about their fears.
- Provide general supportive measures (food, water, shelter).
- Treatment of contamination before and after exposure will decrease symptoms and reduce mortality. Prevention of anthrax may be accomplished through vaccination. Anthrax exposure may be treated with ciprofloxacin, doxycycline, or penicillin. Organophosphate contamination may be treated with atropine and pralidoxime (Protopam) (http://www.atsdr.cdc.gov/MMG/MMG.asp?id=1140&tid=246); (http://www.ahrq.gov/research/cbmprophyl/index.html).

Specific Interventions

Prevention

- Identify community risk factors and develop programs to prevent disasters from occurring.

Preparedness

- Plan for communication, evacuation, rescue, and victim care.
- Schedule mass casualty and disaster readiness drills.

Response

- Identify contaminants in the environment.
- Educate community about the environmental contaminant.
- Collaborate with other agencies (local health department, emergency medical services, state and federal agencies).
- Rescue, triage, stabilize, transport, and treat affected community members.

Recovery

- Act to repair, rebuild, or relocate; mental health services should assist in psychological recovery (adapted from Allender & Spradley, 2006).

Decontamination Procedure

- Primary decontamination of exposed personnel is agent specific.
- Remove contaminated clothing.
- Use copious amounts of water and soap or diluted (0.5%) sodium hypochlorite.
- Secondary decontamination from clothing or equipment of those exposed; use proper physical protection.
- Employ appropriate isolation precautions (universal, airborne, droplet, and contact isolation).

Risk for Community Contamination

NANDA-I Definition

At risk for exposure to environmental contaminants in doses sufficient to cause adverse health effects

Risk Factors

Refer to Related Factors under *Community Contamination*.

NOC

Community Disaster Readiness, Community Health Status, Community Risk Control: Communicable Disease; see *Community Contamination* for other possible NOC outcomes

Goals

- Community will use health surveillance data system to monitor for contamination incidents.
- Community will participate in mass casualty and disaster readiness drills.
- Community will remain free of contamination-related health effects.

NIC

Environmental Management, Environmental Risk Protection, Community Health Development, Bioterrorism Preparedness, Communicable Disease Management, Community Disaster Preparedness, Health Education, Health Policy Monitoring, Surveillance: Community

Interventions

Monitor for Contamination Incidents Using Health Surveillance Data

Provide Accurate Information About Risks Involved and Preventive Measures

- Encourage community members to talk to others about their fears.

Specific Interventions

Identify Community Risk Factors and Develop Programs to Prevent Disasters from Occurring

- Notify agencies authorized to protect the environment from contaminants in the area.
- Modify the environment to minimize risk.

INEFFECTIVE COPING

Ineffective Coping

Defensive Coping

Ineffective Impulse Control

Ineffective Denial

NANDA-I Definition

Inability to form a valid appraisal of the stressors, inadequate choices of practiced responses, and/or inability to use available resources

Defining Characteristics

Verbalization of inability to
  cope or ask for help*
Inappropriate use of defense
  mechanisms
Inability to meet role
  expectations*
Chronic worry, anxiety
Sleep disturbance*
Fatigue*
High illness rate*
Reported difficulty with life
  stressors
Poor concentration*
Difficulty organizing
  information*

Decreased use of social
  support*
Inadequate problem-solving*
Impaired social participation
Use of forms of coping that
  impede adaptive behavior*
Risk taking*
Lack of goal-directed behavior*
Destructive behavior toward
  self or others*
Change in usual communica-
  tion patterns*
High incidence of accidents
Substance abuse*

Related Factors

Pathophysiologic

Related to chronicity of condition

Related to biochemical changes in brain secondary to:
Bipolar disorder
Chemical dependency
Schizophrenia

Personality disorder
Attention-deficit disorders

Related to complex self-care regimens

Related to neurologic changes in brain secondary to:
Stroke
Alzheimer's disease

Multiple sclerosis
End-stage diseases

Related to changes in body integrity secondary to:
Loss of body part

Disfigurement secondary
  to trauma

Related to altered affect caused by changes secondary to:
Body chemistry
Tumor (brain)

Intake of mood-altering
  substance
Mental retardation

Treatment Related

Related to separation from family and home (e.g., hospitalization, nursing home)

Related to disfigurement caused by surgery

Related to altered appearance from drugs, radiation, or other treatment

Situational (Personal, Environmental)

Related to poor impulse control and frustration tolerance

Related to disturbed relationship with parent/caregiver

Related to disorganized family system

Related to ineffective problem-solving skills

Related to increased food consumption in response to stressors

Related to changes in physical environment secondary to:

War	Poverty	Natural disaster
Homelessness	Relocation	Inadequate finances
Seasonal work		

Related to disruption of emotional bonds secondary to:

Death	Institutionalization	Relocation
Desertion	Separation or divorce	Orphanage/foster care
Jail	Educational institution	

Related to unsatisfactory support system

Related to sensory overload secondary to:

Factory environment	Urbanization: crowding, noise pollution, excessive activity

Related to inadequate psychological resources secondary to:

Poor self-esteem	Helplessness
Excessive negative beliefs about self	Lack of motivation to respond
Negative role modeling	

Related to culturally related conflicts with (specify):

Premarital sex	Abortion

Maturational

Child/Adolescent
Related to:

Poor impulse control	Repressed anxiety	Peer rejection
Parental substance abuse	Panic	Parental rejection
Inconsistent methods of discipline	Childhood trauma	Fear of failure
	Poor social skills	

Adolescent
Related to inadequate psychological resources to adapt to:
Physical and emotional changes   Sexual relationships
Educational demands   Independence from family
Sexual awareness   Career choices

Young Adult
Related to inadequate psychological resources to adapt to:
Career choices   Marriage   Educational demands
Parenthood   Leaving home

Middle Adult
Related to inadequate psychological resources to adapt to:
Physical signs of aging   Child-rearing problems
Social status needs   Career pressures
Problems with relatives   Aging parents

Older Adult
Related to inadequate psychological resources to adapt to:
Physical changes   Changes in residence
Response of others   Changes in financial status
Retirement

Author's Note

Ineffective Coping describes a person who is experiencing difficulty adapting to stressful event(s). *Ineffective Coping* can be a recent, episodic problem or a chronic problem. Usual effective coping mechanisms may be inappropriate or ineffective, or the person may have a poor history of coping with stressors.

If the event is recent, *Ineffective Coping* may be a premature judgment. For example, a person may respond to overwhelming stress with a grief response such as denial, anger, or sadness, making a *Grieving* diagnosis appropriate.

Impaired Adjustment may be more useful than *Ineffective Coping* in the initial period after a stressful event. *Ineffective Coping* and its related diagnoses may be more applicable to prolonged or chronic coping problems, such as *Defensive Coping* for a person with a long-standing pattern of ineffective coping.

NOC

Coping, Self-Esteem, Social Interaction Skills

Goals

The person will make decisions and follow through with appropriate actions to change provocative situations in the personal environment as evidenced by the following indicators:

- Verbalize feelings related to emotional state.
- Focus on the present.
- Identify response patterns and the consequences of resulting behavior.
- Identify personal strengths and accept support through the nursing relationship.

NIC

Coping Enhancement, Counseling, Emotional Support, Active Listening, Assertiveness Training, Behavior Modification

Interventions

Assess Causative and Contributing Factors (Lyon, 2002)

Refer to Related Factors.

Establish Rapport

- Spend time with the client. Provide supportive companionship.
- Avoid being overly cheerful and cliché such as, "Things will get better."
- Convey honesty and empathy.
- Offer support. Encourage expression of feelings. Let the client know you understand his or her feelings. Do not argue with expressions of worthlessness by saying things such as, "How can you say that? Look at all you accomplished in life."
- Offer matter-of-fact appraisals. Be realistic.
- Allow extra time for the client to respond.

Assess Present Coping Status

- Determine the onset of feelings and symptoms and their correlation with events and life changes.
- Assess the ability to relate facts.
- Listen carefully as the client speaks to collect facts; observe facial expressions, gestures, eye contact, body positioning, and tone and intensity of voice.
- Determine the risk of the client's inflicting self-harm; intervene appropriately.
- Assess for signs of potential suicide:
  - History of previous attempts or threats (overt and covert)
  - Changes in personality, behavior, sex life, appetite, and sleep habits

- Preparations for death (putting things in order, making a will, giving away personal possessions, acquiring a weapon)
- Sudden elevation in mood
- See *Risk for Suicide* for additional information on suicide prevention.

Assess Level of Depression

- Refer depressed people to specialists.

Assist the Client in Developing Appropriate Problem-Solving Strategies

- Ask the client to describe previous encounters with conflict and how he or she resolved them.
- Evaluate whether his or her stress response is "fight or flight" or "tend and befriend."
- Encourage the client to evaluate his or her behavior.
- "Did that work for you?" "How did it help?" "What did you learn from that experience?"
- Discuss possible alternatives (i.e., talk over the problem with those involved, try to change the situation, or do nothing and accept the consequences).
- Assist the client in identifying problems that he or she cannot control directly; help the client to practice stress-reducing activities for control (e.g., exercise, yoga).
- Be supportive of functional coping behaviors.
- "The way you handled this situation 2 years ago worked well then. Can you do it now?"
- Give options; however, leave the decision-making to the client.
- Mobilize the client to gradually increase activity:
  - Identify activities that were previously gratifying but have been neglected: personal grooming or dress habits, shopping, hobbies, athletic endeavors, and arts and crafts.
  - Encourage the client to include these activities in the daily routine for a set time span (e.g., "I will play the piano for 30 minutes every afternoon").
- Explore outlets that foster feelings of personal achievement and self-esteem:
  - Make time for relaxing activities (e.g., dancing, exercising, sewing, woodworking).
  - Find a helper to take over responsibilities occasionally (e.g., sitter).
  - Learn to compartmentalize (do not carry problems around with you always; enjoy free time).
  - Encourage longer vacations (not just a few days here and there).
  - Provide opportunities to learn and use stress management techniques (e.g., jogging, yoga).

- Facilitate emotional support from others:
  - Seek out people who share a common challenge: establish telephone contact, initiate friendships within the clinical setting, develop and institute educational and support groups.
  - Establish a network of people who understand your situation.
  - Decide who can best act as a support system (do not expect empathy from people who themselves are overwhelmed with their own problems).
  - Make time to share personal feelings and concern with coworkers (encourage expression; frequently people who share the same circumstances help one another).
  - Maintain a sense of humor.
  - Allow tears.
- Teach self-monitoring tools (Finkelman, 2000):
  - Develop a daily schedule to monitor for signs of improvement or worsening.
  - Discuss reasonable goals for present relationships.
  - Write down what is done when in control, depressed, confused, angry, and happy.
  - Identify activities tried, would like to try, or should do more.
  - Create a warning sign checklist that indicates worsening and how to access help.

Teach Problem-Solving Techniques

- *Goal setting* is consciously setting time limits on behaviors, which is useful when goals are attainable and manageable. It may become stress-inducing if unrealistic or short-sighted.
- *Information seeking* is learning about all aspects of a problem, which provides perspective and, in some cases, reinforces self-control.
- *Mastery* is learning new procedures or skills, which facilitates self-esteem and self-control (e.g., self-care of colostomies, insulin injection, or catheter care).

Initiate Health Teaching and Referrals, as Indicated

- Prepare for problems that may occur after discharge:
  - Medications—schedule, cost, misuse, side effects
  - Increased anxiety
  - Sleep problems
  - Eating problems—access, decreased appetite
  - Inability to structure time
  - Family/significant other conflicts
  - Follow-up—forgetting, access, difficulty organizing time

- Instruct the client in relaxation techniques; emphasize the importance of setting 15 to 20 minutes aside each day to practice relaxation:
  1. Find a comfortable position in a chair or on the floor.
  2. Close the eyes.
  3. Keep noise to a minimum (only very soft music, if desired).
  4. Concentrate on breathing slowly and deeply.
  5. Feel the heaviness of all extremities.
  6. If muscles are tense, tighten, then relax each one from toes to scalp.
- Teach assertiveness skills.
- Teach use of cognitive therapy techniques.

Pediatric Interventions

- Assess for signs of attention difficulties.
- Persistent pattern of inattention and/or hyperactivity.
- Clear evidence that behavior interferes with developmentally appropriate social, academic, or occupational functioning.
- Cannot be accounted for by another mental disorder.
- Some hyperactive/inattentive symptoms must be present before the age of 7.
- Establish eye contact before giving instructions.
- Set firm, responsible limits.
- State rules simply; do not lecture.
- Maintain regular routine.
- Advise parents to avoid disagreeing with each other in child's presence.
- Maintain a calm, simple environment.
- If hyperactive, provide for periods of activity using large muscles.
- Provide immediate and constant feedback.
- Advise parents to consult with educational professionals for educational programming.

Geriatric Interventions

- Assess for risk factors for ineffective coping in older adults (Miller, 2009):
  - Inadequate economic resources
  - Immature developmental level
  - Unanticipated stressful events
  - Several major events in short period
  - Unrealistic goals

Defensive Coping

NANDA-I Definition

Repeated projection of falsely positive self-evaluation based on a self-protective pattern that defends against underlying perceived threats to positive self-regard.

Defining Characteristics*

Denial of obvious problems/weaknesses
Projection of blame/responsibility
Rationalization of failures
Hypersensitivity to slight and/or criticism
Grandiosity
Superior attitude toward others
Difficulty establishing/maintaining relationships
Hostile laughter or ridicule of others
Difficulty testing perceptions against reality testing
Lack of follow-through or participation in treatment or therapy
Reality distortion
Lack of participation in therapy

Related Factors*

Related to:

Conflict between self-
  perception and value system
Deficient support system
Fear of failure
Fear of humiliation
Fear of repercussions
Lack of resilience
Low level of confidence in
  others
Low level of self-confidence
Uncertainty
Unrealistic expectations of self

🌀 Author's Note

In selecting this diagnosis, it is important to consider the potentially related diagnoses of *Chronic Low Self-Esteem*, *Powerlessness*, and *Impaired Social Interaction*. They may express how the person established, or why he or she maintains, the defensive pattern.

  Defensive Coping is the "repeated projection of falsely-positive self-evaluation based on a self-protection pattern that defends against perceived threats to positive self-regard" (Varcarolis, 2011). When a defensive pattern is a barrier to effective relationships, *Defensive Coping* is a useful diagnosis.

NOC

Acceptance: Health Status, Coping, Self-Esteem, Social Interaction Skills

Goals

The client will demonstrate appropriate interactions with others and report that they feel safe and are more in control as evidenced by the following indicators:

- Adheres to treatment, for example medications, therapy, and goals.
- Uses newly learned constructive methods to deal with stress and promote feelings of control.
- Removes self from situations that increase their anxiety.

The child/adolescent will comply "with requests and limits on behavior in absence of arguments, tantrums, or other acting-out behaviors" as evidenced by the following indicators (Varcarolis, 2011):

- Demonstrate increased impulse control within (specify time).
- Demonstrate ability to tolerate frustration and delay gratification within (specify time).
- Demonstrate an absence of tantrums, rage reactions, or other acting-out behaviors within (specify time).
- Describe the behavior limits and rationale to an authority figure.
- Acknowledge responsibility for misbehaviors, increased impulse control within (specify time).

NIC

Coping Enhancement, Emotional Support, Self-Awareness Enhancement, Environment Management, Presence, Active Listening

Interventions

Reduce Demands on the Client if Stress Levels Increase

- Modify the level of or remove environmental stimuli (e.g., noise, activity).
- Decrease (or limit) contacts with others (e.g., visitors, other clients, staff) as required.
- Clearly articulate minimal expectations for activities. Decrease or increase as tolerated.
- Identify stressors placing demands on the client's coping resources; develop plans to deal with them. The general goal is to freeze, reduce, or eliminate stress; more specifically, it is to target and deal with those stressors most exacerbating the defensive pattern.

Establish a Therapeutic Relationship

- Maintain a neutral, matter-of-fact tone with a consistent positive regard. Ensure that all staff relate in a consistent fashion, with consistent expectations.
- Focus on simple, here-and-now, goal-directed topics when encountering the client's defenses.
- Do not react to, defend, or dwell on the client's negative projections or displacements; also do not challenge distortions or unrealistic/grandiose self-expressions. Try instead to shift to more neutral, positive, or goal-directed topics.
- Avoid control issues; attempt to present positive options to the client, which allows a measure of choice.
- To promote learning from the client's own actions (i.e., "natural consequences"), identify those actions that have interfered with the achievement of established goals.
- Reinforce more adaptive coping patterns (e.g., formal problem solving, rationalization) that assist the person in achieving established goals.
- Evaluate interactions, progress, and approach with other team members to ensure consistency within the treatment milieu.

Promote Dialogue to Decrease Paranoia and Permit a More Direct Addressing of Underlying Related Factors (see also *Chronic Low Self-Esteem*)

- Validate the client's reluctance to trust in the beginning. Over time, reinforce the consistency of your statements, responses, and actions. Give special attention to your meeting of (reasonable) requests or your following through with plans and agreements.
- Use clear, simple language. Explain activities before you do them.
- Be honest, nonjudgmental, and nondefensive; take a neutral approach.
- Do not whisper, laugh, or engage in behavior that can be misinterpreted.
- Engage the client in diversional, nongoal-directed, noncompetitive activities (e.g., relaxation therapy, games, and outings).
- Initially, provide solitary, noncompetitive activities (Varcarolis, 2011).
- Encourage self-expression of neutral themes, positive reminiscences, and so forth.
- Encourage other means for self-expression (e.g., writing, art) if verbal interaction is difficult or if this is an area of personal strength.

- Listen passively to *some* grandiose or negative self-expression to reinforce your positive regard. If this does not lead to more positive self-expression or activity, then such listening may prove counterproductive.
- Establish an ego-support role for yourself by assisting the client in reviewing and examining his interactive patterns with others.

Pediatric Interventions

- If attention disorders are present, explain their etiology and behavioral manifestations to the child and caregivers.
- Help the child to understand he or she is not "bad" or "dumb."
- Establish target behaviors with the child and caregivers.
- Avoid repetitive lecturing.
- Work with parents and teachers to learn more effective behavioral strategies to support success:
  - Establish eye contact before giving instructions.
  - Set firm, responsible limits.
  - Avoid lectures; simply state rules.
- Maintain routines as much as possible.
- Attempt to keep a calm and simple environment.
- Reinforce appropriate behavior with a positive reinforcer (e.g., praise, hug).
- Monitor for rising levels of frustration. Intervene early to calm child.
- Avoid power struggles and no-win situation. Look for a compromise.
- Allow child to discuss the requests within reason. Provide simple explanation. Provide periodic rewards for positive behaviors.
- Assist the child in improving play with peers (Johnson, 1995):
  - Start with short play periods.
  - Use simple, concrete games.
  - Begin with sympathetic siblings or family members.
  - Initially, select a quieter and less demanding peer as playmate.
  - Provide immediate and instant feedback (e.g., "I see you are being distracted"; "You are playing nicely").
- Initiate health teaching and referrals as needed:
  - Provide information about medication therapy if indicated.
  - Consult with specialists as needed (e.g., psychological, learning specialists).

Ineffective Impulse Control

NANDA-I Definition

A pattern of performing rapid, unplanned reactions to internal or external stimuli without regard to negative consequences of these reactions to the impulsive individual or to others

Defining Characteristics*

Acting without thinking
Irritability
Anorexia
Pathologic gambling
Asking questions of others
    despite their discomfort
Sensation seeking
Bulimia

Sexual promiscuity
Inability to save money or
    regulate finances
Sharing personal details
    inappropriately
Temper outbursts
Too familiar with strangers
Violence

Related Factors

Alcohol dependence
Disorder of cognition*
Anger*
Disorder of development*
Co-dependency*
Disorder of mood*
Compunction*
Disorder of personality*
Delusion*
Disorder of body image
Denial*
Substance abuse (drugs)
Disorder of brain function

Environment that might cause
    irritation or frustration*
Fatigue*
Hopelessness*
Ineffective coping*
Insomnia*
Low self-esteem
Poor
Smoker*
Social isolation*
Stress vulnerability*
Suicidal feelings*
Unpleasant physical symptoms*

 Author's Note

Ineffective Impulse Control is a new NANDA-I nursing diagnosis that represents a behavior that can cause a variety of problems in the individual or to others such as substance abuse, violence, sexual promiscuity, etc. It is a component of the DSM IV-TR diagnosis *Personality Disorders*.

It may be more clinically useful to view *Ineffective Impulse Control* as behavior that contributes to a nursing diagnosis and/or a manifestation rather than as the response or nursing diagnosis. For example, *Risk for Other-Directed Violence, Ineffective Coping, Dysfunctional Family Processes, Defensive Coping, Self-Mutilation, Impaired Social Interactions, Loneliness, Noncompliance, Ineffective Health Maintenance,* and *Stress Overload* all can have a component of poor impulse control that contributes to the diagnosis.

An example would be *Ineffective Coping* related to inadequate psychological resources as manifested by poor impulse control (Varcarolis, 2011).

The clinician can choose to use *Ineffective Impulse Control* as a nursing diagnosis or can use a more specific nursing diagnosis as discussed in this Author's Note. The following interventions can also be used with the aforementioned diagnoses.

NOC

Impulse Self-Control

Goals

The client will consistently demonstrate the use of effective coping responses as evidenced by the following indicators:

- Identifies consequences of impulsive behavior.
- Identifies feelings that precede impulsive behavior.
- Controls impulsive behavior.

NIC

Self-Awareness Enhancement, Presence, Counseling, Behavioral Modification

Interventions

"In a Respectful, Neutral Manner, Explain Expected Client Behaviors, Limits, and Responsibilities" (Varcarolis, 2011)

Assist the Client to Identify Problematic Situations

- Explore possible responses/actions and their benefits and consequences.
- Role play acceptable social skills.

Approach the Client in a Consistent Manner in all Interactions (Varcarolis, 2011)

Teach Strategies to Help Reduce Tension and Negative Feelings (e.g., Assertiveness, Quieting Oneself)

- Be realistic. Begin in small steps.

Encourage Participation in Group Therapy

- Avoid:
  - Giving attention to inappropriate behaviors.
  - Showing own frustration.
  - Accepting gift giving, flattery, seductive behaviors, and instilling guilt by clients (Varcarolis, 2011).

Provide and Encourage the Use of Other Services (e.g., Social Services, Vocational Rehabilitation, Legal Services)

Ineffective Denial

NANDA-I Definition

Conscious or unconscious attempt to disavow the knowledge or meaning of an event to reduce anxiety and/or fear, leading to the detriment of health

Defining Characteristics**

Major* (Must Be Present)

Delays seeking or refuses health care attention
Does not perceive personal relevance of symptoms or danger

Minor (May Be Present)

Uses home remedies (self-treatment) to relieve symptoms
Does not admit fear of death or invalidism*
Minimizes symptoms*
Displaces the source of symptoms to other areas of the body
Cannot admit the effects of the disease on life pattern
Makes dismissive gestures when speaking of distressing events*
Displaces the fear of effects of the condition
Displays inappropriate affect*

** Source: Lynch, C. S., & Phillips, M. W. (1989). Nursing diagnosis: Ineffective denial. In R. M. Carroll-Johnson (Ed.), *Classification of nursing diagnosis: Proceedings of the eighth conference*. Philadelphia, PA: J. B. Lippincott.

Related Factors

Pathophysiologic

Related to inability to tolerate consciously the consequences of (any chronic or terminal illness) secondary to:

AIDS
Cancer
HIV infection

Progressive debilitating disorders (e.g., multiple sclerosis, myasthenia gravis)

Treatment Related

Related to prolonged treatment with no positive results

Psychological

Related to inability to tolerate consciously the consequences of:

Loss of a job
Financial crisis
Negative self-concept, inadequacy, guilt, loneliness, despair, sense of failure

Smoking
Obesity
Loss of spouse/significant other
Domestic abuse

Related to physical and emotional dependence on (Varcarolis, 2011):

Alcohol
Cocaine, crack
Stimulants
Opiates

Cannabis
Barbiturates/sedatives
Hallucinogens

Related to long-term self-destructive patterns of behavior and lifestyle (Varcarolis, 2011)

Related to feelings of increased anxiety/stress, need to escape personal problems, anger, and frustration

Related to feelings of omnipotence

Related to culturally permissive attitudes toward alcohol/drug use

Related to genetic origins of alcoholism

 Author's Note

Ineffective Denial differs from denial in response to loss. Denial in response to illness or loss is necessary and beneficial to maintain psychological equilibrium. Ineffective Denial is not beneficial when the person will not participate in regimens to improve health or the situation (e.g., denies substance abuse). If the cause is not known, Ineffective Denial related to unknown etiology can be used, such as Ineffective Denial related to unknown etiology as evidenced by repetitive refusal to admit barbiturate use is a problem.

NOC

Acceptance: Health Status, Anxiety Self-Control, Fear Self-Control, Health Beliefs: Perceived Threat

Goal

The client will use alternative coping mechanism in response to stressor instead of denial as evidenced by the following indicators:

- Acknowledge the source of anxiety or stress.
- Use problem-focused coping skills.

NIC

Teaching: Disease Process, Anxiety Reduction, Counseling, Active Listening

Interventions

Initiate a Therapeutic Relationship

- Assess effectiveness of denial.
- Avoid confronting the client that he or she is using denial.
- Approach the client directly, matter-of-factly, and nonjudgmentally.

Encourage the Client to Share Perceptions of the Situation (e.g., Fears, Anxieties)

- Focus on the feelings shared.
- Use reflection to encourage more sharing.

When Appropriate, Help the Client With Problem Solving

- Attempt to elicit from the client a description of the problem.

Assist the Client to Understand Addictions

- Be nonjudgmental.
- Assist the client to gain an intellectual understanding that this is an illness, not a moral problem.
- Provide opportunities to perform successfully; gradually increase responsibility.
- Provide educational information about the progressive nature of substance abuse and its effects on the body and interpersonal relationships.
- Explain that "addiction does not cure itself" and that it requires abstinence and treatment of the underlying issues. (Varcarolis, 2011, p. 336).
- Provide opportunities to share fears and anxieties.

- Focus on present response.
- Assist in lowering anxiety level (see *Anxiety* for additional interventions).
- Avoid confronting person on use of denial.
- Carefully explore with person his or her interpretation of the situation:
  - Reflect self-reported cues used to minimize the situation (e.g., "a little," "only").
  - Identify recent detrimental behavior and discuss the effects of this behavior on health.
- Emphasize strengths and past successful coping.
- Provide positive reinforcement for any expressions of insight.
- Do not accept rationalization or projection. Be polite, caring, but firm.
- If substance abuse is present:
  - Review observations and findings with client and family.
  - Present evidence of damage (e.g., physical, social, financial, spiritual, familial).
  - Establish goals.
  - Provide self-help manuals or other pamphlets.
  - Acquire commitment to keep daily log of alcohol/drug use.
- At next visit:
  - Review log.
  - Review progress.
  - Refer those who are dependent and desire to continue abstinence.
  - Explain why women are more affected by alcohol than are men.
- "Expect sobriety. Reinforce for individuals to view their commitment to one day at a time" (Varcarolis, 2011, p. 339).
- Refer the client to AA, Al-Anon, or Alateen.
- Refer the client to a treatment facility for a structured treatment program.
- Reinforce healthy living choices (e.g., balanced diet, exercise, recreation, rest).

INEFFECTIVE COMMUNITY COPING

NANDA-I Definition

Pattern of community activities for adaptation and problem solving that is unsatisfactory for meeting the demands or needs of the community

Defining Characteristics*

Community does not meet its own expectations
Deficits in community participation
Excessive community conflicts
Reports of community powerlessness
Reports of community vulnerability
High rates of illness
Increased social problems (e.g., homicides, vandalism, arson,
    terrorism, robbery, infanticide, abuse, divorce, unemploy-
    ment, poverty, militancy, mental illness)
Stressors perceived as excessive

Risk Factors

Presence of Risk Factors (see Related Factors)

Related Factors

Situational

*Related to ineffective or nonexistent community systems (e.g., lack of
emergency medical system, transportation system, disaster planning
system)***

Related to lack of knowledge of resources

Related to inadequate communication patterns

Related to inadequate community cohesiveness

Related to inadequate resources for problem solving**

Related to natural disasters** *secondary to:*
Flood   Epidemic
Hurricane   Avalanche
Earthquake

Related to traumatic effects of**:
Airplane crash   Environmental accident
Industrial disaster   Earthquake
Large fire

*Related to threat to community safety (e.g., murder, rape, kidnapping,
robberies)***

Related to sudden rise in community unemployment

** These represent risk factors for *Risk for Ineffective Community Coping.* Refer
to Author's Note for additional clarification.

Maturational

Related to inadequate resources for:

Children   Adolescents

Working parents   Older adults

🔵 Author's Note

Ineffective Community Coping is a diagnosis of a community that does not have a constructive system in place to cope with events or changes that occur. The focus of interventions is to improve community dialogue, planning, and resource identification.

When a community has experienced a natural disaster (e.g., hurricane, flood), a threat to safety (e.g., murder, violence, rape), or a man-made disaster (e.g., airplane crash, large fire), the focus should be on preventive strategies. The diagnosis *Risk for Ineffective Community Coping* is more appropriate when the community has been a victim of a disaster or a violent crime.

NOC

Community Competence, Community Health Status, Community Risk Control

Goal

The community will engage in effective problem solving, as evidenced by the following indicators:

- Identify problem.
- Access information to improve coping.
- Use communication channels to access assistance.

NIC

Community Health Development, Environmental Risk Protection, Program Development, Risk Identification

Interventions

Assess for Causative or Contributing Factors

- Refer to Related Factors.

Provide Opportunities for Community Members (e.g., Schools, Churches, Synagogues, Town Hall) to Meet and Discuss the Situation

- Demonstrate acceptance of community members' anger, withdrawal, or denial.
- Correct misinformation as needed.
- Discourage blaming.

Provide for Effective Communication (Allender, Rector, & Warner, 2010)

- Allow for and address questions.
- Convey the facts.
- Convey seriousness.
- Be clear, simple, and repetitive.
- Present solutions and suggestions.
- Address real and perceived needs.

Promote Community Competence in Coping

- Focus on community goals, not individuals' goals.
- Engage subgroups in group discussions and planning.
- Ensure access to resources for all members (e.g., flexible hours for working members).
- Devise a method for formal disagreements.
- Evaluate each decision's impact on all community members.

Establish a Community Information Center at the Local Library to Access Information and Support (e.g., Telephone, Online)

Identify the Collaborative Resources That Can Be Accessed in the Health Department, Faith-Based Organization, Social Services, and Health Care Provider Agencies

Use the Community Information Center (e.g., Local Library) to Inform Residents of Ongoing Activities and Progress

COMPROMISED FAMILY COPING

NANDA-I Definition

A usually supportive primary person (family member, significant other, or close friend) provides insufficient, ineffective, or compromised support, comfort, assistance, or encouragement that may be needed by the client to manage or master adaptive tasks related to his or her health challenge

Defining Characteristics*

Subjective Data

Client reports a concern about significant person's response to health problem.
Significant person reports preoccupation with personal reaction (e.g., fear, anticipatory grief, guilt, anxiety) to client's need

Significant person reports inadequate understanding, which interferes with effective supportive behaviors

Objective Data

Significant person attempts assistive or supportive behaviors with unsatisfactory results

Significant person enters into limited personal communication with the client

Significant person displays protective behavior disproportionate to client's need for autonomy

Related Factors

Refer to *Interrupted Family Processes*.

 Author's Note

This nursing diagnosis describes situations similar to the diagnosis *Interrupted Family Processes* or *Risk for Interrupted Family Processes*. Until clinical research differentiates this diagnosis from the aforementioned diagnosis, use *Interrupted Family Processes*.

DISABLED FAMILY COPING

Definition

Behavior of primary person (family member, significant other, or close friend) that disables his or her capacities and the client's capacities to effectively address tasks essential to either person's adaptation to the health challenge (NANDA-I).

The state in which a family demonstrates, or is at risk to demonstrate, destructive behavior in response to an inability to manage internal or external stressors due to inadequate resources (physical, psychological, cognitive)**

Defining Characteristics

Decisions/actions that is detrimental to family well-being**
Neglectful care of client in regard to basic human needs*
Neglectful care of client in regard to illness treatment*

** This definition and characteristic have been added by the author for clarity and usefulness.

Neglectful relationships with other family members*
Family behaviors that are detrimental to well-being*
Distortion of reality regarding the client's health problem*

Rejection*	Intolerance*
Agitation*	Abandonment*
Aggression*	Depression*
Impaired restructuring of a family unit	Hostility*

Related Factors

Biopathophysiologic

Related to impaired ability to fulfill role responsibilities secondary to:
Any acute or chronic illness

Situational (Personal, Environmental)

Related to impaired ability to constructively manage stressors secondary to:
Substance abuse (e.g., alcoholism)
Negative role modeling
History of ineffective relationship with own parents
History of abusive relationship with parents

Related to unrealistic expectations of child by parent

Related to unrealistic expectations of parent by child

Related to unmet psychosocial needs of child by parent

Related to unmet psychosocial needs of parent by child

Related to marital stressors secondary to:

Financial difficulties	Problematic children
Separation	Problematic relatives
Infidelities	

 Author's Note

Disabled Family Coping describes a family with a history of overt or covert destructive behavior or responses to stressors. This diagnosis necessitates long-term care from a nurse therapist with advanced specialization in family systems and abuse.

The use of this diagnosis in this book focuses on nursing interventions appropriate for a nurse generalist in a short-term relationship (e.g., emergency unit, nonpsychiatric in-house unit) and for any nurse in the position to prevent *Disabled Family Coping* through teaching, counseling, or referrals.

NOC

Caregiver Emotional Health, Caregiver Stressors, Family Coping, Family Normalization

Goals

Each family member will set short- and long-term goals for change, as evidenced by the following indicators:

* Appraise unhealthy coping behaviors of family members.
* Relate expectations for self and family.
* Relate community resources available.

NIC

Caregiver Support, Referral, Emotional Support, Family Therapy, Family Involvement Promotion

Interventions

Identify With Each Family Member Their Strengths

Identify With Each Family Member Their Stressors

Assist Members to Appraise Family Behaviors (Effective, Ineffective, Destructive)

Discuss the Effects of Behaviors on Individuals and Family Unit

* Emotions
* Roles
* Support
* Performance

Assist Family to Set Short-Term and Long-Term Goals

Promote Family Resilience

* Ask each family member to identify one activity he or she would like to add to their family.

Promote Adaption to Stressors and Crises (Kaakinen et al., 2010)

* Identify stressors that can be reduced or eliminated.
* Engage the family members to discuss the situation.
* Allow each member to share their thoughts and suggestions for improving the situation.
* Negotiate necessary changes.
* Identify available resources.
* Ask each family member to identify one behavior he or she could control. Begin to help members to work through resentments of the past.

Improve Family Cohesiveness

• Determine family recreational activities that include all members and are enjoyable.

Provide Anticipatory Guidance (Kaakinen et al., 2010)

• Identify relevant life changes that will occur in this family (e.g., birth of child, relocation, empty nest). Discuss necessary adjustments in the family routines.
• Identify family member's responsibilities. Evaluate the balance of responsibilities.
• Initiate referrals, as needed.
• Support groups, family therapy, economic support.

Encourage Decision-Making If Domestic Abuse Is Suspected

• Provide an opportunity to validate abuse and talk about feelings; if the acutely injured client is accompanied by a spouse/caregiver who is persistent about staying, make an attempt to see the client alone (e.g., tell her that you need a urine specimen and accompany her to the bathroom).
• Be direct and nonjudgmental:
  • How do you handle stress?
  • How does your partner or caregiver handle stress?
  • How do you and your partner argue?
  • Are you afraid of him?
  • Have you ever been hit, pushed, or injured by your partner?
• Provide options but allow client to make a decision at her own pace.
• Encourage a realistic appraisal of the situation; dispel guilt and myths.
  • Violence is not normal for most families.
  • Violence may stop, but it usually becomes increasingly worse.
  • The victim is not responsible for the violence.

Provide Legal and Referral Information

• Discreetly inform of community agencies available to victim and abuser (emergency and long-term).
  • Hotlines
  • Legal services
  • Shelters
  • Counseling agencies
• Discuss mandatory reporting.
• Discuss the availability of the social service department for assistance.

- Consult with legal resources in the community and familiarize the victim with state laws regarding:
  - Abuse
  - Eviction of abuser
  - Counseling
  - Temporary support
  - Protection orders
  - Criminal law
  - Types of police interventions
- Document findings and dialogue (Carlson & Smith-DiJulio, 2006).
- Refer for individual, group, or couples counseling.
- Explore strategies to reduce stress and more constructively manage stressors (e.g., relaxation exercises, walking, and assertiveness training).

Pediatric Interventions

Report Suspected Cases of Child Abuse

- Know your state's child abuse laws and procedures for reporting child abuse (e.g., Bureau of Child Welfare, Department of Social Services, and Child Protective Services).
- Maintain an objective record (Cowen, 1999):
  - Health history, including accidental or environmental injuries
  - Detailed description of physical examination (nutritional status, hygiene, growth and development, cognitive and functional status)
  - Environmental assessment of home (if in community)
  - Description of injuries
  - Verbal conversations with parents and child in quotes
  - Description of behaviors, not interpretation (e.g., avoid "angry father," instead, "Father screamed at child, 'If you weren't so bad this wouldn't have happened.'")
  - Description of parent–child's interactions (e.g., "shies away from mother's touch")

Promote a Therapeutic Environment

Provide the Child With Acceptance and Affection
- Show child attention without reinforcing inappropriate behavior.
- Use play therapy to allow child's self-expression.
- Provide consistent caregivers and reasonable limits on behavior; avoid pity.
- Avoid asking too many questions and criticizing parent's actions.
- Ensure that play and educational needs are met.
- Explain in detail all routines and procedures in age-appropriate language.

Assist Child With Grieving If Placement in Foster Home Is Necessary
- Acknowledge that child will not want to leave parents despite severity of abuse.
- Allow opportunities for child to express feelings.
- Explain reasons for not allowing child to return home; dispel belief it is a punishment.
- Encourage foster parents to visit child in hospital.

Provide Interventions That Promote Parent's Self-Esteem and Sense of Trust
- Tell them it was good that they brought the child to the hospital.
- Welcome parents to the unit and orient them to activities.
- Promote their confidence by presenting a warm, helpful attitude and acknowledging any competent parenting activities.
- Provide opportunities for parents to participate in child's care (e.g., feeding, bathing).

Initiate Health Teaching and Referrals, as Indicated

- Provide anticipatory guidance for families at risk.
- Disseminate information to the community about child abuse (e.g., parent–school organizations, radio, television, newspaper).

Geriatric Interventions

Identify Suspected Cases of Elder Abuse (Fulmer & Paveza, 1998)

- Signs include:
  - Failure to adhere to therapeutic regimens, which can pose threats to life (e.g., insulin administration, ulcerated conditions)
  - Evidence of malnutrition, dehydration, elimination problems
  - Bruises, swelling, lacerations, burns, bites
  - Pressure ulcers
  - Caregiver not allowing nurse to be alone with elder

Report Suspected Cases

- Consult with supervisor for procedures for reporting suspected cases of abuse.
- Maintain an objective record, including:
  - Description of injuries
  - Conversations with elder and caregiver(s)
  - Description of behaviors
  - Nutritional, hydration status
- Consider the elder's right to choose to live at risk of harm, providing he or she is capable of making that choice.

- Do not initiate an action that could increase the elder's risk of harm or antagonize the abuser.
- Respect the elder's right to secrecy and the right for self-determination.

Initiate Health Teaching and Referrals, as Indicated

- Refer high-risk families to a home health nursing agency to assess
- Refer elder for counseling to explore choices. Reassure him or her that they did nothing wrong to deserve maltreatment (Varcarolis, 2011).
- Explore support services (e.g., respite, home health aide, homemaker services).
- Disseminate information to community regarding prevention.

DECISIONAL CONFLICT

NANDA-I Definition

Uncertainty about course of action to be taken when choice among competing actions involves risk, loss, or challenge to values and beliefs

Defining Characteristics*

Verbalized uncertainty about choices
Verbalizes undesired consequences of alternatives being considered
Vacillation among alternative choices
Delayed decision-making
Self-focusing
Verbalizes feeling of distress while attempting a decision
Physical signs of distress or tension (e.g., increased heart rate, increased muscle tension, restlessness)
Questioning of personal values and/or beliefs while attempting to make a decision
Questioning moral values while attempting a decision
Questioning moral rules while attempting a decision
Questioning moral principles while attempting a decision

Related Factors

Many situations can contribute to decisional conflict, particularly those that involve complex medical interventions of great risk. Any decisional situation can precipitate conflict for a client; thus, the examples listed below are not exhaustive, but reflect situations that may be problematic and possess factors that increase the difficulty.

Treatment Related

Related to lack of relevant information

Related to risks versus the benefits of (specify test, treatment):

Surgery	Cataract removal	Enteral feedings
Tumor removal	Cesarean section	Intravenous
Cosmetic surgery	Diagnostics	hydration
Amputation	Amniocentesis	Use of preterm
Transplant	X-rays	labor medications
Orchiectomy	Ultrasound	Participation in
Prostatectomy	Chemotherapy	treatment study
Hysterectomy	Radiation	trials
Laminectomy	Dialysis	HIV antiviral
Mastectomy	Mechanical	therapy
Joint replacement	ventilation	

Situational (Personal, Environmental)

Related to perceived threat to value system

Related to risks versus the benefits of:

Personal	Institutionalization
Marriage	(child, parent)
Breast versus bottle feeding	Contraception
Parenthood	Nursing home placement
Sterilization	Foster home placement
In vitro fertilization	Separation
Transport from rural facilities	Work/task
Circumcision	Career change
Divorce	Professional ethics
Abortion	Business investments
Artificial insemination	Relocation
Adoption	

Related to:
Lack of relevant information*
Confusing information

Related to:
Disagreement within support systems
Inexperience with decision-making
Unclear personal values/beliefs*
Conflict with personal values/beliefs
Family history of poor prognosis
Hospital paternalism—loss of control
Ethical or moral dilemmas of:

Quality of life	Organ transplant
Cessation of life-support systems	Selective termination with multiple-gestation
"Do not resuscitate" orders	pregnancies
Termination of pregnancy	

Maturational

Related to risks versus benefits of:

Adolescent

Peer pressure	Career choice
Alcohol/drug use	Use of birth control

Adult

College	Relocation
Whether to continue a relationship	Retirement
	Sexual activity
Career change	Illegal/dangerous situations

Older Adult

Retirement	Nursing home placement

🔘 Author's Note

The nurse has an important role in assisting clients and families with making decisions. Because nurses usually do not benefit financially from decisions made regarding treatments and transfers, they are in an ideal position to assist with decisions. Although, according to Davis (1989), "Nursing or medical expertise does not enable health care professionals to know the values of patients or what patients think is best for themselves," nursing expertise enables nurses to facilitate systematic decision-making that considers all possible alternatives and possible outcomes, as well as individual beliefs and values. The focus is on assisting with logical decision-making, not on promoting a certain decision.

When people are making a treatment decision of considerable risk, they do not necessarily experience conflict. In situations where the treatment option is "choosing life," individual perception may be one of submitting to fate and be relatively unconflicted. Because of this, nurses must be cautious in labeling patients with the nursing diagnosis of "Decisional Conflict" without sufficient validating cues (Soholt, 1990).

NOC

Decision-Making, Information Processing, Participation: Health Care Decisions

Goal

The client/group will make an informed choice as evidenced by the following indicators:

- Relate the advantages and disadvantages of choices.
- Share fears and concerns regarding choices and responses of others.
- Define what would be most helpful to support the decision-making process.

NIC

Decision-Making Support, Mutual Goal Setting, Learning Facilitation, Health System Guidance, Anticipatory Guidance, Patient Right Protection, Values Clarification, Anxiety Reduction

Interventions

Assess Causative/Contributing Factors

Refer to Related Factors.

Reduce or Eliminate Causative or Contributing Factors

Internal

Lack of Experience With or Ineffective Decision-Making
- Review past decisions and the steps that were taken to help the client decide.
- Facilitate logical decision-making:
  - Assist the client in recognizing the problem and clearly identifying the needed decision.
  - Generate a list of all possible alternatives or options.
  - Help identify the probable outcomes of the various alternatives.
  - Aid in evaluating the alternatives based on actual or potential threats to beliefs/values.
  - Encourage the client to make a decision.
- Encourage significant others to be involved in the entire decision-making process.

- Suggest the client use significant others as a sounding board when considering alternatives.
- Respect and support the role that the client desires in the decision, whether it is active, collaborative, or passive.
- Be available to review the needed decision and the various alternatives.
- Facilitate refocusing on the needed decision when the client experiences fragmented thinking during high anxiety.
- Encourage the client to take time in deciding.
- With adolescents, focus on the present—what will happen versus what will not. Help identify the important things because they do not have extensive past experiences on which to base decisions.

Value Conflict (Also Refer to *Spiritual Distress*)
- Use values clarification techniques to assist the client in reviewing the parts of his or her life that reflect his or her beliefs.
  - Help the client to identify his or her most prized and cherished activities.
  - Ask reflective statements that lead to further clarification.
  - Review past decisions in which the client needed to publicly affirm opinions and beliefs.
  - Evaluate the stands the client has taken on controversial subjects. Does he or she view them in black-and-white terms, or various shades of gray?
  - Identify values the client is proud of. Rank them in order of importance.

Fear of Outcome/Response of Others (Also Refer to *Fear*)
- Provide clarification regarding potential outcomes and correct misconceptions.
- Explore with the client what the risks of not deciding would be.
- Encourage expression of feelings.
- Promote self-worth.
- Encourage the client to face fears.
- Encourage the client to share fears with significant others.
- Actively reassure the client that the decision is his or hers to make and that he or she has the right to do so.
- Assist the client in recognizing that it is his or her life; if he or she is comfortable with the decision, others will respect the conviction.
- Reassure the client that individuality is acceptable.

External

Insufficient or Inconsistent Information
- Provide information comprehensively and sensitively.
- Correct misinformation.

- Give concise information that covers the major points when the decision must be made quickly.
- Inform the client of his or her right to know.
- Enable the client to determine the amount of information that he or she desires.
- Encourage verbalization to determine the client's perception of choices.
- Ensure that the client clearly understands what is involved in the decision and the various alternatives (i.e., informed choice).
- Encourage the client to seek second professional opinions regarding health.
- Collaborate with other health care members/significant others to determine appropriate timing for truthfulness.

Controversy with Support System

- Reassure the client that he or she does not have to give in to pressure from others, whether family, friends, or health professionals.
- Advocate for the client's wishes if others attempt to undermine his or her ability to make the decision personally.
- Identify leaders within the support system and provide information.
- Advocate for the client if the family/significant others are excluding him or her from decision-making.
- Recognize that the client may become ambivalent about "choosing" when putting the needs of the support system above his or her own.

Unsatisfactory Health Care Environment

- Establish a trusting and meaningful relationship that promotes mutual understanding and caring.
- Provide a quiet environment for thought and reduce sensory stimulation.
- Allow uninterrupted periods with significant others.
- Promote accepting, nonjudgmental attitudes.
- Reduce the number of small decisions that the client must make to facilitate focusing on the decision in conflict.

Confer With Client and Family Facing Decisions Regarding Cancer Treatments

- Establish a pretreatment quality of life using a tested instrument (Halyard & Ferrans, 2008).
- Explore how cancer treatment decisions will affect quality of life (Yarbro, Wujcik, & Gobel, 2011).
- Consult with others if needed for necessary data. Avoid relinquishing your responsibility to the client and family to others.

- What are the long-term negative effects when survival is long?
- Is a supportive care only better than therapeutic regimen when survival time is short (6–12 months) or median?
- Is a new therapy preferable?
- What are the side effects of all the proposed therapies?

Explore End-of-Life Decisions

- Explore with the client and family whether they have discussed and recorded their end-of-life decisions.
- Describe the possible future dilemmas when these discussions are avoided.
- Instruct the client and the family to provide directives in the following areas:
  - Person to contact in emergency
  - Person the client trusts most with personal decisions
  - Decision to be kept alive if the client will be mentally incompetent or terminally ill
  - Preference to die at home, hospital, or no preference
  - Desire to sign a living will
  - Decision regarding organ donation
  - Funeral arrangements and burial or cremation
  - Circumstances (if any) when information should be withheld from the client
- Document these decisions and make two copies (retain one and give one to the person who is designated to be the decision-maker in an emergency).
- Discuss the purpose of a living will. Provide information when requested. To obtain a copy of your state's living will, visit www.livingwillid.com/state.html.

Initiate Referrals as Needed

Refer Families to Social Service for Assistance With Decisions Regarding Care of a Family Member

 Pediatric Interventions

- Include children and adolescents in decision-making process.

 Geriatric Interventions

- Ensure that older adult is involved in decisions.
- Facilitate communication among the elder, family, and professionals.
- If needed, use simple explanations and provide the pros and cons of the decision.

DIARRHEA

NANDA-I Definition

Passage of loose, unformed stools

Defining Characteristics*

Major (Must Be Present)*

At least three loose, liquid stools per day

Minor (May Be Present)*

Urgency
Cramping/abdominal pain
Hyperactive bowel sounds

Related Factors

Pathophysiologic

Related to malabsorption or inflammation* secondary to:*
Colon cancer   Celiac disease (sprue)
Diverticulitis   Gastritis
Irritable bowel   Spastic colon
Crohn's disease   Ulcerative colitis
Peptic ulcer

Related to lactose deficiency, dumping syndrome

Related to increased peristalsis secondary to increased metabolic rate (hyperthyroidism)

Related to infectious processes secondary to:*
Trichinosis   Shigellosis   Dysentery
Typhoid fever   Cholera   Infectious hepatitis
Malaria   Microsporidia   Cryptosporidium

Related to excessive secretion of fats in stool secondary to liver dysfunction

Related to inflammation and ulceration of gastrointestinal mucosa secondary to high levels of nitrogenous wastes (renal failure)

Treatment Related

Related to malabsorption or inflammation secondary to surgical intervention of the bowel

Related to adverse effects of pharmaceutical agents* of (specify):

Thyroid agents	Chemotherapy	Antacids
Analgesics	Laxatives	Cimetidine
Stool softeners	Iron sulfate	Antibiotics

Related to tube feedings

Situational (Personal, Environmental)

Related to stress or anxiety*

Related to irritating foods (fruits, bran cereals) or increase in caffeine consumption

Related to changes in water and food secondary to travel*

Related to change in bacteria in water

Related to bacteria, virus, or parasite to which no immunity is present

 Author's Note

See *Constipation*.

NOC

Bowel Elimination, Electrolyte & Acid–Base Balance, Fluid Balance, Hydration, Symptom Control

Goal

The client/parent will report less diarrhea as evidenced by the following indicators:

• Describe contributing factors when known.

NIC

Bowel Management, Diarrhea Management, Fluid/Electrolyte Management, Nutrition Management, Enteral Tube Feeding

Interventions

Assess Causative Contributing Factors

- Tube feedings
- Dietetic foods
- Foreign travel
- Dietary indiscretions/contaminated foods
- Food allergies
- Medications

Eliminate or Reduce Contributing Factors

Side Effects of Tube Feeding (Fuhrman, 1999)
- Control the infusion rate (depending on delivery set).
- Administer smaller, more frequent feedings.
- Change to continuous-drip tube feedings.
- Administer more slowly if signs of gastrointestinal intolerance occur.
- Control temperature.
- If formula has been refrigerated, warm it in hot water to room temperature.
- Dilute the strength of feeding temporarily.
- Follow the standard procedure for administration of tube feeding.
- Follow tube feeding with the specified amount of water to ensure hydration.
- Be careful of contamination/spoilage (unused but opened formula should not be used after 24 hours; keep unused portion refrigerated).

Contaminated Foods (possible sources)
- Raw seafood
- Raw milk
- Shellfish
- Restaurants
- Excess milk consumption
- Improperly cooked/stored food

Dietetic Foods: Eliminate Foods Containing Large Amounts of the Hexitol, Sorbitol, and Mannitol That Are Used as Sugar Substitutes in Dietetic Foods, Candy, and Chewing Gum

Reduce Diarrhea

- Advise not to stop eating or from withholding food from children (Sack et al., 2004).
- Avoid milk (lactose) products, fat, whole grains, fried and spicy foods, and fresh fruits and vegetables.

- Gradually add semisolids and solids (crackers, yogurt, rice, bananas, applesauce).
- Instruct the client to seek medical care if blood and mucous are in stool and fever greater than 101° F.

Replace Fluids and Electrolytes

- Increase oral intake to maintain a normal urine specific gravity (light yellow in color).
- Encourage liquids (tea, water, apple juice, flat ginger ale).
- When diarrhea is severe, use an over-the-counter oral rehydration solution.
- Teach the client to monitor the color of urine to determine hydration needs. Increase fluids if urine color is amber or dark yellow.
- Caution against the use of very hot or cold liquids.
- See *Deficient Fluid Volume* for additional interventions.

Conduct Health Teaching as Indicated

- Explain safe food handling (e.g., required temperature storage, washing of food preparation objects after use with raw food, frequent hand washing).
- Explain the interventions required to prevent future episodes and effects of diarrhea on hydration.
- Consult with primary health care provider for prophylactic use of bismuth subsalicylate (e.g., Pepto-Bismol) 30 to 60 mL or 2 tablets qid during travel and 2 days after return; or antimicrobials for prevention of traveler's diarrhea.
- Advise not to treat traveler's diarrhea with antimotility agents (e.g., Lomotil, Imodium).
- Teach precautions to take when traveling to foreign lands:
  - Avoid salads, milk, fresh cheese, cold cuts, and salsa.
  - Drink carbonated or bottled beverages; avoid ice.
  - Peel fresh fruits and vegetables.
  - Avoid foods not stored at proper temperature.
  - Advise not to treat traveler's diarrhea with antimotility agents (e.g., Lomotil, Imodium), which can delay the clearance of organisms and thus can increase the severity of traveler's diarrhea with complications (e.g., sepsis, toxic megacolon; CDC, 2006).
- Explain how to prevent food-borne diseases at home:
  - Refrigerate all perishable foods.
  - Cook all food at high temperature or boil (212° F) for at least 15 minutes before serving.
  - Avoid allowing food to stand at warm temperatures for several hours.
  - Caution about foods at picnics in hot summer.

- Thoroughly clean kitchen equipment after contact with perishable foods (e.g., meats, dairy, fish).
- Explain that a diet primarily made up of dietetic foods containing sugar substitutes (hexitol, sorbitol, and mannitol) can cause diarrhea.
- Teach the client to gently clean the anal area after bowel movements; lubricants (e.g., petroleum jelly) can protect skin.

Pediatric Interventions

Monitor Fluid and Electrolyte Losses

- Fluid volume lost
- Urine color and output
- Skin color
- Mucous membranes
- Capillary refill time

Consult With Primary Care Provider If:

- Diarrhea persists.
- Blood or mucus is in stools.
- Child is lethargic.
- Urine output is scanty.
- Stools suddenly increase.
- Child is vomiting.

Reduce Diarrhea

- Avoid milk (lactose) products, fat, whole grains, and fresh fruits and vegetables.
- Avoid high-carbohydrate fluids (e.g., soft drinks), gelatin, fruit juices, caffeinated drinks, and chicken or beef broths.

Provide Oral Rehydration

- Use oral rehydration solutions (e.g., Pedialyte, Lytren, Ricelyte, Resol [Larson, 2000]).
- Determine fluid loss by body weight loss. If less than 5% of total weight is lost, 50 mL/kg of fluids will be needed during the next 3 to 6 hours (Pillitteri, 2010).
- For more than a 5% weight loss, consult with the primary care provider for fluid replacement.
- Fluids must be given to replace losses and continuing losses until diarrhea improves (Pillitteri, 2010).

Reintroduce Food

- Begin with bananas, rice, cereal, and crackers in small quantities.
- Gradually return to regular diet (except milk products) after 36 to 48 hours; after 3 to 5 days, gradually add milk products

(half-strength skim milk to skim milk to half-strength milk (whole or 1%).
- Gradually introduce formula (half-strength formula to full-strength formula).

For Breast-Fed Infants

- Continue breast-feeding.
- Use oral rehydration therapy if needed.

Protect Skin From Irritation With Non–Water-Soluble Cream (e.g., Petroleum Jelly)

Initiate Health Teaching as Needed

Teach Parents Signs to Report:
- Sunken eyes
- Dry mucous membranes
- Rapid, thready pulse
- Rapid breathing
- Lethargy
- Diarrhea increases

✺ Geriatric Interventions

- Determine if impaction is present; if so, remove it (refer to *Constipation* for specific interventions).
- Monitor closely for hypovolemia and electrolyte imbalances (e.g., potassium, sodium).
- Advise individual to seek medical care if diarrhea continues over 24 hours.

RISK FOR DISUSE SYNDROME

NANDA-I Definition

At risk for deterioration of body systems as the result of prescribed or unavoidable musculoskeletal inactivity

Defining Characteristics

Presence of a cluster of actual or risk nursing diagnoses related to inactivity:

Risk for Impaired Skin Integrity
Risk for Constipation
Risk for Altered Respiratory Function

Risk for Ineffective Peripheral Tissue Perfusion
Risk for Infection
Risk for Activity Intolerance
Risk for Impaired Physical Mobility
Risk for Injury
Powerlessness
Disturbed Body Image

Related Factors

(Optional) Refer to Author's Notes

Pathophysiologic

Related to:

Decreased sensorium	Unconsciousness

Neuromuscular impairment secondary to:

Multiple sclerosis	Partial/total paralysis
Muscular dystrophy	Guillain–Barré syndrome
Parkinsonism	Spinal cord injury

Musculoskeletal impairment secondary to:

Fractures	Rheumatic diseases

End-stage disease

AIDS	Renal
Cardiac	

Cancer

Psychiatric/Mental Health Disorders

Major depression	Severe phobias
Catatonic state	

Treatment Related

Related to:

Surgery (amputation, skeletal)	Invasive vascular lines
Mechanical ventilation	Prescribed immobility
Traction/casts/splints	

Situational (Personal, Environmental)

Related to:

Depression	Fatigue
Debilitated state	Pain

Maturational

Newborn/Infant/Child/Adolescent
Related to:

Down syndrome

Juvenile arthritis

Cerebral palsy

Risser-Turnbuckle jacket

Osteogenesis imperfecta

Mental/physical disability

Legg–Calvé–Perthes disease

Autism

Spina bifida

Older Adult
Related to:

Decreased motor agility

Muscle weakness

Presenile dementia

 Author's Note

Risk for Disuse Syndrome describes a client at risk for the adverse effects of immobility. *Risk for Disuse Syndrome* identifies vulnerability to certain complications and also altered functioning in a health pattern. As a syndrome diagnosis, its etiology or contributing factor is within the diagnostic label (*Disuse*); a "related to" statement is not necessary. As discussed in Chapter 2, a syndrome diagnosis comprises a cluster of predicted actual or risk nursing diagnoses because of the situation. Eleven risk or actual nursing diagnoses are clustered under *Disuse Syndrome* (see Defining Characteristics).

The nurse no longer needs to use separate diagnoses, such as *Risk for Ineffective Respiratory Function* or *Risk for Impaired Skin Integrity*, because they are incorporated into the syndrome category. If an immobile client manifests signs or symptoms of impaired skin integrity or another diagnosis, however, the nurse should use the specific diagnosis. He or she should continue to use *Risk for Disuse Syndrome* so other body systems do not deteriorate.

NOC

Endurance, Immobility Consequences: Physiologic, Immobility Consequences: Psycho-Cognitive, Mobility Level Joint Movement

Goal

The client will not experience complications of immobility as evidenced by the following indicators:

- Intact skin/tissue integrity
- Maximum pulmonary function
- Maximum peripheral blood flow

- Full range of motion
- Bowel, bladder, and renal functioning within normal limits
- Uses of social contacts and activities when possible
- Explain rationale for treatments
- Make decisions regarding care when possible
- Share feelings regarding immobile state

NIC

Activity Therapy, Energy Management, Mutual Goal Settings, Exercise Therapy, Fall Prevention, Pressure Ulcer Prevention, Body Mechanics Correction, Skin Surveillance, Positioning, Coping Enhancement, Decision-Making, Support Therapeutic Play

Interventions

Identify Causative and Contributing Factors

- Pain; refer also to *Impaired Comfort*
- Fatigue; refer also to *Fatigue*
- Decreased motivation; refer also to *Activity Intolerance*
- Depression; refer also to *Ineffective Coping*

Promote Optimal Respiratory Function

- Vary the position of the bed, thus gradually changing the horizontal and vertical position of the thorax, unless contraindicated.
- Assist the client to reposition, turning frequently from side-to-side (hourly if possible).
- Encourage deep breathing and controlled coughing exercises 5 times every hour.
- Teach the client to use a blow bottle or incentive spirometer every hour when awake (with severe neuromuscular impairment, the client also may have to be awakened at night).
- For a child, use colored water in the blow bottle; have him or her blow up balloons, soap bubbles, or cotton balls with straw.
- Auscultate lung fields every 8 hours; increase frequency if breath sounds are altered.
- Encourage small, frequent feedings to prevent abdominal distention.

Maintain Usual Pattern of Bowel Elimination

- Refer to *Constipation* for specific interventions.

Prevent Pressure Ulcers

- Use repositioning schedule that relieves vulnerable area most often (e.g., if vulnerable area is the back, the turning schedule would be left side to back, back to right side, right side to left side, and left side to back); post "turn clock" at bedside.

- Turn the client or instruct him or her to turn or shift weight every 30 minutes to 2 hours, depending on other causative factors and the ability of the skin to recover from pressure.
- Frequency of turning schedule should increase if any reddened areas that appear do not disappear within 1 hour after turning.
- Position the client in normal or neutral position with body weight evenly distributed.
- Keep the bed as flat as possible to reduce shearing forces; limit Fowler's position to only 30 minutes at a time.
- Use foam blocks or pillows to provide a bridging effect to support the body above and below the high-risk or ulcerated area so affected area does not touch the bed surface; do not use foam donuts or inflatable rings because they increase the area of pressure.
- Alternate or reduce the pressure on the skin surface with:
  - Foam mattresses
  - Air mattresses
  - Air-fluidized beds
  - Vascular boots to suspend heels
- Use enough personnel to lift the client up in bed or a chair rather than pull or slide skin surfaces; use protectors to reduce friction on elbows and heels.
- To reduce shearing forces, support feet with a footboard to prevent sliding.
- Promote optimum circulation when the client is sitting.
- Limit time spent sitting for the client at high risk for ulcer development.
- Instruct the client to lift self, using chair arms every 10 minutes if possible, or assist the client to rise from the chair every 10 to 20 minutes, depending on risk factors.
- Inspect areas at risk for ulcers with each position change: Ears, occiput, heels, sacrum, scrotum, elbows, trochanter, ischia, scapula.
- Observe for erythema and blanching and palpate for warmth and tissue sponginess with each position change.
- Massage nonreddened, vulnerable areas gently with each position change.
- Refer to *Impaired Skin Integrity* for additional interventions.

Promote Factors That Improve Venous Blood Flow

- Elevate extremity above the level of the heart (may be contra-indicated in cases of severe cardiac or respiratory disease).

- Ensure the client avoids standing or sitting with legs dependent for long periods.
- Consider the use of below-knee elastic stockings to prevent venous stasis.
- Reduce or remove external venous compression, which impedes venous flow.
- Avoid pillows behind the knees or suggest a bed that is elevated at the knees.
- Tell the client to avoid crossing the legs.
- Remind the client to change positions, move extremities, or wiggle fingers and toes every hour.
- Ensure the client avoids garters and tight elastic stockings above the knees.
- Monitor legs for edema, tissue warmth, and redness daily.

Maintain Limb Mobility and Prevent Contractures (Maher et al., 1998)

Increase Limb Mobility

- Perform range-of-motion exercises (frequency to be determined by the client's condition).
- Support extremity with pillows to prevent or reduce swelling.
- Encourage the client to perform exercise regimens for specific joints as prescribed by physician or physical therapist.

Position the Client in Alignment to Prevent Complications

- Point toes and knees toward ceiling when the client is supine. Keep them flat when in a chair.
- Use footboard.
- Instruct the client to wiggle toes, point them up and downward, rotate their ankles inward and outward every hour.
- Avoid placing pillows under the knee; support calf instead.
- Avoid prolonged periods of hip flexion (i.e., sitting position).
- To position hips, place rolled towel lateral to the hip to prevent external rotation.
- Keep arms abducted from the body with pillows.
- Keep elbows in slight flexion.
- Keep wrist neutral, with fingers slightly flexed and thumb abducted and slightly flexed.
- Change position of shoulder joints during the day (e.g., abduction, adduction, range of circular motion).

Provide or Assist in Range-of-Motion Exercises Every 8 Hours

Prevent Urinary Stasis and Calculi Formation

- Provide a daily fluid intake of 2,000 mL or more (unless contraindicated); see *Deficient Fluid Volume* for specific interventions.

- Maintain urine pH below 6.0 (acidic) with acid ash foods (cereals, meats, poultry, fish, cranberry juice, apple juice).
- Teach the client to avoid foods high in calcium and oxalate (*very high):
  - Milk, milk products, and cheese
  - Bran cereals
  - *Spinach, cranberries, plums, raspberries, and gooseberries
  - Sardines, shrimp, oysters, legumes, and whole-grain rice
  - Asparagus, rhubarb, kale, Swiss chard, turnip greens, mustard greens, broccoli, and beet greens; also, peanut butter, ripe olives, and chocolate

Reduce and Monitor Bone Demineralization

- Monitor for hypercalcemia.
- Monitor serum levels.
- Monitor for nausea/vomiting, polydipsia, polyuria, lethargy.
- Promote weight-bearing when possible (tilt-table).
- Maintain vigorous hydration. Adults: 2,000 mL/day. Adolescents: 3,000 to 4,000 mL/day.

Promote Sharing and a Sense of Well-Being

- Encourage the client to share feelings and fears regarding restricted movement.
- Encourage the client to wear own clothes, rather than pajamas, and unique adornments (e.g., baseball caps, colorful socks) to express individuality.

Reduce the Monotony of Immobility
- Vary daily routine when possible (e.g., give a bath in the afternoon so the client can watch a special show or talk with a visitor during the morning).

Include the Client in Planning Daily Schedule
- Allow the client to make as many decisions as possible.
- Make daily routine as normal as possible (e.g., have the client wear street clothes during the day, if feasible).
- Encourage the client to make a schedule for visitors so everyone does not come at once or at inconvenient times.
- Spend quality time with the client (i.e., not time that is task oriented; rather, sit down and talk).

Be Creative; Vary the Physical Environment and Daily Routine When Possible
- Update bulletin boards, change pictures on the walls, and move furniture within the room.
- Maintain a pleasant, cheerful environment (e.g., plenty of light, flowers).

- Place the client near a window, if possible.
- Provide reading material (print or audio), radio, and television.
- Plan an activity daily to give the client something to look forward to; always keep promises.
- Discourage the use of television as the primary source of recreation unless it is highly desired.
- Consider using a volunteer to spend time reading to the client or helping with an activity.
- Encourage suggestions and new ideas (e.g., "Can you think of things you might like to do?").

Pediatric Interventions

Plan Appropriate Activities for Children

- Provide an environment with accessible toys that suit the child's developmental age; ensure they are well within reach.
- Encourage the family to bring in the child's favorite toys, including items from nature that will keep the "real world" alive (e.g., goldfish, leaves in fall).

Use Play Therapy (Pillitteri, 2010)

- As an energy release:
  - Pound pegs
  - Cut wood with pretend saw
  - Pound clay
  - Punch a balloon
- As dramatic play:
  - Provide health care equipment as dolls, doll beds, play stethoscopes, IV equipment, syringes, masks, and gowns.
  - Allow the child to choose the objects.
  - Allow the child opportunities to play and express their feelings.
  - Use opportunities to ask the child questions.
  - Reflect only what the child expresses.
  - Do not criticize.
- As creative play:
  - Provide opportunities to draw pictures.
  - Ask the child to describe the picture.
- Vary the environment.
- Transport child outside the room as much as possible.

DEFICIENT DIVERSIONAL ACTIVITY

NANDA-I Definition

Decreased stimulation from, (or interest or engagement in) recreational or leisure activities

Defining Characteristics

Observed and/or statements of boredom due to inactivity

Related Factors

Pathophysiologic

Related to difficulty accessing or participating in usual activities secondary to:
Communicable disease   Pain

Situational (Personal, Environmental)

Related to unsatisfactory social behaviors

Related to no peers or friends

Related to monotonous environment

Related to long-term hospitalization or confinement

Related to lack of motivation

Related to difficulty accessing or participating in usual activities secondary to:
Excessive stressful work
No time for leisure activities
Career changes (e.g., new job, retirement)
Children leaving home ("empty nest")
Immobility
Decreased sensory perception
Multiple role responsibilities

Maturational

Infant/Child
Related to lack of appropriate stimulation toys/peers

Older Adult
Related to difficulty accessing or participating in usual activities secondary to:

Sensory/motor deficits	Lack of peer group
Lack of transportation	Limited finances
Fear of crime	Confusion

Author's Note

Only the client can express a deficit in diversional activities based on his or her determination that types and amounts of activity are desired. Miller (2009) writes that activities associated with various roles affirm a client's self-concept.

To validate *Deficient Diversional Activity*, explore the etiology of factors amenable to nursing interventions, keeping your main focus on improving the quality of leisure activities. For a client with personality problems that hinder relationships and decrease social activities, *Impaired Social Interactions* is more valid. In this case, focus on helping the client identify behavior that imposes barriers to socialization.

NOC

Leisure Participation, Social Involvement

Goal

The client will rate that he or she is more satisfied with current activity level as evidenced by the following indicators:

- Relate methods of coping with anger or depression resulting from boredom.
- Report participation in one enjoyable activity each day.

NIC

Recreation Therapy, Socialization Enhancement, Self-Esteem Enhancement, Therapeutic Play

Interventions

Assess Causative Factors

Refer to Related Factors.

Reduce or Eliminate Causative Factors

Monotony
- Refer to Interventions, "Reduce the monotony of immobility," under *Disuse Syndrome*.

- Provide opportunities for reminiscence individually or in groups (e.g., past trips, hobbies).
- Provide music therapy with audiocassette players with light-weight headphones. For group music therapy (Rantz, 1991), the following is recommended:
  - Introduce a topic.
  - Play related music.
  - Develop the topic with discussion.
  - Discuss responses.
- Consider using holistic and complementary therapies (e.g., aromatherapy, pet therapy, therapeutic touch). For pet therapy (Rantz, 1991), the following is recommended:
  - Animals must be well groomed, healthy, and clean.
  - Animals should be relaxed with strangers.
  - Animals should eliminate before entering the facility.
  - Sponsors always should ask the client if he or she likes the type of animal before approaching the client.

Lack of Motivation

- Stimulate motivation by showing interest and encouraging sharing of feelings and experiences.
- Explore fears and concerns about participating in activities.
- Discuss likes and dislikes.
- Encourage sharing of feelings of present and past experiences.
- Spend time with the client purposefully talking about other topics (e.g., "I just got back from the shore. Have you ever gone there?").
- Point out the need to "get going" and try something new.
- Help the client work through feelings of anger and grief:
  - Allow him or her to express feelings.
  - Take the time to be a good listener.
  - See *Anxiety* for additional interventions.
- Encourage the client to join a group of possible interest or help. (He or she may have to participate by way of intercom or special arrangement.)
- Consider the use of music therapy or reminiscence therapy.

Inability to Concentrate

- Plan a simple daily routine with concrete activities (e.g., walking, drawing, folding linens).
- If the client is anxious, suggest solitary, noncompetitive activities (e.g., puzzles, photography).

Identify Factors That Promote Activity and Socialization

Encourage Socialization With Peers and All Age Groups (Frequently Very Young and Very Old Clients Mutually Benefit From Interactions)

Acquire Assistance to Increase the Client's Ability to Travel
- Arrange transportation to activities if necessary.
- Acquire aids for safety (e.g., wheelchair for shopping, walker for ambulating in hallways).

Increase the Client's Feelings of Productivity and Self-Worth
- Encourage the client to use strengths to help others and self (e.g., assign him or her tasks to perform in a general project). Acknowledge these efforts (e.g., "Thank you for helping Mr. Jones with his dinner").
- Encourage open communication; value the client's opinion ("Mr. Jones, what do you think about _____?").
- Encourage the client to challenge him or herself to learn a new skill or pursue a new interest.
- Provide opportunities to interact with nature and animals.

Refer to Social Isolation for Additional Interventions

Pediatric Interventions

- Provide an environment with accessible toys that suit the child's developmental age; ensure that they are well within reach.
- Keep toys in all waiting areas.
- Encourage the family to bring in the child's favorite toys, including items from nature that will help to keep the "real world" alive (e.g., goldfish, leaves in fall).
- Consult a child life specialist as indicated.
- Refer to the Pediatric Intervention in the Nursing Diagnosis *Disuse Syndrome* on for specifics on how to engage in therapeutic play.

Geriatric Interventions

- Explore interests and the feasibility of trying a new activity (e.g., mobility).
- Arrange for someone to accompany or orient the client during initial encounters.
- Explore possible volunteer opportunities (e.g., Red Cross, hospitals).
- Initiate referrals, if indicated.
  - Suggest joining the American Association of Retired Persons (AARP).
  - Write local health and welfare council or agencies.
  - Provide a list of associations/clubs with senior citizen activities (i.e., YMCA) such as Sixty Plus Club, Churches, XYZ

Group (Extra Years of Zest), Golden Age Club, Young at Heart Club, SOS (Senior Outreach Services), Encore Club, Leisure Hour Group, MORA (Men of Retirement Age), Gray Panthers.

AUTONOMIC DYSREFLEXIA

Autonomic Dysreflexia

Risk for Autonomic Dysreflexia

NANDA-I Definition

Life-threatening, uninhibited sympathetic response of the nervous system to a noxious stimulus after a spinal cord injury at T7 or above

Defining Characteristics

Major (Must Be Present)

The client with spinal cord injury (T6 or above) with:

Paroxysmal hypertension* (sudden periodic elevated blood pressure in which systolic pressure is above 140 mm Hg and diastolic is above 90 mm Hg)
Bradycardia or tachycardia* (pulse rate less than 60 or more than 100 beats/min)
Diaphoresis (above the injury)*
Red splotches on skin (above the injury)*
Pallor (below the injury)*
Headache (a diffuse pain in different portions of the head and not confined to any nerve distribution area)*
Apprehension
Dilated pupils

Minor (May Be Present)

Chilling*
Conjunctival congestion*
Horner's syndrome* (pupillary contraction; partial ptosis of the eyelid; enophthalmos; sometimes, loss of sweating over the affected side of the face)
Paresthesia*

Pilomotor reflex* (gooseflesh)
Blurred vision*
Chest pain*
Metallic taste in mouth*
Nasal congestion*
Penile erection and semen emission

Related Factors

Pathophysiologic

Related to visceral stretching and irritation secondary to:

Gastrointestinal
Gastric distention   Hemorrhoids
Constipation   Acute abdominal condition
Gastric ulceration   Anal fissure
Fecal impaction

Urologic
Bladder distension*   Urinary calculi   Urinary tract infection

Skin Irritation*
Pressure ulcers   Burns   Sunburn
Insect bites   Ingrown toenails   Blister

Reproductive
Menstruation   Uterine contraction
Epididymitis   Vaginal infection
Pregnancy or delivery   Vaginal dilation

Related to fracture

Related to stimulation of skin (abdominal, thigh)

Related to spastic sphincter

Related to deep vein thrombosis

Related to pain

Treatment Related

Related to visceral stretching secondary to:
Removal of fecal impaction
Clogged or nonpatent catheter
Visceral stretching and irritation secondary to surgical incision,
    enemas
Catheterization, enema

Situational (Personal, Environmental)

Related to deficient client knowledge* of prevention or treatment

Related to visceral stretching secondary to:
"Boosting" (Binding legs and distending bladder to boost norepi-
    nephrine production; McClain et al., 1999).
Sexual activity
Menstruation
Pregnancy or delivery

Related to neural stimulation secondary to immersion in cold water

 Author's Note

Autonomic Dysreflexia represents a life-threatening situation that nurse-
prescribed interventions can prevent or treat. Prevention involves
teaching the client to reduce sympathetic nervous system stimulation
and not using interventions that can cause such stimulation. Treatment
focuses on reducing or eliminating noxious stimuli (e.g., fecal impaction,
urinary retention). If nursing actions do not resolve symptoms, initiation
of medical intervention is critical. When a client requires medical treatment for all or most episodes of dysreflexia, the situation can be labeled
a collaborative problem: *RC of Dysreflexia.*

NOC

Neurologic Status, Neurologic Status: Autonomic, Vital Signs Status

Goal

The client/family will respond to early signs/symptoms. The cli-
ent/family will take action to prevent dysreflexia as evidenced by
the following indicators:

- State factors that cause dysreflexia.
- Describe the treatment for dysreflexia.
- Relate indications for emergency treatment.

NIC

Dysreflexia Management, Vital Signs Monitoring, Emergency Care, Medication
Administration

Interventions

Assess for Causative or Contributing Factors

See Related Factors.

Proceed as Follows If Signs of Dysreflexia Occur

- Stand or sit the client up.
- Lower the client's legs.
- Loosen all the client's constrictive clothing or appliances.

Check for Distended Bladder

If the Client Is Catheterized:
- Check the catheter for kinks or compression.
- Irrigate the catheter with only 30 mL of saline, very slowly.
- Replace the catheter if it will not drain.

If the Client Is Not Catheterized:
- Insert the catheter using dibucaine hydrochloride ointment (Nupercainal).
- Remove 500 mL, then clamp for 15 minutes.
- Repeat the cycle until the bladder is drained.

Check for Fecal Impaction

- First apply Nupercainal to the anus and into the rectum for 1 inch (2.54 cm).
- Gently check the rectum with a well-lubricated glove using your index finger.
- Insert rectal suppository or gently remove impaction.

Check for Skin Irritation

- Spray the skin lesion that is triggering the dysreflexia with a topical anesthetic agent.
- Remove support hose.

Continue to Monitor Blood Pressure Every 3 to 5 Minutes

Immediately Consult Physician for Pharmacologic Treatment If Hypertension Is Double Baseline or Noxious Stimuli Are Unable to Be Eliminated

Initiate Health Teaching and Referrals as Indicated

- Teach the signs, symptoms, and treatment of dysreflexia to the client and family.
- Teach the indications that warrant immediate medical intervention.
- Explain situations that trigger dysreflexia (menstrual cycle, sexual activity, elimination).
- Teach the client to watch for early signs and to intervene immediately.
- Teach the client to observe for early signs of bladder infections and skin lesions (pressure ulcers, ingrown toenails).

- Advise consultation with a physician for long-term pharmacologic management if the client is very vulnerable.
- Document the frequency of episodes and precipitating factor(s).
- Provide printed instructions to guide actions during the crisis or to show to other health care personnel (e.g., dentists, gynecologists; Kavchak-Keyes, 2000).
- Advise athletes with high spinal cord injury about the danger of boosting.
- Explain that failure to reverse dysreflexia can result in status epilepticus, stroke, and death. However, avoidance of noxious triggers can "prevent the episode entirely" (Somani, 2009).

Risk for Autonomic Dysreflexia

NANDA-I Definition

Refer to *Autonomic Dysreflexia*.

Risk Factors

Refer to *Autonomic Dysreflexia—Related Factors*.

Goals

Refer to *Autonomic Dysreflexia*.

Interventions

Refer to *Autonomic Dysreflexia*.

RISK FOR ELECTROLYTE IMBALANCE

See also *Risk for Complications of Electrolyte Imbalance* on http://thePoint.lww.com/CarpenitoHB14e.

NANDA-I Definition

At risk for a change in serum electrolyte levels that may compromise health

Risk Factors*

Endocrine dysfunction
Diarrhea
Fluid imbalance (e.g., dehydration, water intoxication)
Impaired regulatory mechanisms (e.g., diabetes insipidus, syn-
    drome of inappropriate secretion of antidiuretic hormones)
Renal dysfunction
Treatment related side effects (e.g., medications, drains)
Vomiting

 Author's Note

This NANDA-I diagnosis is a collaborative problem. Refer to http://thePoint.
lww.com/CarpenitoHB14e for *Risk for Complications of Electrolyte Imbalances.*

DISTURBED ENERGY FIELD

NANDA-I Definition

Disruption of the flow of energy surrounding a person's being that
results in disharmony of the body, mind, and/or spirit

Defining Characteristics*

Perception of changes in patterns of the energy flow, such as:
Temperature change (warmth, coolness)
Visual changes (image, color)
Disruption of the field (vacant, hole, spike, bulge, obstruction,
    congestion, diminished flow in energy field)
Movement (wave, spike, tingling, dense, flowing)
Sounds (tone, word)

Related Factors

Pathophysiologic

Related to slowing or blocking of energy flows secondary to:
Illness (specify)   Pregnancy   Injury

Treatment Related

Related to slowing or blocking of energy flow secondary to:
Immobility*   Labor and delivery*
Perioperative experience*   Chemotherapy

Situational (Personal, Environmental)

Related to slowing or blocking of energy flow secondary to:
Pain*   Fear*
Grieving*   Anxiety*

Maturational

Related to age-related developmental difficulties or crises (specify)*

 Author's Note

This diagnosis is unique for two reasons: (1) it represents a specific theory (human energy field theory) and (2) its interventions require specialized instruction and supervised practice. Meehan (1991) recommends the following preparation:

- At least 6 months of professional practice in an acute care setting
- Guided learning by a nurse with at least 2 years of experience
- Conformance with practice guidelines
- Thirty hours of instruction in the theory and practice
- Thirty hours of supervised practice with relatively healthy people
- Successful completion of written and practice evaluations

Some may consider this diagnosis unconventional. Nurses may need to be reminded that there are many theories, philosophies, and frameworks of nursing practice, just as there are many definitions of clients and practice settings. Some nurses practice on street corners with homeless people, whereas others practice in offices attached to their homes. Nursing diagnosis should not represent only mainstream nursing (acute care, long-term care, home health). Nurses should celebrate diversity despite opinions that this diagnosis has little applicability. Fundamentally, nurses are all connected through the quest to improve the condition of individuals, families, groups, and communities.

 NOC

Spiritual Health

Goal

The client will report relief of symptoms after therapeutic touch as evidenced by the following indicators:

* Report increased sense of relaxation.
* Report decreased pain, using a scale of 0 to 10 before and after therapies.
* Have slower, deeper respirations.

Therapeutic Touch, Spiritual Support, Presence

Interventions

Note: The following phases of therapeutic touch are learned separately but rendered concurrently. Presentation of these interventions is to describe the process for nurses who do not practice therapeutic touch. This discussion may help them to support colleagues who practice therapeutic touch and also to initiate referrals. As discussed before, preparation for therapeutic touch requires specialized instruction, which is beyond the scope of this book. Refer to the reference Nurse Healers Professional Associates International for Standards.

Prepare the Client and Environment for Therapeutic Touch (TT)

* Provide as much privacy as possible.
* Explain therapeutic touch and obtain verbal permission to perform it.
* Give the client permission to stop the therapy at any time.
* Allow the client to assume a comfortable position (e.g., lying on a bed, sitting on a couch).

Shift From a Direct Focus on the Environment to an Inner Focus

* Perceived as the center of life within the nurse (centering).

Assess the Client

* Scan the client's energy field for openness and symmetry (Krieger, 1987).
* Move the palms of your hands toward the client, at a distance of 2 to 4 inches over his or her body, from head to feet in a smooth, light movement.
* Use calm and rhythmic hand movements.
* Sense the cues to energy imbalance (e.g., warmth, coolness, tightness, heaviness, tingling, and emptiness).

Facilitate a Rhythmic Flow of Energy

• Moving hands vigorously from head to toe (unruffling/clearing).

Focus Intent on the Specific Repatterning of Areas of Imbalance
and Impeded Flow

• Using your hands as focal points, move them gently, sweeping
  from head to feet one time.
• Note the energy flow over lower legs and feet.
• If the energy flow is not open in this area, continue to move
  your hands or hold the feet physically to facilitate energy flow.
• Briefly shake your hands to dispel congestion from the field if
  needed.
• When therapeutic touch is complete, place your hands over
  the solar plexus area (just above the waist) and focus on facilitating the flow of healing energy to the client.
• Provide the client with an opportunity to rest.

Encourage the Client to Provide Feedback

• Assess if the client exhibits a relaxation response. Signs include
  drops of several decibels in voice volume; slower, deeper
  respirations; audible sign of relaxation; and a peripheral flush
  perceived on face.

Document Both the Procedure and the Feedback

• Provide therapeutic touch to:
  • Reduce agitation in individuals with dementia (Woods et. al.,
    2009).
  • Promote sleep (Heidt, 1991).
  • Promotes physiologic defense mechanisms (e.g., fibroblast
    proliferation) (Gronowicz, 2006), hemoglobin increases
    (Movaffaghi et al., 2006), and increased CD 4 cell concentra-
    tion (Turner et al., 1998).

IMPAIRED ENVIRONMENTAL INTERPRETATION SYNDROME

NANDA-I Definition

Consistent lack of orientation to person, place, time, or circumstances over more than 3 to 6 months necessitating a protective
environment

Defining Characteristics*

Major (Must Be Present, One or More)

Consistent disorientation   Chronic confusional states

Minor (May Be Present)

Loss of occupation   Inability to reason
Loss of social functioning   Inability to follow simple
Slow in responding to questions   directions
Inability to concentrate

Related Factors

Dementia* (Alzheimer's disease, multi-infarct dementia, Pick's
    disease, AIDS dementia)
Parkinson's disease
Huntington's disease*
Depression*
Alcoholism

 Author's Note

Environmental Interpretation Syndrome describes an individual who needs
a protective environment because of consistent lack of orientation to
person, place, time, or circumstances. This diagnosis is described under
Chronic Confusion, Wandering, and *Risk for Injury.* Interventions focus on
maintaining maximum level of independence and preventing injury. Until
clinical research differentiates this diagnosis from the aforementioned
diagnoses, use *Chronic Confusion, Wandering,* or *Risk for Injury,* depending
on the data presented.

INTERRUPTED FAMILY PROCESSES

Interrupted Family Processes

Dysfunctional Family Processes

Definition

Change in family relationships and/or functioning (NANDA-I)

State in which a usually supportive family experiences, or is at risk to experience, a stressor that challenges its previously effective functioning**

Defining Characteristics

Major (Must Be Present)

Family system cannot or does not:
Adapt constructively to crisis
Communicate openly and effectively between family members

Minor (May Be Present)

Family system cannot or does not:
Meet physical needs of all its members
Meet emotional needs of all its members
Meet spiritual needs of all its members
Express or accept a wide range of feelings
Seek or accept help appropriately

Related Factors

Any factor can contribute to *Interrupted Family Processes.* Common factors are listed below.

Treatment Related

Related to:
Disruption of family routines because of time-consuming treatments (e.g., home dialysis)
Physical changes because of treatments of ill family member
Emotional changes in all family members because of treatments of ill family member
Financial burden of treatments for ill family member
Hospitalization of ill family member

** This definition has been added by the author for clarity and usefulness.

Situational (Personal, Environmental)

Related to loss of family member:

Death	Separation
Incarceration	Hospitalization
Going away to school	Divorce
Desertion	

Related to addition of new family member:

Birth	Adoption
Marriage	Elderly relative

Related to losses associated with:

Poverty	Birth of child with defect
Economic crisis	Relocation
Change in family roles	Disaster
(e.g., retirement)	

Related to conflict (moral, goal, cultural)

Related to breach of trust between members

Related to social deviance by family member (e.g., crime)

🕐 Author's Note

Interrupted Family Processes describes a family that reports usual constructive function but is experiencing an alteration from a current stress-related challenge. The family is viewed as a system, with interdependence among members. Thus, life challenges for individual members also challenge the family system. Certain situations may negatively influence family functioning; examples include illness, an older relative moving in, relocation, separation, and divorce. *Risk for Interrupted Family Processes* can represent such a situation.

  Interrupted Family Processes differs from *Caregiver Role Strain*. Certain situations require one or more family members to assume a caregiver role for a relative. Caregiver role responsibilities can vary from ensuring an older parent has three balanced meals daily to providing for all hygiene and self-care activities for an adult or child. *Caregiver Role Strain* describes the mental and physical burden that the caregiver role places on individuals, which influences all their concurrent relationships and role responsibilities. It focuses specifically on the individual or individuals with multiple direct caregiver responsibilities.

NOC

Family Coping, Family Environment: Internal, Family Normalization, Parenting

Goal

The family will maintain functional system of mutual support for one another, as evidenced by the following indicators:

* Frequently verbalize feelings to professional nurse and one another.
* Identify appropriate external resources available.

NIC

Family Involvement Promotion, Coping Enhancement, Family Integrity Promotion, Family Therapy, Counseling, Referral

Interventions

Assess Causative and Contributing Factors

Illness-Related Factors
* Sudden, unexpected nature of illness
* Burdensome, chronic problems
* Potentially disabling nature of illness
* Symptoms creating disfiguring change in physical appearance
* Social stigma associated with illness
* Financial burden

Factors Related to Behavior of Ill Family Member
* Refuses to cooperate with necessary interventions
* Engages in socially deviant behavior associated with illness (e.g., suicide attempts, violence, substance abuse)
* Isolates self from family
* Acts out or is verbally abusive to health professionals and family members

Factors Related to Overall Family Functioning
* Unresolved guilt, blame, hostility, jealousy
* Inability to solve problems
* Ineffective communication patterns among members
* Changes in role expectations and resulting tension
* Unclear role boundaries

Factors Related to Illness in Family (See Also Caregiver Role Strain)

Factors Related to the Community
* Lack of support from spiritual resources (philosophical, religious, or both)
* Lack of relevant health education resources
* Lack of supportive friends
* Lack of adequate community health care resources (e.g., long-term follow up, hospice, respite)

Promote Cohesiveness

- Approach the family with warmth, respect, and support.
- Keep family members abreast of changes in ill family member's condition when appropriate.
- Avoid discussing what caused the problem or blaming.
- Encourage verbalization of guilt, anger, blame, and hostility and subsequent recognition of own feelings in family members.
- Explain the importance of functional communications, which uses verbal and nonverbal communication to teach behavior, share feelings and values, and evolve decisions about family health practices (Kaakinen et al., 2010).

Assist Family to Appraise the Situation

- What is at stake? Encourage family to have a realistic perspective by providing accurate information and answers to questions. Ensure all family members have input.
- What are the choices? Assist family to reorganize roles at home and set priorities to maintain family integrity and reduce stress.
- Initiate discussions regarding stressors of home care (physical, emotional, environmental, and financial).
- "Family-oriented approaches that include helping a family gain insight and make behavioral changes are most successful" (Varcarolis, Carson, & Shoemaker, 2010).

Promote Clear Boundaries Between Individuals in Family

- Ensure that all family members share their concerns.
- Elicit the responsibilities of each member.
- Acknowledge the differences.

Initiate Health Teaching and Referrals, as Necessary

- Include family members in group education sessions.
- Refer families to lay support and self-help groups.
  - Al-Anon
  - Lupus Foundation of America
  - Syn-Anon
  - Arthritis Foundation
  - Alcoholics Anonymous
  - National Multiple Sclerosis Society
  - Sharing and Caring
  - American Cancer Society
  - American Hospital Association
  - American Heart Association
  - American Diabetes Association
  - Ostomy Association

- American Lung Association
- Reach for Recovery
- Alzheimer's Disease and Related Disorders Association
- Facilitate family involvement with social supports.
- Assist family members to identify reliable friends (e.g., clergy, significant others); encourage seeking help (emotional, technical) when appropriate.
- Enlist help of other professionals (social work, therapist, psychiatrist, school nurse).

Dysfunctional Family Processes

Related to destructive family response patterns to alcohol abuse.

NANDA-I Definition

Psychosocial, spiritual, and physiologic functions of the family unit are chronically disorganized, which leads to conflict, denial of problems, resistance to change, ineffective problem-solving, and a series of self-perpetuating crises

Defining Characteristics†

Major (Must Be Present)

Behaviors

Inappropriate expression of anger*	Alcohol abuse
	Rationalization*
Inadequate understanding or knowledge of alcoholism	Enabling behaviors
	Blaming*
Manipulation*	Ineffective problem solving*
Denial of problems*	Inability to meet emotional
Dependency*	needs
Loss of control of drinking	Broken promises*
Refusal to get help*	Criticizing*
Impaired communication*	

Feelings*

Hopelessness	Emotional isolation
Anger	Worthlessness
Guilt	Vulnerability
Powerlessness	Suppressed rage

† Lindeman, Hokanson, & Batek, 1994

Repressed emotions
Anxiety
Shame
Mistrust

Loneliness
Responsible for alcoholic's
  behavior
Embarrassment

Roles and Relationships

Deteriorated family
  relationships
Inconsistent parenting
Disturbed family dynamics
Closed communication systems
Family denial

Marital problems
Ineffective spouse
  communication
Intimacy dysfunction
Disruption of family roles

Minor (May Be Present)

Behaviors

Inability to accept a wide range
  of feelings*
Inability to get or receive help
  appropriately*
Orientation toward tension
  relief rather than goal
  achievement*
Ineffective decision-making
Failure to deal with conflict
Contradictory, paradoxical
  communication*
Family's special occasions are
  alcohol centered*
Harsh self-judgment*
Escalating conflict*
Isolation
Lying*
Failure to send clear messages
Difficulty having fun*

Immaturity*
Disturbances in concentration*
Chaos*
Inability to adapt to change*
Power struggles*
Substance abuse other than
  alcohol
Difficulty with life-cycle
  transitions*
Verbal abuse of spouse or
  parent*
Stress-related physical
  illnesses*
Failure to accomplish current
  or past developmental tasks*
Lack of reliability*
Disturbances in academic
  performance in children*

Feelings

Being different from other
  people*
Lack of identity*
Unresolved grief
Feelings misunderstood
Loss*
Depression*
Fear*
Hostility*
Abandonment*

Moodiness*
Confused love and pity
Emotional control by others*
Dissatisfaction*
Confusion*
Failure*
Being unloved*
Self-blaming

Roles and Relationships
Triangulating family relationships*
Inability to meet spiritual needs of members
Reduced ability to relate to one another for mutual growth and
    maturation*
Lack of skills necessary for relationships*
Lack of cohesiveness*
Disrupted family rituals or no family rituals*
Inability to meet security needs of members
Does not demonstrate respect for individuality of its members
Decreased sexual communication and individuality of its
    members
Low perception of parental support*
Pattern of rejection
Neglected obligations*

Related Factors

*Related to inadequate coping skills and/or inadequate problem-solving
skills secondary to:*

Alcohol abuse	Compromised cognitive
Substance abuse*	function
Mental illness	

🜂 Author's Note

Alcoholism is a family disease. This nursing diagnosis can represent the
consequences of the disturbed family dynamics related to alcohol abuse
by a family member. In addition, the individual with substance abuse will
also have a specific nursing diagnosis of *Ineffective Coping* or *Ineffective
Denial.*

NOC

Family Coping, Family Functioning, Substance Addiction Consequences

Goals

The family will acknowledge the alcoholism in the family and
will set short- and long-term goals, as evidenced by the following
indicators:

* Relate the effects of alcoholism on the family unit and indi-
  viduals.
* Identify destructive response patterns.
* Describe resources available for individual and family therapy.

Coping Enhancements, Referral, Family Process Maintenance, Substance Use Treatment, Family Integrity Promotion, Limit Setting, Support Group

Interventions

Establish a Trusting Relationship

- Be consistent; keep promises.
- Be accepting and noncritical.
- Do not pass judgment on what is revealed.
- Focus on family members' responses.

Allow Family Members as Individuals and a Group to Share Pent-Up Feelings

- Validate feelings as normal.
- Correct inaccurate beliefs.

Emphasize That Family Members Are Not Responsible for the Client's Drinking (Starling & Martin, 1990; Carlson, Smith, & Julio, 2006)

- Explain that emotional difficulties are relationship-based rather than "psychiatric."
- Instruct that their feelings and experiences are associated frequently with family alcoholism.

Explore the Family's Beliefs About Situation and Goals

- Discuss characteristics of alcoholism; review a screening test (e.g., MAST, CAGE) that outlines characteristics of alcoholism.
- Discuss causes and correct misinformation.
- Assist to establish short- and long-term goals.

Assist the Family to Gain Insight Into Behavior; Discuss Ineffective Methods Families Use

- Hiding alcohol or car keys
- Anger, silence, threats, crying
- Making excuses for work, family, or friends
- Bailing the client out of jail
- Does not stop drinking
- Increases family anger
- Removes the responsibility for drinking from the client
- Prevents the client from suffering the consequences of his or her drinking behavior

Emphasize to Family That Helping the Alcoholic Means First Helping Themselves

- Focus on changing their response.
- Allow the client to be responsible for his or her drinking behavior.
- Describe activities that will improve their lives, as individuals and a family.
- Initiate one stress management technique (e.g., aerobic exercise, assertiveness course, meditation).
- Plan time as a family together outside the home (e.g., museum, zoos, and picnic). If the alcoholic is included, he or she must contract not to drink during the activity and agree on a consequence if he or she does.

Discuss With Family That Recovery Will Dramatically Change Usual Family Dynamics

- The alcoholic is removed from the center of attention.
- All family roles will be challenged.
- Family members will have to focus on themselves instead of the alcoholic client.
- Family members will have to assume responsibility for their behavior, rather than blaming others.
- Behavioral problems of children serve a purpose for the family.

Discuss Possibility of and Contributing Factors to Relapse

If Additional Family or Individual Nursing Diagnoses Exist, Refer to Specific Diagnosis (e.g., Child Abuse, Domestic Violence)

Initiate Health Teaching Regarding Community Resources and Referrals, as Indicated

- Al-Anon
- Alcoholics Anonymous family therapy
- Individual therapy
- Self-help groups

FATIGUE

NANDA-I Definition

An overwhelming sustained sense of exhaustion and decreased capacity for physical and mental work at the usual level

Defining Characteristics*

Reports an unremitting and overwhelming lack of energy
Perceived need for additional energy to accomplish routine tasks
Reports inability to maintain usual routines
Reports feeling tired
Compromised concentration
Compromised libido
Increased physical complaints
Decreased performance
Disinterest in surroundings
Lethargic; drowsy
Reports inability to maintain usual level of physical activity
Increase in physical complaints
Increase in rest requirements
Reports guilt for not keeping up with responsibilities
Reports inability to restore energy even after sleep
Introspection
Listlessness

Related Factors

Many factors can cause fatigue; combining related factors may be useful (e.g., *Related to muscle weakness, accumulated waste products, inflammation, and infections secondary to hepatitis*).

Bio-Pathophysiologic

Related to hypermetabolic state secondary to:
Viruses (e.g., Epstein–Barr)   Pregnancy*
Fever

Related to inadequate tissue oxygenation secondary to:
Chronic obstructive lung   Anemia*
    disease   Peripheral vascular disease
Congestive heart failure

Related to biochemical changes secondary to:

Endocrine/Metabolic Disorders
Diabetes mellitus   Hypothyroidism
Pituitary disorders   Addison's disease
Acquired immunodeficiency
    syndrome (AIDS)

Chronic Diseases
Renal failure   Lyme disease
Cirrhosis

Related to muscular weakness/wasting secondary to:

Myasthenia gravis | AIDS
Parkinson's disease | Amyotrophic lateral sclerosis
Multiple sclerosis

Related to hypermetabolic state, competition between body and tumor for nutrients, anemia, and stressors associated with cancer

Related to malnutrition*

Related to nutritional deficits* or changes in nutrient metabolism secondary to:

Nausea | Gastric surgery
Side effects of medications | Diarrhea
Vomiting | Diabetes mellitus

Related to chronic inflammatory process secondary to:

AIDS | Lupus erythematosus
Cirrhosis | Renal failure
Arthritis | Hepatitis
Inflammatory bowel disease | Lyme disease

Treatment Related

Biochemical changes secondary to:

Chemotherapy | Side effects of (specify)
Radiation therapy

Related to surgical damage to tissue and anesthesia

Related to increased energy expenditure secondary to:

Amputation | Use of walker, crutches
Gait disorder

Situational (Personal, Environmental)

Related to prolonged decreased activity and deconditioning secondary to:

Anxiety* | Diarrhea
Social isolation | Depression
Fever | Pain
Nausea/vomiting | Obesity

Related to excessive role demands

Related to overwhelming emotional demands

Related to extreme stress*

Related to sleep disturbance

Maturational

Child/Adolescent
Related to hypermetabolic state secondary to:
Mononucleosis   Fever

Related to chronic insufficient nutrients secondary to:
Obesity   Eating disorders
Excessive dieting

Related to effects of newborn care on sleep patterns and need for continuous attention

Related to hypermetabolic state during first trimester

 Author's Note

Fatigue as a nursing diagnosis differs from acute tiredness. Tiredness is a transient, temporary state (Rhoten, 1982) caused by lack of sleep, improper nutrition, increased stress, sedentary lifestyle, or temporarily increased work or social responsibilities. Fatigue is a pervasive, subjective, drained feeling that cannot be eliminated; however, the nurse can assist the person to adapt to it. Activity intolerance differs from fatigue in that the nurse will assist the person with activity intolerance to increase endurance and activity.

The focus for the person with fatigue is not on increasing endurance. If the cause resolves or abates (e.g., acute infection, chemotherapy, radiation), *Fatigue* as a diagnosis is discontinued and *Activity Intolerance* can be initiated to focus on improving the deconditioned state.

NOC
Activity Tolerance, Endurance, Energy Conservation

Goals

The person will participate in activities that stimulate and balance physical, cognitive, affective, and social domains as evidenced by the following indicators:

- Discuss the causes of fatigue.
- Share feelings regarding the effects of fatigue on life.
- Establish priorities for daily and weekly activities.

NIC
Energy Management, Environmental Management, Mutual Goal Setting, Socialization Enhancement

Interventions

Nursing interventions for this diagnosis are for people with fatigue regardless of etiology that cannot be eliminated. The focus is to assist the client and family to adapt to the fatigue state.

Assess Causative or Contributing Factors

- If fatigue has related factors that can be treated, refer to the specific Nursing Diagnosis as:
  - Lack of sleep; refer to *Disturbed Sleep Pattern*
  - Poor nutrition; refer to *Imbalanced Nutrition*
  - Sedentary lifestyle; refer to *Sedentary Lifestyle*
  - Inadequate stress management; refer to *Stress Overload*
  - Chronic excessive role or social demands; refer to *Ineffective Coping*

Explain the Causes of Fatigue

Allow Expression of Feelings Regarding the Effects of Fatigue on Life

- Identify difficult activities.
- Help the client verbalize how fatigue interferes with role responsibilities.
- Encourage the client to convey how fatigue causes frustration.

Assist the Client to Identify Strengths, Abilities, and Interests

- Identify values and interests.
- Identify areas of success and usefulness; emphasize past accomplishments.
- Use information to develop goals with the client.
- Assist the client in identifying sources of hope (e.g., relationships, faith, things to accomplish).
- Assist the client in developing realistic short- and long-term goals (progress from simple to more complex; use a "goals poster" to indicate type and time for achieving specific goals).

Assist the Client to Identify Energy Patterns

Instruct the Client to Record Fatigue Levels Every Hour Over 24 Hours; Select a Usual Day

- Ask the client to rate fatigue using the Rhoten fatigue scale (0 = not tired, peppy; 10 = total exhaustion).
- Record the activities during each rating.

Analyze Together the 24-Hour Fatigue Levels

- Times of peak energy
- Times of exhaustion
- Activities associated with increasing fatigue

Explain Benefits of Exercise and Discuss What Is Realistic

Explain the Purpose of Pacing and Prioritization

- Explore what activities the client views as important to maintain self-esteem.
- Attempt to divide vital activities or tasks into components (e.g., preparing menu, shopping, storing, cooking, serving, cleaning up); the client can delegate some parts and retain others.
- Plan important tasks during periods of high energy (e.g., prepare all meals in the morning).
- Assist client in identifying priorities and to eliminate nonessential activities.
- Plan each day to avoid energy- and time-consuming, nonessential decision-making.
- Distribute difficult tasks throughout the week.
- Rest before difficult tasks and stop before fatigue ensues.

Teach Energy Conservation Techniques

- Modify the environment.
  - Replace steps with ramps.
  - Install grab rails.
  - Elevate chairs 3 to 4 inches.
  - Organize kitchen or work areas.
  - Reduce trips up and down stairs (e.g., put a commode on the first floor).
  - Use a taxi instead of driving self.
  - Delegate housework (e.g., employ a high-school student for a few hours after school).
- Discuss with individual some type of appropriate exercise component that could be integrated into their life.

Promote Socialization With Family and Friends (Dzurec, 2000)

- Encourage the client to participate in one social activity, weekly.
- Explain that feelings of connectedness decrease fatigue.

Explain the Effects of Conflict and Stress on Energy Levels

- Teach the importance of mutuality in sharing concerns.
- Explain the benefits of distraction from negative events.
- Teach and assist with relaxation techniques before anticipated stressful events. Encourage mental imagery to promote positive thought processes.
- Allow the client time to reminisce to gain insight into past experiences.
- Teach the client to maximize aesthetic experiences (e.g., smell of coffee, feeling warmth of the sun).

- Teach the client to anticipate experiences he or she takes delight in each day (e.g., walking, reading favorite book, writing a letter).
- Help the client identify how he or she can help others. Listening to clients' problems, using the computer to access information, and making phone calls

Provide Significant Others Opportunities to Discuss Feelings in Private Regarding:

- Changes in person with fatigue
- Caretaking responsibilities
- Financial issues
- Changes in lifestyle, role responsibilities, and relationships
- See *Caregiver Role Strain* for additional strategies for caregivers.

Initiate Health Teaching and Referrals, as Indicated

- Counseling
- Community services (Meals On Wheels, housekeeper)
- Financial assistance

Maternal Interventions

- Explain the reasons for fatigue in first and third trimesters:
  - Increased basal metabolic rate
  - Changes in hormonal levels
  - Anemia
  - Increased cardiac output (third trimester)
- Emphasize the need for naps and 8 hours of sleep each night.
- Discuss the importance of exercise (e.g., walking).
- For postpartum women, discuss factors that increase fatigue:
  - Labor more than 30 hours
  - Pre-existing chronic disease
  - Hemoglobin less than 10 g/dL or postpartum hemorrhage
  - Episiotomy, tear, or cesarean section
  - Sleeping difficulties
  - Ill newborn or a congenital anomaly
  - Dependent children at home
  - Child care problems
  - Unrealistic expectations
  - No daytime rest periods

Geriatric Interventions

- Consider if chronic fatigue is the consequence of late-life depression.
- Refer the client with suspected depression for evaluation.

FEAR

NANDA-I Definition

Response to perceived threat that is consciously recognized as a danger

Defining Characteristics

Verbal Reports of Panic*
Alarm*
Aggression
Apprehension*
Avoidance behaviors*
Being scared*
Decreased self-assurance*
Dread*

Excitement*
Impulsiveness*
Increased alertness*/tension
Narrowed focus on source of the fear*
Panic
Terror*

Visceral–Somatic Activity

Musculoskeletal
Shortness of breath
Fatigue*/limb weakness
Muscle tightness*
Respiratory
Increased rate*
Trembling
Cardiovascular
Palpitations
Rapid pulse*
Increased systolic blood pressure*
Skin
Flush/pallor*
Increased perspiration*
Paresthesia

Gastrointestinal
Anorexia*
Nausea/vomiting
Diarrhea*/urge to defecate
Dry mouth*/throat
Central Nervous System (CNS)/Perceptual
Syncope
Irritability
Insomnia
Absentmindedness
Lack of concentration
Nightmares
Pupil dilation*
Diminished problem-solving ability*
Genitourinary
Urinary frequency/urgency

Related Factors

Fear can be a response to various health problems, situations, or conflicts. Some common sources are indicated in the following.

Pathophysiologic

Related to perceived immediate and long-term effects of:

Cognitive impairment   Loss of body function or part
Disabling illness   Sensory impairment
Long-term disability   Terminal disease

Treatment Related

Related to loss of control and unpredictable outcome secondary to:

Hospitalization   Radiation
Invasive procedures   Anesthesia
Surgery and its outcome

Situational (Personal, Environmental)

Related to loss of control and unpredictable outcome secondary to:

Change or loss of significant   Divorce
  other   Lack of knowledge
Pain   Failure
New environment   Related to potential loss
New people   of income
Success

Maturational

Preschool (2 to 5 years)

Related to:

Age-related fears   Dark, strangers, ghosts
Animals   Not being liked
Being alone   Separation from parents, peers
Bodily harm   Strangers

School-Age (6 to 12 years)

Related to:

Being lost   Bad dreams
Being in trouble   Weapons
Thunder, lightning

Adolescent (13 to 18 years)

Related to uncertainty of:

Appearance
Scholastic success
Peer support

Adult
Related to uncertainty of:

Marriage	Effects of aging
Job security	Parenthood
Pregnancy	

Older Adult
Related to anticipated dependence:

Prolonged suffering	Vulnerability to crime
Financial insecurity	Abandonment

 Author's Note

See *Anxiety*.

NOC

Anxiety Self-Control, Fear Self-Control

Goals

The adult will relate increased psychological and physiologic comfort as evidenced by the following indicators:

- Show decreased visceral response (pulse, respirations).
- Differentiate real from imagined situations.
- Describe effective and ineffective coping patterns.
- Identify own coping responses.

The child will exhibit or relate increased psychological and physiologic comfort as evidenced by the following indicators:

- Discuss fears.
- Exhibit less crying.

NIC

Anxiety Reduction, Coping Enhancement; Presence, Counseling, Relaxation Therapy

Interventions

Nursing interventions for *Fear* represent interventions for any client with fear regardless of the etiologic or contributing factors.

Assess Possible Contributing Factors

Refer to Related Factors.

Reduce or Eliminate Contributing Factors

Unfamiliar Environment
- Orient client to environment using simple explanations.
- Speak slowly and calmly.
- Avoid surprises and painful stimuli.
- Use soft lights and music.
- Remove threatening stimulus.
- Plan one-day-at-a-time, familiar routine.
- Encourage gradual mastery of a situation.
- Provide a transitional object with symbolic safeness (security blanket, religious medal).

Intrusion on Personal Space
- Allow personal space.
- Move the client away from the stimulus.
- Remain with the client until fear subsides (listen, use silence).
- Later, establish frequent and consistent contacts; use family members and significant others to stay with the client.
- Use touch as tolerated (sometimes holding the client firmly helps him or her maintain control).

Threat to Self-Esteem
- Support preferred coping style when client uses adaptive mechanisms.
- Initially, decrease the client's number of choices.
- Use simple, direct statements (avoid detail).
- Give direct suggestions to manage everyday events (some prefer details; others like general explanations).
- Encourage expression of feelings (helplessness, anger).
- Give feedback about expressed feelings (support realistic assessments).
- Refocus interaction on areas of capability rather than dysfunction.
- Encourage normal coping mechanisms.
- Encourage sharing common problems with others.
- Give feedback of effect the client's behavior has on others.
- Encourage the client to face the fear.

When Intensity of Feelings Has Decreased, Assist With Insight and Controlling Response

- Bring behavioral cues into the client's awareness.
- Ask to write their fears in narrative form.
- Teach how to solve problems.
  - What is the problem?
  - Who or what is responsible?
  - What are the options?
  - What are the advantages and disadvantages of each option?

Initiate Health Teaching and Referrals as Indicated

- Progressive relaxation technique
- Reading, music, breathing exercises
- Desensitization, self-coaching
- Thought stopping, guided fantasy
- Yoga, hypnosis, assertiveness training

⚜ Pediatric Interventions

Participate in Community Functions to Teach Parents Age-
Related Fears and Constructive Interventions (e.g., Parent–School
Organizations, Newsletters, Civic Groups)

- Provide child opportunities to talk and write about fears and to learn healthy outlets for anger or sadness, such as play therapy.
- Acknowledge illness, death, and pain as real; refrain from protecting children from the reality of existence; encourage open, honest sharing that is age-appropriate.
- Never make fun of the child. Share with child that these fears are okay.
- Fear of imaginary animals and intruders (e.g., "I don't see a lion in your room, but I will leave the light on for you, and, if you need me again, please call.")
- Fear of parent being late (establish a contingency plan [e.g., "If you come home from school and Mommy is not here, go to Mrs. S next door."]).
- Fear of vanishing down a toilet or bathtub drain:
  - Wait until child is out of the tub before releasing the drain.
  - Wait until child is off the toilet before flushing.
  - Leave toys in bathtub and demonstrate how they do not go down the drain.
- Fear of dogs and cats:
  - Allow child to watch a child and a dog playing from a distance.
  - Do not force child to touch the animal.
- Fear of death
- Fear of pain (see Pediatric Interventions for *Pain*)
- Refusal to go to sleep:
  - Establish a realistic hour for retiring.
  - Contract for a reward if the child is successful.
  - Do not sleep with the child or take the child to the parent's room.
- Discuss with parents the normality of fears in children; explain the necessity of acceptance and the negative outcomes of punishment, shaming, or of forcing the child to overcome the fear.

- Provide the child with the opportunity to observe other children cope successfully with the feared object.
- Demonstrate strength and self-confidence.
- Take child's hand and gently guide into shallow water.
- Allow child to watch you pet a dog.

Maternal Interventions

- Provide opportunities to express fears during each trimester.
- Provide opportunities for expectant father to share his concerns and fears.

DEFICIENT FLUID VOLUME

Deficient Fluid Volume

Risk for Deficient Fluid Volume

NANDA-I Definition

Decreased intravascular, interstitial, and/or intracellular fluid. This refers to dehydration, water loss alone without change in sodium.

Defining Characteristics

Major (Must Be Present, One or More)

Insufficient oral fluid intake
Dry skin*/mucous membranes*
Negative balance of intake and output
Weight loss

Minor (May Be Present)

Increased serum sodium
Thirst*/nausea/anorexia
Concentrated urine or urinary frequency
Decreased urine output* or excessive urine output

Related Factors

Pathophysiologic

Related to excessive urinary output:
Uncontrolled diabetes
Diabetes insipidus (inadequate antidiuretic hormone)

Related to increased capillary permeability and evaporative loss from burn wound (nonacute)

Related to losses secondary to:
Abnormal drainage
Diarrhea
Excessive menses
Fever or increased metabolic rate
Peritonitis
Wound

Situational (Personal, Environmental)

Related to vomiting/nausea

Related to decreased motivation to drink liquids secondary to:
Depression   Fatigue

Related to fad diets/fasting

Related to high-solute tube feedings

Related to difficulty swallowing or feeding self secondary to:
Oral or throat pain   Fatigue

Related to extreme heat/sun/dryness

Related to excessive loss through:
Indwelling catheters   Drains

Related to insufficient fluids for exercise effort or weather conditions

Related to excessive use of:
Laxatives or enemas
Diuretics, alcohol, or caffeine

Maturational

Infant/Child
Related to increased vulnerability secondary to:
Decreased fluid reserve and decreased ability to concentrate
   urine

Older Adult

Related to increased vulnerability secondary to:
Decreased fluid reserve and decreased sensation of thirst

 Author's Note

Deficient Fluid Volume frequently is used to describe people who are NPO, in hypovolemic shock, or experiencing bleeding. This author recommends its use only when a client can drink but has an insufficient intake for metabolic needs. If the client cannot drink or needs intravenous therapy, refer to the collaborative problems on http://thePoint.lww.com/CarpenitoHB14e: *Risk for Complications of Hypovolemia and Risk for Complications of Electrolyte Imbalances.*

   Should *Deficient Fluid Volume* be used to represent such clinical situations as shock, renal failure, or thermal injury? Most nurses would agree that these are collaborative problems to report to the physician for collaborative treatments.

NOC

Electrolyte and Acid/Base Balance, Fluid Balance, Hydration

Goal

The client will maintain urine-specific gravity within normal range as evidenced by the following indicators:

- Increase fluid intake to a specified amount according to age and metabolic needs.
- Identify risk factors for fluid deficit and relate need for increased fluid intake as indicated.
- Demonstrate no signs and symptoms of dehydration.

NIC

Fluid/Electrolyte Management, Fluid Monitoring

Interventions

Assess Causative Factors

Prevent Dehydration in High-Risk Clients

- Monitor client intake; ensure at least 2,000 mL of oral fluids every 24 hours unless contraindicated. Offer fluids that are desired hourly.
- Teach the client to avoid coffee, tea, grapefruit juice, sugared drinks, and alcohol.

- Monitor output; ensure at least 5 mg/kg per hour.
- Weigh the client daily in the same clothes, at the same time. A 2% to 4% weight loss indicates mild dehydration; 5% to 9% weight loss indicates moderate dehydration.
- Monitor urine and serum electrolytes, blood urea nitrogen, osmolality, creatinine, hematocrit, and hemoglobin.
- For older people scheduled to fast before diagnostic studies, advise them to increase fluid intake 8 hours before fasting.
- Review the client's medications. Do they contribute to dehydration (e.g., diuretics)? Do they require increased fluid intake (e.g., lithium)?

Initiate Health Teaching, as Indicated

- Give verbal and written directions for desired fluids and amounts.
- Include the client/family in keeping a written record of fluid intake, output, and daily weight.
- Provide a list of alternative fluids (e.g., ice cream, pudding).
- Explain the need to increase fluids during exercise, fever, infection, and hot weather.
- Teach the client/family how to observe for dehydration (especially in infants, elderly) and to intervene by increasing fluid intake (see Subjective and Objective Data for signs of dehydration).
- For athletes, stress the need to hydrate before and during exercise, preferably with a high–sodium-content beverage. (Refer to *Hyperthermia* for additional interventions.)

Pediatric Interventions

To Increase Fluid Intake, Offer:

- Appealing fluids (popsicles, frozen juice bars, snow cones, water, milk, Jell-O); let the child help make them
- Use unusual containers (colorful cups, straws)
- A game or activity
  - On a chart, have the child cross out the number of cups he or she drank each day.
  - Read a book to the child and have him or her drink a sip when turning a page, or have a tea party.
  - Have child take a drink when it is his or her turn in a game.
  - Set a schedule for supplementary liquids to promote the habit of in-between–meal fluids (e.g., juice or Kool-Aid at 10 AM and 2 PM each day).
  - Decorate straws.
  - Let the child fill small cups with a syringe.
  - Make a progress poster; use stickers or stars to indicate fluid goals met.

- Older children usually respond to the challenge of meeting a specific intake goal.
- Rewards and contracts are also effective (e.g., a sticker for drinking a certain amount).
- Young children usually respond to games that integrate drinking fluids.

Take Measures for Fever in Children Younger Than 5 Years

- Work to attain a temperature below 101° F (38.4° C) with medication (acetaminophen or ibuprofen) only. Instruct parents to closely follow instructions for age.
- Overdose of these medications can cause liver toxicity.
- Dress children in lightweight pajamas and infant in diapers only.
- Should a seizure occur; instruct the parents to:
  - Not give oral medications.
  - Place cool washcloths on forehead, axillary, and groin areas.
  - Transport the child to the emergency room.

For Fluid Replacement, Refer to Pediatric Interventions Under Diarrhea

Geriatric Interventions

- Monitor for signs of dehydration, dizziness, and weakness; mucous membrane; and intake versus output.
- Avoid caffeine, alcohol, and high-sugar foods and drinks.
- Explain to the client the need to drink fluids and to use a system for reminding himself or herself not to rely on thirst.
- Incorporate strategies to prompt fluid intake:
  - Fill a large pitcher of water in the morning to monitor intake.
  - Drink an extra glass of water with medications.
  - In care facilities, structure a schedule with a beverage cart with choices.

Risk for Deficient Fluid Volume

NANDA-I Definition

At risk for experiencing decreased intravascular, interstitial, and/or intracellular fluid. This refers to dehydration, water loss alone without change in sodium

Risk Factors*

Deviations affecting access to fluids
Deviations affecting intake of fluids
Deviations affecting absorption of fluids
Excessive losses through normal routes (e.g., diarrhea)
Extremes of age
Extremes of weight
Factors influencing fluid needs (e.g., hypermetabolic state)
Loss of fluid through abnormal routes (e.g., indwelling tubes)
Deficient knowledge
Pharmaceutical agents (e.g., diuretics)

 Author's Note

If the individual is NPO, refer to the collaborative problem *Risk for Complications of Hypovolemia.* If the person can drink, refer to *Deficient Fluid Volume* for interventions.

 NOC

Refer to *Deficient Fluid Volume.*

Goals

The individual will demonstrate continued hydrated state with a urine output >5 mL/kg/hour.

EXCESS FLUID VOLUME

NANDA-I Definition

Increased isotonic fluid retention

Defining Characteristics

Major (Must Be Present, One or More)

Edema (peripheral, sacral)
Taut, shiny skin

Minor (May Be Present)

Intake greater than output
Weight gain

Related Factors

Pathophysiologic

Related to compromised regulatory mechanisms secondary to:
Renal failure (acute or chronic)
Systemic and metabolic abnormalities
Endocrine dysfunction
Lipedema

Related to portal hypertension, lower plasma colloidal osmotic pressure, and sodium retention secondary to:

Liver disease	Ascites
Cirrhosis	Cancer

Related to venous and arterial abnormalities secondary to:

Varicose veins	Trauma
Phlebitis	Thrombus
Infection	Lymphedema
Peripheral vascular disease	Neoplasms
Immobility	

Treatment Related

Related to sodium and water retention secondary to corticosteroid therapy

Related to inadequate lymphatic drainage secondary to mastectomy

Situational (Personal, Environmental)

Related to excessive sodium intake/fluid intake

Related to low protein intake:

Fad diets	Malnutrition

Related to dependent venous pooling/venostasis secondary to:
Standing or sitting for long periods
Immobility
Tight cast or bandage

Related to venous compression from pregnant uterus

Maturational

Older Adult

Related to impaired venous return secondary to increased peripheral resistance and decreased efficiency of valves

 Author's Note

Excess Fluid Volume is frequently used to describe pulmonary edema, ascites, or renal failure. These are all collaborative problems that should not be renamed as *Excess Fluid Volume. Refer to http://thePoint.lww.com/ CarpenitoHB14e for collaborative problems related to renal failure, pulmo- nary edema, and hepatic dysfunction.* This diagnosis represents a situa- tion for which nurses can prescribe if the focus is on peripheral edema. Nursing interventions center on teaching the client or family how to minimize edema and protect tissue.

NOC

Electrolyte Balance, Fluid Balance, Hydration

Goals

The client will exhibit decreased edema (specify site), as evidenced by the following indicators:

- Relate causative factors.
- Relate methods of preventing edema.

NIC

Electrolyte Management, Fluid Management, Fluid Monitoring, Skin Surveillance

Interventions

Identify Contributing and Causative Factors

Refer to Related Factors.

Reduce or Eliminate Causative and Contributing Factors

Improper Diet
- Assess dietary intake and habits that may contribute to fluid retention.
- Be specific; record daily and weekly intake of food and fluids.

- Assess weekly diet for inadequate protein or excessive sodium intake.
  - Discuss likes and dislikes of foods that provide protein.
  - Teach the client to plan a weekly menu that provides protein at an affordable price.
  - Teach the client to decrease salt intake.
  - Read labels for sodium content.
  - Avoid convenience and canned and frozen foods.
  - Cook without salt; use spices (lemon, basil, tarragon, mint) to add flavor.
  - Use vinegar in place of salt to flavor soups, stews, etc. (e.g., 2 to 3 teaspoons of vinegar per 4 to 6 quarts, according to taste).
  - Ascertain whether the client may use salt substitute (caution that he or she must use the exact substitute prescribed).

Dependent Venous Pooling

- Assess for evidence of dependent venous pooling or venous stasis.
- Encourage alternating periods of horizontal rest (legs elevated) with vertical activity (standing); this may be contraindicated in congestive heart failure.
  - Keep the edematous extremity elevated above the level of the heart whenever possible (unless contraindicated by heart failure).
  - Keep the edematous arms elevated on two pillows or with IV pole sling.
  - Elevate the legs whenever possible, using pillows under them (avoid pressure points, especially behind the knees).
  - Discourage leg and ankle crossing.
- Reduce constriction of vessels.
  - Assess clothing for proper fit and constrictive areas.
  - Instruct the client to avoid panty girdles/garters, knee-high stockings, and leg crossing and to practice elevating the legs when possible.
- Consider using antiembolism stockings or Ace bandages; measure the legs carefully for stockings/support hose.*
- Measure circumference of the calf and thigh. Consider both measurements when choosing stockings, matching measurements with a size requirement chart that accompanies the stockings.
- Apply stockings while lying down (e.g., in the morning before arising).
- Check extremities frequently for adequate circulation and evidence of constrictive areas.

Venous Pressure Points
- Assess for venous pressure points associated with casts, bandages, and tight stockings.
  - Observe circulation at edges of casts, bandages, and stockings.
  - For casts, insert soft material to cushion pressure points at the edges.
- Check circulation frequently.
- Shift body weight in the cast to redistribute weight within (unless contraindicated).
  - Encourage client to do this every 15 to 30 minutes while awake to prevent venostasis.
  - Encourage wiggling of fingers or toes and isometric exercise of unaffected muscles within the cast.
  - If the client cannot do this alone, assist him or her at least hourly to shift body weight.
- See *Impaired Physical Mobility*.

Inadequate Lymphatic Drainage
- Keep the extremity elevated on pillows.
  - If the edema is marked, the arm should be elevated *but not in adduction* (this position may constrict the axilla).
  - The elbow should be higher than the shoulder.
  - The hand should be higher than the elbow.
- Measure blood pressure in the unaffected arm.
- Do not give injections or start IV fluids in the affected arm.
- Protect the affected limb from injury.
- Teach the client to avoid using strong detergents, carrying heavy bags, holding cigarettes, injuring cuticles or hangnails, reaching into hot ovens, wearing jewelry or a wristwatch, or using Ace bandages.
- Advise the client to apply lanolin or a similar cream, often daily, to prevent dry, flaky skin.
- Encourage the client to wear a Medic-Alert tag engraved with *Caution: lymphedema arm—no tests/no needle injections*.
- Caution the client to visit a physician if the arm becomes red, swollen, or unusually hard.
- After a mastectomy, encourage range-of-motion (ROM) exercises and use of the affected arm to facilitate development of a collateral lymphatic drainage system (explain that lymphedema often decreases within 1 month, but that the client should continue massaging, exercising, and elevating the arm for 3 to 4 months after surgery).

Immobility/Neurologic Deficit
- Plan passive or active ROM exercises for all extremities every 4 hours, including dorsiflexion of the foot to massage veins.

- Change the client's position at least every 2 hours, using the four positions (left side, right side, back, abdomen) if not contraindicated (see *Impaired Skin Integrity*).
- If the client must remain in high Fowler's position, assess for edema of buttocks and sacral area; help the client shift body weight every 2 hours to prevent pressure on edematous tissue.

Protect Edematous Skin From Injury

- Inspect skin for redness and blanching.
- Reduce pressure on skin areas; pad chairs; use knee-high stockings and footstools.
- Prevent dry skin.
- Use soap sparingly.
- Rinse off soap completely.
- Use a lotion to moisten skin.
- See *Impaired Skin Integrity* for additional information about preventing injury.

Initiate Health Teaching and Referrals, as Indicated

- Give clear verbal and written instructions for all medications: what, when, how often, why, side effects; pay special attention to drugs that directly influence fluid balance (e.g., diuretics, steroids).
- Write down instructions for diet, activity, and use of Ace bandages, stockings, and so forth.
- Have the client demonstrate the instructions.
- With severe fluctuations in edema, have the client weigh himself or herself every morning and before bedtime daily; instruct the client to keep a written record of weights. For less severe illness, the client may need to weigh him or herself only once daily and record the weight.
- Caution the client to call a physician for excessive edema/weight gain (greater than 2 lb/day) or increased shortness of breath at night or upon exertion. Explain that these signs may indicate early heart problems and may require medication to prevent them from worsening.
- Consider home care or visiting nurses referral to follow at home.
- Provide literature concerning low-salt diets; consult with a dietitian if necessary.

⚕ Maternal Interventions

- Explain the cause of edema of ankles and fingers.
- Advise the client to limit salt intake moderately (e.g., eliminate processed meats, chips) and to maintain water intake of 8 to 10 glasses daily unless contraindicated.

- Consult with an advanced practice nurse or physician if client has elevated blood pressure, proteinuria, facial puffiness, sacral or pitting edema, or weight gain of more than 2 lb in 1 week.
- Advise the client to avoid reclining on her back, sitting for prolonged periods without elevating feet, or standing for prolonged periods (Davis, 1996).
- Instruct the client to lie on the left side for short periods several times a day and to take a warm tub bath daily.

RISK FOR IMBALANCED FLUID VOLUME

NANDA-I Definition

At risk for a decrease, increase, or rapid shift from one to the other of intravascular, interstitial, and/or intracellular fluid that may compromise health. This refers to body fluid loss, gain, or both.

Risk Factors*

Abdominal surgery
Ascites
Burns
Intestinal obstruction
Pancreatitis

Receiving apheresis
Sepsis
Traumatic injury
  (e.g., fractured hip)

Author's Note

This diagnosis can represent several clinical conditions, such as edema, hemorrhage, dehydration, and compartmental syndrome. If the nurse is monitoring a client for imbalanced fluid volume, labeling the specific imbalance as a collaborative problem, such as hypovolemia, compartment syndrome, increased intracranial pressure, gastrointestinal bleeding, or postpartum hemorrhage, would be more useful clinically. For example, most intraoperative clients would be monitored for hypovolemia. If the procedure was neurosurgery, then cranial pressure would also be monitored. If the procedure were orthopedic, compartment syndrome would be addressed. Refer to http://thePoint.lww.com/CarpenitoHB14e for specific collaborative problems and interventions.

DYSFUNCTIONAL GASTROINTESTINAL MOTILITY

Dysfunctional Gastrointestinal Motility

Risk for Dysfunctional Gastrointestinal Motility

See also *Risk for Complications of Paralytic Ileus* on http://thePoint. lww.com/CarpenitoHB14e.

NANDA-I Definition

Increased, decreased, ineffective, or lack of peristaltic activity within the gastrointestinal system

Defining Characteristics*

Absence of flatus
Abdominal cramping or pain
Abdominal distention
Accelerated gastric emptying
Bile-colored gastric residual
Change in bowel sounds
(e.g., absent, hypoactive, hyperactive)

Diarrhea
Dry stool difficulty passing stools
Hard stools
Increased gastric residual
Nausea
Regurgitation, vomiting

Related Factors*

Aging
Anxiety
Enteral feedings
Food intolerance (e.g., gluten lactose)
Immobility
Ingestion of contaminates (e.g., food, water)

Malnutrition
Pharmaceutical agents
(e.g., narcotics/opiates, antibiotics, laxatives, anesthesia)
Prematurity, sedentary lifestyle
Surgery

🌐 Author's Note

This NANDA-I diagnosis is too broad for clinical usefulness. It represents collaborative problems and some nursing diagnoses such as *Diarrhea*, *Constipation*. Refer to http://thePoint.lww.com/CarpenitoHB14e for more specific collaborative problems as *Risk for Complications of Gastrointestinal Dysfunction*, *Risk for Complications of Paralytic Ileus*, and *Risk for Complications for GI Bleeding*.

Goals/Interventions

The nurse should examine the assessment data to determine the focus.

- To monitor for physiologic complications that require nursing and medical interventions as *Risk for Complications of Paralytic Ileus or GI Bleeding* (collaborative problem). Refer to http://thePoint.lww.com/CarpenitoHB14e.
- To prevent or treat a physiologic dysfunction as constipation, diarrhea, fluid imbalance, compromised nutrition, or complications of immobility as *Risk for Imbalanced Nutrition, Deficient Fluid Volume, Diarrhea, Disuse Syndrome,* or *Risk for Constipation* (nursing diagnoses). Refer to Section 1.

Risk for Dysfunctional Gastrointestinal Motility

See also *Risk for Complications of Gastrointestinal Dysfunction* on http://thePoint.lww.com/CarpenitoHB14e.

NANDA-I Definition

At risk for increased, decreased, ineffective, or lack of peristaltic activity within the gastrointestinal system

Risk Factors*

Abdominal Surgery
Aging
Anxiety
Change in food or water
Decreased gastrointestinal circulation
Diabetes mellitus
Food intolerance (gluten, lactose)
Gastroesophageal reflux disease (GERD)

Immobility
Infection (e.g., bacteria parasitic, viral)
Pharmaceutical agents (e.g., antibiotics, laxatives, narcotics/opiates, proton pump inhibitors)
Prematurity
Sedentary lifestyle
Stress
Unsanitary food preparation

Author's Note

This NANDA-I diagnosis is too broad for clinical use. This diagnosis represents some collaborative problems such as *Risk for Complications of Gastrointestinal Dysfunction*, *Risk for Complications of GI Bleeding*, *Risk for Complications of Paralytic Ileus* and nursing diagnoses such as *Risk for Diarrhea*, *Risk for Constipation*, and *Risk for Infection*. Refer to http://thePoint.lww.com/CarpenitoHB14e.

Examine the risk factors in the client and determine if the focus of nursing interventions is prevention; if yes, use *Risk for Infection*, *Risk for Diarrhea*, or *Risk for Constipation*. If the focus is to monitor gastrointestinal function for complications that require medical and nursing interventions, use a collaborative problem as *Risk for Complications of* (specify).

GRIEVING

Grieving

Anticipatory Grieving

Complicated Grieving

Risk for Complicated Grieving

NANDA-I Definition

A normal complex process that includes emotional, physical, spiritual, social, and intellectual responses and behaviors by which individuals, families, and communities, incorporate an actual, anticipated, or perceived loss into their daily lives.

Defining Characteristics

Major (Must Be Present)

The client reports an actual or perceived loss (person, pet, object, function, status, or relationship) with varied responses such as:

Denial	In sleep patterns*
Suicidal thoughts	Blame*
Guilt	Detachment*
Crying	Anergia
Anger*	Disorganization*
Sorrow	Feelings of worthlessness
Despair*	Numbness
Longing/searching behaviors	Disbelief
Inability to concentrate	Anxiety
Alterations	Helplessness

Related Factors

Many situations can contribute to feelings of loss. Some common situations follow.

Pathophysiologic

Related to loss of function or independence secondary to:

Neurologic	Sensory
Digestive	Renal
Cardiovascular	Musculoskeletal
Respiratory	Trauma

Treatment Related

Related to losses associated with:
Long-term dialysis
Surgery (e.g., mastectomy)

Situational (Personal, Environmental)

Related to the negative effects and losses secondary to:

Chronic pain	Terminal illness
Death	

Related to losses in lifestyle associated with:

Childbirth	Divorce
Child leaving home	Separation
Marriage	Role function

Related to loss of normalcy secondary to:

Handicap	Scars
Illness	

Maturational

Related to changes attributed to aging:

Friends	Occupation
Function	Sexual performance
Home	

Related to loss of hope, dreams

 Author's Note

Grieving, Anticipatory, and *Complicated Grieving* represent three types of responses of individuals or families experiencing a loss. *Grieving* describes normal grieving after a loss and participation in grief work. *Anticipatory Grieving* describes engaging in grief work before an expected loss. *Complicated Grieving* represents a maladaptive process in which grief work is suppressed or absent or a client exhibits prolonged exaggerated responses. For all three diagnoses, the goal of nursing is to promote grief work. In addition, for *Complicated Grieving*, the nurse directs interventions to reduce excessive, prolonged, problematic responses.

In many clinical situations, the nurse expects a grief response (e.g., loss of body part, death of significant other). Other situations that evoke strong grief responses are sometimes ignored or minimized (e.g., abortion, newborn death, death of one twin or triplet, death of secreted lover, suicide, loss of children to foster homes, or adoption).

NOC

Coping, Family Coping, Grief Resolution, Psychosocial Adjustment, Life Change

Goals

- The client will express his or her grief.
- Grief will be freely expressed.

Indicators:
- Describe the meaning of the death or loss to him or her.
- Share his or her grief with significant others.

NIC

Family Support, Grief Work Facilitation, Coping Enhancement, Anticipatory Guidance, Emotional Support

Interventions

Assess for Factors That May Delay Grief Work

- Unavailable or no support system
- Dependency
- Previous emotional illness
- Uncertain loss (e.g., missing child)
- Inability to grieve
- Early object loss
- Failure to grieve for past loss
- Personality structure
- Nature of relationship
- Multiple losses

Reduce or Eliminate Factors, If Possible

Promote a Trust Relationship
- Promote feelings of self-worth through one-on-one or group sessions.
- Allow for established time to meet and discuss feelings.
- Communicate clearly, simply, and to the point.
- Never try to lessen the loss (e.g., "She didn't suffer long"; or "You can have another baby").
- Use feedback to assess what the client and the family are learning.
- Offer support and reassurance.
- Create a therapeutic milieu (convey that you care).
- Establish a safe, secure, and private environment.
- Demonstrate respect for the client's culture, religion, race, and values.
- Provide privacy but be careful not to isolate the client or family inadvertently.
- Provide a presence of simply "being" with the bereaved.

Support Grief Reactions
- Explain grief reactions: shock and disbelief, developing awareness, and resolution.
- Describe varied acceptable expressions:
  - Elated or manic behavior as a defense against depression
  - Elation and hyperactivity as a reaction of love and protection from depression
  - Various states of depression
- Various somatic manifestations (weight loss or gain, indigestion, dizziness)
- Assess for past experiences with loss (e.g., losses in childhood and later life).

Determine Whether Family Has Special Requests Regarding Viewing the Deceased (Vanezis & McGee, 1999)
- Prepare them for possible body changes.
- Remove all equipment; change soiled linen.
- Support their request (e.g., holding, washing, touching, kissing).

Promote Family Cohesiveness
- Support the family at its level of functioning.
- Encourage self-exploration of feelings with family members.
- Explain the need to discuss behaviors that interfere with relationships.
- Recognize and reinforce the strengths of each family member.
- Encourage family members to evaluate their feelings and support one another.

Promote Grief Work with Each Response

Denial
- Recognize that response is useful and necessary.
- Explain the use of denial by one family member to the other members.
- Do not push client to move past denial without emotional readiness.

Isolation
- Convey acceptance by acknowledging grief.
- Create open, honest communication to promote sharing.
- Reinforce the client's self-worth by providing privacy.
- Encourage client/family to increase social activities (e.g., support groups, church groups) gradually.
- Prepare client/family that they may experience avoidance from some friends and family who may not be comfortable with their situation of loss or their grief responses.
- Encourage client/family to let significant others know their needs (e.g., support, privacy, permission to share their experience).

Depression
- Reinforce the client's self-esteem.
- Identify the level of depression and develop the approach accordingly.
- Use empathic sharing; acknowledge grief ("It must be very difficult").
- Identify any indications of suicidal behavior (frequent statements of intent, revealed plan).
- See *Risk for Self-Harm* for additional information.

Anger
- Acknowledge the client's anger as a coping mechanism.
- Explain to the family that anger serves to try to control one's environment more closely because of an inability to control loss.
- Stress that the illness or death did not result from being bad or because the well child wished it.

Identify Clients at High Risk for Complicated Grieving Reactions
- Length of relationship: more than 55 years, less than 5 years; consider significance and quality of relationship to the survivor
- Medical issues: pending treatments or surgeries; history of acute or chronic illness
- Mental health history or treatment: outpatient counseling/ follow-up; psychiatric medications (depression, anxiety, sleep, etc.); psychiatric hospitalizations; suicide attempts; suicidal ideations
- Substance abuse: alcohol or drug abuse treatment

- Suicidality: in family history, suicidal ideation or potential for it
- Family dynamics: alliances, conflicts
- Children: 17 years or younger, either in home or with significant relationship to deceased (e.g., grandparent who lived in the same home)
- Multiple losses: deaths, moves, retirement, divorce
- Traumatic death: circumstances of death, sudden or unexpected, as perceived by bereaved
- Isolation: geographical, social, emotional

Teach the Client/Family Signs of Pathologic Grieving, Especially Those at Risk
- Continued searching for the deceased (frequent moves/relocations)
- Delusions
- Isolation
- Egocentricity
- Overt hostility (usually toward a family member)

Promote Physical Well-Being: Nutrition, Sleep/Rest, Exercise for Survivors of Suicide
- Encourage them to see a primary care professional.
- Elicit their interpretation of the event. Clarify distortions.
- Discuss plans for the funeral and notification of friends and relatives.
- Discuss the hazards of secrecy.
- Allow for expression of guilt, rage, and blame (e.g., of professionals).
- Follow-up with telephone contacts to family.
- Refer all survivors to counseling, especially those at high risk (surviving children; those with inadequate support; those who respond with blaming, scapegoating, or secrecy).

Provide Health Teaching and Referrals, as Indicated

Teach the Client and the Family Signs of Resolution
- Grieving client no longer lives in the past but is future oriented and establishes new goals.
- Grieving client redefines relationship with the lost object/person.
- Grieving client begins to resocialize.

Identify Agencies That May Be Helpful (e.g., Community Agencies, Religious Groups)

Pediatric Interventions

Explain What Caused the Death

- Clarify child's perceptions.
- Openly clarify that the child did not cause the death.

Openly Discuss Possible Responses (Hooyman & Kramer, 2006)

- "Sometimes when someone dies we feel bad if we said or did something bad to them."
- "Sometimes we feel glad we didn't die and then feel bad because _____ did."
- "When someone dies, we can become afraid that we may die also."
- "I remember when _____ said or did _____. What do you remember?"

Explain Rituals (e.g., Read Children's Book About Death)

Assist Family With the Decision About the Child Attending the Funeral and Determine If the Following Are Present (Hooyman & Kramer, 2006; Boyd, 2005)

- Child has a basic understanding of death and good coping skills.
- Child is not afraid of adults' emotional responses.
- The ethnic group approaches death openly (e.g., children commonly attend funerals).
- A familiar adult who is coping well with his or her own grief is available to monitor the child's needs.
- Child expresses a desire to attend and has a basic understanding of what will happen.

Explore the Child's Modified Involvement in Funeral Activities (e.g., Visit Funeral Home Before Guests Come, Attend After-Service Gathering)

Allow Child to Grieve at Own Pace. Give Adolescents Permission to Grieve Openly. Consider a Sibling Support Group, If Indicated

Maternal Interventions

Assist Parents of a Deceased Infant, Newborn, or Fetus With Grief Work (Mina, 1985; Hockenberry & Wilson, 2009)

Promote Grieving
- Use baby's name when discussing the loss.
- Allow parents to share the hopes and dreams they had for the child.
- Provide parents with access to a hospital chaplain or religious leader of their choice.
- Encourage parents to see and to hold their infant to validate the reality of the loss.
- Design a method to communicate to auxiliary departments that the parents are in mourning (e.g., rose sticker on door, chart).

- Prepare a memory packet wrapped in a clean baby blanket (photograph [Polaroid], ID bracelet, footprints with birth certificate, lock of hair, crib card, fetal monitor strip, infant's blanket). Encourage them to take the memory packet home. If they prefer not to, keep the packet on file in case they change their minds later.
- Encourage parents to share the experience with their other children at home (refer to pertinent literature for consumers).
- Provide for follow-up support and referral services (e.g., support group) after discharge.

Assist Others to Comfort Grieving Parents
- Stress the importance of openly acknowledging the death.
- If the baby or fetus was named, use the name in discussions.
- Never try to lessen the loss with discussions of future pregnancies or other healthy siblings.
- Send sympathy cards. Create a remembrance (e.g., plant a tree).
- Be sensitive to the gravity of the loss for both the mother and the father.

Anticipatory Grieving**

Definition

State in which a client/group experiences reactions in response to an expected significant loss

Defining Characteristics

Major (Must Be Present)

Expressed distress at potential loss

Minor (May Be Present)

Anger
Change in communication patterns, eating habits, sleep patterns, and/or social patterns
Decreased libido

** This diagnosis is not presently on the NANDA-I list but has been added for clarity and usefulness.

Denial   Sorrow
Guilt   Withdrawal

Related Factors

See *Grieving*.

 NOC

See also *Grieving*

Goal

Client will identify expected loss, and grief reactions will be freely expressed, as evidenced by the following indicators:

- Participate in decision-making for the future.
- Share concerns with significant others.

 NIC

See also *Grieving*

Interventions

Assess for Causative and Contributing Factors of Anticipated or Potential Loss

- Aging
- Body image, self-esteem, or role changes
- Impending retirement
- Terminal illness
- Separation (divorce, hospitalization, marriage, relocation, job)
- Socioeconomic status

Assess Individual Response

- Denial
- Anger
- Isolation
- Fear
- Shock
- Bargaining
- Guilt
- Sadness
- Rejection
- Depression
- Helplessness/hopelessness
- Anxiety

Encourage the Client to Share Concerns

- Use open-ended questions and reflection ("What are your thoughts today?" "How do you feel?").
- Acknowledge the value of the client and his or her grief by using touch, sitting with him or her, and verbalizing your concern ("This must be very difficult," "What is most important to you now?").
- Recognize that some people may choose not to share their concerns, but convey that you are available if they desire to do so later ("What do you hope for?").

Assist the Client and the Family to Identify Strengths

- "What do you do well?"
- "What are you willing to do to address this issue?"
- "Is religion/spirituality a source of strength for you?"
- "Do you have close friends?"
- "Whom do you turn to in times of need?"
- "What does this person do for you?"
- "What sources of strength have you called upon successfully in the past?"

Promote Integrity of the Client and the Family by Acknowledging Strengths

- "Your brother looks forward to your visit."
- "Your family is so concerned for you."

Support the Client and the Family With Grief Reactions

- Prepare them for possible grief reactions.
- Explain possible grief reactions.
- Focus on the current situation until the client or family indicates the desire to discuss the future.

Promote Family Cohesiveness

Identify Availability of a Support System
- Meet consistently with family members.
- Identify family member roles, strengths, and weaknesses.

Identify Communication Patterns Within the Family Unit
- Assess positive and negative feedback, verbal and nonverbal communication, and body language.
- Listen and clarify messages being sent.

Provide for the Concept of Hope
- Supply accurate information.
- Resist the temptation to give false hope.
- Discuss concerns willingly.
- Help the family reframe hope (i.e., for a peaceful death)

Promote Group Decision Making to Enhance Group Autonomy
- Establish consistent times to meet with the client and the family.
- Encourage members to talk directly with and to listen to one another.

Promote Grief Work With Each Response

Isolation
- Listen and spend designated time consistently with client and family.
- Offer the client and the family opportunity to explore their emotions.
- Reflect on past losses and acknowledge loss behavior (past and present).

Depression
- Begin with simple problem solving and move toward acceptance.
- Enhance self-worth through positive reinforcement.
- Identify level of depression and indications of suicidal behavior or ideas.
- Be consistent and establish times daily to speak with client and family.

Anger
- Support crying as a release of this energy.
- Listen to and communicate concern.
- Encourage concerned support from significant others as well as professionals.

Guilt
- Listen and communicate concern.
- Promote more direct expression of feelings.
- Explore methods to resolve guilt, such as ritual forgiveness.

Fear
- Help the client and the family to recognize the feeling.
- Explain that fear is a normal aspect of grieving.
- Explore attitudes about loss, death, and so forth.
- Explore methods of coping.

Rejection
- Allow for verbal expression of this feeling to diminish the emotional strain.
- Recognize that expression of anger may cause rejection by significant others.

Provide for Expression of Grief

- Encourage emotional expressions of grieving.
- Caution the client about use of sedatives and tranquilizers, which may prevent or delay expressions.
- Encourage verbalization by clients of all age groups and families.
  - Support family cohesiveness.
  - Promote and verbalize strengths of the family group.
- Encourage the client and the family to engage in life review.
  - Focus and support the social network relationships.
  - Reevaluate past life experiences and integrate them into a new meaning.
  - Convey empathic understanding.
  - Explore unfinished business.

Identify Potential Complicated Grieving Reactions

- Suicidal indications
- Delusions
- Hallucinations
- Difficulty crying
- Difficulty controlling crying
- Phobias
- Obsessions
- Isolation
- Conversion hysteria
- Agitated depression
- Restrictions of pleasure
- Delay in grief work
- Intense longing or pining (longer than 12 to 18 months with few signs of relief)
- Loss of control of environment leading to hopelessness/ helplessness

Provide Health Teaching and Referrals, as Indicated

Refer the Client With Potential for Dysfunctional Grieving Responses for Counseling (Psychiatrist, Nurse Therapist, Counselor, Psychologist)

Explain What to Expect:
- Anger
- Fear
- Feelings of aloneness
- Feeling of "going crazy"
- Guilt
- Labile emotions
- Sadness
- Rejection

Teach the Client and the Family Signs of Resolution
- Grieving client no longer lives in the past but establishes new goals for life.
- Grieving client redefines relationship with the lost object/person.
- Grieving client begins to resocialize.

Teach Signs of Complicated Responses and Referrals Needed
- Defenses used in uncomplicated grief work that become exaggerated or maladaptive responses
- Persistent absence of any emotion
- Prolonged intense reactions of anxiety, anger, fear, guilt, and helplessness

Identify Agencies That May Enhance Grief Work:
- Self-help groups
- Widow-to-widow groups
- Parents of deceased children
- Single-parent groups
- Bereavement groups

Complicated Grieving

NANDA-I Definition

A disorder that occurs after the death of a significant other, in which the experience of distress accompanying bereavement fails to follow normative expectations and manifests in functional impairment.

Defining Characteristics

Major (Must Be Present, One or More)

Unsuccessful adaptation to loss
Prolonged denial, depression
Delayed emotional reaction
Inability to assume normal patterns of living
Grief avoidance*
Yearning*

Minor (May Be Present)

Social isolation or withdrawal
Inability to develop new relationships/interests
Inability to restructure life after loss

Rumination*
Self-blame*
Verbalizes persistent painful memories*

Related Factors

See *Grieving*.

 Author's Note

How one responds to loss is highly individual. Responses to acute loss should not be labeled dysfunctional, regardless of the severity. *Complicated Grieving* is characterized by its sustained or prolonged detrimental response in the grieving person. The validation of *Complicated Grieving* cannot occur until several months or 1 to 2 years after the death. Careful assessment with the grieving person can help to determine if the grieving process is being integrated into his or her life or if it is damaging his or her life. In many clinical settings, the diagnosis of *Risk for Complicated Grieving* for individuals at risk for unsuccessful reintegration after a loss may be more useful.

NOC

See also *Grieving*

Goal

The client will verbalize intent to seek professional assistance, as evidenced by the following indicators:

• Acknowledge the loss.
• Acknowledge an unresolved grief process.

NIC

See also *Grieving*

Interventions

Assess for Causative and Contributing Factors

• Unavailable (or lack of) support system
• History of dependency on deceased
• History of a difficult relationship with the lost person or object
• Multiple past losses
• Ineffective coping strategies

- Unexpected or traumatic death
- Expectations to "be strong"

Promote a Trust Relationship

- Implement the General Interventions under *Grieving*.

Support the Client's and the Family's Grief Reactions

- Implement the General Interventions under *Grieving*.

Promote Family Cohesiveness

- Implement the General Interventions under *Grieving*.
- Slowly and carefully identify the reality of the situation (e.g., "After your husband died, who helped you most?").

Promote Grief Work With Each Response

- Explain the use of denial by one family member to the other members.
- Do not force the client to move past denial without emotional readiness.

Isolation
- Convey a feeling of acceptance by allowing grief.
- Create open, honest communication to promote sharing.
- Reinforce the client's self-worth by allowing privacy.
- Encourage the client/family gradually to increase social activities (e.g., support or church groups).

Depression
- Implement the General Interventions under *Grieving*.

Anger
- Understand that this feeling usually replaces denial.
- Explain to the family that anger serves to try to control one's environment more closely because of the inability to control loss.
- Encourage verbalization of the anger.
- See *Anxiety* for additional information for anger.

Guilt/Ambivalence
- Acknowledge the client's expressed self-view.
- Role play to allow the client to "express" to dead person what he or she wants to say or how he or she feels.
- Encourage the client to identify positive contributions/aspects of the relationship.
- Avoid arguing and participating in the client's system of shoulds and should nots.
- Discuss the client's preoccupation with dead person and attempt to move verbally beyond the present.

Fear
- Focus on the present and maintain a safe and secure environment.
- Help the client to explore reasons for a meaning of the behavior.
- Consider alternative ways of expressing his or her feelings.

Provide Health Teaching and Referrals, as Indicated

Teach the Client and the Family Signs of Resolution
- Grieving client no longer lives in the past but is future oriented and is establishing new goals.
- Grieving client redefines the relationship with the lost object/person.
- Grieving client begins to resocialize; seeks new relationships, experiences.

Teach the Client/Family to Recognize Signs of Complicated Grieving, Especially for People Who Are at Risk, and to Seek Professional Counseling:
- Continued searching for deceased
- Prolonged depression
- Denial
- Living in past
- Prolonged hallucinations
- Delusions
- Isolation
- Egocentricity
- Overthostility

Identify Agencies That May Be Helpful:
- Support groups
- Mental health agencies
- Psychotherapists
- Grief specialists
- Faith communities

Risk for Complicated Grieving

NANDA-I Definition

At risk for a disorder that occurs after the death of a significant other, in which the experience or distress accompanying bereavement fails to follow normative expectations and manifests in functional impairment

Risk Factors*

Death of significant other
Lack of support
Significant loss or losses (e.g., divorce, termination, natural
    disaster, war)

Goals

Refer to *Grieving*

Interventions

- Identify clients at high risk for complicated grieving response:
  - Length of relationship: more than 55 years, less than 5 years
  - Medical issues: pending treatments, surgeries, history of
    acute or chronic illness
  - Significant mental health issues of deceased or grieving
    person
  - Substance abuse
  - Suicide in family history, potential for suicide
  - Family conflicts
- Refer also to *Complicated Grieving*.

DELAYED GROWTH AND DEVELOPMENT

Delayed Growth and Development

Risk for Delayed Development

Risk for Disproportionate Growth

Adult Failure to Thrive

NANDA-I Definition

Deviations from age-group norms

Defining Characteristics

Inability or difficulty performing skills or behaviors typical of
    his or her age group* (e.g., motor, personal/social, language/
    cognition; Table II.2)

Table 11.2	AGE-RELATED DEVELOPMENTAL TASKS	
Developmental Tasks/Needs	**Parental Guidance**	**Implications for Nursing**

Birth to 1 Year

Personal/Social Learns to trust and anticipate satisfaction Sends cues to mother/caretaker Begins understanding self as separate from others (body image) *Motor* Responds to sound Social smile Reaches for objects Begins to sit, creep, pull up, and stand with support Attempting to walk *Language/Cognition* Learns to signal wants/needs with sounds, crying Begins to vocalize with meaning (two-syllable words: Dada, Mama) Comprehends some verbal/nonverbal messages (no, yes, bye-bye) Learns about words through senses *Fears* Loud noises Falling	Encourage parent to respond to cry, meet infant's need *consistently* Teach parent not to be afraid of spoiling infant with too much attention Talk and sing to child; hold and cuddle often Provide variety of stimulation Allow infant to feed self (cereal, etc.) Do not prop bottle *Toys* Brightly colored crib toys, mobiles Stuffed toys of varied textures Music boxes *Safety* Be aware of rapidly changing loco-motive ability (e.g., childproof kitchen, stairways; small objects within reach; tub safety)	Encourage parent to participate in care: Bathing Feeding Holding Teach parent guidance information Provide ongoing stimula-tion while confined through use of toys, mirrors, mobiles, music Hold, speak to infant, maintain eye contact Investigate crying Do not restrain

Developmental Tasks/Needs	Parental Guidance	Implications for Nursing
1 to 3 Years		
Personal/Social	Provide child with peer companionship	Allow child to take liquids from a cup (including medicines)
Establishes self-control, decision-making, self-independence (autonomy)	Allow for brief periods of separation under familiar surroundings	Allow child to perform some self-care tasks:
Extremely curious, prefers to do things himself	Practice safety measures that guard against child's increased motor ability and curiosity (poisoning, falls)	Wash face and arms
		Brush teeth
Demonstrates independence through negativism		Expect resistant behavior to treatments; reinforce treatments, not punishments
Very egocentric: believes he controls the world		Use firm, direct approach and provide child with choices only when possible
Learns about words through senses	Tell the truth	Restrain child when needed
Motor	Disciplining child for violation of safety rules:	Explain to parents methods for disciplining child:
Begins to walk and run well	Running in street	Slap hand once (for dangerous touching, [e.g., stove])
Drinks from cup, feeds self	Touching electrical wires	
Develops fine motor control	Allow child some control over fears:	Sit in chair for 2 min (if child gets up, put him back and reset timer)
Climbs	Favorite toy	
Begins self-toileting	Night light	
Language/Cognition	Allow exploration within safe limits	Explain the need for consistency
Has poor time sense	Explain as simply as possible why things happen	Allow expression of fear, pain, displeasure
Increasingly verbal (4- to 5-word sentences by age 3½)	Allow child to explain why he thinks things are happening	Assign consistent caregiver
Talks to self/others	Correct misconceptions	Let child play with simple equipment (stethoscope)
Misconceptions about cause/effect	Include child in domestic activities when possible:	Provide materials for play (favorite toy)
Fears	Dusting	Be honest about procedure
Loss/separation from parents	Cleaning spoons	
Darkness		
Machines/equipment		
Intrusive procedures		

(continued)

Table 11.2 AGE-RELATED DEVELOPMENTAL TASKS (continued)

Developmental Tasks/Needs	Parental Guidance	Implications for Nursing
	Discuss differences in opinions (between parents) in front of child	Praise child for helping you: Holding still Holding the Band-Aid
	Do not threaten child with what will happen if he does not behave	Give child choices whenever possible
	Always follow through with punishment	Tell child he can cry or squeeze your hand, but you expect him to hold still
	Toys	Have parents present for procedures when at all possible
	Manipulative toys	Explore with child his fantasies of the situation:
	Puzzles	Use play therapy
	Bright-colored, simple books	Explain the procedure immediately beforehand if short (e.g., injection) and when appropriate if longer or intrusive (e.g., x-ray, IV insertion)
	Large-muscle devices (gym sets, etc.)	
	Music (songs, records)	Follow home routines when possible

3 to 5 Years

Personal/Social

Attempts to establish self as like his parents, but independent	Teach parents to listen to child's fears, feelings	Encourage expressing of fears
Explores environment on his own initiative	Encourage hugs, touch as expressions of acceptance	Reinforce reality of body image
Boasts, brags, has feelings of indestructibility	Provide simple explanations	Encourage self-care, decision-making when possible
		Involve parents in teaching

Developmental Tasks/Needs	Parental Guidance	Implications for Nursing
Family is primary group	Limit stimulation from television to avoid intense material	Provide peer stimulation
Peers increasingly important	Focus on positive behaviors	Limit physical restraint
Assumes sex roles	Allow child to help as much as possible	Provide play opportunities for acting out fantasy, story-telling
Aggressive	Provide child with regular contact with other children (e.g., nursery school)	Explain to child how he can cooperate (e.g., hold still), and expect that he will
Motor		
Locomotion skills increase, and coordinates easier		
Rides tricycle/bicycle	Explain that television, movies are make-believe	Use play therapy to allow child free expression
Throws ball, but has difficulty catching	Practice definite limit-setting behavior	Explain all procedures: Use equipment if possible; allow therapeutic play
Language/Cognition	Offer child choices	
Egocentric	Allow child to express anger verbally but limit motor aggression ("You may slam a door but you may not throw a toy")	Encourage child to ask questions
Language skills flourish		Tell child the exact body parts that will be affected
Generates many questions: how, why, what?		Use models, pictures
Simple problem solving; uses fantasy to understand, problem solve	Discipline (examples): Sit in chair 5 minutes	Explain when procedure will occur in relation to daily schedule (e.g., after lunch, after bath)
Fears	Forbid a favorite pastime (no bicycle riding for 2 h)	
Mutilation		
Castration		
Dark		
Unknown	Be consistent and firm	
Inanimate, unfamiliar objects	Teach safety precautions about strangers	
	Toys and Games	
	"Make-believe" play (play house, toy models, etc.)	
	Simple games with others, books, puzzles, coloring	

(continued)

Table 11.2	AGE-RELATED DEVELOPMENTAL TASKS (continued)	
Developmental Tasks/Needs	**Parental Guidance**	**Implications for Nursing**
5 to 11 Years	Teach appropriate foods needed each day; provide choices	Promote family and peer interactions (e.g., visiting, telephone)
Personal/Social		
Learns to include values and skills of school, neighborhood, peers	Encourage interaction outside home	Explain all procedures and impact on body
Peer relationships important	Include cooking and cleaning in home activities	Encourage questioning, *active* participation in care
Focuses more on reality, less on fantasy	Teach safety (bicycle, street, playground equipment, fire, water, strangers)	Be direct about explanation of procedures (e.g., body part involved, use anatomic names, pictures, etc.); explain step by step
Family is main base of security and identity		
Sensitive to reactions of others	Maintain limit-setting and discipline	
Seeks approval, recognition	Prepare child for bodily changes of pubescence and provide with concrete sex education information (late childhood)	Be honest
Enthusiastic, noisy, imaginative, desires to explore		Reassure child that he is liked
Likes to complete a task		Provide privacy
Enjoys helping		Involve parents but make direction of care the child's decision
Motor		
Moves constantly		Reason and explain
Physical play prevalent (sports, swimming, skating, etc.)	Expect fluctuations between immature and mature behavior	Encourage continuance of school work, activities if condition permits (e.g., homework, contact with classmates)
Language/Cognition	Respect peer relationships but do not compromise your values (e.g., "But, Mom, all the other girls are wearing makeup!")	Encourage continuance of hobbies, interests
Organized, stable thought		
Concepts more complicated		
Focuses on concrete understanding		

Developmental Tasks/Needs	Parental Guidance	Implications for Nursing
Fears Rejections, failures Immobility Mutilation Death	Promote responsibility, contribution to family (e.g., duties for helping, etc.) Promote exploration and development of skills (e.g., joining clubs, sports, hobbies, etc.) *Toys and Games* Group games, board games, art activities, crafts, video games, reading	
11 to 15 Years *Personal/Social* Family values continue to be significant influence Peer group values have increasing significance Early adolescence: outgoing and enthusiastic Emotions are extreme: mood swings, introspection Sexual identity fully mature Wants privacy/independence Develops interests not shared with family Concern with physical self Explores adult roles	Encourage independent problem solving, decision-making within established values Be available Compliment child's achievements Listen to interests, likes, dislikes without passing judgment Respect privacy Allow independence while maintaining safety limits Provide concrete information about sexuality, function, bodily changes Teach about: Auto safety Drug abuse	Respect privacy Accept expression of feelings Direct discussions of care and condition to child Ask for opinions, allow input into decisions Be flexible with routines; explain all procedures/treatments Encourage continuance of peer relationships Listen actively Identify impact of illness on body image, future functioning Correct misconceptions Encourage continuance of schoolwork, hobbies, interests

(continued)

Table 11.2	AGE-RELATED DEVELOPMENTAL TASKS (continued)	
Developmental Tasks/Needs	**Parental Guidance**	**Implications for Nursing**
Motor	Alcohol hazards	
Well developed	Tobacco hazards	
Rapid physical growth	Mechanical safety	
Secondary sex characteristics	Sexuality relations	
	Dating	
Language/Cognition	*Games/Interests*	
Plans for future career	Intellectual games	
Able to abstract solutions and solve problems in future tense	Reading	
	Arts, crafts, hobbies	
	Video games	
	Problem-solving games	
Fears	Computers	
Mutilation		
Disruption in body image		
Rejection from peers		

Altered physical growth*; weight lagging behind height by two
standard deviations; pattern of height and weight percentiles
indicate a drop in pattern
Inability to perform self-care or self-control activities appropriate
for age* (see Table II.2)
Flat affect*
Listlessness*
Decreased response time*
Slow social responses
Limited signs of satisfaction to caregiver
Limited eye contact
Difficulty feeding
Decreased appetite
Lethargy
Irritability
Negative mood
Regression in self-toileting
Regression in self-feeding
Infants: watchfulness, interrupted sleep pattern

Related Factors

Pathophysiologic

Related to compromised physical ability and dependence secondary to:
Disability related to trauma, mental health issues, Autism spectrum, genetic syndromes, child abuse and neglect, unknown causes
Cardiovascular defects or disease
Central nervous system dysfunction
Congenital anomalies of extremities
Cystic fibrosis
GI dysfunction
Inadequate nutritional intake
Malabsorption syndrome
Muscular dystrophy
Prolonged pain
Repeated acute or chronic illness or disability

Treatment Related

Related to separation from significant others or school, or inadequate sensory stimulation secondary to:
Confinement for ongoing treatment
Isolation from disease
Prolonged bed rest
Prolonged, painful treatment
Traction or casts
Repeat or prolonged hospitalizations

Situational (Personal and Environmental)

Related to parental stressor secondary to:
Insufficient knowledge of child care, development, and growth
Change in usual environment
Separation from significant others (parents, primary caretaker)
School-related conflicts
Loss of significant other
Loss of control over environment (established rituals, activities, established hours of contact with family)
Related to inadequate, inappropriate parental support (neglect, abuse)
Related to inadequate sensory stimulation (neglect, isolation)
Related to cultural beliefs and practices

Maturational

Infant–Toddler (Birth to 3 Years)

Related to limited opportunities to meet social, play, or educational needs secondary to:

Separation from parents/ significant others	Inability to trust significant other
Inadequate parental support	Multiple caregivers
Inability to communicate (e.g., deafness)	Decreased sensory functions (e.g., vision, hearing)
Restriction of activities of daily living, to (specify)	Excessive painful experiences

Preschool Age (4 to 6 Years)

Related to limited opportunities to meet self-care, social, play, or educational needs secondary to:
Loss of ability to communicate
Lack of significant other
Lack of stimulation

Related to loss of significant other (death, divorce)

Related to loss of peer group

Related to removal from home environment

School Age (6 to 11 Years)

Related to limited opportunities to develop skills to achieve success in school, social environment, or their physical abilities secondary to (specify):

Related to loss of significant others:
Peer group
Strange environment

Adolescent (12 to 18 Years)

Related to loss of independence and autonomy secondary to (specify):

Related to disruption of peer relationships

Related to disruption of body image

Related to loss of significant others

Author's Note

Specific developmental tasks are associated with various age groups (e.g., to gain autonomy and self-control [e.g., toileting] from 1 to 3 years of age and to establish lasting relationships from 18 to 30 years of age). An adult's failure to accomplish a developmental task may cause or contribute to a change in functioning in a functional health pattern (e.g., *Impaired Social Interactions, Powerlessness*). Because nursing interventions focus on altered functioning rather than achievement of past developmental tasks, the diagnosis *Delayed Growth and Development* has limited uses for adults. It is most useful for a child or adolescent experiencing difficulty achieving a developmental task.

NOC

Child Development (specify age)

Goal

The child will demonstrate increased age-appropriate behaviors as evidenced by the following indicators (specify for age):

- Socialization
- Language
- Motor skills
- Self-care
- Cognitive skills

NIC

Development Enhancement, Parenting Promotion, Infant/Child Care

Interventions

Assess Causative or Contributing Factors

Refer to Related Factors.

Teach Parents Age-Related Developmental Tasks and Anticipatory Guidance Information (see Table II.2)

Carefully Assess Child's Level of Development in All Areas of Functioning by Using Specific Assessment Tools (e.g., Brazelton Assessment Table, DDST)

Provide Opportunities for an Ill Child to Meet Age-Related Developmental Tasks (see Implications for Nursing in Table II.2 to Assist With Designing Interventions)

Birth to 1 Year
- Encourage parental visits, calls, and, if possible, involvement in care.
- Demonstrate methods that allow parents/family to participate in child's care.
- Provide child with age-appropriate communication and preparation regarding procedures.
- Consider cultural practices and beliefs.
- Increase stimulation by using various-colored toys in crib (e.g., mobiles, musical toys, stuffed toys of varied textures) and frequently holding and speaking to the infant.
- Hold the infant while feeding him or her slowly and in a relaxed environment.
- Provide rest periods before feeding.
- Observe mother and child during interaction, especially during feeding.
- Investigate crying promptly and consistently.
- Assign a consistent caregiver and/or provide clear communication to relay a consistent method of care-giving.
- Allow the infant's hands and feet to be free, if possible.

1 to 3 Years
- Encourage and support parental or caregiver presence.
- Demonstrate methods that allow parents/family to participate in child's care.
- Provide child with age-appropriate communication and preparation regarding procedures.
- Assign a consistent caregiver and/or provide clear communication to relay a consistent method of care-giving.
- Consider cultural practices and beliefs.
- Encourage self-care activities (e.g., self-feeding, self-dressing, and bathing).
- Reinforce word development by repeating words the child uses, naming objects, and speaking to the child often.
- Provide frequent periods of play with peers and various toys (puzzles, books with pictures, manipulative toys, trucks, cars, blocks, and bright colors).
- Demonstrate all procedures on a doll before you do them to the child.

- Provide a safe area where the child can move around.
- Provide comfort measures after painful procedures.

3 to 5 Years
- Encourage and support parental or caregiver presence.
- Demonstrate methods that allow parents/family to participate in child's care.
- Provide child with age-appropriate communication and preparation regarding procedures.
- Assign a consistent caregiver and/or provide clear communication to relay a consistent method of care-giving.
- Consider cultural practices and beliefs.
- Encourage self-care: self-grooming, self-dressing, mouth care, hair care.
- Offer appropriate choices (e.g. "Which arm shall we put the medicine in?")
- Provide frequent playtime with others and various toys (e.g., models, musical toys, dolls, puppets, books, mini-slides, wagons, tricycles).
- Read stories aloud. Ask for verbal responses and requests.
- Say words for equipment, objects, and people; ask the child to repeat them.
- Allow time for individual play and exploration of play environment.
- Monitor use of television.
- Use familiar routines to help child understand time (e.g. "After breakfast your mother will be here").

5 to 11 Years
- Encourage and support parental or caregiver presence.
- Demonstrate methods that allow parents/family to participate in child's care.
- Provide child with age-appropriate communication and preparation regarding procedures.
- Assign a consistent caregiver and/or provide clear communication to relay a consistent method of care-giving.
- Consider cultural practices and beliefs.
- Allow the child to wear his or her own clothes if possible.
- Provide periods of interaction with other children.
- Provide craft projects that the child can complete each day or week.
- Continue schoolwork at intervals each day.
- Praise positive behaviors.
- Read stories and provide several independent games, puzzles, books, video games, and art projects.

- Introduce the child by name to people involved in their care.
- Encourage visits with or telephone calls from parents, siblings, and peers.

11 to 15 Years

- Encourage and support parental or caregiver presence.
- Demonstrate methods that allow parents/family to participate in child's care.
- Provide child with age-appropriate communication and preparation regarding procedures.
- Assign a consistent caregiver and/or provide clear communication to relay a consistent method of care-giving.
- Consider cultural practices and beliefs.
- Speak frequently with child about feelings, ideas, and concerns about condition or care.
- Provide an opportunity for interaction with others of the same age.
- Identify an interest or a hobby that the unit can support, and support it daily.
- Allow the health care facility routine to be altered to suit the child's schedule.
- Allow the child to wear his or her own clothes if possible.
- Involve the child in decisions about his or her care.
- Provide an opportunity for involvement in several activities (e.g., reading, video games, movies, board games, art, and trips outside or to other areas).
- Encourage visits or telephone calls from parents, siblings, and peers.

Initiate Health Teaching and Referrals, When Indicated

- Provide anticipatory guidance for parents regarding constructive handling of developmental problems and support of developmental process (see Table II.2 and *Impaired Parenting*).
- Refer the family to the appropriate agency for counseling or follow-up treatment of abuse, parent–child conflict, chemical dependency, and so forth (see *Disabled Family Coping*).
- Refer the family to the appropriate agency for structured, ongoing stimulation program (e.g., schooling) when functioning is likely to be impaired permanently.
- Refer the family to community programs specific to contributing factors (e.g., Women, Infants, and Children Program [WIC], social services, family services, counseling).
- Provide a list of parent support groups (e.g., Down Syndrome Awareness, Muscular Dystrophy Association, National Epilepsy Association).

Risk for Delayed Development

NANDA-I Definition

At risk for delay of 25% or more in one or more of the areas of social or self-regulatory behavior or in cognitive, language, gross, or fine motor skills

RISK FACTORS

Refer to *Delayed Growth and Development*—Related Factors.

Child Development (specify age)

Goal

The child/adolescent will continue to demonstrate appropriate behavior, as evidenced by the following indicators (specify for age):

- Self-care
- Social skills
- Language
- Cognitive skills
- Motor skills

Interventions

Refer to *Delayed Growth and Development*.

Risk for Disproportionate Growth

NANDA-I Definition

At risk for growth above the 97th percentile or below the third percentile for age, crossing two percentile channels

Risk Factors

Refer to *Delayed Growth and Development*—Related Factors.

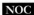
NOC
Child Development (specify age)

Goal

The child/adolescent will continue to demonstrate age-appropriate growth.

• Height
• Weight
• Head circumference

Interventions

• Refer to *Delayed Growth and Development*.

Adult Failure to Thrive

Definition

Progressive functional deterioration of a physical and cognitive nature. The individual's ability to live with multisystem diseases, cope with ensuing problems, and manage his or her care is remarkably diminished (NANDA-I).

State in which a client experiences insidious and progressive physical and psychosocial deterioration characterized by limited coping and diminished resilience in response to deteriorations in health.**

Defining Characteristics

Major (Must Be Present, One or More)

Altered mood state*
Anorexia*
Apathy*
Cognitive decline*
Consumption of minimal to no food at most meals*
Decreased social skills*

** This definition has been added by Lynda Juall Carpentino, the author, for clarity and usefulness.

Denial of symptom(s)
Depression
Expresses loss of interest in pleasurable outlets*
Giving up
Loneliness
Neglect of home environment
Physical decline* (e.g., fatigue, dehydration, incontinence
   of bowel and bladder)
Social withdrawal*
Self-care deficit*
Unintentional weight loss* (e.g., 5% in 1 month, 10% in
   6 months)

Related Factors

The cause of failure to thrive in adults (usually older adults) is unknown (Kimball & Williams-Burgess, 1995; Murray, Zentner, &
Yakimo, 2009). Researchers have identified some possible contributing factors, listed below.

Situational (Personal, Environmental)

Related to diminished coping abilities

Related to limited ability to adapt to effects of aging

Related to loss of social skills and resultant social isolation

Related to loss of social relatedness

Related to increasing dependency and feelings of helplessness

NOC

Physical Aging, Psychological Adjustment, Life Change, Will to Live

Goal

The client will participate to increase functioning, as evidenced by
the following indicators:

• Increase social relatedness.
• Maintain or increase present weight.

Coping Enhancement, Hope Instillment, Spiritual Support, Social Enhancement, Family Support, Referral

Interventions

Consult With a Therapist to Evaluate Client for Depression

Assess for Malnutrition, Renal Failure, Dementia, and Dehydration

Promote Socialization (Refer to *Risk for Loneliness*)

- Attempt to identify one activity that provides enjoyment.
- Provide opportunities to increase social relatedness, such as music therapy, recreation therapy, and reminiscence therapy.
- Engage in useful and meaningful conversations about likes, dislikes, interests, hobbies, and work history.
- Speak as one adult to another. Use average volume, appropriate eye contact, and slow rate of speech.
- Encourage the client to be as independent as possible.

Assist Client to Adapt to Changes

- Elicit unpleasant experiences and promote discussion of them.
- Encourage reminiscing about strengths and successes.
- Validate that adaptation to these changes is difficult.

Provide Respect and Promote Sharing

- Pay attention to what the client is saying.
- Pick out meaningful comments and continue talking.
- Call the client by name and introduce yourself each time you make contact; use touch if welcomed.

Advise the Family of the Condition and the Need to Monitor Social Interactions for Cognitive Changes and Nutrition

Institute Health Teaching and Referrals, as Indicated (e.g., Consult With Home Health Agency for a Home Assessment)

- Advise on the need to go outside the house at least weekly, if possible (Kono et al., 2004).
- Refer also to *Chronic Confusion* for additional interventions.
- For specific problems, refer to other nursing diagnoses, such as *Imbalanced Nutrition*, *Self-Care Deficits*, *Ineffective Coping*, *Confusion*, and *Risk for Loneliness*.

DEFICIENT COMMUNITY HEALTH

NANDA-I Definition

Presence of one or more health problems or factors that deter wellness or increase the risk of health problems experienced by an aggregate

Defining Characteristics*

Incidence of risks relating to hospitalization experienced by aggregates or populations
Incidence of risks relating to physiologic states experienced by aggregates or populations
Incidence of risks relating to psychological states experienced by aggregates or populations
Incidence of health problems experienced by aggregates or populations
No program available to enhance wellness for aggregates or populations**
No program available to prevent one or more health problems for aggregates or populations**
No program available to reduce one or more health problems for aggregates or populations**
No program available to eliminate one or more health problems for aggregates or populations**

Related Factors*

Lack of access to public health care providers
Lack of community experts
Limited resources
Program has inadequate budget
Program has inadequate community support
Program has inadequate consumer satisfaction
Program has inadequate evaluation
Program has inadequate outcome data
Program partly addresses health problem

** These four defining characteristics do not define community health but instead are related factors that contribute to *Deficient Community Health*.

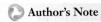 **Author's Note**

This NANDA-I nursing diagnosis describes a community that has health problems that need assessment and program development. The programs must be accessible, affordable, available, and realistic for optimal outcomes to be achieved.

This diagnosis, although different from *Ineffective Self-health Management*, shares the same focus of community assessment and program development.

NOC

Refer to *Ineffective Community Self-Health Management*.

Goals

Refer to *Ineffective Community Self-Health Management*.

NIC

Refer to *Ineffective Community Self-Health Management*.

Interventions

Refer to *Ineffective Community Self-Health Management*.

RISK-PRONE HEALTH BEHAVIOR

Definition

Impaired ability to modify lifestyle/behaviors in a manner that improves health status (NANDA-I)

State in which a person has an inability to modify lifestyle/behavior in a manner consistent with a change in health status**

Defining Characteristics*

Demonstrates nonacceptance of health status change
Failure to achieve optimal sense of control
Minimizes health status change
Failure to take action that prevents health problems

** This definition has been added by Lynda Juall Carpenito, the author, for clarity and usefulness.

Related Factors

Situational (Personal, Environmental)

Related to:
Low self-efficacy*
Negative attitude toward health care*
Multiple stressors
Inadequate social support*
Inadequate resources
Inadequate finances
Multiple responsibilities
Related to unhealthy lifestyle choices (e.g., tobacco use, excessive
   alcohol use, overweight)

Related to impaired ability to understand secondary to:
Low literacy   Language barriers

 Author's Note

This nursing diagnosis replaces the NANDA diagnosis *Impaired
Adjustment*. *Risk-Prone Health Behavior* has some commonalities with
Ineffective Health Maintenance and *Noncompliance*. This author recommends that *Ineffective Health Maintenance* be used to describe a person
with an unhealthy lifestyle that puts him or her at risk for a chronic
health problem or disease. *Noncompliance* applies to a person who
wants to comply, but factors are present that deter adherence.

   Risk-Prone Health Behavior describes a person with a health problem
who is not participating in management of the health problem because
of lack of motivation, comprehension, or personal barriers.

NOC

Adherence Behavior, Symptom Control, Health Beliefs, Treatment Behavior, Illness/
Injury

Goal

The client will verbalize intent to modify one behavior to manage
health problem, as evidenced by the following indicators:

* Describe the health problem.
* Describe the relationship of present practices/behavior to
   decreased health.
* Engage in goal setting.

Health Education, Mutual Goal Setting, Self-responsibility, Teaching: Disease Process, Decision-Making Process

Interventions

If Low Literacy Is Suspected, Start With What the Client Is Most Stressed About

- Speak simply.
- Repeat and ask client to repeat.
- Use pictures.
- Use appropriate examples.
- Demonstrate and ask for a return demonstration.
- Use videotapes and audiotapes.

Engage in Collaborative Negotiation (Tyler & Horner, 2008)

- Ask client: "How can you be healthier?" Focus on the area they choose.
- Do not provide unsolicited advice.
- Accept that only the client can make the change.
- Accept resistance.

For example: Diabetes

- Exercise
- Healthy eating
- Medication
- Blood glucose monitoring
- Client-defined choice

Clients Are Responsible for Day-to-Day Decisions (Bodenheimer et al., 2005)

Provide information as directed by the client:

- Ask: What do you want to know about _____?
- Provide information the client wants to know.
- Ask the client if he or she understood.
- Ask if there are other questions.

Ask the Client to Repeat the Goal, Behavior, or Activity

Assess Readiness to Change

- Determine how important the client thinks the behavior change is. For example:
  - How important is it to you to increase your activity? Rate from 0–10 (0 = not important, 10 = important).

Determine How Confident the Client Is to Make the Change

- For example:
  - How confident are you that you can get more exercise? Rate from 0–10.
  - Determine if the client is ready for change.
  - If the importance level is 7 or above, assess confidence level. If the importance level is low, provide more information regarding the risks of not changing behavior.
  - If the level of confidence is 4 or less, ask the client why it is not a 1.
  - Ask client what is needed to change the low score to an 8.

Collaboratively, Set a Realistic Goal and Action Plan

- *For example:* How often each week could you walk around the block two times?

Establish a Follow-up Plan. Ask the Client If You Can Call Him or Her in 2 Weeks to See How He or She Is Doing. Gradually Extend the Time to Monthly Calls.

INEFFECTIVE HEALTH MAINTENANCE

Definition

Inability to identify, manage, and/or seek out help to maintain health (NANDA-I)

State in which a person experiences or is at risk of experiencing a disruption in health because of lack of knowledge to manage a condition or basic health requirements**

Defining Characteristics*

Demonstrated lack of adaptive behaviors to environmental changes
Demonstrated lack of knowledge about basic health practices
Lack of expressed interest in improving health behaviors
History of lack of health-seeking behaviors
Inability to take responsibility for meeting basic health practices
Impairment of personal support systems

** This definition has been added by Lynda Juall Carpenito, the author, for clarity and usefulness.

Related Factors

Various factors can produce *Ineffective Health Maintenance*. Common causes are listed in the following.

Situational (Personal, Environmental)

Related to:

Misinterpretation of information	Deficient communication skills*
Insufficient resources*	Lack of access to adequate health care services
Lack of motivation	Cognitive impairments*
Lack of education or readiness	Perceptual impairment*

Maturational

Related to insufficient of knowledge of age-related risk factors. Examples include the following:

Child

Sexuality and sexual development	Substance abuse
	Poor nutrition
Inactivity	Safety hazards

Adolescent

Same as children practices	Vehicle safety

Adult

Parenthood	Sexual function
Safety practices	

Older Adult

Effects of aging	Sensory deficits

🌀 Author's Note

The nursing diagnosis *Ineffective Health Maintenance* applies to both well and ill populations. Health is a dynamic, ever-changing state defined by the individual based on his or her perception of highest level of functioning (e.g., a marathon runner's definition of health will differ from that of a paraplegic). Because clients are responsible for their own health, an important associated nursing responsibility involves raising client consciousness that better health is possible.

The nursing diagnosis *Risk for Ineffective Health Maintenance* is useful to describe a person who needs teaching or referrals before discharge from an acute care center to prevent problems with health maintenance after discharge or in community settings.

As focus shifts from an illness/treatment-oriented to a health-oriented health care system, *Ineffective Health Maintenance* and

Readiness for Enhanced Diagnoses are becoming increasingly significant. The increasingly high acuity and shortened lengths of stay in hospitals require nurses to be creative in addressing health promotion (e.g., by using printed materials, television instruction, and community-based programs).

NOC

Health Promoting Behavior, Health-Seeking Behaviors, Knowledge: Health Promotion, Knowledge: Health Resources, Participation: Health Care Decisions, Risk Detection

Goal

The client or caregiver will verbalize intent to engage in health maintenance behaviors, as evidenced by the following indicator:

• Identify barriers to health maintenance.

NIC

Health Education, Self-Responsibility Facilitation, Health Screening, Risk Identification, Family Involvement Promotion, Nutrition Counseling, Weight Reduction Assistance

Interventions

Assess for Barriers to Health Maintenance

Refer to Related Factors.

Determine the Person's or Family's Knowledge or Perception

• Life cycle challenges (e.g., marriage, parenting, aging, finances).
• Need to maintain responsible relationships with health care providers.
• Ability to attain a higher level of health through anticipatory planning for life cycle events (e.g., financial planning).
• Need to provide and nurture reciprocity in social support.

Determine the Person's or Family's Past Patterns of Health Care

• Expectations
• Interactions with health care system or providers
• Influences of family, cultural group, peer group, mass media

Provide Specific Information Concerning Age-Related Health Promotion (see Table II.3)

Table II.3 PRIMARY AND SECONDARY PREVENTION FOR AGE-RELATED CONDITIONS (1,4,5)

Developmental Level	Primary Prevention	Secondary Prevention

Infancy (0–1 year)	Parent education
	Infant safety
	Nutrition
	Breast feeding
	Sensory stimulation
	  Infant massage and touch
	  Visual stimulation
	    Activity
	    Colors
	  Auditory stimulation
	    Verbal
	    Music
	Immunizations
	  DPT or DTaP
	  IPV, Hib
	  Hepatitis B (3-dose series)
	  Hepatitis A (2)
	  Rotavirus (RV)
	  Pneumococcal (PCV)**
	  Meningococcal
	  Influenza (yearly)
	Oral hygiene
		Complete physical examination every 2–3 months
		Screening at birth
		  Congenital hip dysplasia
		  PKU
		  G-6-PD deficiency in blacks, Mediterranean,
		    and Far Eastern origin children
		  Sickle cell
		  Hemoglobin or hematocrit (for anemia)
		  Cystic fibrosis
		  Vision (startle reflex)
		Hearing (response to and localization of sounds)
		TB test at 12 months
		Developmental assessments
		Screen and intervene for high risk
		  Low birth weight
		  Maternal substance abuse during pregnancy
		    Alcohol: fetal alcohol syndrome
		    Cigarettes: SIDS
		    Drugs: addicted neonate, AIDS
		  Maternal infections during pregnancy

Preschool (1–5 years)

Teething biscuits
Fluoride (if needed >6 months)
Avoid sugared food and drink
Parent education
  Teething
  Discipline
  Nutrition
  Accident prevention
  Normal growth and development
Child education
  Dental self-care
  Dressing
  Bathing with assistance
  Feeding self-care
Immunizations
  DTaP
  IPV
  MMR
  HIB
  H. Influenzae (yearly)
  Varicella
  Hepatitis A (2)(2-dose series)

Complete physical examination between 2 and 3 years
  and preschool (UA, CBC)
TB test at 3 years
Development assessments (annual)
  Speech development
  Hearing
  Vision
Screen and intervene
  Lead poisoning
  Developmental lag
  Neglect or abuse
Strong family history of
  arteriosclerotic diseases (e.g., MI, CVA, peripheral
  vascular disease), diabetes, hypertension, gout,
  or hyperlipidemia—fasting serum cholesterol at
  age 2 years, then every 3–5 years if normal
  Strabismus
  Hearing deficit
  Vision deficit
  Autism

(continued)

Table II.3   PRIMARY AND SECONDARY PREVENTION FOR AGE-RELATED CONDITIONS (1,4,5) (continued)

Developmental Level	Primary Prevention	Secondary Prevention

School age (6–11 years)	Pneumococcal**
	 Hepatitis B (3-dose series)
	 Dental/oral hygiene
	 Fluoride treatments
	 Fluoridated water
	 Health education of child
	 "Basic 4" nutrition
	 Accident prevention
	 Outdoor safety
	 Substance abuse counsel
	 Anticipatory guidance for physical changes at puberty
	 Immunizations
	 Tdap age 11–12
	 MMR (2 lifetime doses)
	 OPV/IPV (4 lifetime doses)
	 Hepatitis B 3-dose series if needed
	 Hepatitis A (2)
	 Pneumococcal (3)
	 Varicella (at age 11–12 if no history of infection)
		Complete physical examination
		 TB test every 3 years (at ages 6 and 9)
		 Developmental assessments
		   Language
		   Vision: Snellen charts at school
		     6–8 years, use "E" chart
		     Older than 8 years, use alphabet chart
		   Hearing: audiogram
		 Cholesterol profile, if high risk, every 3–5 years
		 Serum cholesterol one time (not high risk)

Adolescence (12–19 years)

Gardasil (HPV) series of three for girls
9–26 years, for boys age 9–18 years
Dental hygiene every 6–12 months
Continue fluoridation
Complete physical examination
Health education
Proper nutrition and healthful diets
Calcium 100mg & Vitamin D 400 units
daily
Sex education
Choices
Risks
Precautions
Sexually transmitted diseases
Safe driving skills
Adult challenges
Seeking employment and career choices
Dating and marriage
Confrontation with substance abuse
Safety in athletics, water
Skin care
Dental hygiene every 6–12 months

Complete physical exam yearly
Blood pressure
Cholesterol profile
PPD test at 12 years and yearly if high risk
RPR, CBC, U/A
Female: breast self-exam (BSE)
Male: testicular self-exam (TSE)
Female, Pap and pelvic exam yearly after 3 years of
onset of sexual activity or at age 21
Urine gonorrhea and chlamydia tests with yearly PE's
Screening
Depression
Suicide
Tobacco use
Eating disorders
Substance abuse
Pregnancy
Family history of alcoholism or domestic violence
Sexually Transmitted Infections

(continued)

Table II.3 PRIMARY AND SECONDARY PREVENTION FOR AGE-RELATED CONDITIONS (1,4,5) (continued)

Developmental Level	Primary Prevention	Secondary Prevention

	Immunizations
	  Tdap if not received then Td every
	    10 years thereafter
	  Hepatitis B 3-dose series if needed,
	  Hepatitis A series (2) 2-dose series
	  TOPV (if needed to complete 4-dose
	    series)
	  Gardasil (HPV) (series of three for girls
	    ages 11–26, for boys ages 9–18)
	  Pneumococcal (3)	

Young adult (20–39 years)	Health education
	  Weight management with good
	    nutrition as BMR changes
	  Low-cholesterol diet
	  Calcium 100 mg daily (females)
	  Vitamin D 400 units daily (females)
	Lifestyle counseling
	  Stress management skills
	  Safe driving
	  Family planning
	  Divorce
	  Sexual practices
		Complete physical exam at about 20 years, then every
		  5–6 years
		Female: BSE monthly, Pap 1–2 years unless high risk
		Male: TSE monthly
		Parents-to-be: high-risk screening for Down syndrome,
		  Tay-Sachs
		Female pregnant: RPR, rubella titer, Rh factor, amniocen-
		  tesis for women 35 years or older (if desired)
		All females: baseline mammography between ages 35
		  and 40

Parenting skills
Regular exercise
Environmental health choices
Alcohol, drug use
Use of hearing protection devices
Dental hygiene every 6–12 months

Immunizations
If needed one time dose of Tdap, then Td every 10 years thereafter
Influenza yearly
Pneumovax (3)
Varicella (2-dose series for those with no evidence of immunity)
Female: rubella, if serum negative for antibodies
Hepatitis B 3-dose series
Hepatitis A (2)
Gardasil (3-dose series for females from age 11–26)
MMR (If born in 1957 or later 1 or more doses)
Pneumococcal**
diabetes mellitus

If high risk, female with previous breast cancer: annual mammography at 35 years and yearly after, a female with mother or sister who has had breast cancer, same as above
Family history colorectal cancer or high risk: annual stool guaiac, digital rectal, and colonoscopy at intervals determined after baseline colonoscopy.
PPD if high risk
Glaucoma screening at 35 years and along with routine physical exams
Cholesterol profile every 5 years, if normal
Cholesterol profile every year if borderline
Screening (Refer to adolescent section)

Middle-aged adult (40–59 years)

Health education: continue with young adult

Complete physical exam every 5–6 years with complete laboratory evaluation (serum/urine tests, x-ray, ECG)

(continued)

Table II.3 PRIMARY AND SECONDARY PREVENTION FOR AGE-RELATED CONDITIONS (1,4,5) (continued)

Developmental Level	Primary Prevention	Secondary Prevention
	Calcium 1000–1500 mg daily Vitamin D 400 units daily Midlife changes, male and female counseling (see also Young adult) "Empty nest syndrome" Anticipatory guidance for retirement Menopause Grandparenting Dental hygiene every 6–12 months Immunizations Hepatitis B 3-dose series Hepatitis A (2) If needed one time dose of Tdap, then Td every 10 years thereafter Influenza—yearly Pneumococcal (3) at age 65 for all those who were not high risk for vaccine prior	DEXA scan (screening for high-risk men and women for osteoporosis) once then as needed Female: BSE monthly Male: TSE monthly PSA yearly after age 40 for African Americans and Hispanics and after age 50 for others All females: mammogram every 1–2 years (40–49 years) then annual mammography 50 years and older Screening (Refer to adolescent section) Schiotz's tonometry (glaucoma) every 3–5 years Colonoscopy at 50 and 51, then at intervals determined after baseline colonoscopy. Stool guaiac annually at 50 and yearly after
Older adult (60–74 years)	Health education: continue with previous counseling Home safety Retirement Loss of spouse, relatives, friends	Complete physical exam every 2 years with laboratory assessments Blood pressure annually Female: BSE monthly, Pap every 1–3 years annual mammogram Male: TSE monthly, PSA yearly

Special health needs
Calcium 1000–1500 mg daily
Vitamin D 400 units daily
Changes in hearing or vision
Dental/oral hygiene every
6–12 months

Immunizations
Tdap one dose then Td every
10 years
Influenza—annual
Hepatitis B 3-dose series
Hepatitis A (2)
Pneumococcal (3)
Herpes Zoster 60 years or older
unless a live vaccine is
contraindicated

Annual stool guaiac
Colonoscopy (interval determined by baseline results)
Complete eye exam yearly
DEXA scan once and as needed
Screen for high-risk
Depression
Suicide
Alcohol/drug abuse
"Elder abuse"

Old-age adult (75 years and older)
Dental/oral hygiene
every 6–12 months

Immunizations
Tetanus every 10 years
Influenza—annual
Pneumococcal—if not already
received

Discuss Client's Food Choices and Assist as He or She Identifies New Goals for Health Promotion

- Assist in the selection of foods to sustain life and facilitate body functioning.
- Discuss the risk of excess intake of:
  - Salt
  - Starches (e.g., bread, pasta, rice, potatoes)
  - Snack foods
  - Fried foods
  - Processed meats
  - Fats
  - Soda, fruit drinks
- Provide information, when needed, about developmental considerations for dependents.
- Healthful diet (e.g., "basic four," low fat and salt, high complex carbohydrate, sufficient intake of vitamins, minerals, 2 to 3 quarts of water daily).

Discuss the Benefits of a Regular Exercise Program

Advise all Tobacco Users to Quit

Discuss the Elements of Constructive Stress Management

- Assertiveness training
- Problem solving
- Relaxation techniques

Discuss Strategies for Developing Positive Social Networks

Promote Self-Actualization in the Client Who Is Seeking to Promote Health

- Demonstrate an interested but nonjudgmental attitude.
- View the client–nurse relationship as collaborative; the client remains in control of choices, actions, and evaluations.
- Facilitate adoption of new behaviors rather than defining them.
- Listen, reflect, and converse to clarify the client's current behavior patterns and desired goals.
- Enhance the client's strengths, empower with choices and self-control, and always demonstrate respect for those choices.

Assess Knowledge of Primary Prevention

- Safety—accident prevention (e.g., car, machinery, outdoor safety, occupational)
- Weight control
- Avoidance of substance abuse (e.g., alcohol, drugs, tobacco)
- Avoidance of sexually transmitted diseases
- Dental/oral hygiene (e.g., daily, dentist)
- Immunizations

Determine Knowledge Needed to Manage Condition

- Causes
- Treatments
- Medications
- Diet
- Activity
- Risk factors
- Signs/symptoms of complications
- Restrictions
- Follow-up care

Assess If Needed At-Home Resources Are Available

- Caregiver
- Finances
- Equipment

Determine If Referrals Are Indicated (e.g., Social Services, Housekeeping Services, Home Health)

Identify Strategies to Improve Access for the Vulnerable Populations (e.g., Uninsured, Displaced, Homeless, Poor)

- Community centers, school-based clinics, Planned Parenthood, faith-based clinics
- Pharmaceutical companies' assistance programs, generic alternative medications

IMPAIRED HOME MAINTENANCE

NANDA-I Definition

Inability to independently maintain a safe growth-promoting immediate environment

Defining Characteristics

Major (Must Be Present, One or More)

Expressions or observations of:
Difficulty maintaining home hygiene
Difficulty maintaining a safe home
Inability to keep up home
Lack of sufficient finances

Minor (May Be Present)

Repeated infections   Unwashed utensils
Infestations   Offensive odors
Accumulated wastes   Overcrowding

Related Factors

Pathophysiologic

Related to impaired functional ability* secondary to chronic debilitating disease*

Diabetes mellitus   Congestive heart failure
Arthritis   Cerebrovascular accident
Chronic obstructive pulmonary Parkinson's disease
  disease (COPD)   Muscular dystrophy
Multiple sclerosis   Cancer

Situational (Personal, Environmental)

Related to change in functional ability of (specify family member) secondary to:
Injury* (fractured limb, spinal cord injury)
Surgery (amputation, ostomy)
Impaired mental status (memory lapses, depression, anxiety–
  severe panic)
Substance abuse (alcohol, drugs)

Related to inadequate support system*

Related to loss of family member

Related to deficient knowledge

Related to insufficient finances*

Related to unfamiliarity with neighborhood resources*

Maturational

Infant
Related to multiple care requirements secondary to:
High-risk newborn

Older Adult
Related to multiple care requirements secondary to:
Family member with deficits (cognitive, motor, sensory)

Author's Note

With rising life expectancy and declining mortality rates, the number of older adults is steadily increasing, with many living alone at home. Eighty percent of people 65 years or older report one or more chronic diseases. Of adults 65 to 74 years of age, 20% report activity limitations, and 15% cannot perform at least one activity of daily living (ADL) independently (Miller, 2009). The shift from health care primarily in hospitals to reduced lengths of stay has resulted in the discharge of many functionally compromised people to their homes. Often a false assumption is that someone will assume the management of household responsibilities until the client has recovered.

Impaired Home Maintenance describes situations in which a client or family needs teaching, supervision, or assistance to manage the household. Usually, a community health nurse is the best professional to complete an assessment of the home and the client's functioning there. Nurses in acute settings can make referrals for home visits for assessment.

A nurse who diagnoses a need for teaching to prevent household problems may use *Risk for Impaired Home Maintenance* related to insufficient knowledge of (specify).

NOC

Family Functioning

Goal

The client or caretaker will express satisfaction with home situation, as evidenced by the following indicators:

- Identify factors that restrict self-care and home management.
- Demonstrate ability to perform skills necessary for care of the home.

NIC

Home Maintenance Assistance, Environmental Management: Safety, Environmental Management

Interventions

The following interventions apply to many with impaired home maintenance, regardless of etiology.

Assess for Causative or Contributing Factors

- Lack of knowledge
- Insufficient funds

- Lack of necessary equipment or aids
- Inability (illness, sensory deficits, motor deficits) to perform household activities
- Impaired cognitive functioning
- Impaired emotional functioning

Reduce or Eliminate Causative or Contributing Factors, If Possible.

Lack of Knowledge

- Determine with client and family the information they need to learn:
  - Monitoring skills (pulse, circulation, urine)
  - Medication administration (procedure, side effects, precautions)
  - Treatment/procedures
  - Equipment use/maintenance
  - Safety issues (e.g., environmental)
  - Community resources
  - Follow-up care
  - Anticipatory guidance (e.g., emotional and social needs, alternatives to home care)
  - Initiate teaching; give detailed written instruction.

Insufficient Funds

- Consult with social service department for assistance.
- Consult with service organizations (e.g., American Heart Association, The Lung Association, American Cancer Society) for assistance.

Lack of Necessary Equipment or Aids

- Determine type of equipment needed, considering availability, cost, and durability.
- Seek assistance from agencies that rent or loan supplies.
  - Teach care and maintenance of supplies to increase length of use.
  - Consider adapting equipment to reduce cost.

Inability to Perform Household Activities

- Determine type of assistance needed (e.g., meals, housework, transportation); assist client to obtain it.

Meals

- Discuss with relatives the possibility of freezing complete meals that require only heating (e.g., small containers of soup, stews, casseroles).
- Determine availability of meal services for ill people (e.g., Meals on Wheels, church groups).
- Teach people about nutritious foods that are easily prepared (e.g., hard-boiled eggs, tuna fish, peanut butter).

Housework

- Encourage client to contract with an adolescent for light housekeeping.
- Refer client to community agency for assistance.

Transportation

- Determine availability of transportation for shopping and health care.
- Suggest client request rides with neighbors to places they drive routinely.

Impaired Cognitive Functioning

- Assess client's ability to maintain a safe household.
- Refer to *Risk for Injury* related to lack of awareness of hazards.
- Initiate appropriate referrals.

Impaired Emotional Functioning

- Assess severity of the dysfunction.
- Refer to *Ineffective Coping* for additional assessment and interventions.

Initiate Health Teaching and Referrals, as Indicated

- Refer to community nursing agency for a home visit.
- Provide information about how to make the home environment safe and clean (Bulechek, Butcher, & Dochterman, 2008).
- Refer to community agencies (e.g., visitors, meal programs, homemakers, adult day care).
- Refer to support groups (e.g., local Alzheimer's Association, American Cancer Society).

HOPELESSNESS

NANDA-I Definition

Subjective state in which an individual sees limited or no alternatives or personal choices available and is unable to mobilize energy on own behalf

Defining Characteristics

Major (Must Be Present, One or More)

Expresses profound, overwhelming, sustained apathy in response to a situation perceived as impossible.
States "My future seems dark to me" (Yip & Chang, 2006).

Physiologic
Increased sleep   Decreased response to stimuli*
Lack of energy

Emotional
Person Feels:
As though they do not receive any breaks and there is no reason
    to believe they will in the future
Empty or drained
Demoralized
Helpless
Incompetent or trapped
Lack of meaning or purpose in life
Sense of loss and deprivation
Unable to seek good fortune, luck, God's favor

Person Exhibits:
Passivity* and lack of   Inability to accomplish
    involvement in care   anything
Decreased affect*   Slowed thought processes
Giving up–given up complex   Demoralization
Lack of responsibility for   Fatigue
    decisions and life   Participation in health related
Isolating behaviors   risk-taking behaviors such
Negative present and future   as failure to wear seat belt,
    comments   helmet, or driving while
Decreased verbalization*   intoxicated
Lack of ambition, initiative*,
    and interest

Cognitive
Focus on past and future, not here and now
Decreased flexibility in thought processes
Rigidity (e.g., all-or-none thinking)
Lack of imagination and wishing capabilities
Inability to identify or accomplish desired objectives and goals
Inability to plan, organize, make decisions, or problem-solve
Inability to recognize sources of hope
Suicidal thoughts

Minor (May Be Present)

Physiologic
Anorexia   Weight loss

Emotional

Person Feels:

A lump in the throat

Tense

Discouraged

Overwhelmed and exhausted

At the end of his or her rope

Loss of gratification from roles
and relationships

Vulnerable

Person Exhibits:

Poor eye contact

Decreased motivation

Sighing

Regression

Resignation

Fatigue (Hammell, Miller,
Forwell, Forman, &
Jacobson, 2009)

Cognitive

Decreased ability to integrate information received

Loss of time perception (past, present, and future)

Decreased ability to recall from the past

Inability to communicate effectively

Distorted thought perceptions and associations or confusion

Unreasonable judgment

Related Factors

Pathophysiologic

Any chronic or terminal illness (e.g., heart disease, diabetes, kidney disease, cancer, acquired immunodeficiency syndrome [AIDS]) can cause or contribute to hopelessness.

Related to impaired ability to cope secondary to the following:

Failing or deteriorating physiologic condition

New and unexpected signs or symptoms of previously diagnosed disease process (i.e., recurrence of cancer) (Brothers and Anderson, 2009).

Prolonged pain, discomfort, and weakness

Impaired functional abilities (walking, elimination, eating, dressing, bathing, speaking, writing)

Treatment Related

Related to:

Prolonged treatments (e.g., chemotherapy, radiation) that cause pain, nausea, and discomfort

Treatments that alter body image (e.g., surgery, chemotherapy)

Prolonged diagnostic studies

Prolonged dependence on equipment for life support (e.g., dialysis, respirator)
Prolonged dependence on equipment for monitoring bodily functions (e.g., telemetry)

Situational (Personal, Environmental)

Related to:
Prolonged activity restriction (e.g., fractures, spinal cord injury, imprisonment)
Prolonged isolation (e.g., infectious diseases, reverse isolation for suppressed immune system)
Abandonment by, separation from, or isolation from significant others (Brothers and Anderson, 2009)
Inability to achieve valued goals in life (marriage, education, children)
Inability to participate in desired activities (walking, sports, work)
Loss of something or someone valued (spouse, children, friend, financial resources)
Prolonged caretaking responsibilities (spouse, child, parent)
Recurrence of breast cancer
Exposure to long-term physiologic or psychological stress
Recurrence of breast cancer (Brothers & Anderson, 2009)
Loss of belief in transcendent values/God
Ongoing, repetitive losses in community related to AIDS
Repetitive nature disasters (hurricanes, tornadoes, flooding, fires)
Prolonged exposure to violence and war

Maturational

Child
Loss of autonomy related to illness (e.g., fracture)
Loss of bodily functions
Loss of caregiver
Loss of trust in significant other
Inability to achieve developmental tasks (trust, autonomy, initiative, industry)
Rejection, abuse, or abandonment by caregivers

Adolescent
Change in body image
Inability to achieve developmental task (role identity)
Loss of bodily functions
Loss of significant other (peer, family)
Rejection by family

Adult
Abortion
Impaired bodily functions, loss of body part
Impaired relationships (separation, divorce)
Inability to achieve developmental tasks (intimacy, commitment, productivity)
Loss of job, career
Loss of significant others (death of spouse, child)
Miscarriage

Older Adult

Cognitive deficits
Inability to achieve developmental tasks
Loss of independence

Loss of significant others, things (in general)
Motor deficits
Sensory deficits

Author's Note

Hopelessness describes a person who sees no possibility that his or her life will improve and maintains that no one can do anything to help. *Hopelessness* differs from *Powerlessness* in that a hopeless person sees no solution or no way to achieve what is desired, even if he or she feels in control. In contrast, a powerless person may see an alternative or answer, yet be unable to do anything about it because of lack of control or resources. Sustained feelings of powerlessness may lead to hopelessness. Hopelessness is commonly related to grief, depression, and suicide. For a person at risk for suicide, the nurse should also use the diagnosis *Risk for Suicide*. A study by Brothers and Anderson (2009) supported the view that hopelessness is a distinct concept and not merely a symptom of depression.

NOC

Decision-Making, Depression Control, Hope, Quality of Life

Goals

- Demonstrate increased energy, as evidenced by an increase in activities (e.g., self-care, exercise, hobbies).
- Express desirable expectations for the near future. Describe one's own meaning and purpose in life.
- Demonstrate initiative, self-direction, and autonomy in decision-making. Demonstrate effective problem-solving strategies.
- Redefine the future, setting realistic goals with expectation to meet these goals.
- Exhibit peace and comfort with situation.

The client will strive for the goals listed above as evidenced by the following indicators:

- Shares suffering openly and constructively with others.
- Reminisces and reviews life positively.
- Considers values and the meaning of life.
- Expresses optimism about the present.
- Practices energy conservation.
- Develops, improves, and maintains positive relationships with others.
- Participates in a significant role.
- Expresses spiritual beliefs.

NIC

Hope Instillation, Values Classification, Decision-Making Support, Spiritual Support, Support System Enhancement

Interventions

Assist Client to Identify and Express Feelings

- Listen actively, treat the client as an individual, and accept his or her feelings. Convey empathy to promote verbalization of doubts, fears, and concerns.
- Validate and reflect impressions with the person. It is important to realize that clients with cancer often have their own reality, which may differ from the nurse's.
- Encourage expressions of how hope is uncertain and areas in which hope has failed the client.
- Assist the client in recognizing that hopelessness is part of everyone's life and demands recognition. The client can use it as a source of energy, imagination, and freedom to consider alternatives. Hopelessness can lead to self-discovery.
- Assist the client to understand that he or she can deal with the hopeless aspects of life by separating them from the hopeful aspects. Help the client to identify and to acknowledge areas of hopelessness. Help the client to distinguish between the possible and impossible.
- The nurse mobilizes a client's internal and external resources to promote and instill hope. Assist clients to identify their personal reasons for living that provide meaning and purpose to their lives.

Assess and Mobilize the Client's Internal Resources (Autonomy, Independence, Rationality, Cognitive Thinking, Flexibility, Spirituality)

- Emphasize strengths, not weaknesses.
- Compliment the client on appearance or efforts as appropriate.
- Promote motivation.
  - Identify reasons for living.
  - Identify client's perception of hope.
- Identify areas of success and usefulness; emphasize past accomplishments. Use this information to develop goals with the client.
- Assist the client in identifying things he or she has fun doing and perceives as humorous. Such activities can serve as distractions to discomfort and allow the client to progress to cognitive comfort (Hinds, Martin & Vogel, 1987).
- Assist the client in identifying sources of hope (e.g., relationships, faith, things to accomplish).
- Assist the client in adjusting and developing realistic short- and long-term goals (progress from simple to more complex; may use a "goals poster" to indicate type and time for achieving specific goals). Attainable expectations promote hope.
- Inspire hope by reflecting on the following metaphors of hope:
  - Living in hope is a living dimension
  - Hoping for something is a doing dimension
  - Hope as a light on the horizon is a becoming dimension
  - Hope as a human-to-human relationship is a relational dimension
  - Hope versus hopelessness: two sides of the same coin is a dialectic dimension
  - Hope as a weathering storm is a situational and dynamic dimension
- Teach the client to monitor specific signs of progress to use as self-reinforcement.
- Encourage "means–end" thinking in positive terms (i.e., "If I do this, then I'll be able to…").
- Foster lightheartedness and the sharing of uplifting memories.

Assist the Client With Problem Solving and Decision-Making

- Respect the client as a competent decision-maker; treat his or her decisions and desires with respect.
- Encourage verbalization to determine the client's perception of choices.
- Clarify the client's values to determine what is important.
- Correct misinformation.

- Assist the client in identifying those problems he or she cannot resolve to advance to problems he or she can. In other words, assist the client to move away from dwelling on the impossible and hopeless and to begin to deal with realistic and hopeful matters.
- Assess the client's perceptions of self and others in relation to size. (People with hopelessness often perceive others as large and difficult to deal with and themselves as small.) If perceptions are unrealistic, assist the client to reassess them to restore proper scale.
- Promote flexibility. Encourage the client to try alternatives and take risks.

Assist Client to Learn Effective Coping Skills

- Assist the client with setting realistic, attainable short- and long-term goals.
- Teach the importance of mutuality in sharing concerns.
- Teach the value of confronting issues.
- Allow the client time to reminisce to gain insight into past experiences.
- Explain the benefits of distraction from negative events.
- Teach and assist with relaxation techniques before anticipated stressful events.
- Encourage mental imagery to promote positive thought processes.
- Teach the client to "hope to be" the best person possible today and to appreciate the fullness of each moment.
- Teach the client to maximize aesthetic experiences (e.g., smell of coffee, back rub, feeling warmth of the sun, or a breeze) that can inspire hope.
- Teach the client to anticipate experiences he or she delights in daily (e.g., walking, reading favorite book, writing a letter).
- Assist the client to express spiritual beliefs (Jennings, 1997).
- Teach the client ways to conserve and generate energy through moderate physical exercise.
- Encourage music therapy, aromatherapy, and message with essential oils to improve the client's physical and mental status.

Assess and Mobilize the Client's External Resources

Family or Significant Others
- Involve the family and significant others in plan of care.
- Encourage the client to spend increased time or thoughts with loved ones in healthy relationships.
- Teach the family members their role in sustaining hope through supportive, positive relationships.

- Discuss the client's attainable goals with family.
- Empower clients who have chronic disease by instilling hope through the bolstering of support systems.
- Convey hope, information, and confidence to the family because they will convey their feelings to the client.
- Use touch and closeness with the client to demonstrate to the family its acceptability (provide privacy).
- Herth (1993) found the following strategies to foster hope in caregivers of terminally ill people:
  - *Cognitive reframing*—positive self-talk, praying/meditating, and envisioning hopeful images (this may involve letting go of expectations for things to be different)
  - *Time refocusing*—focusing less on the future and more on living one day at a time
  - Belief in a power greater than self—empowering the caregiver's hope
  - *Balancing available energy*—listening to music or other favorite activities to empower the caregiver's hope through uplifting energy

Health Care Team
- Develop a positive, trusting nurse–client relationship by:
  - Answering questions
  - Respecting client's feelings
  - Providing consistent care
  - Following through on requests
  - Touching
  - Providing comfort
  - Being honest
  - Conveying positive attitude
- Convey attitude of "We care too much about you to let you just give up," or "I can help you."
- Hold conferences and share the client's goals with staff.
- Share advances in technology and research for treatment of diseases.
- Have available a list of laughter resources (e.g., books, films).
- Provide nurses and caregivers support in times of disaster.

Support Groups
- Encourage the client to share concerns with others who have had a similar problem or disease and positive experiences from coping effectively with it.
- Provide information on self-help groups (e.g., "Make today count"—40 chapters in the United States and Canada; "I can cope"—series for clients with cancer; "We Can Weekend"—for families of clients with cancer).

God or Higher Powers
- Assess the client's belief support system (value, past experiences, religious activities, relationship with God, meaning and purpose of prayer; refer to *Spiritual Distress*).
- Create an environment in which the client feels free to express spirituality.
- Allow the client time and opportunities to reflect on the meaning of suffering, death, and dying.
- Accept, respect, and support the client's hope in God.

Pediatric Interventions (Adolescent)

- Provide truthful explanations.
- Engage in activities.
- If appropriate, discuss knowledge of survivors.
- Focus on future.
- Discuss topics interesting to the child.
- Use humor if appropriate.

RISK FOR COMPROMISED HUMAN DIGNITY

NANDA-I Definition

At risk for perceived loss of respect and honor

Risk Factors

Treatment Related

Related to multiple factors associated with hospitalization, institutionalization, supervised group living environments, or any health care environment.

Examples of factors are as follows:

- Unfamiliar procedures
- Intrusions for clinical procedures
- Multiple, unfamiliar personnel
- Assistance needed for personal hygiene
- Painful procedures
- Unfamiliar terminology

Situational (Personal, Environmental)

Related to the nature of restrictions and environment of incarceration.

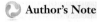 **Author's Note**

Risk for compromised human dignity was accepted by NANDA-I in 2006.

This nursing diagnosis presents a new application for nursing practice. All clients are at risk for this diagnosis. Providing respect and honor to all clients, families, and communities is a critical core element of professional nursing. Prevention of compromised human dignity must be a focus of all nursing interventions. It is the central concept of a caring profession.

This diagnosis can also apply to prisoners, who as part of their penalty will be deprived of some rights, for example, privacy and movement. Prisoners, however, should always be treated with respect and not be tortured or humiliated. Nurses have the obligation to honor and "do no harm" in all settings in which they practice.

This author recommends that this diagnosis be developed and integrated into a Standard Care of the Nursing Department for all clients and families. The outcomes and interventions apply to all individuals, families, and groups. This Department of Nursing Standards of Practice could also include *Risk for Infection*, *Risk for Infection Transmission*, *Risk for Falls*, and *Risk for Compromised Family Coping*.

NOC

Abuse Protection, Comfort Level, Dignified Dying, Information Processing, Knowledge: Illness Care, Self-Esteem, Spiritual Well-Being

Goals

The client will report respectful and considerate care as evidenced by the following indicators:

- Respect for privacy
- Consideration of emotions
- Anticipation of feelings
- Given options and control
- Asked for permission
- Given explanations
- Minimization of body part exposure
- No involvement of unnecessary personnel during stressful procedures

NIC

Patient Rights Protection, Anticipatory Guidance, Counseling, Emotional Support, Preparatory Sensory Information, Family Support, Humor, Mutual Goal Setting, and Teaching: Procedure/Treatment, Touch

Interventions

- Determine and accept your own moral responsibility.
- Determine if the agency has a policy for prevention of compromised human dignity (Note: this type of policy or standard may be titled differently).
- Review the policy: Does it include (Walsh & Kowanko, 2002):
  - Protection of privacy and private space
  - Acquiring permission continuously
  - Providing time for decision-making
  - Advocating for the client
- Ensure that there are clear guidelines regarding the number of personnel (e.g., students, nurses, physicians, residents, interns) that can be present when confidential and/or stressful information is discussed.
- Reduce exposure of the client's body with the use of drapes and limit the gaze of others who are not needed.
- Provide care to each client and family as you would expect or demand for your family, partner, child, friend, or colleague.
- When performing a procedure, engage the client in a conversation; act as if the situation is a matter-of-fact for you in order to reduce embarrassment; use humor if appropriate; talk to the client even if he or she is unresponsive.
- Explain the procedure to the client during painful or embarrassing procedures and explain what he or she will feel.
- Determine if unnecessary personnel are present before a vulnerable or stressful event is initiated (e.g., code or a painful or embarrassing procedure); advise them that they are not needed.
- Allow the client an opportunity to share his or her feelings after a difficult situation and maintain privacy for the client's information and emotional responses.
- Role-model and advocate to maintain client dignity after death.
- Discuss with involved personnel an incident that was disrespectful to a client or family and report any incident that may be a violation of a client's dignity to the appropriate person.
- Engage in a dialogue with the client and family regarding their pre-emptions of the present plan of care, and decisions that may need to be explained.
- When extreme measures that are futile are planned for or are being provided for a client, refer to *Moral Distress*.
- Practice expecting that honoring and protecting the dignity of a client/group is not a value, but a way of being.

DISORGANIZED INFANT BEHAVIOR

Disorganized Infant Behavior
Risk for Disorganized Infant Behavior

NANDA-I Definition

Disintegrated physiologic and neurobehavioral responses of infant to the environment

Defining Characteristics**

Autonomic System

Cardiac
Increased rate

Respiration
Pauses   Gasping
Tachypnea

Skin Color Changes*
Paling around nostrils   Cyanosis
Perioral duskiness   Grayness
Mottling   Flushing/ruddiness

Visceral
Hiccuping*   Grunting
Straining as if producing   Spitting up
  a bowel movement   Gagging

Motor
Seizures   Twitches*
Sneezing*   Sighing*
Tremors/startles*   Coughing*
Yawning

Motor System

Fluctuating Tone
Flaccidity of:
Trunk   Extremities
Face

** Vandenberg (1990); Hockenberry & Wilson (2009)

Hypertonicity
Extending legs
Arching
Saluting
Splaying fingers*

Airplaning
Extending tongue
Sitting on air
Fisting*

Hyperflexions
Trunk
Fetal tuck

Extremities

Frantic Diffuse Activity

State System (Range)

Difficulty maintaining state control
Difficulty in transitions from one state to another

Sleep
Twitches*
Whimpers
Makes sounds
Grimaces

Makes jerky movements
Fusses in sleep
Has irregular respirations

Awake
Eyes floating
Panicky, worried*, dull look
Glassy eyes
Weak cry
Strain, fussiness

Irritability*
Staring*
Abrupt state changes
Gaze aversion*

Attention–Interaction System

Attempts at engaging behaviors elicit stress
Impaired ability to orient, attend, engage in reciprocal social
   interactions
Difficulty consoling

Related Factors**

Pathophysiologic

*Related to immature or altered central nervous system (CNS)
secondary to:*
Prematurity*
Perinatal factors
Hyperbilirubinemia
Hypoglycemia

Infection
Intraventricular hemorrhage
Congenital anomalies

** Askin & Wilson (2007)

Prenatal exposure to drugs/
   alcohol

Decreased oxygen saturation
Respiratory distress

Related to nutritional deficits secondary to:

Reflux

Feeding intolerance*

Swallowing problems

Emesis

Colic

Poor Suck/Swallow
   coordination

Related to excess stimulation secondary to:

Oral hypersensitivity

Frequent handling and position changes

Treatment Related

Related to excess stimulation secondary to:

Invasive procedures*

Movement

Lights

Medication administration

Restraints

Noise (e.g., prolonged alarm,
   voices, environment)

Chest physical therapy

Feeding

Tubes, tape

Related to inability to see caregivers secondary to eye patches

Situational (Personal, Environmental)

Related to unpredictable interactions secondary to multiple caregivers

Related to imbalance of task touch and consoling touch

Related to decreased ability to self-regulate secondary to:
(Holditch-Davis & Blackburn, 2007)

Sudden movement

Noise

Prematurity*

Disrupted sleep–wake cycles

Fatigue

Stimulation that exceeds the
   infant's tolerance threshold

Environmental demands

Author's Note

Disorganized Infant Behavior describes an infant who has difficulty regulating and adapting to external stimuli due to immature neurobehavioral development and increased environmental stimuli associated with neonatal units. When an infant is overstimulated or stressed, he or she uses energy to adapt; this depletes the supply of energy available for physiologic growth. The goal of nursing care is to assist the infant to conserve energy by reducing environmental stimuli, allowing the infant sufficient time to adapt to handling, and providing sensory input appropriate to the infant's physiologic and neurobehavioral status.

NOC

Neurologic Status, Preterm Infant Organization, Sleep, Comfort Level

Goal

The infant will demonstrate increase signs of stability as evidenced by the following indicators:

- Exhibit smooth, stable respirations; pink, stable color; consistent tone; improve posture; calm, focused alertness; well-modulated sleep; responsive to visual and social stimuli.
- Demonstrate self-regulatory skills as sucking, hand to mouth, grasping, hand holding, hand and foot clasping, tucking.

The parent(s)/caregiver(s) will describe techniques to reduce environmental stress in agency, at home, or both.

- Describe situations that stress infant.
- Describe signs/symptoms of stress in infant.
- Describe ways to support infant's efforts to self-calm (VandenBerg, 2007).

NIC

Environmental Management, Neurologic Monitoring, Sleep Enhancement, Newborn Care, Parent Education: Newborn Positioning

Interventions

See Related Factors.

Reduce or Eliminate Contributing Factors, If Possible

Pain
- Observe for responses that are different from baseline and have been associated with neonatal pain responses (Bozzette, 1993):
  - Facial responses (open mouth, brow bulge, grimace, chin quiver, nasolabial furrow, taut tongue)
  - Motor responses (flinch, muscle rigidity, clenched hands, withdrawal) (AAP, 2006)
  - Pain management requires routine assessment using a reliable pain-assessment tool which measures both physiologic and behavioral indicators of pain.
  - Develop strategies to minimize the number and frequency of painful or stressful procedures in the NICU.

- Provide pharmacologic and/or nonpharmacologic pain relief for all painful procedures, such as gavage tube placement, tape removal, needle insertions, heel sticks, insertion and removal of chest tubes, intubation, prolonged mechanical ventilation, eye exams, circumcision, and surgery.
- Pharmacologic implications:
  - Doses of effective medications to reduce pain may be close to doses that cause toxicity in the neonate.
  - Early administration of pain medication may reduce the effective dose needed and thereby reduce toxicity.
  - Treatment of pain must be guided by ongoing pain assessments.
  - Pain relief for circumcisions should be provided.
  - Topical anesthetics can reduce pain for some procedures such as venipuncture, lumbar puncture, and IV insertion. Due to a risk of methemoglobinemia, in certain situations, use should be on intact skin only, no more than once a day, and not with other drugs known to cause methemoglobinemia.
- Nonpharmacologic interventions:
  - Developmental care that includes attention to behavioral cues and reducing environmental stimuli, has shown to be effective in reducing pain from minor procedures.
  - Facilitated tuck
  - Swaddling
  - Supportive bedding
  - Side-lying position
  - Kangaroo care
  - Nonnutritive suck
  - Oral sucrose solution combined with sucking has proved effective at reducing pain from many minor procedures.

Disrupted 24-hour Diurnal Cycles
- Evaluate the need for and frequency of each intervention.
- Consider 24-hour caregiving assignment and primary caregiving to provide consistent caregiving throughout the day and night for the infant from the onset of admission. This is important in terms of responding to increasingly more mature sleep cycles, feeding ability, and especially emotional development.
- Consider supporting the infant's transition to and maintenance of sleep by avoiding peaks of frenzy and overexhaustion; continuously maintaining a calm, regular environment and schedule; and establishing a reliable, repeatable pattern of gradual transition into sleep in prone and side-lying positions in the isolette or crib.

Problematic Feeding Experiences
- Observe and record infant's readiness for participation with feeding.

Hunger Cues

- Transitioning to drowsy or alert state
- Mouthing, rooting, or sucking
- Bringing hands to mouth
- Crying that is not relieved with pacifier or nonnutritive sucking alone

Physiologic Stability

- Look for regulated breathing patterns, stable color, and stable digestion.
- Promote nurturing environment in support of a coregulatory feeding experience.
- Decrease environmental stimulation.
- Provide comfortable seating (be especially sensitive to the needs of postpartum mothers: e.g., soft cushions, small stool to elevate legs, supportive pillows for nursing).
- Encourage softly swaddling the infant to facilitate flexion and balanced tone during feeding.
- Explore feeding methods that meet the goals of both infant and family (e.g., breastfeeding, bottle-feeding, gavage).

Support the Infant's Self-Regulatory Efforts

- When administering painful or stressful procedures, consider actions to enhance calmness.
- Support the flexed position with another caregiver.
- Provide opportunities to feed while shielding the infant from other stresses.
- Consider the efficient execution of necessary manipulations while supporting the infant's behavioral organization.
- Consider *unhurried* reorganization and stabilization of the infant's regulation (e.g., position prone, give opportunities to hold onto caregiver's finger and suck, encase trunk and back of head in caregiver's hand, provide inhibition to soles of feet).
- Consider removing extraneous stimulation (e.g., stroking, talking, shifting position) to institute restabilization. Consider spending 15 to 20 minutes after manipulation; over time, the infant's self-regulatory abilities will improve, making the caregiver's intervention less important.
- Consider supporting the infant's transition to and maintenance of sleep by avoiding peaks of frenzy and over-exhaustion; by continuously maintaining a calm, regular environment and schedule; and by establishing a reliable, repeatable pattern of gradual transition into sleep in prone and side-lying positions in the isolette or crib.
- Consider initiating calming on the caregiver's body and then transferring the baby to the crib as necessary. For other infants,

this may be too arousing, and transition is accomplished more easily in the isolette with the provision of steady boundaries and encasing without any stimulation.

- A nonstimulating sleep space with minimal exciting visual targets, social inputs, and so forth, may need to be made available to facilitate relaxation before sleep. A regular sleep routine helps many infants.

Reduce Environmental Stimuli

Noise (Merenstein & Gardner, 1998; Thomas, 1989)

- Do not tap on incubator.
- Place a folded blanket on top of the incubator if it is the only work surface available.
- Slowly open and close porthole.
- Pad incubator doors to reduce banging.
- Use plastic instead of metal waste cans.
- Remove water from ventilator tubing.
- Speak softly at the bedside and only when necessary.
- Slowly drop the head of the mattress.
- Eliminate radios.
- Close doors slowly.
- Position the infant's bed away from sources of noise (e.g., telephone, intercom, unit equipment).
- Consider the following methods to reduce unnecessary noise in the NICU:
  - Perform rounds away from the bedsides.
  - Adapt large equipment to eliminate noise and clutter.
  - Alert staff when the decibel level in the unit exceeds 60 db (e.g., by a light attached to a sound meter). Institute quiet time for 10 minutes to lower noise.
  - Move more vulnerable infants out of unit traffic patterns.

Lights

- Use full-spectrum instead of white light at bedside. Avoid fluorescent lights.
- Cover cribs, incubators, and radiant warmers completely during sleep and partially during awake periods.
- Install dimmer switches, shades, and curtains. Avoid bright lights.
- Shade infants' eyes with a blanket tent or cutout box.
- Avoid visual stimuli on cribs.
- Shield eyes from bright procedure lights. Avoid patches unless for phototherapy.

Position Infant in Postures That Permit Flexion and Minimize Flailing

- Consider gentle, *unhurried* reorganization and stabilization of infant's regulation by supporting the infant in softly tucked prone position, giving opportunities to hold onto caregiver's finger and suck, encasing trunk and back of head in caregiver's hand, and providing inhibition to soles of feet.
- Use the prone/side-lying position.
- Avoid the supine position.
- Swaddle baby, if possible, to maintain flexion.
- Create a nest using soft bedding (e.g., natural sheepskin, soft cotton, flannel).
- Avoid oversized diapers to allow you to perceive normal hip alignment.
- Avoid tension on lines or tubing.

Reduce the Stress Associated With Handling

- When moving or lifting the infant, contain him or her with your hands by wrapping or placing rolled blankets around the body.
- Maintain containment during procedures and caregiving activities.
- Handle slowly and gently. Avoid stroking.
- Initiate all interactions and treatments with one sense stimulus at a time (e.g., touch), then slowly progress to visual, auditory, and movement.
- Assess child for cues for readiness, impending disorganization, or stability; respond to cues.
- Support minimal disruption of the infant's own evolving 24-hour sleep–wake cycles.
- Use PRN instead of routine suctioning or postural drainage.
- Use minimal adhesive tape. Remove any carefully.

Reduce Disorganized Behavior During Active Interventions and Transport

- Have a plan for transport, with assigned roles for each team member.
- Establish behavior cues of stress on this infant with the primary nurse before transport.
- Minimize sensory input:
  - Use calm, quiet voices.
  - Shade the infant's eyes from light.
  - Protect infant from unnecessary touch.
- Support the infant's softly tucked postures with your hands and offer something to grasp (your finger or corner of a soft blanket or cloth).
- Swaddle the infant or place him or her in a nest made of blankets.

- Ensure that the transport equipment (e.g., ventilator) is ready. Warm mattress or use sheepskin.
- Carefully and smoothly move the infant. Avoid talking, if possible.
- Consider conducting caregiving routines while parent(s) or designated caregiver hold infant, whenever possible.
- Reposition in 2 to 3 hours or sooner if infant behavior suggests discomfort.

Engage Parents in Planning Care

- Encourage them to share their feelings, fears, and expectations.
- Consider involving parents in creating the family's developmental plan:
  - My strengths are:
  - Time-out signals:
  - These things stress me:
  - How you can help me:
- Teach caregivers to continually observe the changing capabilities to determine the appropriate positioning and bedding options, for example infant may fight containment (Hockenberry & Wilson, 2009).

Initiate Health Teaching and Referrals as Indicated

Review the Following Information Relating to Growth and Development of the Infant and Family in Anticipatory Guidance for Home

Health Concerns

- Feeding
- Hygiene
- Illness
- Infection
- Safety
- Temperature
- Growth and development

State Modulation

- Appropriate stimulation
- Sleep–wake patterns

Parent–Infant Interaction

- Behavior cues
- Signs of stress

Infant's Environment

- Animate, inanimate stimulation
- Playing with infant
- Role of father and siblings

Parental Coping and Support

• Support network
• Challenges
• Problem solving

Discuss Transition to Community Supports (Nursing Respite, Social and Civic Groups, Religious Affiliations)

Refer for Follow-Up Home Visits

Risk for Disorganized Infant Behavior

NANDA-I Definition

At risk for alteration in integrating and modulation of the physiologic and behavioral systems of functioning (i.e., autonomic, motor, state-organization, self-regulatory, and attentional-interactional systems

Risk Factors

Refer to Related Factors.

Related Factors

Refer to *Disorganized Infant Behavior*.

Interventions

Refer to *Disorganized Infant Behavior*.

RISK FOR INFECTION

NANDA-I Definition

At risk for being invaded by pathogenic organisms

Risk Factors

See Related Factors.

Related Factors

Various health problems and situations can create favorable conditions that would encourage the development of infections. Some common factors follow.

Pathophysiologic

Related to compromised host defenses secondary to:
Cancer
Altered or insufficient
   leukocytes
Arthritis
Respiratory disorders
Periodontal disease
Renal failure
Hematologic disorders

Hepatic disorders
Diabetes mellitus*
Acquired immunodeficiency
   syndrome (AIDS)
Alcoholism
Immunosuppression*
Immunodeficiency
   secondary to: specify

Related to compromised circulation secondary to:
Lymphedema
Obesity*

Peripheral vascular disease

Treatment Related

Related to a site for organism invasion secondary to:
Surgery
Invasive lines
Dialysis

Intubation
Total parenteral nutrition
Enteral feedings

Related to compromised host defenses secondary to:
Radiation therapy
Organ transplant
Medication therapy (specify; e.g., chemotherapy,
   immunosuppressants)

Situational (Personal, Environmental)

Related to compromised host defenses secondary to:
History of infections
Malnutrition*
Prolonged immobility

Stress
Increased hospital stay
Smoking

Related to a site for organism invasion secondary to:
Trauma (accidental, intentional)
Postpartum period
Bites (animal, insect, human)
Thermal injuries
Warm, moist, dark environment (skin folds, casts)

Related to contact with contagious agents (nosocomial or community acquired)

Maturational

Newborns
Related to increased vulnerability of infant secondary to:
HIV positive mother
Lack of maternal antibodies (dependent on maternal exposures)
Lack of normal flora
Maternal substance addiction
Open wounds (umbilical, circumcision)
Immature immune system

Infant/Child
Related to lack of immunization

Adolescent
Related to lack of immunization

Related to multiple sex partners

Older Adult
Related to increased vulnerability secondary to:
Diminished immune response   Chronic diseases
Debilitated condition

 Author's Note

All people are at risk for infection. Secretion control, environmental control, and hand washing before and after client care reduce the risk of transmission of organisms. Included in the population of those at risk for infection is a smaller group who are at high risk for infection. *Risk for Infection* describes a person whose host defenses are compromised, thus increasing susceptibility to environmental pathogens or his or her own endogenous flora (e.g., a person with chronic liver dysfunction or with an invasive line). Nursing interventions for such a person focus on minimizing introduction of organisms and increasing resistance to infection (e.g., improving nutritional status). For a person with an infection, the situation is best described by the collaborative problem *RC of Sepsis*.

  Risk for Infection Transmission describes a person at high risk for transferring an infectious agent to others. Some people are at high risk both for acquiring opportunistic agents and for transmitting infecting organisms, warranting the use of both *Risk for Infection* and *Risk for Infection Transmission*.

Infection Status, Wound Healing: Primary Intention, Immune Status

Goal

The person will report risk factors associated with infection and precautions needed as evidenced by the following indicators:

- Demonstrate meticulous hand washing technique by the time of discharge.
- Describe methods of transmission of infection.
- Describe the influence of nutrition on prevention of infection.

NIC

Infection Control, Wound Care, Incision Site Care, Health Education

Interventions

Identify Clients at High Risk for Nosocomial Infections (Owen & Grier, 1987)

Use Appropriate Universal Precautions for All Body Fluids

- Wash hands before and after all contact with client or specimen.
- Handle the blood of all clients as potentially infectious.
- Wear gloves for potential contact with blood and body fluids.
- Handle all linen soiled with blood or body secretions as potentially infectious.
- Process all laboratory specimens as potentially infectious.
- Place used syringes immediately in a nearby impermeable container; do not recap or manipulate the needle in any way! Use retractable needle syringes when possible.
- Wear protective eyewear and mask if splatter with blood or body fluids is possible (e.g., bronchoscopy, oral surgery).

Consider Those With the Following Factors at High Risk for Delayed Wound Healing:

- Malnourishment
- Tobacco use
- Obesity
- Anemia
- Diabetes
- Cancer
- Corticosteroid therapy
- Renal insufficiency

- Hypovolemia
- Hypoxia
- Surgery >3 hours
- Night or emergency surgery
- Zinc, copper, magnesium deficiency
- Immune system compromise

Use Universal Precautions

Reduce Client's Susceptibility to Infection

- Encourage and maintain caloric and protein intake in diet (see *Imbalanced Nutrition*).
- Assess client for adequate immunizations against childhood diseases, bacterial infections (e.g., pneumonia, *Haemophilus influenzae*), and other viral infections (e.g., influenza). (Refer to Altered Health Maintenance on http://thePoint.lww.com/CarpenitoHB14e.)
- Administer prescribed antimicrobial therapy within 15 minutes of schedule.
- Minimize length of stay in hospital.
- Observe for superinfection in clients receiving antimicrobial therapy.

Reduce Entry of Organisms into Clients (Owen & Grier, 1987)

Surgical Wound

- Monitor temperature every 4 hours; notify physician if temperature is greater than 100.8° F.
- Assess wound site every 24 hours and during dressing changes; document any abnormal findings.
- Evaluate all abnormal laboratory findings, especially culture/sensitivities and complete blood count (CBC).
- Assess nutritional status to provide adequate protein and caloric intake for healing.

Urinary Tract

- Evaluate all abnormal laboratory findings, especially cultures/sensitivities and CBC.
- Assess for abnormal signs and symptoms after any urologic procedure, including frequency, urgency, burning, abnormal color, and odor.
- Monitor client's temperature at least every 24 hours for elevation; notify physician if temperature is greater than 100.8° F.
- Encourage fluids when appropriate.
- Use aseptic technique when emptying any urinary drainage device; keep bag off the floor, but below bladder or clamped during transport.
- Reassess need for indwelling urinary catheter daily.

Circulatory

- Assess all invasive lines every 24 hours for redness, inflammation, drainage, and tenderness.
- Monitor client's temperature at least every 24 hours; notify physician if greater than 100.8° F.
- Maintain aseptic technique for all invasive devices, changing sites, dressings, tubing, and solutions per policy schedule.
- Evaluate all abnormal laboratory findings, especially cultures/sensitivities and CBC.
- Assess client's nutritional status.

Respiratory Tract

- Evaluate risk for infection after any instrumentation of the respiratory tract for at least 48 hours after procedure.
- Monitor temperature at least every 8 hours and notify physician if greater than 100.8° F.
- Evaluate sputum characteristics for frequency, purulence, blood, and odor.
- Evaluate sputum and blood cultures, if done, for significant findings.
- Assess lung sounds every 8 hours or PRN.
- If client has abdominal/thoracic surgery, instruct before surgery on importance of coughing, turning, and deep breathing.
- Prompt to cough and deep breathe hourly.
- If client has had anesthesia, monitor for appropriate clearing of secretions in lung fields.
- Evaluate need for suctioning if client cannot clear secretions adequately.
- Assess for risk of aspiration, keeping head of bed elevated 30 degrees unless otherwise contraindicated.
- Ensure optimal pain management.

Protect the Client With Immune Deficiency From Infection

- Place client in private room.
- Instruct client to ask all visitors and personnel to wash their hands before approaching.
- Limit visitors when appropriate.
- Screen all visitors for known infections or exposure to infections.
- Limit invasive devices to those that are necessary.
- Teach client and family members signs and symptoms of infection.
- Evaluate client's personal hygiene habits.

Initiate Health Teaching and Referrals, as Indicated

- Instruct client and family regarding the causes, risks, and communicability of the infection.
- Have family demonstrate use of equipment or treatment procedure.
- Collaborate with nurse epidemiologist on needs of client and family.

Pediatric Interventions

- Monitor for signs of infection (e.g., lethargy, feeding difficulties, vomiting, temperature instability, subtle color changes).
- Provide umbilical cord care. Teach cord care and signs of infection (e.g., increased redness, purulent drainage).
- Teach signs of infection of circumcised area (e.g., bleeding, increased redness, or unusual swelling).

Maternal Interventions

- Explain the increased vulnerability to infection during pregnancy.
- Teach how to prevent urinary tract infections during pregnancy:
  - Drink at least eight 8-oz glasses of water.
  - Void frequently.
  - Void before and after intercourse (Reeder et al., 1997).
- Teach how to prevent infection postpartum:
  - Wipe from front to back.
  - Clean perineal area after voiding or defecating (e.g., sitz bath, squirt bottle).
  - Change perineal pads after each voiding.
  - Teach proper breast care.
- Identify risk factors for postpartum infections:
  - Anemia
  - Poor nutrition
  - Lack of prenatal care
  - Obesity
  - Intercourse after membrane rupture
  - Immunosuppression
  - Prolonged labor
  - Prolonged membrane rupture
  - Intrauterine fetal monitoring (in high-risk mothers)
  - Bleeding
- Instruct on signs and symptoms of infection (e.g., fever, purulent drainage), and report promptly.

Geriatric Considerations

- Explain that the usual signs of infection may not be present (e.g., fever, chills).
- Assess for anorexia, weakness, change in mental status, or hypothermia.
- Monitor skin and urinary system for signs of fungal, viral, or mycobacterial pathogens.

RISK FOR INFECTION TRANSMISSION**

Definition

The state in which an individual is at risk for transferring an opportunistic or pathogenic agent to others

Risk Factors

Presence of risk factors (see Related Factors).

Related Factors

Pathophysiologic

Related to:
Colonization with highly antibiotic-resistant organism
Airborne transmission exposure (sneezing, coughing, spitting)
Contact transmission exposure (direct, indirect, contact droplet)
Vehicle transmission exposure (food, water, contaminated drugs or blood, contaminated sites [IV, catheter])
Vector-borne transmission exposure (animals, rodents, insects)

Treatment Related

Related to exposure to a contaminated wound
Related to devices with contaminated drainage:
Urinary, chest, endotracheal   Suction equipment
   tubes

Situational (Personal, Environmental)

Related to:
Unsanitary living conditions (sewage, personal hygiene)
Areas considered high risk for vector-borne diseases (malaria, rabies, bubonic plague)
Areas considered high risk for vehicle-borne disease (hepatitis A, *Shigella*, *Salmonella*)

** This diagnosis is not currently on the NANDA list but has been included for clarity or usefulness.

Exposures to sources of infection as:
  Intravenous/intranasal/intradermal drug use (sharing of
    needles, drug paraphernalia straws)
  Contaminated sex paraphernalia
  Multiple sex partners
  Natural disaster (e.g., flood, hurricane)
  Disaster with hazardous infectious material

Maturational

Newborn

Related to birth outside hospital setting in uncontrolled environment

*Related to exposure during prenatal or perinatal period to communi-
cable disease through mother*

Infection Status, Risk Control, Risk Detection

Goal

The client will describe the mode of transmission of disease by the
time of discharge as evidenced by the following indicators:

• Relate the need to be isolated until noninfectious (e.g., TB)
• Relate factors that contribute to the transmission of the infection
• Relate methods to reduce or prevent infection transmission
• Demonstrate meticulous hand washing

NIC

Teaching: Disease Process, Infection Control Infection Protection

Interventions

Identify People Who Are Susceptible Hosts Based on Focus
Assessment for Risk for Infection and History of Exposure

Identify the Mode of Transmission Based on Infecting Agent

• Airborne
• Contact:
  • Direct
  • Indirect
  • Contact droplet
• Vehicle-borne
• Vector-borne

Reduce the Transfer of Pathogens

- Isolate clients with airborne communicable infections (Table II.4).
- Secure appropriate room assignment depending on the type of infection and hygienic practices of the infected client.
- Use universal precautions to prevent transmission to self or other susceptible host.

Table II.4	AIRBORNE COMMUNICABLE DISEASES	
Disease	**Apply Airborne Precautions for How Long**	**Comments**
Anthrax, inhalation	Duration of illness	Promptly report to infection control office
Chickenpox (varicella)	Until all lesions are crusted	Immune person does not need to wear a mask. Exposed susceptible clients should be placed in a private special airflow room on STOP SIGN alert status beginning 10 days after initial exposure until 21 days after last exposure Report to epidemiology
Diphtheria, pharyngeal	Until two cultures from both nose and throat taken at least 24 h after cessation of antimicrobial therapy are negative for *Corynebacterium diphtheriae*	Promptly report to epidemiology
Epiglottis, due to *Haemophilus influenzae*	For 24 h after cessation of antimicrobial therapy	Report to epidemiology
Erythema infectiosum	For 7 days after onset	Report to epidemiology

(continued)

Table II.4	AIRBORNE COMMUNICABLE DISEASES (continued)	
Disease	**Apply Airborne Precautions for How Long**	**Comments**
Hemorrhagic fevers	Duration of illness	Call epidemiology office immediately. May call the State Health Department and Centers for Disease Control and Prevention for advice about management of a suspected case
Herpes zoster (varicella zoster), disseminated	Duration of illness	Localized; does not require STOP SIGN
Lassa fever	Duration of illness	Call epidemiology office immediately
Marburg virus disease		May call the State Health Department and Centers for Disease Control and Prevention for advice about management of a suspected case
Measles (rubeola)	For 4 days after start of rash, except in immunocompromised clients, for whom precautions should be maintained for duration of illness	Immune people do not need to wear a mask. Exposed susceptible clients should be placed in a private special air flow room on STOP SIGN alert status beginning the 5th day after exposure until 21 days after last exposure
Meningitis *Haemophilus influenzae* known or suspected	For 24 h after start of effective antibiotic therapy	Call epidemiology to report

Disease	Apply Airborne Precautions for How Long	Comments
Neisseria meningitidis (meningococci) known or suspected	For 24 h after start of effective antibiotic therapy	Promptly report to epidemiology
Meningococcal pneumonia	For 24 h after start of effective antibiotic therapy	Promptly report to epidemiology
Meningococcemia	For 24 h after start of effective antibiotic therapy	Consult with epidemiology
Multiply resistant organisms	Until culture negative or as determined by epidemiology	Consult with epidemiology
Mumps (infectious parotitis)	For 9 days after onset of swelling	People with history do not need to wear a mask. Call epidemiology office to report
Pertussis (whooping cough)	For 7 days after start of effective therapy	Call epidemiology to report
Plague, pneumonic	For 3 days after start of effective therapy	Promptly report to epidemiology
Pneumonia, *Haemophilus* in infants and children any age	For 24 h after start of effective therapy	Call epidemiology
Pneumonia, meningococcal	For 24 h after start of effective antibiotic therapy	Promptly report to epidemiology
Rubella (German measles)	For 7 days after onset of rash	Immune people do not need to wear a mask. Promptly report to epidemiology

(continued)

Table II.4	AIRBORNE COMMUNICABLE DISEASES (continued)	
Disease	**Apply Airborne Precautions for How Long**	**Comments**
Tuberculosis, bronchial, laryngeal, pulmonary, confirmed or suspect	Clients are not considered infectious if they meet all these criteria: Adequate therapy received for 2–3 weeks	Call epidemiology to report; prompt use of effective antituberculosis drugs is the most effective means of limiting transmission
	Favorable clinical response to therapy Three consecutive negative sputum smear results from sputum collected on different days	
Varicella (chickenpox)	Until all lesions crusted over	See chickenpox

Source: Centers for Disease Control and Prevention. www.cdc.gov.

Initiate Health Education and Referrals as Indicated and Discuss the Mode of Transmission of Infection With the Client, Family, and Significant Others

RISK FOR INJURY

Risk for Injury
Risk for Aspiration
Risk for Falls
Risk for Poisoning
Risk for Suffocation
Risk for Thermal Injury

Risk for Trauma

Risk for Perioperative Positioning Injury

NANDA-I Definition

At risk for injury as a result of environmental conditions interacting with the individual's adaptive and defensive resources

Risk Factors

Presence of risk factor (see Related Factors).

Related Factors

Pathophysiologic

Related to altered cerebral function secondary to hypoxia
Related to syncope
Related to vertigo or dizziness

Related to impaired mobility secondary to:
Cerebrovascular accident
Arthritis
Parkinsonism

Related to loss of limb

Related to impaired vision

Related to hearing impairment

Related to fatigue

Related to orthostatic hypotension

Related to vestibular disorders

Related to lack of awareness of environmental hazards secondary to:
Confusion

Related to tonic–clonic movements secondary to:
Seizures

Treatment Related

Related to prolonged bed rest

Related to effects of (specify) or sensorium

Examples:
Sedatives   Hypoglycemics   Diuretics
Phenothiazine   Antispasmodics   Antihypertensives

Pain medications   Psychotropics
Vasodilators   Muscle relaxants

Related to casts/crutches, canes, walkers

Situational (Personal, Environmental)

Related to decrease in or loss of short-term memory

Related to faulty judgment secondary to:
Stress   Dehydration
Alcohol, drugs*   Depression

Related to household hazards (specify):
Unsafe walkways   Improperly stored poisons
Slippery floors   Unsafe toys
Bathrooms (tubs, toilets) Faulty electric wires
Stairs   Throw Rugs
Inadequate lighting

Related to automotive hazards:
Lack of use of seat belts or child seats
Mechanically unsafe vehicle

Related to fire hazards

Related to unfamiliar setting (hospital, nursing home)

Related to improper footwear

Related to inattentive caretaker

Related to improper use of aids (crutches, canes, walkers, wheelchairs)

Related to history of accidents

Related to unstable gait

Maturational

Infant/Child
Related to lack of awareness of hazards

Older Adult

Related to faulty judgments, secondary cognitive deficits

Related to sedentary lifestyle and loss of muscle strength

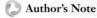 **Author's Note**

This diagnosis has five subcategories: *Risk for Aspiration, Poisoning, Suffocation, Risk for Thermal Injury,* and *Trauma.* Interventions to prevent poisoning, suffocation, falls, and trauma are included under the general category *Risk for Injury.* Should the nurse choose to isolate interventions only for prevention of poisoning, suffocation, or trauma, then the diagnosis *Risk for Poisoning, Risk for Suffocation, Risk for Falls,* or *Risk for Trauma* would be useful.

Nursing interventions related to *Risk for Injury* focus on protecting a client from injury and teaching precautions to reduce the risk of injury. When the nurse is teaching a client or family safety measures to prevent injury but is not providing on-site protection (as in the community or outpatient department, or for discharge planning), the diagnosis *Risk for Injury related to insufficient knowledge of safety precautions* may be more appropriate.

NOC

Risk Control, Safe Home Environment, Falls Occurrence, Fall Prevention Behavior

Goal

The client will relate fewer or no injuries as evidenced by the following indicators:

- Identify factors that increase risk for injury.
- Relate intent to use safety measures to prevent injury (e.g., remove or anchor throw rugs).
- Relate intent to practice selected prevention measures (e.g., wear sunglasses to reduce glare).
- Increase daily activity, if feasible.

NIC

Fall Prevention, Environmental Management: Safety, Health Education, Surveillance: Safety, Risk Identification

Interventions

Refer to Related Factors

Reduce or Eliminate Causative or Contributing Factors, If Possible

Unfamiliar Surroundings

- Orient each client to surroundings on admission; explain the call system, and assess client's ability to use it.
- Closely supervise the client during the first few nights to assess safety.
- Use a night-light.
- Encourage the client to request assistance during the night.
- Teach about side effects of certain drugs (e.g., dizziness, fatigue).
- Keep bed at lowest level during the night.
- Consider use of a movement detection monitor (bed-based alarm or personal alarm), if needed.

Impaired Vision
- Provide safe illumination and teach client to:
  - Ensure adequate lighting in all rooms, with soft light at night.
  - Have a light switch easily accessible, next to the bed.
  - Provide background light that is soft.
- Teach the client how to reduce glare:
  - Avoid glossy surfaces (e.g., glass, highly polished floors).
  - Use diffuse rather than direct light; use shades that darken the room.
  - Turn the head away when switching on a bright light.
  - Wear sunglasses or hats with brims, or carry umbrellas, to reduce glare outside.
  - Avoid looking directly at bright lights (e.g., headlights).
- Teach the client or family to provide sufficient color contrast for visual discrimination and to avoid green and blue:
  - Color-code edges of steps (e.g., with colored tape).
  - Avoid white walls, dishes, and counters.
  - Avoid clear glasses (i.e., use smoked glass).
  - Choose objects colored black on white (e.g., black phone).
  - Avoid colors that merge (e.g., beige switches on beige walls).
  - Paint doorknobs with bright colors.

Decreased Tactile Sensitivity
- Teach preventive measures:
  - Assess temperature of bath water and heating pads before use.
  - Use bath thermometers.
  - Assess extremities daily for undetected injuries.
  - Keep the feet warm and dry and skin softened with emollient lotion (lanolin, mineral oil). (NOTE: Use socks with grips after just putting on lotion to prevent slips/falls).
- See *Ineffective Peripheral Tissue Perfusion* for additional interventions.

Orthostatic Hypotension
- See *Risk for Injury Related to Vertigo Secondary to Orthostatic Hypotension* for additional interventions.

Decreased Strength/Flexibility
- Perform ankle-strengthening exercises daily (Schoenfelder, 2000):
  - Stand behind a straight chair, with feet slightly apart.
  - Slowly raise both heels until body weight is on the balls of the feet; hold for a count of 3 (e.g., 1 Mississippi, 2 Mississippi, 3 Mississippi).
  - Do 5 to 10 repetitions; increase repetitions as strength increases.

- Walk at least two or three times a week.
  - Use ankle exercises as a warm-up before walking.
  - Begin walking with someone at side, if needed, for 10 minutes.
  - Increase time and speed according to capabilities.

Hazardous Environmental Factors

- Teach the client to:
  - Eliminate throw rugs, litter, and highly polished floors.
  - Ensure nonslip surfaces in bathtub or shower by applying commercially available traction tapes.
  - Install handgrips in bathroom.
  - Install railings in hallways and on stairs.
  - Remove protruding objects (e.g., coat hooks, shelves, light fixtures) from stairway walls.
- Instruct staff to:
  - Keep side rails on bed in place and bed at the lowest position when the client is left unattended.
  - Keep the bed at the lowest position with wheels locked when stationary.
  - Teach the client in the wheelchair to lock and unlock the wheels.
  - Ensure that client's shoes or slippers have nonskid soles.
- If cognitively impaired, Refer to *Wandering*.

Pediatric Interventions

- Teach parents to expect frequent changes in infants' and children's ability and to take precautions (e.g., infant who suddenly rolls over for the first time might be on a changing table unattended).
- Discuss with parents the necessity of constant monitoring of small children.
- Provide parents with information to assist them in selecting a babysitter.
  - Determine previous experiences and knowledge of emergency measures.
  - Observe the interaction of the sitter with the child.
- Teach parents to expect children to mimic them and to teach their children what they can do with or without supervision (e.g., seat belts, helmets, safe driving).
- Explain and expect compliance with certain rules (depending on age) concerning:
  - Streets
  - Playground equipment
  - Water (e.g., pools, bathtubs)
  - Bicycles

- Fire
- Animals
- Strangers
- Instruct how to "child-proof" the home.
- Explain why children should not ride in front (air bags).
- Refer to local fire department for assistance in staging home fire drills.
- Encourage parents to learn basic life-saving skills (e.g., CPR, Heimlich maneuver).
- Teach children how to dial 911.
- Teach parents to assist their children in handling peer pressure that involves risk-taking behavior.

Geriatric Interventions

- Assess for orthostatic hypotension. Compare brachial blood pressure (e.g., supine, standing).
- Discuss physiology of orthostatic hypotension with client.
- Teach techniques to reduce orthostatic hypotension.
  - Change positions slowly.
  - Move from lying to an upright position in stages.
  - During day, rest in a recliner rather than in bed.
  - Avoid prolonged standing.
- Teach to avoid dehydration and vasodilation (e.g., hot tubs).
- Teach exercises to increase strength and flexibility.
- Perform ankle-strengthening exercises daily (Schoenfelder, 2000).
  - Stand behind a straight chair, with feet slightly apart.
  - Slowly raise both heels until body weight is on balls of feet; hold for count of 3 (e.g., "1 Mississippi, 2 Mississippi, 3 Mississippi").
  - Do 5 to 10 repetitions; increase repetitions as strength increases.
- Walk at least two or three times a week.
  - Use ankle exercises as a warm-up before walking.
  - Begin walking with someone at side if needed for 10 minutes.
  - Increase time and speed according to capabilities.

Risk for Aspiration

NANDA-I Definition

At risk for entry of gastrointestinal secretions, solids, or fluids into the tracheobronchial passages

Risk Factors

Pathophysiologic

Related to reduced level of consciousness secondary to:
Presenile dementia   Alcohol- or drug-induced
Head injury   Coma
Cerebrovascular accident   Seizures
Parkinson's disease   Anesthesia

Related to depressed cough/gag reflexes

Related to increased intragastric pressure secondary to:
Lithotomy position   Obesity
Ascites   Enlarged uterus

Related to impaired swallowing or decreased laryngeal and glottic reflexes secondary to:
Achalasia   Debilitating conditions
Cerebrovascular accident   Multiple sclerosis
Myasthenia gravis   Scleroderma
Catatonia   Parkinson's disease
Muscular dystrophy   Guillain–Barré syndrome
Esophageal strictures

Related to tracheoesophageal fistula

Related to impaired protective reflexes secondary to:
Facial/oral/neck surgery or trauma*
Paraplegia or hemiplegia

Treatment Related

Related to depressed laryngeal and glottic reflexes secondary to:
Tracheostomy/endotracheal tube*
Sedation
Tube feedings

Related to impaired ability to cough secondary to:
Wired jaw*
Imposed prone position

Situational (Personal, Environmental)

Related to inability/impaired ability to elevate upper body

Related to eating when intoxicated

Maturational

Premature
Related to impaired sucking/swallowing reflexes

Neonate
Related to decreased muscle tone of inferior esophageal sphincter

Older Adult
Related to poor dentition

Author's Note

Risk for Aspiration is a clinically useful diagnosis for people at high risk for aspiration because of reduced level of consciousness, structural deficits, mechanical devices, and neurologic and gastrointestinal disorders. People with swallowing difficulties often are at risk for aspiration; the nursing diagnosis *Impaired Swallowing* should be used to describe a client with difficulty swallowing who is also at risk for aspiration. *Risk for Aspiration* should be used to describe people who require nursing interventions to prevent aspiration, but do not have a swallowing problem.

NOC
Aspiration Control

Goals

The client will not experience aspiration as evidenced by the following indicators:

• Relate measures to prevent aspiration.
• Name foods or fluids that are high risk for causing aspiration.

The parent will reduce opportunities for aspirations as evidenced by the following indicators:

• Remove small objects from child's reach.
• Inspect toys for removable small objects.
• Discourage the child from putting objects in his or her mouth.

NIC
Aspiration Precautions, Airway Management, Positioning, Airway Suctioning

Interventions

Assess Causative or Contributing Factors

Refer to Related Factors.

Reduce the Risk of Aspiration in:

Clients With Decreased Strength, Decreased Sensorium, or Autonomic Disorders

- Maintain a side-lying position if not contraindicated by injury.
- If the client cannot be positioned on the side, open the oropharyngeal airway by lifting the mandible up and forward and tilting the head backward. (For a small infant, hyperextension of the neck may not be effective.)
- Assess for position of the tongue, ensuring it has not dropped backward, occluding the airway.
- Keep the head of the bed elevated, if not contraindicated by hypotension or injury.
- Maintain good oral hygiene. Clean teeth and use mouthwash on cotton swab; apply petroleum jelly to lips; removing encrustations gently.
- Clear secretions from mouth and throat with a tissue or gentle suction.
- Reassess frequently for obstructive material in mouth and throat.
- Reevaluate frequently for good anatomic positioning.
- Maintain side-lying position after feedings.
- Positions are maintained to reduce aspiration.

Clients With Tracheostomy or Endotracheal Tubes

- Inflate cuff:
  - During continuous mechanical ventilation
  - During and after eating
  - During an 1 hour after tube feedings
  - During intermittent positive-pressure breathing treatments
- Suction every 1 to 2 hours and PRN and provide oral care.

Clients With Gastrointestinal Tubes and Feedings

- Confirm that tube placement has been verified by radiography or aspiration of greenish fluid (check hospital/organizational policy for preferred method).
- Confirm that tube position has not changed since it was inserted and verified.
- Elevate the head of the bed for 30 to 45 minutes during feeding periods and 1 hour after to prevent reflux by use of reverse gravity.

- Aspirate for residual contents before each feeding for tubes positioned gastrically.
- Administer feeding if residual contents are less than 150 mL (intermittent), or administer feeding if residual is no greater than 150 mL at 10% to 20% of hourly rate (continuous).
- Regulate gastric feedings using an intermittent schedule, allowing periods for stomach emptying between feeding intervals.

For an Older Adult With Difficulties Chewing and Swallowing (See Impaired Swallowing)

Initiate Health Teaching and Referrals, as Indicated

- Instruct the client and family on causes and prevention of aspiration.
- Maintain oral hygiene to prevent pneumonia related to oral bacteria aspiration.
- Have the family demonstrate tube-feeding technique.
- Refer the family to a community nursing agency for assistance at home.
- Teach the client about the danger of eating when under the influence of alcohol.
- Teach the Heimlich or abdominal thrust maneuver to remove aspirated foreign bodies.

Pediatric Interventions

For Newborns With Cleft Lip, Palate, or Both
- Position infant's head upright.
- Use a special feeding device for infants with cleft lip/cleft palate such as a cleft lip/cleft palate nurser, the Haberman feeder, or a gravity flow nipple.
- If nipple feeding is unsuccessful, use a rubber-tipped syringe to deposit the formula on the back of the tongue.
- Observe for signs to stop feeding momentarily, such as elevated eyebrows and wrinkled forehead.
- Do not position the nipple through the cleft.
- Position the nipple so it is compressed by the infant's tongue and existing palate.
- Apply gentle counterpressure on the base of the bottle to assist the infant with tongue and palate control of the milk flow.
- Burp frequently because of excessive air swallowing.

Risk for Falls

NANDA-I Definition

At risk for increased susceptibility to falling that may cause physical harm

Risk Factors

Presence of risk factors (see Risk Factors for *Risk for Injury*).

 Author's Note

This new nursing diagnosis can be used to specify a client at risk for falls. If the client is at risk for various types of injuries (e.g., a cognitively impaired client), the broader diagnosis *Risk for Injury* is more useful.

NOC
Refer to *Risk for Injury*

Goal

The client will relate controlled falls or no falls as evidenced by the following indicators:

- Relate the intent to use safety measures to prevent falls.
- Demonstrate selective prevention measures.

NIC
Refer to *Risk for Injury*

Interventions

Orient the Client to Environment and Safety Measures

- Advise the client on the location of the bathroom.
- Educate the client on the bed controls and call bell.
- Leave the bathroom light on.
- Remove obstacles to the bathroom.
- Evaluate if side rails are hazardous.
- Keep the bed position at low.
- Instruct the client to wear nonslip shoes or socks with grips.

Identify Clients Who Are at High Risk for Falling to All Personnel

- Sticker on headboard
- Brightly colored arm band
- Sign on door
- "Red Slipper Program" (May be yellow or alternate color as designated by the facility.)
- Specific programs to alert staff to high-risk clients are effective.

Implement Safety Measures for Clients Who Are Cognitively Impaired

- Place an alarm pad (or personal alarm) on the bed.
- Clients can be place in small groups with intense, focused supervision.
- Intense supervision is effective in preventing falls.

Ensure Proper Use of Assistive Devices

- Consult with physical therapist.

Engage the Client in Exercise Routines

- Assess the client's fear of falling.
- Encourage group classes if feasible (e.g., Tai chi, water classes).
- Provide opportunities for exercise walking.
- Engage in exercises specifically to improve gait, balance, and ankle strength.
- Initiate health teaching and referrals as needed.
- Refer the client to Home Health Nursing Agency for a home assessment.
- Ensure that family is aware of issues related to safety and risk for falls.
- Refer to *Risk for Injury*.

Risk for Poisoning

NANDA-I Definition

At risk of accidental exposure to or ingestion of drugs or dangerous products in sufficient doses that may compromise health

Risk Factors

Presence of risk factors (see Risk Factors for *Risk for Injury*).

Risk for Suffocation

NANDA-I Definition

At risk of accidental suffocation (inadequate air available for inhalation)

Risk Factors

Presence of risk factors (see Risk Factors for *Risk for Injury*).

Risk for Thermal Injury

NANDA-I Definition

At risk for damage to skin and mucous membranes due to extreme temperatures

Risk Factors*

Cognitive impairment (e.g., dementia, psychoses)
Developmental level (infants, aged)
Exposure to extreme temperatures
Fatigue
Inadequate supervision
Inattentiveness
Intoxication (alcohol, drug)
Lack of knowledge (client, caregiver)
Lack of protective clothing (e.g., flame-retardant sleepwear, gloves, ear covering)
Neuromuscular impairment (e.g., stroke, amyotrophic lateral sclerosis, multiple sclerosis)
Neuropathy
Smoking
Treatment-related side effects (e.g., pharmaceutical agents)
Unsafe environment

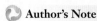 **Author's Note**

Risk for Thermal Injury is a new NANDA-I diagnosis that focuses on thermal injury only. The risk factors listed represent those related to most type of injuries. It is probably more useful to use *Risk for Injury*, to cover all the types of injury including thermal. Individuals who are at risk for thermal injury are also at risk for a multitude of injuries. *Risk for Thermal Injury* could be used in a standard of care to emphasize environmental hazards such as combustibles, fireworks, heaters, fires.

Goals

Refer to *Risk for Injury related to lack of awareness of environmental hazards.*

Interventions

Refer to *Risk for Injury related to lack of awareness of environmental hazards.*

Risk for Trauma

NANDA-I Definition

At risk of accidental tissue injury (e.g., wound, burns, fracture)

Risk Factors

Presence of risk factors (see Risk Factors for *Risk for Injury*).

Risk for Perioperative Positioning Injury

NANDA-I Definition

At risk for inadvertent anatomical and physical changes as a result of posture or equipment used during an invasive/surgical procedure

Risk Factors

Presence of risk factors (see Related Factors).

Related Factors

Pathophysiologic

Related to increased vulnerability secondary to:

Chronic disease	Osteoporosis
Cancer	Compromised immune system
Thin body frame	Renal, hepatic dysfunction
Radiation therapy	Infection

Related to compromised tissue perfusion secondary to:

Diabetes mellitus	Dehydration
Anemia	Peripheral vascular disease
Ascites	History of thrombosis
Cardiovascular disease	Edema*
Hypothermia	

Related to vulnerability of stoma during positioning

Related to preexisting contractures or physical impairments secondary to:
Rheumatoid arthritis   Polio

Treatment Related

Related to position requirements and loss of usual sensory protective responses secondary to anesthesia

Related to surgical procedures of 2 hours or longer

Related to vulnerability of implants or prostheses (e.g., pacemakers) during positioning

Situational (Personal, Environmental)

Related to compromised circulation secondary to:

Obesity*	Pregnancy	Cool operating suite
Tobacco use	Infant status	Elder status

Maturational

Related to increased vulnerability to tissue injury secondary to:

 Author's Note

This diagnosis focuses on identifying the vulnerability for tissue, nerve, and joint injury resulting from required positions for surgery. The addition of *perioperative positioning* to *Risk for Injury* adds etiology to the label.

   If a client has no pre-existing risk factors that make him or her more vulnerable to injury, this diagnosis could be used with no related factors because they are evident. If related factors are desired, the statement could read *Risk for Perioperative Positioning Injury related to position requirements for surgery and loss of usual sensory protective measures secondary to anesthesia.*

When a client has pre-existing risk factors, the statement should include these—for example, *Risk for Perioperative Positioning Injuries related to compromised tissue perfusion secondary to peripheral arterial disease.*

NOC

Circulation Status, Neurologic Status, Tissue Perfusion: Peripheral

Goal

The client will have no neuromuscular damage or injury related to the surgical position as evidenced by the following indicators:

- Padding is used as indicated for procedure.
- Limbs are secured when at risk.
- Limbs are flexed when indicated.

NIC

Positioning Intraoperative, Surveillance, Pressure Management

Interventions

Determine Whether the Client Has Pre-existing Risk Factors (Refer to Risk Factors); Communicate Findings to Surgical Team

Before Positioning, Assess and Document:

- Range-of-motion ability
- Physical abnormalities (skin, contractions)
- External/internal prostheses or implants
- Neurovascular status
- Circulatory status

Advise If Any Pre-existing Factors Exist and Determine If the Position Will Be Arranged Before or After Anesthesia

- Discuss with the surgeon the surgical position desired.
- Move the client from the transport stretcher to the operating room (OR) bed.
  - Have a minimum of two people with their hands free (e.g., not holding an IV bag).
  - Explain the transfer to the client. Lock all wheels on the stretcher and bed.

- Ask the client to move slowly to the OR bed. Assist during the move. Do not pull or drag the client.
- When the client is on the OR bed, attach a safety belt a few inches above the knees with a space of three fingerbreadths.
- Check that legs are not crossed and that feet are slightly separated and not over the edge.
- Do not leave the client unattended.
- Always ask the anesthesiologist or nurse anesthetist for permission before moving or repositioning an anesthetized client.
- Reduce vulnerability to injury (soft tissue, joint, nerves, blood vessels).
  - Align the neck and spine at all times.
  - Gently manipulate the joints. Do not abduct more than 90 degrees.
  - Do not let limbs extend off the OR bed. Reposition slowly and gently.
  - Use a draw-sheet above the elbows to tuck in arms at the side or abduct arm on an arm board with padding.
- Protect eyes and ears from injury.
  - Use padding or a special headrest to protect ears, superficial nerves, and blood vessels of the face if the head is on its side.
  - Ensure that the ear is not bent when positioned.
  - If needed, protect eyes from abrasions with an eye patch or shield.
- Depending on the surgical position used, protect vulnerable areas; document position and protection measures used (Rothrock, 2003).

Supine
- Pad the calcaneus, sacrum, coccyx, olecranon process, scapula, ischial tuberosity, and occiput.
- Keep the arms at side, palms down or abducted on an arm board.
- Protect the head and ears if the head is turned to the side.

Trendelenburg
- Use a well-padded shoulder brace over the acromion process, not soft tissue, and away from the neck.

Reverse Trendelenburg
- Use a padded footboard.

Jack-Knife (Modified Prone)
- Use padded arm boards at correct heights to allow elbows to bend comfortably.
- Place a soft pillow under the down ear.
- Cushion hips and thighs with large pillows.

- Cushion breasts.
- Cushion male genitalia in natural position.
- Use a large pillow under the lower legs and ankles to raise the toes off the bed.
- Use additional padding on the shoulder girdle, olecranon, anterosuperior iliac spine, patella, and dorsum of the foot.
- Apply a safety strap across the thighs.

Prone
- Position two large body rolls longitudinally from the acromio-clavicular joint to the iliac crest.
- Refer to jack-knife for additional information.

Laminectomy
- After induction of anesthesia, at least six people help roll the client from the stretcher to the OR bed onto the laminectomy brace.
- Keep body aligned.
- Protect limbs from torsion.
- Place rolled towels in axillary regions.
- Follow precautions for jack-knife.

Lithotomy
- Prepare stirrups with padding.
- Have two people simultaneously and slowly raise the client's legs with slight rotation of the hips. Gently position the knees slightly flexed.
- Position the client's buttocks about 1 inch over the end of the table.
- Use a small lumbar pad and extra padding in the sacral area.
- Cover the legs with cotton boots.
- Position arms on arm boards or loosely over abdomen, supported with a sheet.

Fowler
- Position the neck in straight alignment.
- Use a padded footboard.
- Support the knees with a pillow.
- Cross the arms loosely over the abdomen and tape them on the pillow.

Sims (Lateral)
- Position the client on the side with arms extended on double arm boards.
- Flex the lower leg.
- Use a small pillow under the head.
- Use a rolled towel in the axillary area of the downside arm.
- Elevate and pad the flank.

- Flex the lower leg and place a long pillow the length of the leg to the groin.
- Use a 4-inch strip of adhesive tape attached to one side of the table, over the iliac crest and to the other side.
- Protect ankles and feet from pressure.
- Protect male genitalia, female breasts, and ear as for jack-knife position.
- Hyperextension of the arm on an arm board can injure the brachial plexus (in the arm). Improper positioning of the brace also can injure the brachial plexus.
- Ulnar nerve injuries occur when an elbow slips off the mattress and is compressed between the table and the medial epicondyle.
- Radial nerve injuries occur when the nerve is compressed between the client and the table surface or from striking the table.
- Saphenous and peroneal nerve damage occurs with the use of stirrups with lithotomy—compression of the peroneal nerve against the stirrups or of the saphenous nerve between the metal popliteal knee support stirrup and the medial tibial condyle.
- If feasible, ask the client if he or she feels pain, burning, pressure, or any discomfort after positioning
- Continually assess that team members are not leaning on the client, especially limbs.
- Ensure that the head is lifted slightly every 30 minutes.
- Slowly reposition or return the client to supine position after certain surgical positions (e.g., trendelenburg, lithotomy, reverse trendelenburg, jack-knife, lateral).
- Assess skin condition when surgery is over; document findings; continue to assess and to relieve pressure to vulnerable areas postoperatively.

DECREASED INTRACRANIAL ADAPTIVE CAPACITY

NANDA-I Definition

Intracranial fluid dynamic mechanisms that normally compensate for increases in intracranial volumes are compromised, resulting in repeated disproportionate increases in intracranial pressure (ICP) in response to a variety of noxious and nonnoxious stimuli

Defining Characteristics

Major (Must Be Present)*

Repeated increases of >10 mm Hg for more than 5 minutes following any of a variety of external stimuli.

Minor (May Be Present)

Disproportionate increase in ICP following stimulus
Elevated P2 ICP waveform*
Volume–pressure response test variation (volume: pressure ratio 2, pressure–volume index <10)*
Baseline ICP ≥10 mm Hg*
Wide-amplitude ICP waveform*

 Author's Note

This diagnosis represents increased intracranial pressure. It is a collaborative problem because it requires two disciplines to treat—nursing and medicine. In addition, it requires invasive monitoring for diagnosis. The collaborative problem *Risk for Complications of Increased Intracranial Pressure* represents this clinical situation.

NEONATAL JAUNDICE

Neonatal Jaundice
Risk for Neonatal Jaundice

See also *Risk for Complications of Hyperbilirubinemia* on http://thePoint.lww.com/CarpenitoHB14e.

NANDA-I Definition

The yellow-orange tint of the neonate's skin and mucous membranes that occurs after 24 hours of life as a result of unconjugated bilirubin in the circulation

Defining Characteristics*

Abnormal blood profile (hemolysis; total serum bilirubin greater than 2 mg/dL: inherited disorder; total serum bilirubin in high-risk range on age in hour-specific nomogram)

Abnormal skin bruising
Yellow-orange skin
Yellow sclera

Related Factors*

Abnormal weight loss (>7% to 8% in breastfeeding newborn;
   15% in term infant)
Feeding pattern not well established
Infant experiences difficulty making transition to extrauterine life
Neonate age 1 to 7 days
Stool (meconium) passage delayed

 Author's Note

This NANDA-I diagnosis is a collaborative problem (the reader is
referred to http://thePoint.lww.com/CarpenitoHB14e in the next
sentence) that requires a laboratory test for diagnosis and treatment from medicine and nursing. Refer to *Risk for Complications of
Hyperbilirubinemia* on http://thePoint.lww.com/CarpenitoHB14e for
neonates at risk for or experiencing hyperbilirubinemia.

Risk for Neonatal Jaundice

NANDA-I Definition

At risk for yellow-orange tint of the neonate's skin and mucous
membranes that occurs after 24 hours of life as a result of unconjugated bilirubin in the circulation

Risk Factors*

Abnormal weight loss (>7% to 8% in breastfeeding newborn,
   15% in term infant)
Feeding pattern not well established
Infant experiences difficulty making the transition to extrauter-
   ine life
Neonate aged 1 to 7 days
Prematurity
Stool (meconium) passage delayed

 Author's Note

Refer to Author's Notes under *Neonatal Jaundice.*

DEFICIENT KNOWLEDGE

NANDA-I Definition

Absence or deficiency of cognitive information related to a specific topic

Defining Characteristics

Exaggerated behaviors*
Inappropriate behaviors (e.g., hysterical, hostile, agitated, apathetic)*
Verbalization of a problem
Inaccurate follow-through of instruction*
Inaccurate performance of test*

Related Factors*

Cognitive limitation   Lack of recall
Lack of exposure   Unfamiliarity with information
Information misinterpretation   resources
Lack of interest in learning

 Author's Note

Deficient Knowledge does not represent a human response, alteration, or pattern of dysfunction; rather, it is an etiologic or contributing factor (Jenny, 1987). Lack of knowledge can contribute to a variety of responses (e.g., anxiety, self-care deficits). All nursing diagnoses have related client/family teaching as a part of nursing interventions (e.g., *Impaired Bowel Elimination, Impaired Verbal Communication*). When the teaching relates directly to a specific nursing diagnosis, incorporate the teaching into the plan. When specific teaching is indicated before a procedure, the diagnosis *Anxiety related to unfamiliar environment or procedure* can be used. When information is given to assist a person or family with self-care at home, the diagnosis *Ineffective Therapeutic Regimen Management* may be indicated.

LATEX ALLERGY RESPONSE

Latex Allergy Response

Risk for Latex Allergy Response

NANDA-I Definition

A hypersensitive reaction to natural latex rubber products

Defining Characteristics

Positive skin or serum test to natural rubber latex (NRL) extract.
After exposure to latex protein:

Contact dermatitis progressing to generalized symptoms	Itching
	Edema (e.g., facial, eyelids, tongue)
Flushing	Allergic conjunctivitis
Redness	Asthma
Eczema	Rhinitis
Wheezing	Urticaria

Related Factors

Biopathophysiologic

Related to hypersensitivity response to the protein component of NRL

 NOC

Immune Hypersensitivity Control

Goal

The client will report no exposure to latex, as evidenced by the
following indicators:

- Describe products of NRL.
- Describe strategies to avoid exposure.

Allergy Management, Latex Precautions, Environmental Risk Protection

Interventions

Assess for Causative and Contributing Factors

Eliminate Exposure to Latex Products

Use Nonlatex Alternative Supplies
- Clear disposable amber bags
- Silicone baby nipples
- 2 × 2 gauze pads with silk tape in place of adhesive bandages
- Clear plastic or silastic catheters
- Vinyl or neoprene gloves
- Kling-like gauze

Protect From Exposure to Latex
- Cover the skin with cloth before applying the blood pressure cuff.
- Do not allow rubber stethoscope tubing to touch the client.
- Do not inject through rubber parts (e.g., heparin locks); use syringe and stopcock.
- Change needles after each puncture of rubber stopper.
- Cover rubber parts with tape.

Teach Which Products Are Commonly Made of Latex

Health Care Equipment
- Natural latex rubber gloves, powdered or unpowdered, including those labeled "hypoallergenic"
- Blood pressure cuffs
- Stethoscopes
- Tourniquets
- Electrode pads
- Airways, endotracheal tubes
- Syringe plunges, bulb syringes
- Masks for anesthesia
- Rubber aprons
- Catheters, wound drains
- Injection ports
- Tops of multidose vials
- Adhesive tape
- Ostomy pouches
- Wheelchair cushions
- Briefs with elastic
- Pads for crutches
- Some prefilled syringes

Office/Household Products
- Erasers
- Rubber bands
- Dishwashing gloves
- Balloons
- Condoms, diaphragms
- Baby bottle nipples, pacifiers
- Rubber balls and toys
- Racquet handles
- Cycle grips
- Tires
- Hot water bottles
- Carpeting
- Shoe soles
- Elastic in underwear
- Rubber cement

Initiate Health Teaching as Indicated

- Explain the importance of completely avoiding direct contact with all NRL products.
- Advise that a client with a history of a mild skin reaction to latex is at risk for anaphylaxis.
- Instruct the client to wear a Medic-Alert bracelet stating "Latex Allergy" and to carry auto-injectable epinephrine.
- Instruct the client to warn all health care providers (e.g., dental, medical, surgical) of the allergy.

Risk for Latex Allergy Response

NANDA-I Definition

Risk of hypersensitivity to natural latex rubber products that may compromise health

Risk Factors

Biopathophysiologic

Related to history of atopic eczema

Related to history of allergic rhinitis

*Related to history of asthma**

Treatment Related

*Related to multiple surgical procedures, especially beginning in infancy**

Related to frequent urinary catheterizations

Related to frequent rectal impaction removal

Related to frequent surgical procedures

Related to barium enema (before 1992)

Situational (Personal, Environmental)

*Related to history of allergies**
History of food allergy to banana, kiwi, avocado, chestnuts, trop-
    ical fruits (mango, papaya, passion fruit), poinsettia plants,*
    tomato, raw potato, peach,
History of allergy to gloves, condoms, and so forth
Frequent occupational exposure to NRL,* such as:
    Workers making NRL products
    Food handlers
    Greenhouse workers
    Health care workers
    Housekeepers

 Author's Note

Frequent exposure to airborne latex has contributed to latex allergies.
All individuals who do not have latex allergies should use nonpowdered
latex gloves (De Jong et al., 2011).

 NOC

Immune Hypersensitivity Control

Goal

Refer to *Latex Allergy Response.*

NIC

Allergy Management, Latex Precautions, Environmental Risk Protection

Interventions

Refer to *Latex Allergy Response.*

SEDENTARY LIFESTYLE

NANDA-I Definition

Reports a habit of life that is characterized by a low physical activity level

Defining Characteristics*

Chooses a daily routine lacking physical exercise
Demonstrates physical deconditioning
Verbalized preference for activities low in physical activity

Related Factors*

Pathophysiologic

*Related to decreased endurance secondary to obesity***

Situational (Personal, Environment)

Related to inadequate knowledge of health benefits of physical activity

*Related to inadequate knowledge of exercise routines***

Related to insufficient resources (money, facilities)

Related to perceived lack of time

Related to lack of motivation

Related to lack of interest

Related to lack of training for accomplishment of physical exercise

 Author's Note

This is the first nursing diagnosis submitted by a nurse from another country and accepted by NANDA. Congratulations to J. Adolf Guirao-Goris of Valencia, Spain.

NOC

Knowledge: Health Behaviors, Physical Fitness

** Added by author for clarity.

Goal

The client will verbalize intent to or engage in increased physical activity, as evidenced by the following indicators:

- Set a goal for weekly exercise.
- Identify a desired activity or exercise.

NIC

Exercise Promotion, Exercise Therapy

Interventions

Discuss Benefits of Exercise

- Reduces caloric absorption
- Improves body posture
- Increases metabolic rate
- Preserves lean muscle mass
- Suppresses appetite
- Improves self-esteem
- Reduces depression, anxiety, and stress
- Provides fun, recreation, diversion
- Increases oxygen uptake
- Increases caloric expenditure
- Maintains weight loss
- Increases restful sleep
- Increases resistance to age-related degeneration

Assist Client to Identify Realistic Exercise Program. Consider:

- Physical limitations (consult nurse or physician)
- Personal preferences
- Lifestyle
- Community resources (e.g., safe places to exercise)
- Clients must learn to monitor pulse before, during, and after exercise to assist them to achieve target heart rate and not to exceed maximum advisable heart rate for age.

Age (years)	Maximum Heart Rate (bpm)	Target Heart Rate (bpm)
30	190	133 to 162
40	180	126 to 153
50	170	119 to 145
60	160	112 to 136

- A regular exercise program should be:
  - Enjoyable
  - Use a minimum of 400 calories in each session
  - Sustain a heat rate of approximately 120 to 150 bpm
  - Involve rhythmic, alternating contracting and relaxing of muscles
  - Be integrated into the client's lifestyle of 4 to 5 days/week for at least 30 to 60 minutes

Discuss Aspects of Starting the Exercise Program

- Start slow and easy; obtain clearance from physician.
- Read, consult experts, and talk with friends/coworkers who exercise.
- Plan a daily walking program:
  - Start at 5 to 10 blocks for 0.5 to 1 mile/day; increase 1 block or 0.1 mile/week.
  - Gradually increase rate and length of walk; remember to progress slowly.
  - Avoid straining or pushing too hard and becoming overly fatigued.
  - Stop immediately if any of the following occur:
    - Lightness or pain chest
    - Dizziness, lightheadedness
    - Severe breathlessness
    - Loss of muscle control
    - Nausea
- If pulse is 120 bpm at 4 minutes or 100 bpm at 10 minutes after stopping exercise, or if shortness of breath occurs 10 minutes after exercise, slow down either the rate or the distance of walking for 1 week to point before signs appeared and then start to add 1 block/0.1 mile each week.
- Walk at same rate; time with stopwatch or second hand on watch; after reaching 10 blocks (1 mile), try to increase speed.
- Remember, increase only the rate or the distance of walking at one time.
- Establish a regular time for exercise, with the goal of three to five times/week for 15 to 45 minutes and a heart rate of 80% of stress test or gross calculation (170 bpm for 20 to 29 years of age.) Decrease 10 bpm for each additional decade (e.g., 160 bpm for 30 to 39 years of age, 150 bpm for 40 to 49 years of age).
- Encourage significant others to engage in walking program.
- Add supplemental activity (e.g., parking far from destination, gardening, using stairs, spending weekends at activities that require walking).
- Work up to 1 hour of exercise per day at least 4 days per week.
- Avoid lapses of more than 2 days between exercise sessions.

Assist Client to Increase Interest and Motivation

- Develop a contract listing realistic short- and long-term goals.
- Keep intake/activity records.
- Increase knowledge by reading and talking with health-conscious friends and coworkers.
- Make new friends who are health conscious.
- Get a friend to follow the program or be a source of support.
- Be aware of rationalization (e.g., a lack of time may be a lack of prioritization).
- Keep a list of positive outcomes.

RISK FOR IMPAIRED LIVER FUNCTION

See also *Risk for Complications of Hepatic Dysfunction* on http://thePoint.lww.com/CarpenitoHB14e.

NANDA-I Definition

At risk for a decrease in liver function that may compromise health

Risk Factors*

Hepatotoxic medications (e.g., acetaminophen, statins)
HIV coinfection
Substance abuse (e.g., alcohol, cocaine)
Viral infection (e.g., hepatitis A, hepatitis B, hepatitis C, Epstein–Barr virus)

 Author's Note

This diagnosis represents a situation that requires collaborative intervention with medicine. This author recommends the collaborative problem *Risk for Complications of Hepatic Dysfunction* be used instead. Refer to http://thePoint.lww.com/CarpenitoHB14e for interventions. Students should consult with their faculty for advice on the use of *Risk for Impaired Liver Function* or *Risk for Complications of Hepatic Dysfunction*.

RISK FOR LONELINESS

NANDA-I Definition

At risk for experiencing discomfort associated with a desire or need for more contact with others

Risk Factors

Pathophysiologic

Related to fear of rejection secondary to:
Obesity
Cancer (disfiguring surgery of head or neck, superstition from
    others)
Physical handicaps (paraplegia, amputation, arthritis, hemiplegia)
Emotional handicaps (extreme anxiety, depression, paranoia,
    phobias)
Incontinence (embarrassment, odor)
Communicable diseases (acquired immunodeficiency syndrome
    [AIDS], hepatitis)
Psychiatric illness (schizophrenia, bipolar affective disorder,
    personality disorders)

Related to difficulty accessing social events secondary to:
Debilitating diseases
Physical disabilities

Treatment Related

Related to therapeutic isolation

Situational (Personal, Environmental)

*Related to affectional or cathectic deprivation**

*Related to physical or social isolation**

Related to insufficient planning for retirement

Related to death of a significant other

Related to divorce

Related to visible physical disabilities

Related to fear of rejection secondary to:

Obesity	Extreme poverty
Hospitalization or terminal illness (dying process)	Unemployment

Related to moving to another culture (e.g., unfamiliar language)

Related to history of unsatisfactory social experiences secondary to:

Drug abuse	Delusional thinking
Unacceptable social behavior	Immature behavior
Alcohol abuse	

Related to loss of usual means of transportation

Related to change in usual residence secondary to:
Long-term care   Relocation

Maturational

Child
Related to protective isolation or a communicable disease

Related to autism

Older Adult
Related to loss of usual social contacts secondary to:
Retirement   Relocation
Death of (specify)   Loss of driving ability

Author's Note

Risk for Loneliness was added to the NANDA list in 1994. Currently, *Social Isolation* is also on the NANDA list. *Social Isolation* is a conceptually incorrect diagnosis because it does not represent a response, rather a cause. ElSadr, Noureddine, & Kelley (2009), in a concept analysis of loneliness, found the literature that supports social isolation as a possible cause of loneliness. *Loneliness* and *Risk for Loneliness* better describe the negative state of aloneness.

Loneliness is a subjective state that exists whenever a client says it does and perceives it as imposed by others. Social isolation is *not* the voluntary solitude necessary for personal renewal, nor is it the creative aloneness of the artist or the aloneness—and possible suffering— a client may experience from seeking individualism and independence (e.g., moving to a new city, going away to college).

NOC

Loneliness, Social Involvement

Goal

The client will report decreased feelings of loneliness, as evidenced by the following indicators:

• Identify the reasons for his or her feelings of isolation.
• Discuss ways to increase meaningful relationships.

NIC

Socialization Enhancement, Spiritual Support, Behavior Modification: Social Skills, Presence, Anticipatory Guidance

Interventions

The nursing interventions for various contributing factors that might be associated with *Risk for Loneliness* are similar.

Identify Causative and Contributing Factors (Refer to Related Factors)

Reduce or Eliminate Causative and Contributing Factors

- Promote social interaction.
- Support the client who has experienced a loss as he or she works through grief (refer to *Grieving*).
- Encourage client to talk about feelings of loneliness and their causes.
- Encourage development of a support system or mobilize client's existing family, friends, and neighbors to form one.
- Discuss the importance of high-quality, rather than high-quantity, socialization.
- Refer to social skills teaching (see *Impaired Social Interaction*).
- Offer feedback on how the client presents himself or herself to others (refer to *Impaired Social Interaction*).

Decrease Barriers to Social Contact

- Help identify transportation options.
- Determine available transportation in the community (public, church-related, volunteer).
- Determine if client must learn how to use alternative transportation. Help desensitize client to fear/stigma of using public transportation.
- Assist with the development of alternative means of communication for people with compromised sensory ability (e.g., amplifier on phone, taped instead of written letters; refer to *Impaired Communication*).
- Assist with management of aesthetic problems (e.g., consult enterostomal therapist if ostomy odor is a problem; teach client with cancer to control odor of tumors by packing area with yogurt or pouring in buttermilk, then rinsing well with saline solution).
- Refer to *Impaired Urinary Elimination* for specific interventions to control incontinence.

Identify Strategies to Expand the World of the Isolated

- Senior centers and church groups
- Volunteer assignments (e.g., hospital, church)
- Foster grandparent programs
- Adult day-care centers
- Retirement communities
- House sharing, group homes, community kitchens
- Adult education classes, special interest courses
- Pets
- Regular contact to diminish the need to obtain attention through a crisis (e.g., suicidal gesture)
- Psychiatric day hospital or activity program

Implement the Following for People With Poor or Offensive Social Skills

- Refer to *Impaired Social Interactions*.

Discuss the Anticipatory Effects of Retirement; Assist With Planning

- Prepare for ambivalent feelings and short-term negative effects on self-esteem.

Discuss Those Factors That Contribute to Successful Retirement (Santrock, 2004; Murray, Zentner, & Yakimo, 2009)

- Stable health status
- Adequate income and health benefits
- Active in community, church, or professional organizations
- Higher education level and ability to pursue new goals/activities
- Extended social network, family friends, colleagues
- Satisfied with life before retirement
- Satisfied with living arrangements
- Plan to ensure adequate income
- Decreased time at work the last 2 to 3 years (e.g., shorter days, longer vacations)
- Cultivate friends outside work.
- Develop routines at home to replace work structure.
- Rely on others rather than spouse for leisure activities.
- Cultivate realistic leisure activities (energy, cost).
- Engage in community or church programs or professional organizations.

Initiate Referrals, as Indicated

- Community-based groups that contact the socially isolated
- Self-help groups for clients isolated because of specific medical problems (e.g., Reach to Recovery, United Ostomy Association)
- Wheelchair groups
- Psychiatric consumer rights associations

RISK FOR DISTURBED MATERNAL/ FETAL DYAD

NANDA-I Definition

At risk for disruption of the symbiotic maternal/fetal dyad as a result of comorbid or pregnancy-related conditions

Risk Factors*

Complications of pregnancy (e.g., premature rupture of membranes, placenta previa or abruption, late prenatal care, multiple gestation)

Compromised oxygen transport (e.g., anemia, cardiac disease, asthma, hypertension, seizures, premature labor, hemorrhage)

Impaired glucose metabolism (e.g., diabetes, steroid use)

Physical abuse

Substance abuse (e.g., tobacco, alcohol, drugs)

Treatment-related side effects (e.g., medications, surgery, chemotherapy)

Author's Note

This NANDA-I nursing diagnosis represents numerous situations or factors that can compromise a pregnant woman, her fetus, or both. The primary responsibility of nursing is to monitor the status of the mother, fetus, and pregnancy and to collaborate with medicine for monitoring (e.g., electronic fetal monitoring, Doppler, laboratory tests) and treatments.

Refer to http://thePoint.lww.com/CarpenitoHB14e under *Risk for Complications of Reproductive Dysfunction* for interventions for this generic collaborative problem. More specific collaborative problems such as the following may also apply:

- *Risk for Complications of Preterm Labor*
- *Risk for Complications of Nonreassuring Fetal Status*
- *Risk for Complications of Prenatal Bleeding*
- *Risk for Pregnancy-Associated Hypertension*
- *Risk for Complications of Postpartum Hemorrhage*

For example, if a pregnant woman is using cocaine, the collaborative problem *Risk for Complications of Reproductive Dysfunction secondary to cocaine use* would be valid because cocaine contributes to preterm labor and fetal complications. In another situation such as placenta previa, *Risk for Complications of Prenatal Bleeding* would be valid. In addition, some Nursing Diagnoses may be valid, such as *Ineffective Denial* and *Disabled Family Coping*.

IMPAIRED MEMORY

NANDA-I Definition

Inability to remember or recall bits of information or behavioral skills

Defining Characteristics*

Major (Must Be Present, One or More)

Reports experiences of forgetting
Inability to recall if a behavior was performed
Inability to learn or retain new skills or information
Inability to perform a previously learned skill
Inability to recall factual information
Inability to recall events

Related Factors

Pathophysiologic

Related to neurologic disturbances secondary to:*
Degenerative brain disease   Head injury
Lesion   Cerebrovascular accident

Related to reduced quantity and quality of information processed secondary to:
Visual deficits   Learning habits
Hearing deficits   Intellectual skills
Poor physical fitness   Educational level
Fatigue

Related to nutritional deficiencies (e.g., vitamins C and B_{12}, folate, niacin, thiamine)

Treatment Related

Related to effects of medication (specify) on memory storage

Situational (Personal, Environmental)

Related to self-fulfilling expectations

Related to excessive self-focus and worry secondary to:
Grieving   Depression
Anxiety

Related to alcohol consumption

Related to lack of motivation

Related to lack of stimulation

Related to difficulty concentrating secondary to:

Stress	Lack of intellectual stimulation
Pain	Sleep disturbances
Distractions	

 Author's Note

This diagnosis is useful when the client can be helped to function better because of improved memory. If the client's memory cannot be improved because of cerebral degeneration, this diagnosis is not appropriate. Instead, the nurse should evaluate the effects of impaired memory on functioning, such as *Self-Care Deficits* or *Risk for Injury*. The focus of interventions for these nursing diagnoses would be improving self-care or protection, not improving memory.

NOC

Cognitive Orientation, Memory

Goal

The client will report increased satisfaction with memory, as evidenced by the following indicators:

- Identify three techniques to improve memory.
- Relate factors that deter memory.

NIC

Reality Orientation, Memory Training, Environmental Management

Interventions

Discuss the Client's Beliefs About Memory Deficits

- Correct misinformation.
- Explain that negative expectations can result in memory deficits.

Assess for Factors That May Negatively Affect Memory (e.g., Pathophysiologic, Literacy, Stressors)

If the Client Has Difficulty Concentrating, Explain the Favorable Effects of Relaxation and Imagery

Teach the Client Two or Three of the Following Methods to Improve Memory Skills (Maier-Lorentz, 2000; Miller, 2009):

- Write things down (e.g., use lists, calendars, notebooks).
- Use auditory cues (e.g., timers, alarm clocks) in conjunction with written cues.
- Use environmental cues (e.g., you might remove something from its usual place, then return it to its normal location after it has served its purpose as a reminder).
- Have specific places for specific items; keep items in their proper place (e.g., keep keys on a hook near the door).
- Put reminders in appropriate places (e.g., place shoes to be repaired near the door).
- Use visual images ("A picture is worth a thousand words"). Create a picture in your mind when you want to remember something; the more bizarre the picture, the more likely you will remember.
- Use active observation—pay attention to details around you and be alert to the environment.
- Make associations or mental connections (e.g., "Spring ahead and fall back" for changing clocks to and from daylight savings time).
- Make associations between names and mental images (e.g., Carol and Christmas carol).
- Rehearse items you want to remember by repeating them aloud or writing them on paper.
- Use self-instruction—say things aloud (e.g., "I'm putting my keys on the counter so I remember to turn off the stove before I leave").
- Divide information into small chunks that can be remembered easily (e.g., to remember an address or a zip code, divide it into groups ["seven hundred sixty, fifty-five"]).
- Organize information into logical categories (e.g., shampoo and hair spray, toothpaste and mouthwash, soap and deodorant).
- Use rhyming cues (e.g., "In 1492, Columbus sailed the ocean blue").
- Use first-letter cues and make associations (e.g., to remember to buy carrots, apples, radishes, pickles, eggs, and tea bags, remember the word *carpet*).
- Make word associations (e.g., to remember the letters of your license plate, make a word, such as "camel" for CML).
- Search the alphabet while focusing on what you are trying to remember (e.g., to remember that someone's name is Martin, start with names that begin with "A" and continue naming names through the alphabet until your memory is jogged for the correct one).

- Make up a story to connect things you want to remember (e.g., if you have to go to the cleaners and post office, create a story about mailing a pair of pants).

When Trying to Learn or Remember Something:

- Minimize distractions.
- Do not rush.
- Maintain some form of organization of routine tasks.
- Carry a note pad or calendar or use written cues.

When Teaching (Miller, 2009):

- Determine if there are barriers to learning (e.g., stress, alcohol use/abuse, pain, depression, low literacy).
- Eliminate distractions.
- Present information as concretely as possible.
- Use practical examples.
- Allow learner to pace the learning.
- Use visual, auditory aids.
- Provide advance organizers; outlines, written cues.
- Encourage use of aids.
- Make sure glasses are clean and lights are soft white.
- Correct wrong answers immediately.
- Encourage verbal responses.
- Try to organize self-care activities in the same order and same time each day.

Geriatric Interventions

- Provide accurate information about age-related changes.
- Explain the difference between age-related forgetfulness and dementia.

IMPAIRED PHYSICAL MOBILITY

Impaired Physical Mobility

Impaired Bed Mobility

Impaired Walking

Impaired Wheelchair Mobility

Impaired Transfer Ability

NANDA-I Definition

Limitation in independent, purposeful physical movement of the body or of one or more extremities

Defining Characteristics**

Major (Must Be Present; 80% to 100%)

Compromised ability to move purposefully within the environment (e.g., bed mobility, transfers, ambulation)
Range-of-motion (ROM) limitations

Minor (May Be Present; 50% to 80%)

Imposed restriction of movement
Reluctance to move

Related Factors

Pathophysiologic

Related to decreased muscle strength * and endurance* secondary to:*
Neuromuscular impairment
Autoimmune alterations
  (e.g., multiple sclerosis,
  arthritis)
Nervous system diseases
  (e.g., Parkinson's disease,
  myasthenia gravis)
Respiratory conditions
  (e.g., chronic obstructive
  pulmonary disease [COPD])
Muscular dystrophy
Partial paralysis (spinal cord
  injury, stroke)
Central nervous system (CNS)
  tumor
Trauma
Cancer
Increased intracranial pressure
Sensory deficits
Musculoskeletal impairment
Fractures
Connective tissue disease
  (systemic lupus
  erythematosus)
Cardiac conditions

Related to joint stiffness * or contraction* secondary to:*
Inflammatory joint disease
Post–joint-replacement or spinal surgery
Degenerative joint disease
Degenerative disc disease

Related to edema

** Levin, Krainovitch, Bahrenburg, & Mitchell, 1989.

Treatment Related

Related to external devices (casts or splints, braces, intravenous [IV] tubing)

Related to insufficient strength and endurance for ambulation with (specify):

Prosthesis   Walker
Crutches

Situational (Personal, Environmental)

Related to:
Fatigue   Deconditioning*
Depressive mood state*   Obesity
Decreased motivation   Dyspnea
Sedentary lifestyle*   Cognitive impairment*
Pain*

Maturational

Children
Related to abnormal gait secondary to:
Congenital skeletal deficiencies
Congenital hip dysplasia
Legg–Calvé–Perthes disease
Osteomyelitis

Older Adult
Related to decreased motor agility

*Related to decreased muscle mass and strength**

 Author's Note

Impaired Physical Mobility describes a client with limited use of arm(s) or leg(s) or limited muscle strength. Nurses should not use this diagnosis to describe complete immobility; in this case, *Risk for Disuse Syndrome* is more applicable. Limitation of physical movement can also be the etiology of other nursing diagnoses, such as *Self-Care Deficit* and *Risk for Injury*. Nursing interventions for *Impaired Physical Mobility* focus on strengthening and restoring function and preventing deterioration. If the client can exercise but does not, refer to *Sedentary Lifestyle*. If the client has no limitations in movement but is deconditioned and has reduced endurance, refer to *Activity Intolerance*.

NOC

Ambulation, Joint Movement, Mobility, Fall Prevention Behavior

Goal

The client will report increased strength and endurance of limbs, as evidenced by the following indicators:

• Demonstrate the use of adaptive devices to increase mobility.
• Use safety measures to minimize potential for injury.
• Demonstrate measures to increase mobility.
• Evaluate pain and quality of management

NIC

Exercise Therapy: Joint Mobility, Exercise Promotion: Strength Training, Exercise Therapy: Ambulation, Positioning, Teaching: Prescribed Activity/Exercise, Fall Prevention

Interventions

Assess Causative Factors

Refer to Related Factors.

Consult With Physical Therapy for Evaluation and Development of a Mobility Plan

Promote Optimal Mobility and Movement

Promote Motivation and Adherence (Addams & Clough, 1998)

• Explain the problem and the objective of each exercise.
• Establish short-term goals.
• Ensure that initial exercises are easy and require minimal strength and coordination.
• Progress only if the client is successful at the present exercise.
• Provide written instructions for prescribed exercises after demonstrating and observing return demonstration.
• Document and discuss improvement specifically (e.g., can lift leg 2 inches higher).
• Evaluate level of motivation and depression. Refer to a specialist as needed.

Increase Limb Mobility and Determine Type of ROM Appropriate for the Client (Passive, Active Assistive, Active, Active Resistive)

• Perform passive or active assistive ROM exercises (frequency determined by client's condition):
  • Teach the client to perform active ROM exercises on unaffected limbs at least four times a day, if possible.

- Perform passive ROM on affected limbs. Do the exercises slowly to allow the muscles time to relax, and support the extremity above and below the joint to prevent strain on joints and tissues.
- For passive ROM, the supine position is most effective. The client who performs ROM himself or herself can use a supine or sitting position.
- Do ROM daily with bed bath three or four times daily if there are specific problem areas. Try to incorporate into activities of daily living.
- Support extremity with pillows to prevent or reduce swelling.
- Medicate for pain as needed, especially before activity** (see *Impaired Comfort*).
- Apply heat or cold to reduce pain, inflammation, and hematoma (after 48 hours).**
- Apply cold to reduce swelling after injury (usually first 48 hours).**
- Encourage the client to perform exercise regimens for specific joints as prescribed by physician, nurse practitioner, or physical therapist (e.g., isometric, resistive).

Position in Alignment to Prevent Complications

- Use a footboard.
- Avoid prolonged sitting or lying in the same position.
- Change the position of the shoulder joints every 2 to 4 hours.
- Use a small pillow or no pillow when in Fowler's position.
- Support the hand and wrist in natural alignment.
- If the client is supine or prone, place a rolled towel or small pillow under the lumbar curvature or under the end of the rib cage.
- Place a trochanter roll alongside the hips and upper thighs.
- If the client is in the lateral position, place pillow(s) to support the leg from groin to foot, and use a pillow to flex the shoulder and elbow slightly. If needed, support the lower foot in dorsal flexion with a towel roll or special boot.
- For upper extremities:
  - Arms abducted from the body with pillows
  - Elbows in slight flexion
  - Wrist in a neutral position, with fingers slightly flexed and thumb abducted and slightly flexed
  - Position of shoulder joints changed during the day (e.g., adduction, abduction, range of circular motion)

** May require a primary care professional's order.

Maintain Good Body Alignment When Mechanical Devices Are Used

Traction Devices
- Assess for correct position of traction and alignment of bones.
- Observe for correct amount and position of weights.
- Allow weights to hang freely, with no blankets or sheets on ropes.
- Assess for changes in circulation; check pulse quality, skin temperature, color of extremities, and capillary refill (should be less than 3 seconds).
- Assess for feelings of numbness, tingling, and/or pain.
- Assess for changes in mobility (ability to flex/extend unaffected joints).
- Assess for signs of skin irritation (redness, ulceration, blanching).
- Assess skeletal traction pin sites for loosening, inflammation, ulceration, and drainage; clean pin insertion sites (procedure may vary with type of pin and physician's order).
- Encourage isometrics** and prescribed exercise program.

Casts
- Assess for proper fit of cast (should not be too loose or too tight).
- Assess circulation to the encased area every 2 hours (color and temperature of skin, pulse quality, capillary refill less than 2 seconds).
- Assess for changes in sensation of extremities every 2 hours (numbness, tingling, pain).
- Assess motion of uninvolved joints (ability to flex and extend).
- Assess for skin irritation (redness, ulceration, or complaints of pain under the cast).
- Keep the cast clean and dry; do not allow sharp objects to be inserted under the cast; petal rough edges with adhesive tape; place soft cotton under edges that seem to be causing pressure points.
- Allow the cast to air dry while resting on pillows to prevent dents.
- Observe the cast for areas of softening or indentation.
- Exercise joints above and below the cast if allowed (e.g., wiggle fingers and toes every 2 hours).
- Assist with prescribed exercise regimens and isometrics of muscles enclosed in casts.*
- Keep extremities elevated after cast application to reduce swelling.

** May require a primary professional's order.

Braces
- Assess for correct positioning of braces.
- Observe for signs of skin irritation (redness, ulceration, blanching, itching, pain).
- Assist with exercises as prescribed for specific joints.
- Have the client demonstrate correct application of the brace.

Prosthetic Devices
- Observe for signs of skin irritation of the stump before applying prosthetic device (stump should be clean and dry; Ace bandage should be rewrapped and securely in place).
- Have the client demonstrate correct application of the prosthesis.
- Assess for gait alterations or improper walking technique.
- Proceed with health teaching, if indicated.

Ace Bandages
- Assess for correct position of Ace bandage.
- Apply Ace bandage with even pressure, wrapping from distal to proximal portions and making sure that the bandage is not too tight or too loose.
- Observe for bunching of the bandage.
- Observe for signs of irritation of skin (redness, ulceration, excessive tightness).
- Rewrap Ace bandage twice daily or as needed, unless contra-indicated (e.g., if the bandage is a postoperative compression dressing, it should be left in place).
- When wrapping lower extremity, leave the heel exposed, using figure-8 technique.

Slings
- Assess for correct application; sling should be loose around the neck and should support the elbow and wrist at the level of the heart.
- Remove slings for ROM.**
- Note: Some mechanical devices may be removed for exercises, depending on the nature of the injury or type and purpose of the device. Consult with the physician to ascertain when the client may remove the device.

Provide Progressive Mobilization

- Assist the client slowly to a sitting position.
- Allow the client to dangle legs over the side of the bed for a few minutes before standing.

** May require a primary professional's order.

- Limit time to 15 minutes, three times a day the first few times out of bed.
- Increase time out of bed, as tolerated, by 15-minute increments.
- Progress to ambulation with or without assistive devices.
- If the client cannot walk, assist him or her out of bed to a wheelchair or chair.
- Encourage ambulation for short, frequent walks (at least three times daily), with assistance if unsteady.
- Increase lengths of walks progressively each day.

Encourage Use of Affected Arm When Possible

- Encourage the client to use affected arm for self-care activities (e.g., feeding self, dressing, brushing hair).
- For post-CVA neglect of upper limb, see *Unilateral Neglect*.
- Instruct the client to use the unaffected arm to exercise the affected arm.
- Use appropriate adaptive equipment to enhance the use of arms.
  - Universal cuff for feeding in clients with poor control in both arms and hands
  - Large-handled or padded silverware to assist clients with poor fine-motor skills
  - Dishware with high edges to prevent food from slipping
  - Suction-cup aids to prevent sliding of plate
- Use a warm bath to alleviate early-morning stiffness and improve mobility.
- Encourage the client to practice handwriting skills, if able.
- Allow time to practice using affected limb.
- Determine if other factors are interfering with mobility.
  - If the pain is interfering with mobility, refer to *Acute* or *Chronic Pain*.
  - If depression is interfering with mobility, refer to *Ineffective Individual Coping*.
  - If fatigue is interfering with mobility, refer to *Fatigue*.

Teach Methods of Transfer From Bed to Chair or Commode and to Standing Position

- Refer to *Impaired Transfer Ability* for interventions.

Teach the Client How to Ambulate With Adaptive Equipment (e.g., Crutches, Walkers, Canes)

- Instruct client in weight-bearing status.
- Observe and teach the use of the following equipment.

Crutches

- Do not exert pressure on axilla; use hand strength.
- Type of gait varies with client's diagnosis.
- Measure crutches 2 to 3 inches below axilla and tips 6 inches away from feet.

Walkers
- Use arm strength to support weakness in lower limbs.
- Gait varies with the client's problems.
- Adjust to ensure a slight bend at the elbow when client is standing with hands on the walker.

Prostheses (Teach About the Following)
- Stump wrapping before application of the prosthesis
- Application of the prosthesis
- Principles of stump care
- Importance of cleaning the stump, keeping it dry, and applying the prosthesis only when the stump is dry
- Safety precautions
  - Protect areas of decreased sensation from extremes of heat and cold.
  - Practice falling and how to recover from falls while transferring or ambulating.
  - For decreased perception of lower extremity (post-CVA "neglect"), instruct the client to check where limb is placed when changing positions or going through doorways; also check to make sure both shoelaces are tied, that affected leg is dressed with trousers, and that pants are not dragging.
  - Instruct people who are confined to a wheelchair to shift position and lift up buttocks every 15 minutes to relieve pressure; maneuver curbs, ramps, inclines, and around obstacles; and lock wheelchairs before transferring.
- Practice proper positioning, ROM (active or passive), and prescribed exercises.
- Practice climbing stairs if client's condition permits.
- Refer to physical therapy for continued structured physical therapy.

Initiate Health Teaching and Referrals, as Indicated
- Home health nurse and physical therapist.

Impaired Bed Mobility

NANDA-I Definition

Limitation of independent movement from one bed position to another

Defining Characteristics*

Impaired ability to turn from side to side
Impaired ability to move from supine to sitting to supine
Impaired ability to reposition self in bed
Impaired ability to move from supine to prone or prone to supine
Impaired ability to move from supine to long sitting or long
    sitting to supine

Related Factors

Refer to *Impaired Physical Mobility*.

 Author's Note

Impaired Bed Mobility may be a clinically useful diagnosis when a client
is a candidate for rehabilitation to improve strength, ROM, and movement. The nurse can consult with a physical therapist for a specific plan.
This diagnosis is inappropriate for an unconscious or terminally ill client.

NOC

Ambulation Joint Movement, Mobility, Fall Prevention Behavior

Goals

Refer to *Impaired Physical Mobility*.

NIC

Exercise Therapy: Joint Mobility, Exercise Promotion: Strength Training, Exercise
Therapy: Ambulation, Positioning, Teaching: Prescribed Activity/Exercise, Prosthesis Care

Interventions

Refer to *Impaired Physical Mobility*.

Impaired Walking

NANDA-I Definition

Limitation of independent movement within the environment on
foot

Defining Characteristics*

Impaired ability to climb stairs
Impaired ability to walk required distances
Impaired ability to walk on an incline
Impaired ability to walk on uneven surfaces
Impaired ability to navigate curbs

Related Factors

Refer to *Impaired Physical Mobility*.

Refer to *Impaired Physical Mobility*.

Goal

The client will increase walking distances (specify distance goal) as evidenced by the following indicators:

- Demonstrate safe mobility.
- Use mobility aids correctly.

NIC

Refer to *Impaired Physical Mobility*.

Interventions

Explain That Safe Ambulation Is a Complex Movement Involving the Musculoskeletal, Neurologic, and Cardiovascular Systems and Cognitive Factors Such as Mentation and Orientation

Consult With a Physical Therapist for Evaluation and Planning Prior to Initiation

- Ascertain that client is:
  - Using ambulatory aids (e.g., cane, walker, crutches) correctly and safely:
    - Wears well-fitting shoes
    - Can ambulate on inclines, uneven surfaces, and up and down stairs
    - Is aware of hazards (e.g., wet floors, throw rugs)
- Refer to *Impaired Physical Mobility*.

Provide Progressive Mobilization, If Indicated (Botolfsen et al., 2008)

- Assist the client slowly to a sitting position.
- Allow the client to dangle legs over the side of the bed for a few minutes before standing.

- Limit the time to 15 minutes, three times a day the first few times out of bed.
- Increase time out of bed, as tolerated, by 15-minute increments.
- Progress to ambulation, with or without assistive devices.
- Encourage ambulation for short, frequent walks (at least three times daily), with assistance if unsteady.
  - Increase length of walks progressively each day.
  - Evaluate the client's response to ambulation.
- Refer to *Activity Intolerance*, if needed.
- Refer to *Risk for Falls*.

Impaired Wheelchair Mobility

NANDA-I Definition

Limitation of independent operation of wheelchair within environment

Defining Characteristics*

Impaired ability to operate manual or power wheelchair on an even or uneven surface

Impaired ability to operate manual or power wheelchair on an incline

Impaired ability to operate manual or power wheelchair on a decline

Impaired ability to operate the wheelchair on curbs

Related Factors

Refer to *Impaired Physical Mobility*.

Ambulation: Wheelchair, Fall Prevention Behavior

Goal

The client will report satisfactory, safe wheelchair mobility as evidenced by the following indicators:

- Demonstrate safe use of the wheelchair.
- Demonstrate safe transfer to/from the wheelchair.
- Demonstrate pressure relief and safety principles.

NIC

Exercise Therapy: Ambulation, Exercise Therapy: Balance, Exercise Promotion: Joint Mobility, Exercise Promotion: Strength Training, Muscle Control, Positioning: Wheelchair, Fall Prevention

Interventions

Consult With Physical Therapy for a Collaborative Plan

Monitor Pressure Points of Elbow, Sacrum, Coccyx, Ischial Tuberosities, and Heels of Seated Individuals

If Signs of Pressure Occur, Refer to a Physical Therapist for Evaluation of Wheelchair Seat; Access a Specialist for an individualized Fitting of an Appropriate Wheelchair and Seating Components (Bulechek, Butcher, & Dochterman, 2008)

- Avoid doughnut-type cushions and sheepskin.

Maintain Proper Positioning and Good Alignment

- Reposition a slumped client upward in wheelchair using two-person assisted horizontal lift (Bulechek, Butcher, & Dochterman, 2008).

Instruct on Methods to Shift Weight

- Instruct the client to stand briefly and/or shift weight and lean forward every hour when in the wheelchair.
- Instruct the client to manually tilt the chair backward 45 degrees to 150 degrees for 3 to 5 minutes hourly.
- Instruct the client to lean toward one side of the chair and forward while sitting. The client should push himself or herself up with the hands on armrests to lift the buttocks.
- Instruct the client to put his or her feet on the floor, not the footrests, while sitting.

Refer to Physical Therapy for Instruction on Using the Wheelchair on Flat Surfaces, Curbs, in Elevators, etc.

Refer to Home Health Nurse for Evaluation of Home Environment

Impaired Transfer Ability

NANDA-I Definition

Limitation of independent movement between two nearby surfaces

Defining Characteristics*

Impaired ability to transfer:
From bed to chair and chair to bed
On or off a toilet or commode
In and out of tub or shower
Between uneven levels
From chair to car or car to chair
From chair to floor or floor to chair
From standing to floor or floor to standing
From bed to standing or standing to bed
From chair to standing or standing to chair

Related Factors

Refer to *Impaired Physical Mobility*.

NOC

Transfer Performance, Fall Prevention Behavior

Goal

The client will demonstrate transfer to and from the wheelchair as evidenced by the following indicators:

• Identify when assistance is needed.
• The client will demonstrate ability to transfer in varied situations (e.g., toilet, bed, car, chair, uneven levels).

NIC

Positioning: Wheelchair, Fall Prevention

Interventions

Consult With and Refer to a Physical Therapist to Evaluate the Client's Ability to Transfer

• Consider weight, strength, movement ability, tolerance to position changes, balance, motivation, and cognition.
• Use manual transfer or device-assisted lift.
• Consider ratio of staff to clients.

Proceed With Established Plan to Transfer

• Before transferring the client, assess the number of personnel needed for assistance.
• The client should transfer toward the unaffected side.

- Position the client on the side of the bed. His or her feet should be touching the floor, and he or she should be wearing stable shoes or slippers with nonskid soles.
- For getting in and out of bed, encourage weight-bearing on the uninvolved or stronger side.
- Lock the wheelchair before the transfer. If using a regular chair, be sure it will not move.
- Instruct the client to use the arm of the chair closer to him or her for support while standing.
- Use a gait belt (preferred) or place your arm around the client's rib cage and keep the back straight, with knees slightly bent.
- Tell the client to place his or her arms around your waist or rib cage, *not the neck*.
- Support client's legs by bracing his with yours. (While facing the client, lock his or her knees with your knees.)
- Instruct clients with hemiplegia to pivot on the uninvolved foot.

For Clients With Lower Limb Weakness or Paralysis, a Sliding Board Transfer May Be Used

- The client should wear pajamas so he or she will not stick to the board.
- The client needs good upper extremity strength to be able to slide the buttocks from the bed to the chair or wheelchair. (Wheelchairs should have removable arms.)
- When the client's arms are strong enough, he or she should progress to a sitting transfer without the board if he or she can lift their buttocks enough to clear the bed and chair seat.
- If the client's legs give out, guide him or her gently to the floor and *seek additional assistance*.
- Consult and refer client and family to home health nurses for a home evaluation and to access resources for discharge.

MORAL DISTRESS

Moral Distress
Risk for Moral Distress

Definition

Response to the inability to carry out one's chosen ethical/moral decision/action (NANDA-I)

The state in which a person experiences psychological disequilibrium, physical discomforts, anxiety, and/or anguish that results when a person makes a moral decision but does not follow through with the moral behavior**

Defining Characteristics*

Expresses anguish (e.g., powerlessness, guilt, frustration, anxiety, self-doubt, fear) over difficulty acting on one's moral choice

Related Factors

When *Moral Distress* is used to describe a response in nurses, as explained in this section, related factors are not useful. These diagnoses are not documented but rather represent a response that requires actions by the nurse, unit, and/or institution.

The related factors listed below represent a variety of situations that can precipitate *Moral Distress*.

Situational (Personal, Environmental)

End-of-Life Decisions*

Related to providing treatments that were perceived as futile for terminally ill client (e.g., blood transfusions, chemotherapy, organ transplants, mechanical ventilation)

Related to conflicting attitudes toward advanced directives

Related to participation of life-saving actions when they only prolong dying

Treatment Decisions

Related to the client's/family's refusal of treatments deemed appropriate by the health care team

Related to inability of the family to make the decision to stop ventilator treatment of terminally ill client

Related to a family's wishes to continue life support even though it is not in the best interest of the client

Related to performing a procedure that increases the client's suffering

Related to providing care that does not relieve the client's suffering

---

** This definition has been added by Lynda Juall Carpenito, the author, for clarity and clinical usefulness.

Related to conflicts between wanting to disclose poor medical practice and wanting to maintain trust in the physician

Professional Conflicts
Related to insufficient resources for care (e.g., time, staff)

Related to failure to be included in the decision-making process

Related to more emphasis on technical skills and tasks than relationships and caring

Cultural Conflicts
Related to decisions made for women by male family members

Related to cultural conflicts with the American health care system

 Author's Note

This NANDA-I nursing diagnosis, accepted in 2006, has application in all settings where nurses practice. The literature to support this diagnosis when submitted was focused primarily on moral distress in nursing.

If moral distress occurs in a client or family, this author suggests a referral to a professional expert in this area; for example, a counselor, therapist, or nurse spiritual advisor. Refer also to *Spiritual Distress*. Nurses should expect to experience moral distress as they struggle to make clinical decisions involving conflicting ethical principles (Zuzelo, 2007).

This author will present Moral Distress as a Department of Nursing—Standard of Practice. This standard addresses prevention of moral distress with specific individual nurse, unit, and department interventions. Strategies for addressing moral distress for individual nurses, on units, in the department of nursing and in the institution will be presented.

In this 14th edition, this author has developed and included *Risk for Moral Distress*.

Moral Distress represents proactive strategies for individuals, groups, and institutions to prevent moral distress in nurses. This diagnosis has not yet been submitted to NANDA-I.

Most Americans fear how they will die than death itself (Beckstrand, Callister, Kirchhoff, 2006). Eighty-six percent of Americans polled reported nurses have very high or high ethical standards, ranking nurses at the top of other professions (Gallup poll, 2009).

NOC
Non applicable

Goal

The nurse will relate strategies to address moral distress as evidenced by the following indicators:

- Identify source(s) of moral distress.
- Share their distress with a colleague.
- Identify two strategies to enhance decision-making with clients and family.
- Identify two strategies to enhance discussion of the situation with the physician.

Non applicable

Interventions

Identify Sources of Moral Stress (AACN, 2004)

- Staffing
- Competency of nurses, physicians
- Nurse–physician communication
- Futile care
- Needless pain and suffering
- End-of-life conflicts
- Deception/incomplete information
- Inadequate symptom management
- Disrespectful interactions
- Violence in the workplace

Determine Actions or Strategy Options

- Evaluate the risks and benefits of options.
- Consider the worse possible outcome to your action.
- Consider the risks of doing nothing (personal, client, family, unit).
- Avoid rationalization.

Do Not Try to Avoid or Shrug Off Moral Distress

- Acknowledge your distress.
- Affirm your professional obligation to act.
- Ask for help and clarification.

"Use the Chain of Command to Share and Discuss Issues That Have Escalated Beyond the Problem-Solving Ability and/or Scope of Those Immediately Involved" (LaSala & Bjarnason, 2010)

Explore Moral Work and Action

- Educate yourself about moral distress. Refer to articles on the Bibliography.
- Share your stories of moral distress. Elicit stories from coworkers.
- Read stories of moral action. Refer to Gordon's *Life Support: Three Nurses on the Front Lines* and Kritek's *Reflections on Healing: A Central Construct* (see the Bibliography).

Investigate How Clinical Situations That Are Morally Problematic Are Managed in the Institution; If an Ethics Committee Exists, Determine Its Mission and Procedures

Initiate Dialogue With the Client, If Possible, and Family

- Explore what the perception of the situation is (e.g., How do you think your ___ is doing?)
- Pose questions (e.g., "What options do you have in this situation?") Elicit feelings about the present situation. Does the family know that the client is terminal? Is the client improving?
- Access the physician to clarify misinformation. Stay in the room to promote sharing.
- Encourage the client/family to write down questions for the physician.
- Be present during physician's round to ensure client's/family's understanding.
- Avoid deception or supporting deception.

Gently Explore Client/Family End-of-Life Decisions

- Explain the options (e.g., "If you or your loved one's heart/breathing stops...")
  - Give medications, oxygen
  - Cardio defibrillation (shock)
  - Cardiopulmonary resuscitation
  - Intubation and use of respirator
- Advise the client/family that they can choose all, some, or none of the above.
- Differentiate between prolonging life versus prolonging dying.
- Document the discussion and decisions according to institute on policy.

If Indicated, Explain "No Code" Status and Explain the Focus of Palliative Care That Replaces Aggressive and Futile Care (e.g., Pain Management, Symptom Management, Less or No Intrusive/Painful Procedures)

Seek To Transfer Individual From Intensive Care Unit, If Possible

Dialogue With Unit Colleagues About the Situation That Causes Moral Distress

Seek support and Information From Nurse Manager

Enlist a Colleague as a Coach or Engage as a Coach for a Coworker

- For advice, seek out colleagues who implement actions when they are distressed.

Start With an Approach to Address an Unsatisfactory Moral Clinical Situation That Has a Low Risk; Evaluate the Risks Before Taking Action; Be Realistic

Engage in Open Communication With Involved Physicians or Nurse Manager; Start the Conversation With Your Concern, for Example, "I Am Not Comfortable With...," "The Family Is Asking/ Questioning/Feeling...," "Mr. X Is Asking/Questioning/Feeling..."

Dialogue With Other Professionals: Chaplains, Social Workers, or Ethics Committee

Advocate for End-of-Life Decision Dialogues With All Clients and Their Families, Especially When the Situation Is Not Critical; Direct the Client to Create Written Documents of Their Decisions, and Advise Family About the Document

Integrate Health Promotion and Stress Reduction in Your Lifestyle (e.g. Smoking Cessation, Weight Management, Regular Exercise, Meaningful Leisure Activities)

Risk for Moral Distress

Definition**

The state in which a person is at risk to experience psychological disequilibrium, physical discomforts, anxiety, and/or anguish that results when a person makes a moral decision but does not follow through with the moral behavior

---

** This definition has been added by Lynda Juall Carpenito, the author, for clarity and clinical usefulness.

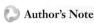 **Author's Note**

Refer to *Moral Distress*.

Risk Factors

Refer to *Moral Distress* Related Factors.

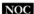 **NOC**

Non applicable

Goal

The nurse will relate strategies to prevent moral distress, as evidenced by the following indicators:

- Identify risk situations for moral distress.
- Share their distress with a colleague.
- Identify two strategies to enhance decision-making with clients and families.
- Identify two strategies to enhance communication patterns with physicians.
- Engage institutional programs to prevent or decrease moral distress.

NIC

Non applicable

Interventions

The following interventions are indicated for the institution and department of nursing.

Create a Just Culture That Fosters Moral Courage (ANA, 2010)

- Commitment to organizational improvement
- Resilience
- Mission, vision, and values that support high-quality client outcomes and increasing situational awareness
- Identifying at-risk behavior creates incentives for healthy behaviors.
- Address the problem of behaviors that threaten the performance of the health care team.
- Make choices that align with organizational values.

Explore Moral Work and Action

- Educate yourself about moral distress. Refer to articles on the Bibliography.
- Share your stories of moral distress. Elicit stories from coworkers.
- Read stories of moral action. Refer to Gordon's *Life Support: Three Nurses on the Front Lines* and Kritek's *Reflections on Healing: A Central Construct* (see the Bibliography).

Investigate How Clinical Situations That Are Morally Problematic Are Managed in the Institution; If an Ethics Committee Exists, Determine Its Mission, Procedures, and Accessibility

Create or Reorganize the Ethics Committee With Membership of Multiple Disciplines (e.g., Medicine, Nursing, Ethics Expert, Administration)

Ensure Accessibility by Health Care Professionals With No Punitive Results for Reporting

The following interventions are indicated for the nursing units and nursing staff.

Clarify the Difference of Medical/Surgical Unit Care, ICUs, and Palliative/Hospice Care

Define and Promote "a Good Death" (Callister & Kirhhoff, 2006). For Example:

- Not allowing client to die alone
- Managing pain and discomforts
- Knowing the client's wishes for end-of-life care
- Following the client's wishes
- Promoting cessation of intrusive treatments sooner rather than later
- Not initiating aggressive or distressing treatments at all
- Communicates effectively as a health care team with the client's choices priority

Advocate for the Client/Family With Their Physician Before Conflicts Arise

- Explore the physician's understanding of the situation, prognosis.
- Elicit the client's and/or family's perception of the situation.
- Explore client's and family's expectations.
- Explore if the client's and/or family's expectations are realistic.
- Offer your observations of the client's/family's understanding of the situation to involved health care professionals (e.g., manager, nurse colleagues, physicians).
- Develop strategies to transition clients from acute care to palliative care.

If Indicated, Explain "No Code" Status and Explain the Focus of Palliative Care That Replaces Aggressive and Futile Care (e.g., Pain Management, Symptom Management, Less or No Intrusive/Painful Procedures)

- Enlist the services of hospice when indicated.
- Seek to transfer client from ICU, if possible.
- If feasible, plan to discharge or transfer the client out of the hospital. Explore the "Going Home Initiative" at Baystate Medical Center, Springfield, Massachusetts (Lusardi et al., 2011).

Develop an On-Unit Process for Individual Nurses to Seek Assistance With Situations That May Precipitate Moral Stress

Establish Formal On-Unit Forums to Discuss Cases That Present Moral Stress or Have Caused Moral Distress; Record Discussions to Share With Other Staff

- Evaluate causes of unsatisfactory outcomes.
- Discuss alternative approach measures.
- Discuss interventions that resulted in optimal outcomes.

Advocate for End-of-Life Decision Dialogues With All Clients and Their Families, Especially When the Situation Is Not Critical. Direct the Client to Create Written Documents of Their Decisions and Advise Family of the Document

Integrate Health Promotion and Stress Reduction in Your Lifestyle (e.g, Smoking Cessation, Weight Management, Regular Exercise, Meaningful Leisure Activities); Refer to *Altered Health Maintenance*

SELF-NEGLECT

NANDA-I Definition

A constellation of culturally framed behaviors involving one or more self-care activities in which there is a failure to maintain a socially accepted standard of health and well-being (Gibbons, Lauder, & Ludwick, 2006)

Defining Characteristics*

Inadequate personal hygiene
Inadequate environmental hygiene
Nonadherence to health activities

Related Factors*

Capgras syndrome
Cognitive impairment
  (e.g., dementia)
Depression
Learning disability
Fear of institutionalization
Frontal lobe dysfunction and
  executive processing ability

Functional impairment
Lifestyle choice
Maintaining control
Malingering
Obsessive-compulsive disorder
Schizotypal personality disorders
Substance abuse
Major life stressor

 Author's Note

This diagnosis focuses on three problems: self-care problems, home hygiene, and noncompliance. Presently, three nursing diagnoses would more specifically describe the focus as *Self-Care Deficit*, *Altered Home Management*, and *Ineffective Self-Health Management*. Refer to these diagnoses in the index.

UNILATERAL NEGLECT

NANDA-I Definition

Impairment in sensory and motor response, mental representation, and special attention of the body, and the corresponding environment characterized by inattention to one side and over-attention to the opposite side. Left-side neglect is more severe and persistent than right side neglect.

Defining Characteristics

Major (Must Be Present, One or More)

Neglect of involved body parts and/or extrapersonal space (hemispatial neglect), and/or denial of the existence of the affected limb or side of body (anosognosia)

Minor (May Be Present)

Difficulty with spatial–perceptual tasks
Hemiplegia (usually of the left side)

Related Factors

Pathophysiologic

Related to brain injury secondary to:
Cerebrovascular accident* Trauma*
Cerebral aneurysms Tumors*
Cerebrovascular problems*

 Author's Note

Unilateral Neglect represents a disturbance in the reciprocal loop that occurs most often in the right hemisphere of the brain. This diagnosis could also be viewed as a syndrome diagnosis, *Unilateral Neglect Syndrome*. As mentioned in Chapter 3, syndrome diagnoses encompass a cluster of nursing diagnoses related to the situation. The nursing interventions for *Unilateral Neglect Syndrome* would focus on *Self-Care Deficit, Anxiety,* and *Risk for Injury.*

NOC

Body Image, Self-Care Assistance

Goal

The client will demonstrate an ability to scan the visual field to compensate for loss of function/sensation in affected limbs as evidenced by the following indicators:

• Identify safety hazards in the environment.
• Describe the deficit and the rationale for treatment.

NIC

Unilateral Neglect Management, Self-Care Assistance

Interventions

Consult With a Neuropsychologist, Physical Therapist, Occupational Therapist, and a Nurse Rehabilitation Specialist to Create a Multidisciplinary Plan With and for the Client

Assist the Client to Recognize the Perceptual Deficit

• Initially adapt the environment to the deficit:
  • Position the client, call light, bedside stand, television, telephone, and personal items on the unaffected side.
  • Position the bed with the unaffected side toward the door.

- Approach and speak to the client from the unaffected side.
- If you must approach the client from the affected side, announce your presence as soon as you enter the room to avoid startling the client.
- When working with the client's affected extremity, position the unaffected side near a wall to minimize distractions.
- Teach the client to scan from left to right frequently.
- Gradually change the client's environment as you teach him or her to compensate and to learn to recognize the forgotten field; move furniture and personal items out of the visual field. Speak to the client from the affected side (after introducing yourself on the unaffected side).
- Provide a simplified, well-lit, uncluttered environment:
  - Provide a moment between activities.
  - Provide concrete cues: "You are on your side facing the wall."
- Provide a full-length mirror to help with vertical orientation and to diminish the distortion of the vertical and horizontal plane, which manifests itself in the client leaning toward the affected side.
- Use verbal instructions rather than mere demonstrations. Keep instructions simple.
- For a client in a wheelchair, obtain a lapboard (preferably Plexiglas); position the affected arm on the lapboard with the fingertips at midline. Encourage the client to look for the arm on the board.
- For an ambulatory client, obtain an arm sling to prevent the arm from dangling and causing shoulder subluxation.
- When the client is in bed, elevate the affected arm on a pillow to prevent dependent edema.
- Constantly cue to the environment.
- Encourage the client to wear a watch, favorite ring, or bracelet on affected arm to draw attention to it.

Assist the Client With Adaptations Needed for Self-Care and Other ADLs

- Encourage the client to wear prescribed corrective lenses or hearing aids for bathing, dressing, and toileting.
- Instruct the client to attend to the affected extremity side first when performing ADLs.
- Instruct the client always to look for the affected extremity when performing ADLs, to know where it is at all times.
- Teach the client to dress and groom in front of a mirror.
- Suggest using color-coded markers sewn or placed inside shoes or clothes to help distinguish right from left.
- Encourage the client to integrate affected extremity during bathing and to feel extremity by rubbing and massaging it.

- Use adaptive equipment as appropriate.
- Refer to *Self-Care Deficit* for additional interventions.
- For feeding:
  - Set up meals with a minimum of dishes, food, and utensils.
  - Instruct the client to eat in small amounts and place food on unaffected side of mouth.
  - Instruct the client to use the tongue to sweep out "pockets" of food from the affected side after every bite.
  - After meals/medications, check oral cavity for pocketed food/medication.
  - Provide oral care t.i.d. and PRN.
  - Initially place food in the client's visual field; gradually move the food out of the field and teach the client to scan entire visual field.
  - Use adaptive feeding equipment as appropriate.
  - Refer to *Self-Care Deficit: Feeding* for additional interventions.
  - Refer to *Imbalanced Nutrition: Less than Body Requirements related to swallowing difficulties* if the client has difficulty chewing and swallowing food.

Teach Measures to Prevent Injury

- Ensure a clutter-free, well-lit environment.
- Retrain the client to scan entire environment.
  - Instruct the client to turn the head past midline to view the scene on the affected side.
  - Perform activities that require turning the head.
  - Remind the client to scan when ambulating or propelling a wheelchair.

Use Tactile Sensation to Reintroduce Affected Arm/Extremity to the Client

- Have the client stroke the involved side with the uninvolved hand and watch the arm or leg while stroking it.
- Rub different-textured materials to stimulate sensations (hot, cold, rough, soft).

Instruct the Client to Keep the Affected Arm and/or Leg in View

- Position the arm on the lapboard. (Plexiglas lapboards allow the client to view the affected leg, thereby helping to integrate the leg into the body schema.)
- Provide an arm sling for an ambulatory client.
- Instruct the client to take extra care around sources of heat or cold and moving machinery or parts to protect the affected side from injury.

Initiate Health Teaching and Referrals

- Ensure that both the client and the family understand the cause of unilateral neglect and the purpose of and rationale for all interventions.
- Proceed with teaching as needed.
- Explain unilateral neglect.
- Instruct the family on how to facilitate the client's relearning techniques (e.g., cueing, scanning visual field).
- Teach use of adaptive equipment, if appropriate.
- Teach principles of maintaining a safe environment.

NONCOMPLIANCE

NANDA-I Definition

Behavior of person and/or caregiver that fails to coincide with a health-promoting or therapeutic plan agreed on by the person (and/or family and/or community) and health care professional. In the presence of an agreed upon, health promoting, or therapeutic plan, the person's or caregiver's behavior is fully or partially nonadherent and may lead to clinically ineffective or partially ineffective outcomes.

Defining Characteristics

Verbalization of noncompliance or nonparticipation or confusion about therapy

Behavior indicative of failure to adhere*
Evidence of development of complications*
Evidence of exacerbation of symptoms*
Failure to keep appointments*
Objective tests provide evidence of failure to adhere* (e.g., physiologic measures, laboratory results, unfilled prescriptions)
Partially used or unused medications
Persistence of symptoms
Progression of disease process
Undesired outcomes (postoperative morbidity, pregnancy, obesity, addiction, regression during rehabilitation)

Related Factors

Pathophysiologic

Related to impaired ability to perform tasks because of disability secondary to:

Poor memory   Motor and sensory deficits

Related to increasing disease-related symptoms despite adherence to advised regimen

Treatment-Related

Related to:

Side effects of therapy   Past unsuccessful experiences
Impersonal aspects of referrals   with advised regimen
Financial cost of therapy   Nontherapeutic environment
                                      Complex, unsupervised,
                                         prolonged therapy

Situational (Personal, Environmental)

Related to barriers to access of care* secondary to:

Mobility problems   Lack of child care
Inclement weather   Financial issues
Transportation problems

Related to concurrent illness of a family member

Nonsupportive family, peers, or community

Related to barriers to care secondary to homelessness

Related to change in employment status

Related to change in health insurance coverage

Related to barriers to comprehension secondary to:

Cognitive deficits   Hearing deficits
Anxiety   Decreased attention span
Visual deficits   Poor memory
Fatigue   Motivation

Author's Note

Compliance depends on various factors, including motivation, perception of vulnerability, and beliefs about controlling or preventing illness; environment; quality of health instruction; and ability to access resources (cost, accessibility). "An important aspect of adherence is recognizing the patient's right to choose whether or not to follow treatment recommendations" (Robinson et al., 2008). The diagnosis *Noncompliance* should describe a client desiring to comply but prevented from doing so by certain factors (e.g., lack of understanding, inadequate finances, overly complex instructions). The nurse must attempt to reduce or eliminate these factors to ensure successful interventions. A nursing diagnosis— *Risk-Prone Health Behavior*—can also be useful to describe a client who is having difficulty modifying behaviors in response to a change in health status.

The process of *informed consent* protects a client's right to self-determination. Informed consent has three conditions: (1) the client must be capable of giving consent, (2) the client must understand the advantages and disadvantages of consent, and (3) the client must not be coerced (Cassells & Redman, 1989). When a client refuses to comply with advice or instructions, it is important for the nurse to assess for and validate the presence of all required elements for informed consent. The nurse is cautioned against using *Noncompliance* to describe a client who has made an informed autonomous decision not to comply. As Cassells and Redman (1989) state, "Human dignity is respected by granting individuals the freedom to make choices in accordance with their own values." When a client must change habits or lifestyle or perform certain activities to manage a health problem, *Risk for Ineffective Self-Health Management* is very useful.

NOC

Adherence Behavior, Compliance Behavior, Symptom Control, Treatment Behavior: Illness/Injury

Goal

The client will report a desire to change or initiate change as evidenced by the following indicators:

• Describe the reasons for the suggested regimen.
• Identify the barriers to adhering to the regimen.

NIC

Health Education, Self-Modification Assistance, Self-Responsibility Facilitation, Coping Enhancement, Decision-Making Support, Health System Guidance, Mutual Goal Setting, Teaching: Disease Process, Teaching: Prescribed Medication

Interventions

Determine the Client Understands:

• Presence of or risk for health problem (prognosis, disability).
• Vulnerability to problem.

- Prevention or treatment measures available.
- Effectiveness of preventive measures.
- Effectiveness of treatment measures.

Explore the Client's Feelings Regarding Their Own Knowledge/ Beliefs of Those of Their Family and Friends

- Determine with the client their confidence (self-efficacy) in his or her ability to make changes in achieving positive outcomes

To Improve Adherence, Use Patient-Centered Practices Such as (Robinson et al., 2008):

- Communication (direct information or sharing).
  - Direct information style to address simple complaints (e.g., take diuretic in morning to prevent sleep interruptions).
  - Sharing style to discuss chronic illness, life-style changes, or stressors (e.g., exploration of pattern of tobacco use and the specific harmful effects present now).
- Shared decision-making.
  - Determines person's goal in treatment.
  - Serves to identify barriers to adherence and solutions.
- Support for self-management.
  - Face-to-face: timely follow-up visits, progress reports, positive feedback.
  - Non face-to-face: print, intranet, telephone calls.
  - Low literacy: visual displays of information.
- Offer praise for honesty about compliance and for sharing reasons. For example:
  - "I'm glad you told me that you stopped taking Motrin because it made your stomach hurt. Now I understand why your hands still ache. Let's talk about other ways we can get you some comfort."
  - "It's good that you told me about your stopping the blood pressure pills. That explains your headaches and higher pressure today. Let's discuss how those pills made you feel."
- *Self-monitoring is useful to determine positive and negative influences on compliance.*
  - Daily records
  - Charts
  - Diary of progress or symptoms, clinical values (e.g., blood pressure), or dietary intake

Review Present Medication Therapy (Prescribed and Over-the-Counter)

- Discuss present therapy (names, dosages, time taken, side effects). Do not ask, "Are you taking your medications?" Ask:
  - "What medications did you take today? Yesterday?"
  - "What time of day is it difficult for you to take your medications?"
  - "Are there times when you decide not to take one of the doses?"
- Determine the client's understanding of the need for medication:
  - Emphasize lifelong therapy when indicated (e.g., hypertension, diabetes mellitus).
  - Explain the complications of unmanaged disease.
- Identify possible adverse interactions among drugs (consult a pharmacist).
- Commit to work with the client to reduce or eliminate side effects (e.g., change agents or dose).
- Help the client identify a reminder to take the medication (e.g., brushing teeth at night, daily favorite TV show, watch timer).
- Ask the client to call the primary provider with problems rather than stopping the medication.
- Emphasize that unavoidable side effects are still better than the consequences of no therapy (e.g., stroke, blindness, renal failure).

Medications for HIV

- Address the benefits of antiviral medications and the risks of nonadherence with HIV medications.
- Emphasize that HIV/AIDS can be a chronic disease.
- Describe the actions of the medications on the virus.
- Explain and track CD4 and viral load counts.
- Explain how resistance to medications occurs (e.g., missed doses).
- Design a system and schedule with the client that will decrease missed doses.
- Advise the client, if he or she is regularly missing doses, to stop all HIV medications and to call the nurse.

Help to Reduce Side Effects

- Address side effects that may occur and encourage the client to report them for evaluation.
- Specify the difference between side effects and adverse events.
- For gastric irritation, administer the drug with milk or food; yogurt may be advisable (unless contraindicated).

- For drowsiness, administer the medication at bedtime or late in the afternoon; consult the primary provider for dose reduction.
- For leg cramps (hypokalemia), increase foods high in potassium (e.g., oranges, raisins, tomatoes, bananas).
- For other side effects, consult pertinent references.
- Use long-acting intramuscular preparations whenever possible; this includes some antibiotics and antipsychotic medications.
- Suggest the use of combination pills if available.
- When appropriate, be sure client is taking the fewest medications possible (check dosages to provide the largest dose available in the fewest number of drugs).
- To decrease the frequency of oral medications, suggest longer-acting drug preparations, such as transdermal patch (e.g., nitroglycerin).
- Management of side effects can increase adherence.

If Indicated, Focus on Emotional Responses That Interfere With Compliance (e.g., Situational Anxiety, Depression, Denial, Relationship Problems)

Initiate Health Teaching and Referrals, as Indicated

Encourage Prescription of Generic Drugs for People With Financial Concerns. Determine If the Client Needs Assistance

- Access specific pharmaceutical assistance programs at www.pparx.org/ or www.rxasst.org/.
- When expensive equipment is involved for treatments at home, make appropriate referrals to social workers and local agencies.
- Teach the importance of adhering to the prescribed regimen.
- Provide written drug information tailored to the client's needs. Include drug names, dosages, number of tablets to take and when, purpose of drugs, potential side effects and adverse reactions, and directions for relief of side effects.
- At discharge from the hospital or outpatient setting, provide the written name and phone number of whom to call with concerns about prescribed drug regimen.

Pediatric Interventions

- Talk with the child to help him or her understand the need for the treatment and the likely problems if it is not followed.
- Keep the information short, simple, and concrete; speak on the family's/child's level.
- Introduce important information first.
- Emphasize visible benefits of compliance.
- Attempt to minimize side effects and/or teach how to manage side effects.

- Design a reminder system with child and family (checklist); write down simple instructions in steps.
- Avoid being punitive; instead, problem-solve with the family to improve compliance.
- Discuss how the child can participate in self-care according to developmental level (Wysocki & Wayne, 1992):
  - Put stars on the child's chart when exercises are completed.
  - Draw up insulin.
  - Select food choices.
- Establish accountability for the child or family members.
- Discuss conflicts (see *Impaired Parenting*).
- Elicit problems in compliance and possible solution or compromises.
- Use age-related behavioral strategies:
  - Earning tokens or stickers
  - Written agreements with positive reinforcers
  - Disciplinary techniques (e.g., time-out for young children, withholding privileges for older children)

IMBALANCED NUTRITION: LESS THAN BODY REQUIREMENTS

Imbalanced Nutrition: Less Than Body Requirements

Impaired Dentition

Impaired Swallowing

Ineffective Infant Feeding Pattern

NANDA-I Definition

Intake of nutrients insufficient to meet metabolic needs

Defining Characteristics

Major (Must Be Present, One or More)

The client who is not NPO reports or is found to have food intake less than the recommended daily allowance (RDA) with or without weight loss

and/or

Actual or potential metabolic needs in excess of intake with weight loss

Minor (May Be Present)

Weight 10% to 20% or more below ideal for height and frame
Triceps skinfold, mid-arm circumference, and mid-arm muscle
    circumference less than 60% standard measurement
Muscle weakness and tenderness
Mental irritability or confusion
Decreased serum albumin
Decreased serum transferrin or iron-binding capacity
Sunken fontanel in infant

Related Factors

Pathophysiologic

*Related to increased caloric requirements and difficulty in ingesting
sufficient calories secondary to:*

Burns (postacute phase)
Cancer
Infection
Trauma
Chemical dependence

Preterm infants
Gastrointestinal (GI)
    complications/deformities
AIDS

Related to dysphagia secondary to:

Cerebrovascular accident
    (CVA)
Parkinson's disease
Möbius syndrome
Muscular dystrophy

Cerebral palsy
Cleft lip/palate
Amyotrophic lateral sclerosis
Neuromuscular disorders

Related to decreased absorption of nutrients secondary to:

Crohn's disease
Lactose intolerance

Necrotizing enterocolitis
Cystic fibrosis

Related to decreased desire to eat secondary to altered level of consciousness

*Related to self-induced vomiting, physical exercise in excess of caloric
intake, or refusal to eat secondary to anorexia nervosa*

*Related to reluctance to eat for fear of poisoning secondary to paranoid
behavior*

*Related to anorexia, excessive physical agitation secondary to bipolar
disorder*

Related to anorexia and diarrhea secondary to protozoal infection

Related to vomiting, anorexia, and impaired digestion secondary to pancreatitis

Related to anorexia, impaired protein and fat metabolism, and impaired storage of vitamins secondary to cirrhosis

Related to anorexia, vomiting, and impaired digestion secondary to GI malformation or necrotizing enterocolitis

Related to anorexia secondary to gastroesophageal reflux

Treatment Related

Related to protein and vitamin requirements for wound healing and decreased intake secondary to:

Surgery	Radiation therapy
Surgical reconstruction of mouth	Medications (chemotherapy)
	Wired jaw

Related to inadequate absorption as a medication side effect of (specify):

Colchicine	Para-aminosalicylic acid
Neomycin	Antacid
Pyrimethamine	

Related to decreased oral intake, mouth discomfort, nausea, and vomiting secondary to:

Radiation therapy	Chemotherapy
Tonsillectomy	Oral trauma

Situational (Personal, Environmental)

Related to decreased desire to eat secondary to:

Anorexia	Nausea and vomiting
Social isolation	Stress
Depression	Allergies

Related to inability to procure food (physical limitation or financial or transportation problems)

Related to inability to chew (damaged or missing teeth, ill-fitting dentures)

Related to diarrhea* secondary to (specify)

Maturational

Infant/Child

Related to inadequate intake secondary to:

Lack of emotional/sensory stimulation	Inadequate production of breast milk
Lack of knowledge of caregiver	

Related to malabsorption, dietary restrictions, and anorexia secondary to:

Celiac disease	Cystic fibrosis
Lactose intolerance	GI malformation
Necrotizing enterocolitis	Gastroesophageal reflux

Related to sucking difficulties (infant) and dysphagia secondary to:

Cerebral palsy	Neurologic impairment
Cleft lip and palate	

Related to inadequate sucking, fatigue, and dyspnea secondary to:

Congenital heart disease	Prematurity
Viral syndrome	Respiratory distress syndrome
Hyperbilirubinemia	Developmental delay

 Author's Note

Nurses are usually the primary diagnosticians and often the prescribers for improving nutritional status. Although *Imbalanced Nutrition* is not a difficult diagnosis to validate, interventions for it can challenge the nurse.

Many factors influence food habits and nutritional status: personal, family, cultural, financial, functional ability, nutritional knowledge, disease and injury, and treatment regimens. *Imbalanced Nutrition: Less Than Body Requirements* describes people who can ingest food but eat an inadequate or imbalanced quality or quantity. For instance, the diet may have insufficient protein or excessive fat. Quantity may be insufficient because of increased metabolic requirements (e.g., cancer, pregnancy, trauma, or interference with nutrient use [e.g., impaired storage of vitamins in cirrhosis]).

The nursing focus for *Imbalanced Nutrition* is assisting the client or family to improve nutritional intake. Nurses should not use this diagnosis to describe clients who are NPO or cannot ingest food. They should use the collaborative problems *RC of Electrolyte Imbalance* or *RC of Negative Nitrogen Balance* to describe those situations.

NOC

Nutritional Status, Teaching: Nutrition, Symptom Control

Goal

The client will ingest daily nutritional requirements in accordance with activity level and metabolic needs, as evidenced by the following indicators:

- Relate importance of good nutrition.
- Identify deficiencies in daily intake.
- Relate methods to increase appetite.

NIC

Nutrition Management, Weight Gain Assistance, Nutritional Counseling

Interventions

Explain the Need for Adequate Consumption of Carbohydrates, Fats, Protein, Vitamins, Minerals, and Fluids

Consult With a Nutritionist to Establish Appropriate Daily Caloric and Food Type Requirements for the Client

Discuss With the Client Possible Causes of Decreased Appetite

Encourage the Client to Rest Before Meals

Offer Frequent, Small Meals Instead of a Few Large Ones; Offer Foods Served Cold

With Decreased Appetite, Restrict Liquids With Meals and Avoid Fluids 1 Hour Before and After Meals

Encourage and Help the Client to Maintain Good Oral Hygiene

Arrange to Have High-Calorie and High-Protein Foods Served at the Times That the Client Usually Feels Most Like Eating

Take Steps to Promote Appetite

- Determine the client's food preferences and arrange to have them provided, as appropriate.
- Eliminate any offensive odors and sights from the eating area.
- Control any pain and nausea before meals.
- Encourage the client's family to bring permitted foods from home, if possible.
- Provide a relaxed atmosphere and some socialization during meals.

Provide for Supplemental Dietary Needs Amplified by Acute Illness

Give the Client Printed Materials Outlining a Nutritious Diet That Includes the Following:

- High intake of complex carbohydrates and fiber
- Decreased intake of sugar, salt, cholesterol, total fat, and saturated fats
- Alcohol use only in moderation
- Proper caloric intake to maintain ideal weight

🍲 Pediatric Interventions

- Teach parents the following regarding infant nutrition:
  - Adequate infant feeding schedule and weight gain requirements for growth: 100 to 120 kcal/kg/day for growth
  - Proper preparation of infant formula
  - Proper storage of breast milk and infant formula
  - Proper elevation of infant's head during and immediately after feedings
  - Proper chin/cheek support techniques for orally compromised infants
- The age-related nutritional needs of their children (consult an appropriate textbook on pediatrics or nutrition for specific recommendations).
- Discuss the importance of limiting snacks high in salt, sugar, or fat (e.g., soda, candy, chips) to limit risks for cardiac disorders, obesity, and diabetes mellitus. Advise families to substitute healthy snacks (e.g., fresh fruits, plain popcorn, frozen fruit juice bars, fresh vegetables).
- Assist families in evaluating their nutritional patterns.
- Discuss strategies to make meals a social event and to avoid struggles (Dudek, 2009; Hockenberry & Wilson, 2009).
- Allow the child to select one type of food he or she does not have to eat.
- Provide small servings (e.g., one tablespoon of each food for every year of age).
- Make snacks as nutritiously important as meals (e.g., hard-boiled eggs, raw vegetable sticks, peanut butter/crackers, fruit juices, cheese, and fresh fruit).
- Offer a variety of foods.
- Encourage all members to share their day.
- Involve the child in monitoring healthy eating (e.g., create a chart where the child checks off intake of healthy foods daily).
- Replace passive television watching with a group activity (e.g., Frisbee tossing, biking, walking).
- Address strategies to improve nutrition when eating fast foods:
  - Drink skim milk.
  - Avoid french fries.
  - Choose grilled foods.
  - Eat salads and vegetables.
- Substitute quick, nutritious fast meals (e.g., frozen dinners).

🤱 Maternal Interventions

- Teach the importance of adequate calorie and fluid intake while breastfeeding in relation to breast milk production.
- Explain physiologic changes and nutritional needs during pregnancy.

- Discuss the effects of alcohol, caffeine, and artificial sweeteners on the developing fetus.
- Explain the different nutritional requirements for pregnant girls 11 to 18 years of age, pregnant young women 19 to 24 years of age, and women older than 25 years.
- Determine if a woman needs more calories because of daily activity.
  - 28.5 kcal/kg for 11 to 14 years
  - 24.9 kcal/kg for 15 to 18 years
  - 23.3 kcal/kg for 19 to 24 years
  - 21.9 kcal/kg for 25 to 50 years
- Multiply resting caloric needs by:
  - 1.5 for light activity
  - 1.6 for moderate activity
  - 1.9 for heavy activity

✹ Geriatric Interventions

Determine the Client's Understanding of Nutritional Needs With:

- Aging
- Medication use
- Illness
- Activity

Assess Whether Any Factors Interfere With Procuring or Ingesting Foods (Miller, 2009)

- Anorexia from medications, grief, depression, or illness
- Impaired mental status leading to inattention to hunger or selecting insufficient kinds/amounts of food
- Impaired mobility or manual dexterity (paresis, tremors, weakness, joint pain, or deformity)
- Voluntary fluid restriction for fear of urinary incontinence
- Small frame or history of undernutrition
- Inadequate income to purchase food
- Lack of transportation to buy food or facility to cook
- New dentures or poor dentition
- Dislike of cooking and eating alone
- Client regularly eats alone
- Client has more than two alcoholic drinks daily

Explain Decline in Sensitivity to Sweet and Salty Tastes; If Indicated, Consult With Home Health Nurse to Evaluate Home Environment (e.g., Cooking Facilities, Food Supply, Cleanliness)

Access Community Agencies as Indicated (e.g., Nutritional Programs, Community Centers, Home-Delivered Grocery Services)

Impaired Dentition

NANDA-I Definition

Disruption in tooth development/eruption patterns or structural integrity of individual teeth

Defining Characteristics*

Excessive plaque
Asymmetric facial expression
Halitosis
Crown or root caries
Toothache
Tooth enamel discoloration
Excessive calculus
Loose teeth

Malocclusion or tooth misalignment
Incomplete eruption for age (may be primary or permanent teeth)
Premature loss of primary teeth
Tooth fracture(s)
Missing teeth or complete absence
Erosion of enamel

Author's Note

Impaired Dentition describes a multitude of problems with teeth. It is unclear how nurses or any health care professional would use this diagnosis. If the client had caries, abscesses, misaligned teeth, or malformed teeth, the nurse should refer the client to a dental professional. If problems with teeth is one that is affecting comfort or nutrition, *Impaired Comfort* or *Imbalanced Nutrition* would be the appropriate nursing diagnosis, instead of *Impaired Dentition*.

Impaired Swallowing

NANDA-I Definition

Abnormal functioning of the swallowing mechanism associated with deficits in oral, pharyngeal, or esophageal structure or function

Defining Characteristics

Major (Must Be Present, One or More)*

Observed evidence of difficulty in swallowing *and/or:*
  Stasis of food in oral cavity
  Coughing before a swallow
  Coughing after food or fluid intake
  Choking
  Gagging

Minor (May Be Present)

Nasal-sounding voice	Vomiting*
Drooling*	Regurgitation*
Slurred speech	Lack of chewing*

Related Factors

Pathophysiologic

Related to decreased/absent gag reflex, mastication difficulties, or decreased sensations secondary to:

Cerebral palsy*	Neoplastic disease affecting brain
Muscular dystrophy	
Poliomyelitis	Right or left hemispheric brain damage
Parkinson's disease	
Guillain–Barré syndrome	Vocal cord paralysis
Myasthenia gravis	Cranial nerve damage (V, VII, IX, X, XI)
Amyotrophic lateral sclerosis	
CVA	

Related to tracheoesophageal tumors, edema

Related to irritated oropharyngeal cavity

Related to decreased saliva

Treatment Related

Related to surgical reconstruction of the mouth, throat, jaw, or nose

Related to decreased consciousness secondary to anesthesia

Related to mechanical obstruction secondary to tracheostomy tube

Related to esophagitis secondary to radiotherapy

Situational (Personal, Environmental)

Related to fatigue

Related to limited awareness, distractibility

Maturational

Infants/Children
Related to decreased sensations or difficulty with mastication

Related to poor suck/swallow/breathe coordination

Older Adult
Related to reduction in saliva, taste

 Author's Note

See *Imbalanced Nutrition: Less Than Body Requirements.*

NOC

Aspiration Control, Swallowing Status

Goal

The client will report improved ability to swallow, as evidenced by the following indicators:

• Describe causative factors when known.
• Describe rationale and procedures for treatment.

NIC

Aspiration Precautions, Swallowing Therapy, Surveillance, Referral, Positioning

Interventions

Assess for Causative or Contributing Factors

Refer to Related Factors.
• Consult with a speech therapist for a bedside swallowing assessment and recommended plan of care.
• Alert all staff that client has impaired swallowing.

Reduce or Eliminate Causative/Contributing Factors in People With:

Mechanical Impairment of Mouth
• Assist client with moving the bolus of food from the anterior to the posterior part of mouth. Place food in the posterior mouth, where swallowing can be ensured, using:
  • A syringe with a short piece of tubing attached
  • A glossectomy spoon
• Soft, moist food of a consistency that can be manipulated by the tongue against the pharynx, such as gelatin, custard, or mashed potatoes.

- Prevent/decrease thick secretions with:
  - Artificial saliva Papain tablets dissolved in mouth 10 minutes before eating
  - Meat tenderizer made from papaya enzyme applied to oral cavity 10 minutes before eating
  - Frequent mouth care
  - Increase fluid intake to 8 glasses of liquid (unless contra-indicated)
- Check medications for potential side effects of dry mouth/decreased salivation
- Use of Haberman or comparable nipple when bottle feeding for infant with cleft lip/palate and Möbius syndrome

Muscle Paralysis or Paresis
- Establish a visual method to communicate with staff at bedside that client is dysphagic.
- Plan meals when client is well rested; ensure that reliable suction equipment is on hand during meals. Discontinue feeding if client is tired.
- If indicated, use modified supraglottic swallow technique (Emick-Herring & Wood, 1990).
  - Position the head of the bed in semi- or high Fowler's position, with the neck flexed forward slightly and chin tilted down.
  - Use cutout cup (remove and round out one third of side of foam cup).
  - Take bolus of food and hold in strongest side of mouth for 1 to 2 seconds, then immediately flex the neck with chin tucked against chest.
  - Without breathing, swallow as many times as needed.
  - When mouth is emptied, raise chin and clear throat.
- Note the consistency of food that is problematic. Select consistencies that are easier to swallow, such as:
  - Highly viscous foods (e.g., mashed bananas, potatoes, gelatin, gravy)
  - Thick liquids (e.g., milkshakes, slushes, nectars, cream soups)
- If drooling is present, use a quick-stretch stimulation just before and toward the end of each meal (Emick-Herring & Wood, 1990):
  - Digitally apply short, rapid, downward strokes to edge of bottom lip, mostly on the affected side.
  - Use a cold washcloth over finger for added stimulation.
- If a bolus of food is pocketed in the affected side, teach client how to use tongue to transfer food or apply external digital pressure to cheek to help remove the trapped bolus (Emick-Herring & Wood, 1990).

Impaired Cognition or Awareness
General
- Remove feeding tube during training if increased gag reflex is present.

- Concentrate on solids rather than liquids because liquids usually are less well tolerated.
- Minimize extraneous stimuli while eating (e.g., no television or radio, no verbal stimuli unless directed at task).
- Have client concentrate on task of swallowing.
- Have client sit up in chair with neck slightly flexed.
- Instruct client to hold breath while swallowing.
- Observe for swallowing and check mouth for emptying.
- Avoid overloading mouth because this decreases swallowing effectiveness.
- Give solids and liquids separately.
- Progress slowly. Limit conversation.
- Provide several small meals to accommodate a short attention span.

Client With Aphasia or Left Hemispheric Damage
- Demonstrate expected behavior.
- Reinforce behaviors with simple, one-word commands.

Client With Apraxia or Right Hemispheric Damage
- Divide task into smallest units possible.
- Assist through each task with verbal commands.
- Allow to complete one unit fully before giving next command.
- Continue verbal assistance at each eating session until no longer needed.
- Incorporate written checklist as a reminder to client.
- *Note:* Client may have both left and right hemispheric damage and require a combination of the above techniques.

Reduce the Possibility of Aspiration

- Before beginning feeding, assess that the client is adequately alert and responsive, can control the mouth, has cough/gag reflex, and can swallow saliva.
- Have suction equipment available and functioning properly.
- Position client correctly:
  - Sit client upright (60 to 90 degrees) in chair or dangle his or her feet at side of bed if possible (prop with pillows if necessary).
  - Client should assume this position 10 to 15 minutes before eating and maintain it for 10 to 15 minutes after finishing eating.
  - Flex client's head forward on the midline about 45 degrees to keep esophagus patent.
  - Keep infant's head elevated during and immediately after feedings
- Keep client focused on task by giving directions until he or she has finished swallowing each mouthful.
  - "Take a breath."
  - "Move food to middle of tongue."

- "Raise tongue to roof of mouth."
- "Think about swallowing."
- "Swallow."
- "Cough to clear airway."
- Reinforce voluntary action.
- Start with small amounts and progress slowly as client learns to handle each step:
  - Ice chips
  - Eyedropper partly filled with water
  - Whole eyedropper filled with water
  - Juice in place of water
  - ¼ teaspoon semisolid food
  - ½ teaspoon semisolid food
  - 1 teaspoon semisolid food
  - Pureed or commercial baby foods
  - One half cracker
  - Soft diet
  - Regular diet; chew food well
- For a client who has had a CVA, place food at back of tongue and on side of face he or she can control:
  - Feed slowly, making certain client has swallowed the previous bite.
  - Some clients do better with foods that hold together (e.g., soft-boiled eggs, ground meat and gravy).
- If the above strategies are unsuccessful, consultation with a physician may be necessary for alternative feeding techniques such as tube feedings or parenteral nutrition.

Initiate Health Teaching and Referrals, as Indicated

Teach Exercises to Strengthen (Grober, 1984):

Lips and Facial Muscles
- Alternate a tight frown with a broad smile with lips closed.
- Puff out cheeks with air and hold.
- Blow out of pursed lips.
- Practice pronouncing *u, m, b, p, w*.
- Suck hard on a popsicle.

Tongue
- Lick a popsicle or lollipop.
- Push tip of tongue against roof and floor of mouth.
- Count teeth with tongue.
- Pronounce *la, la, la; ta, ta, ta; d; n; z; s.*
- See *Impaired Oral Mucous Membranes.*
- See *Imbalanced Nutrition: Less Than Body Requirements.*

Ineffective Infant Feeding Pattern

NANDA-I Definition

Impaired ability of an infant to suck or coordinate the suck/swallow response, resulting in inadequate oral nutrition for metabolic needs

Defining Characteristics

Inability to initiate or sustain an effective suck*
Inability to coordinate sucking, swallowing, and breathing*
Regurgitation or vomiting after feeding

Related Factors

Pathophysiologic

Related to increased caloric need secondary to:
Body temperature instability
Tachypnea with increased
    respiratory effort
Infection
Möbius syndrome
Growth needs
Wound healing
Major organ system disease
    or failure
Cleft lip/palate

Related to muscle weakness/hypotonia secondary to:
Malnutrition
Congenital defects
Prematurity*
Major organ system disease or
    failure
Hyperbilirubinemia
Acute/chronic illness
Neurologic impairment/delay*
Lethargy

Treatment-Related

Related to hypermetabolic state and increased caloric needs secondary to:
Surgery
Painful procedures
Cold stress
Sepsis
Fever

Related to muscle weakness and lethargy secondary to:
Medications
Muscle relaxants (antiseizure medications, past use of paralyzing
    agents, sedatives, narcotics)
Sleep deprivation

*Related to oral hypersensitivity**

Related to previous prolonged NPO state

Situational (Personal, Environmental)

Related to inconsistent caretakers (feeders)

Related to lack of knowledge or commitment of caretaker (feeder) to special feeding needs or regimen

Related to presence of noxious facial stimuli or absence of oral stimuli

Related to inadequate production of breast milk

Author's Note

Ineffective Infant Feeding Pattern describes an infant with sucking or swallowing difficulties. This infant experiences inadequate oral nutrition for growth and development, which is exacerbated when caloric need increases, as with infection, illness, or stress. Nursing interventions assist infants and their caregivers with techniques to achieve nutritional intake needed for weight gain. In addition, the goal is for the intake eventually to be exclusively oral.

Infants with sucking or swallowing problems who have not lost weight need nursing interventions to prevent weight loss. *Ineffective Infant Feeding Pattern* is clinically useful for this situation.

NOC

Muscle Function, Nutritional Status, Swallowing Status

Goal

The infant will receive adequate nutrition for growth appropriate to age and need, as evidenced by the following indicators:

• Parent demonstrates increasing skill.
• Parent identifies techniques that increase effective feeding.

NIC

Nonnutritive Swallowing, Swallowing Therapy, Aspiration, Precautions, Bottle Feeding, Parent Education: Infant

Interventions

Assess the Infant's Feeding Pattern and Nutritional Needs

• Assess volume, duration, and effort during feeding; respiratory rate and effort; signs of fatigue.
• Assess past caloric intake, weight gain, trends in intake and output, renal function, fluid retention.

- Identify physiologic risk factors.
- Identify physiologic ability to feed.
  - Can infant stop breathing when sucking and swallowing?
  - Does infant gasp or choke during feedings?
  - What happens to oxygen level, heart rate, and respiratory rate when sucking/swallowing?
  - Does the infant need rest periods? How long? Are there problems in initiating sucking/swallowing again?
- Assess nipple-feeding skills.
  - Does the infant actively suck with a bottle?
  - Does the infant initiate a swallow in coordination with suck?
  - Does the infant coordinate sucking, swallowing, and breathing?
  - Is the feeding completed in a reasonable time?
- Collaborate with clinical dietitian to set calorie, volume, and weight gain goals.
- Collaborate with occupational therapist, speech therapist to identify oral motor skills and planned intervention, if needed.
- Collaborate with parent(s) about effective techniques used with this infant or other children, temperament, and responses to environmental stimuli.

Provide Specific Interventions to Promote Effective Oral Feeding (Hockenberry & Wilson, 2009)

- Ensure a quiet, calm, and dim environment.
- Eliminate painful procedures prior to feeding.
- Ensure uninterrupted sleep periods.
- Encourage nonnutritive sucking not in response to noxious stimuli.
- Ensure nutritive sucking for an identified period
- Control adverse environmental stimuli and noxious stimuli to face and mouth.
- Specific interventions for facilitating feeding are as follows:
  - Choose nipple according to individual needs and successes; assess effects of changes in formula/breast milk temperature and thickness.
  - Position infant semi-upright, with trunk approximately 45 to 60 degrees. (Do not use a "head-back" position because it makes swallowing and sucking coordination more difficult.)
  - Stroke infant's lips, cheeks, and tongue before feeding.
  - Support cheeks and chin to encourage adequate suck
  - Use nonnutritive sucking before feeding to promote an awake and alert state.
  - Use fingers to provide inward and forward support for infant's cheeks during feeding.
  - Provide support for the base of the tongue (by placing fingers halfway between the chin and the throat, the nurse can provide a slight upward lift under the base of the tongue); *do not* provide strong upward pressure; steady

support is most helpful; avoid moving fingers because it may interfere with the infant's own tongue movements.
- Implement specific interventions for oral motor delays (position, equipment, jaw/mouth manipulation).
- Promote consistency in approach to feeding.
- The following actions hinder feeding:
  - Twisting or turning the nipple
  - Moving the nipple up, down, around in the mouth
  - Putting the nipple in and out of the mouth
  - Putting pressure on the jaw or moving the infant's jaw up and down
  - Placing the infant in a head-back position
  - Caregiver anxiousness and impatience
- Refer to *Risk for Aspiration* for interventions for feeding an infant with cleft lip and/or palate.

Establish Partnership With Parent(s) in All Stages of Plan

- Create a supportive environment for the parents to have the primary role in providing feeding-related intervention, when they are present. Whenever possible, nurses use the parents' approach when a parent is not present. In addition, when parents are not present, nurses can support the parents' role by imitating their approach to the infant, and communicate the infant's responses to the parents at a later time.

Negotiate and Identify Plans for Discharge With Parents and Incorporate Into the Overall Feeding Plan; Provide Ongoing Information About Special Needs and Assist Parents to Establish Needed Resources (Equipment, Nursing Care, Other Caretakers) When Needed

IMBALANCED NUTRITION: MORE THAN BODY REQUIREMENTS

Imbalanced Nutrition: More Than Body Requirements

Risk for Imbalanced Nutrition: More Than Body Requirements

NANDA-I Definition

Intake of nutrients that exceeds metabolic needs

Defining Characteristics

Major (Must Be Present, One or More)

Overweight (weight 10% over ideal for height and frame), or
Obese (weight 20% or more over ideal for height and frame)*
Triceps skinfold greater than 15 mm in men and 25 mm in women*

Minor (May Be Present)

Reported undesirable eating patterns
Intake in excess of metabolic requirements
Sedentary activity patterns

Related Factors

Pathophysiologic

*Related to excessive intake in relation to metabolic needs**

Related to altered satiety patterns secondary to (specify)

Related to decreased sense of taste and smell

Treatment Related

Related to altered satiety secondary to:
Medications (corticosteroids, antihistamines, estrogens)
Radiation (decreased sense of taste and smell)

Situational (Personal, Environmental)

Related to stress

Related to overeating

Related to dysfunctional eating pattern (e.g., pairing with other activities, fast foods)

Related to risk to gain more than 25 to 30 lb when pregnant

Related to lack of basic nutrition knowledge

Maturational

Adult/Older Adult
Related to decreased activity patterns, decreased metabolic needs

 Author's Note

Using this diagnosis to describe people who are overweight or obese places the focus of interventions on nutrition. Obesity is a complex condition with sociocultural, psychological, and metabolic implications. When the focus is primarily on limiting food intake, as with many weight-loss programs, the chance of permanent weight loss is slim. To be successful, a weight-loss program must focus on behavior modification and lifestyle changes.

The nursing diagnosis *Imbalanced Nutrition: More Than Body Requirements* does not describe this focus. Rather, *Risk-Prone Health Behavior related to intake in excess of metabolic requirements* better reflects the need to increase metabolic requirements through exercise and decreased intake. For some people who desire weight loss, *Ineffective Coping related to increased eating in response to stressors* could be useful in addition to *Risk-Prone Health Behavior*.

The nurse should be cautioned against applying a nursing diagnosis for an overweight or obese person who does not want to participate in a weight-loss program. Motivation for weight loss must come from within. Nurses can gently and expertly teach the hazards of obesity but must respect a client's right to choose—the right of self-determination.

Imbalanced Nutrition: More Than Body Requirements does have clinical usefulness for people at risk for or who have experienced weight gain because of pregnancy, taste or smell changes, or medications (e.g., corticosteroids).

NOC
Nutritional Status, Weight Control

Goal

The person will describe why he or she is at risk for weight gain as evidenced by the following indicators:

- Describe reasons for increased intake with taste or olfactory deficits.
- Discuss the nutritional needs during pregnancy.
- Discuss the effects of exercise on weight control.

NIC
Nutritional Management, Weight Management, Teaching: Individual, Behavioral Modification, Exercise Promotion

Interventions

Refer to Related Factors

Explain the Effects of Decreased Sense of Taste and Smell on Perception of Satiety After Eating. Encourage Client to:

- Evaluate intake by calorie counting, not feelings of satiety.
- If not contraindicated, season foods heavily to satisfy decreased sense of taste. Experiment with seasonings (e.g., dill, basil).
- When taste is diminished, concentrate on food smells.

Explain the Rationale for Increased Appetite Owing to Use of Certain Medications (e.g., Steroids, Androgens)

Discuss Nutritional Intake and Weight Gain During Pregnancy

Assist Client to Decrease Calorie Intake

- Request that client write down all the food he or she ate in the past 24 hours.
- Instruct client to keep a diet diary for 1 week that specifies the following:
  - What, when, where, and why eaten
  - Whether he or she was doing anything else (e.g., watching television, cooking) while eating
  - Emotions before eating
  - Others present (e.g., snacking with spouse, children)
- Review the diet diary to point out patterns (e.g., time, place, emotions, foods, persons) that affect food intake.
- Review high- and low-calorie food items.

Teach Behavior Modification Techniques to Decrease Caloric Intake

- Eat only at a specific spot at home (e.g., the kitchen table).
- Do not eat while performing other activities.
- Drink an 8-oz glass of water immediately before a meal.
- Decrease second helpings, fatty foods, sweets, and alcohol.
- Prepare small portions, just enough for one meal, and discard leftovers.
- Use small plates to make portions look bigger.
- Never eat from another person's plate.
- Eat slowly and chew food thoroughly.
- Put down utensils and wait 15 seconds between bites.
- Eat low-calorie snacks that must be chewed to satisfy oral needs (e.g., carrots, celery, apples).

Instruct Client to Increase Activity Level to Burn Calories

- Use the stairs instead of elevators.
- Park at the farthest point in parking lots and walk to buildings.

- Plan a daily walking program with a progressive increase in distance and pace.
- Note: Urge client to consult with a primary provider before beginning any exercise program.

Initiate Referral to a Community Weight Loss Program (e.g., Weight Watchers), If Indicated

Risk for Imbalanced Nutrition: More Than Body Requirements

NANDA-I Definition

At risk for an intake of nutrients that exceeds metabolic needs

Risk Factors*

Parental obesity
Rapid transition across growth percentiles in infants or children
Reported use of solid food as major food source before 5 months of age
Observed use of food as reward or comfort measure
Reported or observed higher baseline weight at beginning of each pregnancy
Dysfunctional eating patterns
Pairing food with other activities
Concentrating food intake at end of day
Eating in response to external cues other than hunger (e.g., time of day, social situation)
Eating in response to internal cues other than hunger (e.g., anxiety)

🔹 Author's Note

This nursing diagnosis is similar to *Risk for Imbalanced Nutrition: More Than Body Requirements*. It describes a person who has a family history of obesity, is demonstrating a pattern of higher weight, or has had a history of excessive weight gain (e.g., previous pregnancy). Until clinical research differentiates this diagnosis from other currently accepted diagnoses, use *Risk for Ineffective Health Maintenance* to direct teaching to assist clients and families to identify unhealthy dietary patterns.

IMPAIRED PARENTING

Impaired Parenting

Risk for Impaired Attachment

Parental Role Conflict

NANDA-I Definition

Inability of the primary caregiver to create, maintain, or regain an environment that promotes the optimum growth and development of the child

Defining Characteristics

The home environment must be assessed for safety before discharge: location of bathroom, access to water, cooking facilities, and environmental barriers (stairs, narrow doorways).

Inappropriate and/or nonnurturing parenting behaviors
Lack of behavior indicating parental attachment
Inconsistent behavior management
Inconsistent care
Frequent verbalization of dissatisfaction or disappointment with infant/child
Verbalization of frustration with role
Verbalization of perceived or actual inadequacy
Diminished or inappropriate visual, tactile, or auditory stimulation of infant
Evidence of abuse or neglect of child
Growth and development challenges in infant/child

Related Factors

Individuals or families who may be at risk for developing or experiencing parenting difficulties

Parent(s)
Financial resources   Abusive
Single   Acutely disabled
Addicted to drugs   Psychiatric disorder
Adolescent   Accident victim
Terminally ill   Alcoholic

Child

Of unwanted pregnancy	Mentally handicapped
With undesired characteristics	Of undesired gender
Terminally ill	Physically handicapped
With hyperactive characteristics	

Situational (Personal, Environmental)

Related to interruption of bonding process secondary to:
Illness (child, parent)
Relocation/change in cultural environment
Incarceration

Related to separation from nuclear family

Related to lack of knowledge

Related to inconsistent caregivers or techniques

Related to relationship problems (specify):

Marital discord	Live-in partner
Stepparents	Separation
Divorce	Relocation

Related to little external support and/or socially isolated family

Related to lack of available role model

Related to ineffective adaptation to stressors associated with:

Illness	Substance abuse
Economic problems	Elder care
New baby	

Maturational

Adolescent Parent

Related to the conflict of meeting own needs over child's

Related to history of ineffective relationships with own parents

Related to parental history of abusive relationship with parents

Related to unrealistic expectations of child by parent

Related to unrealistic expectations of self by parent

Related to unrealistic expectations of parent by child

Related to unmet psychosocial needs of child by parent

Author's Note

The family environment should provide the basic needs for a child's physical growth and development: stimulation of the child's emotional, social, and cognitive potential; consistent, stable reinforcement to learn impulse control; reality testing; freedom to share emotions; and moral stability (Pfeffer, 1981). This environment nurtures a child to develop, as Pfeffer (1981) states, "the ability to disengage from the family constellation as part of a process of lifelong individualization." It is the role of parents to provide such an environment. Most parenting difficulties stem from lack of knowledge or inability to manage stressors constructively. The ability to parent effectively is at high risk when the child or parent has a condition that increases stress on the family unit (e.g., illness, financial problems). "The phenomenon of parenting is relevant to many disciplines, including nursing" (Gage, Everett, & Bullock, 2006).

Impaired Parenting describes a parent experiencing difficulty creating or continuing a nurturing environment for a child. *Parental Role Conflict* describes a parent or parents whose previously effective functioning is challenged by external factors. In certain situations, such as illness, divorce, or remarriage, role confusion and conflict are expected. If parents do not receive assistance in adapting their role to external factors, *Parental Role Conflict* can lead to *Impaired Parenting*. "The family is the primary social institution in which parenting takes place" (Gage, Everert, & Bullock, 2006).

NOC

Child Development (Specify), Family Coping, Family Environment: Internal, Family Functioning, Parent–Infant Attachment

Goal

The parent/primary caregiver demonstrates two effective skills to increase parenting effectiveness, as evidenced by the following indicators:

- Will acknowledge an issue with parenting skills.
- Identify resources available for assistance with improvement of parenting skills that are culturally considerate.

NIC

Parenting Promotion, Developmental Enhancement, Anticipatory Guidance, Parent Education, Behavior Management

Interventions

Encourage Parents to Express Frustrations Regarding Role Responsibilities, Parenting, or Both

- Convey empathy.
- Reserve judgment.
- Convey/offer educational information based on assessment.
- Help foster realistic expectations.
- Encourage discussion of feelings regarding unmet expectations.
- Discuss individualized, achievable, and culturally considerate strategies (e.g., discussing with partner, child; setting personal goals).

Educate Parents About Normal Growth and Development and Age-Related Expected Behaviors (Refer to *Delayed Growth and Development*)

Explore With Parents the Child's Problem Behavior

- Frequency, duration, context (when, where, triggers)
- Consequences (parental attention, discipline, inconsistencies in response)
- Behavior desired by parents

Discuss Positive Parenting Techniques

- Convey to child that he or she is loved.
- Catch child being good; use good eye contact.
- Set aside "special time" when parent guarantees time with child without interruptions.
- Ignore minor transgressions by having no physical contact, eye contact, or discussion of the behavior.
- Practice active listening. Describe what child is saying, reflect back the child's feelings, and do not judge.
- Parents need to identify the difference between discipline and punishment, with parents focusing their communications with children on discipline (Deloian & Berry, 2009).
- Use "I" statements when disapproving of behavior. Focus on the act, not the child, as undesirable.
- Positive reinforcement is an effective and recommended discipline technique for all ages (Banks, 2002). Redirecting is effective for infant to school age, whereas verbal instruction/explanation is most effective for school-age and adolescents (Banks, 2002).
- Different child temperaments may challenge parenting behaviors, as evidenced when an infant is demanding and a parent lacks resilience or when the child's behavior is normal and the parents' expectations are unrealistic (Hagen, Shaw, & Duncan, 2008).

Explain the Discipline Technique of "Time Out," Which Is a Method to Stop Misconduct, Convey Disapproval, and Provide Both Parent and Child Time to Regroup (Christophersen, 1992; Herman-Staab, 1994)

- Time out is most effective for the toddler and school-age child and provides a time for both parent and child to "cool off" (Banks, 2002; Hockenberry, 2011).
- Outline the procedure.
  - Place child in or bring the child to a chair in a quiet place with few distractions (not the child's room or an isolated place).
  - Instruct child to stay in the chair. Set timer for 1 minute of quiet time for each year of age.
  - Start the timer when the child is quiet.
  - If the child misbehaves, cries, or gets off the chair, reset the timer.
  - When the timer goes off, tell the child it is okay to get up.
- Explain to the child.
  - This is not a game.
  - Practice it once when the child is behaving.
  - Explain rules and then ask the child questions to ensure understanding (if older than 3 years).
- Remember:
  - Do not warn child before sending for time out.
  - If time out is appropriate, use it; do not threaten.
  - If child laughs during time out, ignore it.
  - Be sure no television is on or can be seen.
  - Do not look at or talk to or about child during time out.
  - Do not act angry; remain calm.
  - Keep yourself busy; let the child see you and what he or she is missing.
  - Do not give up or give in.

If Additional Sources of Conflict Arise, Refer to the Specific Nursing Diagnosis (e.g., *Caregiver Role Strain, Fatigue*)

Take Opportunities to Model Effective Parenting Skills; If Relevant, Share Some Frustrations You Have Experienced With Your Child to Help Normalize the Frustrations

Acknowledge Cultural Impacts

Clarify the Strengths of the Parents or Family

Role-Play Asking for Help or Disciplining a Child

Provide General Parenting Guidelines

- Routine assessment of parent–child interactions is an important aspect in providing anticipatory guidance about discipline (Banks, 2002; Regalado, Sareen, Inkelas, Wissow, & Halfon, 2004).

- Practice open, honest dialogues. Never threaten with vague parameters (e.g., "If you are bad, I won't take you to the movies").
- Do not lecture. Tell the child he or she was wrong and let it go. Spend time talking about pleasant experiences.
- Compliment children on their achievements. Make each child feel important and special. Especially tell a child when he or she has been good; try not to focus on negative behavior.
- Provide appropriate physical affection to children.
- Set limits and be consistent. Expect cooperation.
- Encourage the child to participate in activities. Let the child help you as much as possible. "Nurses can encourage parents in their roles beyond childbearing, help them to solve problems, perform parenting tasks, and understand what is developmentally appropriate" (Gage, Everett, & Bullock, 2006).
- Discipline the child by restricting activity. Sit a younger child in a chair for 3 to 5 minutes. If the child gets up, reprimand once and put him or her back. Continue until the child sits for the prescribed time. For an older child, restrict bicycle riding or going to the movies (pick an activity that is important to him or her).
- Make sure the discipline corresponds to the unacceptable behavior.
- Allow children opportunities to make mistakes and to express anger verbally.
- Stay in control. Try not to discipline when you are irritated.
- When long explanations are needed, give them after the discipline.
- Remember to examine what you are doing when you are not disciplining your child (e.g., enjoying each other, loving each other).
- Never reprimand a child in front of another person (child or adult). Take the child aside and talk.
- Never decide you cannot control a child's destructive behavior. Examine your present response. Are you threatening? Do you follow through with the punishment or do you give in? Has the child learned you do not mean what you say?
- Be a good model (the child learns from you whether you intend it or not). Never lie to a child even when you think it is better; the child must learn that you will not lie, no matter what.
- Give each child a responsibility suited to his or her age, such as picking up toys, making beds, or drying dishes. Expect the child to complete the task.
- Share your feelings with children (happiness, sadness, anger). Respect and be considerate of the child's feelings and of his or her right to be human.

Initiate Health Teaching and Referrals, as Indicated

- Community resources such as counseling, social services, parenting classes, support groups, self-help, church.
- Support cultural considerations of parenting skills as age appropriate.

Risk for Impaired Attachment

NANDA-I Definition

At risk for disruption of the interactive process between parent/significant other and child that fosters the development of a protective and nurturing reciprocal relationship

Risk Factors

Pathophysiologic

Related to interruption of attachment process secondary to:
Parental illness   Infant illness

Treatment Related

Related to barriers to attachment secondary to:
Lack of privacy*   Equipment-restricted visitation
Intensive care monitoring   Physical barriers*
Ill child*   Separation*
Structured "visitation"   Premature infant*

Situational (Personal, Environmental)

Related to unrealistic expectations (e.g., of child, of self)

Related to unplanned pregnancy

Related to disappointment with infant (e.g., gender, appearance)

Related to ineffective coping associated with new baby and other responsibilities secondary to:
Health issues   Relationship difficulties
Substance abuse   Economic difficulties
Mental illness

Related to lack of knowledge and/or available role model for parental role

Related to physical disabilities of parent (e.g., blindness, paralysis, deafness)

Related to being emotionally unprepared due to premature delivery of infant

Maturational

Adolescent Parent
Related to difficulty delaying own gratification for the gratification of the infant

 Author's Note

This diagnosis describes a parent or caregiver at risk for attachment difficulties with his or her infant. Barriers to attachment can be the environment, knowledge, anxiety, and health of parent or infant. This diagnosis is appropriate as a risk or high-risk diagnosis. If the nurse diagnoses a problem in infant–parent attachment, the diagnosis *Risk for Impaired Parenting* related to difficulties in parent–child attachment would be more useful so that the nurse could focus on improving attachment and preventing destructive parenting patterns.

NOC

Refer to *Impaired Parenting.*

Goal

The parent will demonstrate increased attachment behaviors, such as holding infant close, smiling and talking to infant, and seeking eye contact with infant, as evidenced by the following indicators:

• Be supported in his or her need to be involved in infant's care.
• Begin to verbalize positive feelings regarding infant.
• Engages in infant/child care.

NIC

Refer to *Impaired Parenting.*

Interventions

Assess Causative or Contributing Factors

Maternal
• Unwanted pregnancy
• Prolonged or difficult labor and delivery
• Postpartum pain or fatigue
• Lack of positive support system (mother, spouse, friends)
• Lack of positive role model (mother, relative, neighbor)
• Inability to prepare emotionally (e.g., an unexpected delivery)

Inadequate Coping Patterns (One or Both Parents)
- Financial/economic issues
- Alcoholism
- Drug addiction
- Marital difficulties (separation, divorce, violence)
- Change in lifestyle related to new role
- Adolescent parent
- Career change (e.g., working woman to mother)
- Illness in family

Infant
- Premature, congenital anomalies, ill
- Multiple births

Eliminate or Reduce Contributing Factors, If Possible

Illness, Pain, Fatigue
- Establish with parent/caregiver what infant care activities are feasible.
- Provide parent/caregiver with uninterrupted sleep periods of at least 2 hours during the day and 4 hours at night. Provide relief for discomfort.

Lack of Experience or Positive Parenting Role Model
- Explore parenting feelings and attitudes concerning their own parents.
- Assist parents to identify someone who is a positive parent; encourage parent to seek that person's aid.
- Outline the teaching program available during hospitalization.
- Determine who will assist parent at home initially.
- Identify community programs and reference material that can increase parental learning about child care after discharge (see Bibliography).

Lack of Positive Support System
- Identify parent's support system; assess its strengths and weaknesses.
- Assess the need for counseling.
- Encourage parents to express feelings about the experience and about the future.
- Be an active listener to the parents.
- Observe the parents interacting with the infant.
- Assess for resources (financial, emotional, and cultural) already available to the family.
- Be aware of resources available both within the hospital and in the community.
- Refer to hospital or community services.

Barriers to Practicing Cultural Beliefs That May Affect the Family Unit During Hospitalization
• Support mother–infant–family beliefs.
• Integrate culture and traditions into routine care.
• Identify community resources.

Elimination of Institutional Barriers That Inhibit Individualization of Care
• Sensitize staff to practicing family-centered care.
• Use families to review practice and policies.
• Encourage cultural sensitization of staff.

Provide Opportunities for the Process of Mutual Interaction

Promote Bonding Immediately After Delivery

• Encourage mother to hold infant after birth (may need a short recovery period).
• Provide skin-to-skin contact if desired; keep room warm (72° to 76° F)
• Provide mother with an opportunity to breast-feed immediately after delivery, if desired.
• Give family as much time as they need together with minimum interruption from staff (the "sensitive period" lasts from 30 to 90 minutes).
• Encourage father to hold infant.
• Provide culturally appropriate support to family.

Facilitate the Attachment Process During the Postpartum Phase

• Check mother regularly for signs of fatigue, especially if she received anesthesia.
• Offer flexible rooming-in to the mother; establish with her the care she will assume initially and support her requests for assistance.
• Discuss future involvement of the father in the infant's care (if desired, plan opportunities for father to participate in his child's care during visits).

Provide Support to the Parents

• Listen to the mother's replay of her labor and delivery experience.
• Allow for verbalization of feelings.
• Indicate acceptance of feelings.
• Point out the infant's strengths and individual characteristics to the parents.
• Demonstrate the infant's responses to the parents.
• Have a system of follow-up after discharge, especially for families considered at risk (e.g., telephone call or a home visit by the community health nurse).

- Be aware of resources and support groups available within the hospital and community; refer the family as needed.
- Provide culturally appropriate cares as requested by the family.

Assess the Need to Support the Parents' Emerging Confidence in Child Care

- Observe the parents interacting with the infant.
- Support each parent's strengths.
- Help parents understand infant's cues and temperament.
- Assist each parent in those areas in which he or she is uncomfortable (role modeling).
- Assess for level of knowledge in growth and development; provide information as needed.
- Provide handouts, audiovisual aids, and select Internet resources for parent/family at their level of understanding and language.
- Refer to References/Bibliography for recommended printed material about parenting and child care.

Provide Bonding/Attachment Experiences as Soon as Possible When Immediate Separation Between Parent and Child Is Necessary Because of Prematurity or Illness

- Invite parents to see and touch infant as soon as possible.
- Encourage parents to spend prolonged time with infant.
- Support activities such as skin-to-skin holding, containment of infant with parents' hands in the isolette, and basic caregiving activities.
- If infant is transported to another facility and separated from mother:
  - Have staff make frequent calls to mother.
  - Encourage family to spend time in neonatal intensive care unit; bring back verbal reports and pictures of infant.
  - Explore family and community resources to provide means of rejoining mother and infant as soon as possible.

For Adoptive Parents:

- Counsel adoptive parents that many emotions are normal on first interaction with their children.
- Counsel adoptive parents about the possibility of post adoption depression.
- Encourage adoptive parents to seek parenting classes before receiving their infant.

Initiate Referrals, as Needed

- Consult with community agencies for follow-up visits if indicated.
- Refer parents to pertinent organizations (see Bibliography).

Parental Role Conflict

Definition

Parent experience of role confusion and conflict in response to crisis (NANDA-I)

State in which a parent or primary caregiver experiences or perceives a change in role in response to external factors (e.g., illness, hospitalization, divorce, separation, birth of child with special needs)**

Defining Characteristics

Major (Must Be Present, One or More)*

Parent(s) express(es) concerns about changes in parental role
Demonstrated disruption in care and/or caretaking routines

Minor (May Be Present)

Parent(s) express(es) concerns/feelings of inadequacy to provide for child's physical and emotional needs during hospitalization or in the home
Parent(s) express(es) concerns about the effect of child's illness on other children
Parent(s) express(es) concerns about care of siblings at home
Parent(s) express(es) concern about perceived loss of control over decisions relating to the child*

Related Factors

Situational (Personal, Environmental)

Related to separation from child secondary to:*
Birth of a child with a congenital defect, chronic illness, or both
Hospitalization of a child with an acute or chronic illness
Change in acuity, prognosis, or environment of care (e.g., transfer to or from intensive care unit)

Related to intimidation with invasive or restrictive treatment modalities (e.g., isolation, intubation)

Related to interruption of family life secondary to:*
Home care of a child with special needs* (e.g., apnea monitoring, tracheostomy, gastrostomy, or all three)

** This definition has been added by the author for clarity and usefulness.

Frequent visits to hospital
Addition of new family member (aging relative, newborn)

Related to change in ability to parent secondary to:

Illness of parent	Work responsibilities
Remarriage	Death
Travel requirements	Divorce
Dating	Change in marital status*

 Author's Note

Refer to *Impaired Parenting*.

NOC

Caregiver Adaptation to Child's Hospitalization, Caregiver Home Care Readiness, Coping, Family Environment: Internal Family Functioning, Parenting

Goal

The parent and child will demonstrate control over decision-making, as evidenced by the following indicators:

- Express feelings regarding the situation.
- Identify sources of support.

NIC

Caregiver Support, Role Enhancement, Anticipatory Guidance, Family Involvement Promotion, Counseling Referrals

Interventions

Assess the Present Situation

- Parents' and children's perceptions of and responses to situation
- Parental understanding of the effects of the situation on children and their typical responses
- Changes in parenting practices and daily routines (employment or change in child care arrangements)
- Other related stressors (financial, job related)
- Level of conflict between parents
- Social support for both parents

Encourage the Involvement of Father in Care

- Foster his strengths.
- Provide an appropriate place for discussion of any issues and concerns.

- Encourage the sharing of feelings and concerns as culturally appropriate.
- Include the father in care.

Help Parents With Setting Limits With the Child

- Explain the boundaries of acceptable behavior.
- Offer age-appropriate choices (e.g., "Do you want to take the pill or liquid medicine first? Which arm do you want your shot in?")
- Expect the child to perform age-appropriate self-care activities when able.
- Assign age-appropriate chores.
- Expect the child to participate in his or her care.

Encourage Parents to Address Siblings' Responses

- Help parents talk to siblings about the child's condition.
- Encourage parents to spend special time with siblings, acknowledge that all types of feelings are normal, and allow some participation in the child's care.
- Allow siblings a life outside of caregiving.

Assist Family to Increase Decision-Making Abilities (Dunst, Trivette, Davis, & Cornwell, 1988; Lutz, Anderson, Riesch, Pridham, & Becker, 2009; Smith, 1999)

- Emphasize parental responsibility for meeting needs and solving problems.
- Emphasize building on parental strengths.
- Provide active and reflective listening.
- Offer normative help that is congruent with parental appraisal of need.
- Ensure appropriate cultural and linguistic support through verbal and written resources.
- Promote acquisition of competencies.
- Use parent–professional collaboration as the mechanism for meeting needs.
- Allow locus of control to reside with the parent.
- Accept and support parental decisions.

Support Siblings (Hockenberry & Wilson, 2009)

- Listen to the siblings' feelings. Accept reasonable anger. Praise when they have been patient or helpful.
- Explain their sibling's condition and limit their responsibilities of care taking.

Encourage Expression of Feelings (Hockenberry & Wilson, 2009)

- Describe behavior (e.g., "You seem angry most of the time").
- Provide understanding (e.g., "Being angry is only natural").
- Help focus on feelings ("Do you wonder why this has happened to your child [or siblings]?").

Facilitate Parent–Nurse Partnerships

- Acknowledge the parents' overall competence and their unique expertise.
- Explain everything related to care. Engage parents in team meetings.
- Negotiate differences, be flexible, and offer respite.

Initiate Teaching and Referrals, as Needed

- Ensure that primary health care provider, specialty services, and school nurse are aware of care needs.
- Initiate referrals, as needed (e.g., specialty teaching for cares at home, in home care, day care, respite care).
- Identify local and national disease-oriented organizations, (e.g., National Information Center for children and youth with disabilities [800-695-0285, www.Nichcy.org]).
- Refer to *Caregiver Role Strain* for additional interventions.

POST-TRAUMA SYNDROME

Post-Trauma Syndrome
Risk for Post-Trauma Syndrome
Rape-Trauma Syndrome

NANDA-I Definition

Sustained maladaptive response to a traumatic, overwhelming event

Defining Characteristics

Re-experience of the traumatic event, which may be identified in cognitive, affective, and/or sensory motor activities for more than 1 month such as:

Flashbacks,*intrusive dreams, thoughts*
Repetitive dreams/nightmares
Excessive verbalization of the traumatic event(s)

Survival guilt or guilt* about behavior required for survival
Painful emotion, self-blame, shame*, or sadness
Vulnerability or helplessness, anxiety*, or panic attacks*
Fear* of repetition, death, or loss of bodily control
Anger, rage*
Hypervigilance*Avoidance*
Exaggerated startle response*
Avoidance* of thoughts, feelings or conversations associated with
    trauma
Sleep disturbances
Psychic/emotional numbness
Impaired interpretation of reality, impaired memory
Confusion, dissociation, or psychogenic amnesia*
Vagueness about the traumatic event(s)
Narrowed attention or inattention/daze
Reports of feeling numb* constricted affect
Detachment, alienation*
Reduced interest in significant activities
Submissiveness, passiveness, or dependency
Self-destructiveness (e.g., substance abuse*, suicide attempts,
    reckless driving, illegal activities)
Thrill-seeking activities
Difficulty with interpersonal relationships
Development of phobia regarding trauma
Avoidance of situations or activities that arouse recollection of
    the trauma
Social isolation/withdrawal
Sleep disturbances, emotional disturbances
Enuresis (in children)*
Irritability*, poor impulse control, or explosiveness
Loss of faith in people or the world, feeling of meaninglessness
    in life
Chronic anxiety or chronic depression
Multiple somatic symptoms

Related Factors

Situational (Personal, Environmental)

Related to traumatic events of natural origin, including:

Floods	Avalanches
Earthquakes	Epidemics*
Volcanic eruptions	Disasters*
Storms	

Related to traumatic events of human origin, such as:
Concentration camp confinement
Serious accidents (e.g., industrial, motor vehicle)*

Assault	War*
Torture*	Witnessing mutilation*
Rape	Being held prisoner of war*
Bombing	Criminal victimization*
Large fires	Airplane crashes
Witnessing violent death*	Abuse (e.g., physical,
Terrorist attacks	psychological)*

Related to industrial disasters(nuclear, chemical, or other life-threatening accidents)*

*Related to serious threat or injury to loved ones and/or self**

*Related to tragic occurrence involving multiple deaths**

*Related to events outside the range of unusual human experience**

*Related to sudden destruction of one's home and/ or community**

Author's Note

Post-Trauma Syndrome represents a group of emotional responses to a traumatic event of either natural origin (e.g., floods, volcanic eruptions, earthquakes) or human origin (e.g., war, rape, torture). The emotional responses (e.g., guilt, shame, fear, anger) interfere with interpersonal relationships and can precipitate self-destructive behavior (e.g., substance abuse, suicide). The nurse may find it necessary to use additional diagnoses when specific interventions are indicated (e.g., *Compromised Family Coping, Risk for Self-Harm*).

NANDA-I retired the diagnosis *Rape-Trauma Syndrome* in 2011 because no revisions have been submitted. The author has revised this diagnosis since 1975 and therefore it will be retained in this work.

Rape-Trauma Syndrome was described in 1975 as encompassing an acute phase of disorganization and a long-term phase of reorganization. Based on the most recent definition of syndrome nursing diagnoses as a cluster of associated nursing diagnoses, this diagnosis does not represent a syndrome and would be more accurately labeled *Rape-Trauma Response*. The inclusion of causative or contributing factors with this category is unnecessary, because the etiology is always rape. Thus, the nurse omits the second part of the diagnostic statement; however, he or she can add the client's report of the rape to the statement. For example, *Rape-Trauma Syndrome as evidenced by the report of a sexual assault and sodomy on June 22 and multiple facial bruises* (refer to ER record for description).

NOC

Abuse Recovery, Coping, Fear Control

Goals

In the short term, the client will do the following:

- Acknowledge the traumatic event and begin to work with the trauma.
- Make connections with support persons/resources.
- Engage in activities that reduce stress and improve coping.

As evidenced by the following indicators:

- Talk about the experience and expressing feelings such as fear, anger, and guilt.
- Identify sources of support.
- Identify three coping strategies that may improve their quality of life (e.g., exercise, hobby, nature walks, thought-stopping).

In the long term, the client will assimilate the experience into a meaningful whole and go on to pursue his or her life as evidenced by goal setting and the following indicators:

- Reports a lessening of re-experiencing the trauma or numbing symptoms.
- Reports feelings of support and comfort from individuals and/or support groups (Varcarolis, 2011).
- Reports engaging in regular activities (daily, weekly) that enhance coping.
- Reports cognitive coping strategies that have their improve sense of control.

NIC

Counseling, Anxiety Reduction, Emotional Support, Family Support, Support System Enhancement, Coping Enhancement, Active Listening, Presence, Grief Work, Facilitation, Referral

Interventions

Determine If the Person Has Experienced a Traumatic Event

- During the interview, secure a quiet room where there will be no interruptions but easy access to other staff in case of management problems.
- Be aware that talking about a traumatic experience may cause significant discomfort to the person.

- If the client becomes too anxious, discontinue the assessment and help the client regain control of the distress or provide other appropriate interventions.

Document the Person's Responses

Evaluate the Severity of the Responses and Effects on Current Functioning

- Assess for any suicidal or homicidal thoughts (Varcarolis, 2011).
- Refer to *Risk for Suicide*. Consult with law enforcement if needed.
- Assess for alcohol/drug abuse. Refer for counseling.

Assist Client to Decrease Extremes of Re-experiencing or Numbing Symptoms

- Provide a safe, therapeutic environment where the client can regain control.
- Reassure the client that others who have experienced such traumatic events often experienced these feelings/symptoms.
- Stay with the client and offer support during an episode of high anxiety (see *Anxiety* for additional information).
- Assist client to control impulsive acting-out behavior by setting limits, promoting ventilation, and redirecting excess energy into physical exercise or activity (e.g., walking, jogging). (See *Risk for Self-Harm* and *Risk for Violence* for additional information.)
- Provide techniques to reduce anxiety (e.g., progressive relaxation, deep breathing).

Assist Client to Acknowledge and Begin to Work Through the Trauma by Discussing the Experience and Expressing Feelings Such as Fear, Anger, and Guilt

- Provide a safe, structured setting.
- Explain that talking about the traumatic event may intensify the symptoms (e.g., nightmares, flashbacks, painful emotions, numbness).
- Assist the client to proceed at an individual pace.
- Listen attentively with empathy and an unhurried manner.
- Assist the client to talk about trauma, to understand what has occurred, and to validate the reality of personal involvement.
- Help the client to express feelings associated with the traumatic event and to become aware of the link between the experience and anger, depression, or anxiety.
- Assist the client to differentiate reality from fantasy and to reflect and talk about the areas of his or her life that have changed.
- Recognize and support cultural and religious values in dealing with the traumatic event.

Assist Client to Identify and Make Connections with Support People and Resources

- Help client to identify his or her strength and resources.
- Explore available support systems.
- Assist client to make connections with support and resources according to his or her needs.
- Assist client to resume old activities and explore some new ones such as exercise, nature walks, and hobbies.

Assist Family/Significant Others

- Assist them to understand what is happening to the client.
- Be specific about the various responses the client can display.
- Encourage expression of their feelings.
- Provide counseling sessions or link them with appropriate community resources, as necessary.

Provide Nursing Care Appropriate to Each Client's Traumatic Experience and Needs

Provide or Arrange Follow-Up Treatment in Which the Client Can Continue to Work Through the Trauma and to Integrate the Experience into a New Self-Concept

Pediatric Interventions

- Assist children to understand and to integrate the experience in accordance with their developmental stage.
- Assist them to describe the experience and to express feelings (e.g., fear, guilt, rage) in safe, supportive places, such as play therapy sessions.
- Provide accurate information and explanations in terms the child can understand.
- Provide family counseling to promote understanding of the child's needs.
- Refer to a specialist for on going therapy.

Risk for Post-Trauma Syndrome

NANDA-I Definition

At risk for sustained maladaptive response to a traumatic, overwhelming event

Risk Factors

Refer to Related Factors in *Post-Trauma Syndrome*.

Goal

The client will continue to function appropriately after the traumatic event and relates he or she will seek professional help as evidenced by the following indicators:

- Identify signs or symptoms that necessitate professional consultation.
- Express feelings regarding traumatic event.

Interventions

Refer to *Post-Trauma Syndrome*.

Rape-Trauma Syndrome**

Definition

Sustained maladaptive response to a forced, violent sexual penetration against the victim's will and consent (NANDA-I)

State in which a client experiences a forced, violent sexual assault (vaginal or anal penetration) against his or her will and without his or her consent. The trauma syndrome that develops from this attack or attempted attack includes an acute phase of disorganization of the victim and family's lifestyle and a long-term process of reorganization of lifestyle (Burgess, 1995).***

Defining Characteristics

Major (Must Be Present)

Reports or evidence of sexual assault.

Minor (May Be Present)

If the victim is a child, parents may experience similar responses.

** This diagnosis has been retired by NANDA-I because it has not been revised and updated. The author has revised and updated this diagnosis and thus will retain it for its clinical usefulness.
*** The author has added to the NANDA-I definition to enhance usefulness and clarity.

Acute Phase

Somatic Responses

Physical Trauma (Bruises, Soreness)
Gastrointestinal irritability (nausea, vomiting, anorexia, diarrhea)
Genitourinary discomfort (pain, pruritus, vaginal discharge)
Skeletal muscle tension (spasms, pain, headaches, sleep
   disturbances)

Psychological Responses

Overt
Crying, sobbing   Volatility, anger
Feelings of revenge   Confusion, incoherence,
Change in relationships*   disorientation*
Hyperalertness*

Ambiguous Reaction
Confusion*, incoherence, disorientation*
Masked facies
Calm, numbness
Shock*, numbness, confusion*, or disbelieving
Distractibility and difficulty making decisions

Emotional Reaction
Self-blame
Fear*—of being alone or that the rapist will return (a child victim
   fears punishment, repercussions, abandonment, rejection)
Denial, shock, humiliation, and embarrassment*
Desire for revenge; anger*
Guilt, shame
Fatigue

Sexual Responses
Mistrust of men (if victim is a woman)
Change in sexual behavior, sexual dysfunction*

Long-Term Phase**

Any response of the acute phase may continue if resolution does
not occur. In addition, the following reactions can occur 2 or
more weeks after the assault.

Psychological Responses
Change in relationship(s) associated with nonsupportive parent,
   partner, relative, friend (e.g., blames victim for event, "taking
   too long to get over it")

** Varcarolis, Carlson, & Shoemaker, 2006.

Intrusive thoughts (anger toward assailant, flashbacks of the traumatic event, dreams, insomnia)

Increased motor activity (moving, taking trips, staying some other place)

Increased emotional lability (intense anxiety, mood swings, crying spells, depression)

Fears and phobias (of indoors, or outdoors, where the rape occurred, of being alone, of crowds, of sexual encounters (with partner or potential partners)

Author's Note

See *Post-Trauma Syndrome*.

The author has interacted with numerous girls and women who have shared their sexual assault; some for the first time in their lives. Two themes are woven into their stories: (1) guilt that they contributed to the assault and (2) profound disappointment with their mother's response. Many mothers blamed their daughter for the event and sometimes refuse to believe their daughter if a relative or paramour is involved; or they suggest their daughter provoked the event. Perhaps that was the only reaction a mother could have at the time, because she could not face the truth. I discussed forgiveness with these women. Forgiveness never means you accept what happened only that you are going to release the pain from yourself. It is a gift you give yourself.

Girls and women shared stories that the rape would not have happened if they had not:

Worn that short skirt

Drank too much

Walked home in the dark

Had engaged in kissing and hugging

Had not went somewhere alone with him

I share with each girl or woman this scenario: Instead of being sexually assaulted, imagine that you were hit over the head with a shovel. Would it have mattered what you were wearing, doing, or saying at the time? Sexual assault is not sex, it is a violent act like hitting someone with a shovel. I suggest when thoughts of self-blame surface, these women think of the shovel.

NOC

Abuse Protection, Abuse Recovery, Coping

Goals

The client, parents, spouse, or significant other will return to pre crisis level of functioning and the child will express feelings concerning the assault and the treatment based on the following indicators:

Short-Term Goals
- Share feelings.
- Describe rationale and treatment procedures.
- Identify members of support system and use them appropriately.

Long-Term Goals
- Report sleeping well.
- Report return to former eating pattern.
- Report occasional somatic reactions or none.
- Demonstrate calmness and relaxation.

NIC

Abuse Protection Support, Coping Enhancement, Rape-Trauma Treatment, Support Group, Anxiety Reduction, Presence, Emotional Support, Calming Technique, Active Listening, Family Support, Grief Work Facilitation

Interventions

Assist the Client in Identifying Major Concerns (Psychological, Medical, Legal) and Perception of Help Needed

Explain the Care and Examination

- Provide interventions in an unhurried manner.
- Do not leave the client alone.
- Help the client to meet personal needs (bathing *after* examination and evidence has been acquired).
- Explain every detail before acting and secure permission.

Explain the Legal Issues and Police Investigation (Heinrich, 1987)

Promote a Trusting Relationship

- Stay with the client during acute stage or arrange for other support.
- Brief the client on police and hospital procedures during acute stage.
- Explain that the choice to report the rape is the victim's. Explore pros and cons of reporting.
- Explain the need to collect specimens for future possible court use.

- If this is the client's first pelvic examination, explain the position and the instruments. Explain each step prior to intervention. Have another nurse support the client through the exam.
- If the police interview is permitted:
  - Negotiate with the victim and police for an advantageous time.
  - Explain to the victim what kind of questions will be asked.
  - Remain with the victim during the interview; do not ask questions or offer answers.
- If the officer is insensitive, intimidating, or offensive, or asks improper questions, discuss this with the officer in private. If the behavior continues, use proper channels and make a complaint.
- Initiate play therapy with a child to explain treatments and allow the child to express feelings.
- Play therapy should be an integral part of the treatment regimen for children. The child can act out the assault with dolls of the appropriate sex. Puppets are also beneficial for play therapy (Hockenberry & Wilson, 2009).

Whenever Possible, Provide Crisis Counseling Within
1 Hour of Rape

- Ask permission to contact the rape crisis counselor.
- Be flexible and individualize the approach according to the victim's needs.
- Observe the victim's behavior carefully and record objective data.
- Encourage the victim to verbalize thoughts, feelings, or perceptions of the event.
- Discuss treatment as victim; express empathy.
- Assess the victim's verbal style (expressive, controlled).
- Discuss with the victim previous coping mechanism.
- Explore available support systems; involve significant others if appropriate.
- Assess stress tolerance.
- Reassure the victim about the manner in which she or he reacted.
- Explore with the victim her or his strengths and resources.
- Convey confidence in the victim's ability to return to prior level of functioning.
- Assist the victim in decision-making and problem-solving; involve the victim in own treatment plan.
- Help restore the victim's dignity by calmly exploring together basis for feelings.
- Reassure the victim that rape trauma victims often experience these feelings/symptoms: fear of rapist or death, guilt, loss of control, shame, short attention span, anger, anxiety, phobias, depression, flashbacks, embarrassment, and eating/sleeping pattern disturbances.

- Respect the victim's rights; honor wishes to restrict unwanted visitors; offer privacy when appropriate.
- Explain to the victim that this experience will disrupt his or her life, and that feelings that occurred during acute phase may recur; encourage the victim to proceed at his or her own pace.
- Explain any papers that need to be signed.
- Briefly counsel family and friends at their level.
- Share the immediate needs of the victim for love and support.
- Encourage the victim to express feelings and ask questions.

Fulfill Medical–Legal Responsibilities by Documentation (Ledray, 2001)

- Consult with a sexual assault nurse examiner (SANEs) or clinicians who are specially trained to address the needs of a sexually assault survivor.
- If in the emergency room, consult The Emergency Nurses Association position statement on the role of the nurse in collecting medical and legal evidence at http://www.ena.org/about/position/forensicevidence.asp.

Document

- History of rape (date, time, place).
- Nature of injuries, use of force, weapons used, threats of violence or retribution, restraints used.
- Nature of assault (fondling, oral, anal, vaginal penetration, ejaculation, use of condom).
- Post assault activities (douching, bathing/showering, gargling, urinating, defecating, changing clothes, eating, or drinking).
- Present state (use of drugs, alcohol).
- Medical history, immunization status (tetanus, hepatitis A, B), gynecologic history (last menstrual period, last voluntary intercourse, using a birth control method).
- Emotional state and mental status.
- Examination findings, smears/cultures taken, blood tests, evidence collected, and photographs (if appropriate).
- Document what evidence is delivered and when and to whom.

Explain the Risks of Sexually Transmitted Infections (Ledray, 2001; Centers for Disease Control and Prevention, 2008)

- Sexually transmitted diseases (specimens, blood tests): Gonorrhea, Human immunodeficiency virus (HIV), Trichomoniasis, Syphilis, Hepatitis B, A, C, Chlamydia.
- Consult with protocol or physician/nurse practitioner for prophylaxis for Chlamydia, HIV, Trichomoniasis, and Gonorrhea.
- Vaccinate individuals if needed for tetanus and Hepatitis A, B.
- Determine if the victim is at risk for pregnancy and, if at risk, explain emergency contraceptive pills (ECP).
- No contraceptive use.

- No surgical sterilization.
- Postmenopausal.

Eliminate or Reduce Somatic Symptomatology

Gastrointestinal Irritability

Anorexia
- Offer small, frequent feedings.
- Provide appealing foods.
- Record intake.
- Refer to *Imbalanced Nutrition* if anorexia is prolonged.

Nausea
- Avoid gas-forming foods.
- Restrict carbonated beverages.
- Observe for abdominal distention.
- Offer antiemetic per physician's order.

Genitourinary Discomfort

Pain
- Assess for quality and duration.
- Monitor intake and output.
- Inspect urine and external genitalia for bleeding.
- Listen attentively to the victim's description of pain.
- Give pain medication per physician's order (see *Impaired Comfort*).

Discharge
- Assess amount, color, and odor of discharge.
- Allow the victim time to wash and change garments after initial examination has been completed.

Itching
- Encourage bathing in cool water.
- Avoid use of detergent soaps.
- Avoid touching the area causing discomfort.

Skeletal Muscle Tension

Headaches
- Avoid any sudden change of the victim's position.
- Approach the victim calmly.
- Slightly elevate the bed (unless contraindicated).
- Discuss pain-reducing measures that have been effective in the past.

Fatigue
- Assess present sleeping patterns if altered (see *Disturbed Sleep Pattern*).
- Discuss precipitating factors for sleep disturbance; try to eliminate them, if possible.

- Provide frequent rest periods throughout the day.
- Avoid interruptions during sleep.
- Avoid stress-producing situations.

Emotional Responses
- Provide an emotionally secure environment.
- Discuss the victim's daily routines and adhere to them as much as possible.
- Avoid any sudden movements, and approach the victim in a calm manner.
- Provide frequent quiet periods throughout the day.

Generalized Bruising and Edema
- Avoid constrictive garments.
- Handle affected body parts gently.
- Elevate affected body part if edema is present.
- Apply a cool, moist compress to the edematous area for the first 24 hours, then a warm compress after 24 hours.
- Encourage the victim to verbalize discomfort.
- Record any bruises, lacerations, edema, or abrasions.

Proceed with Health Teaching to Victim and Family

- Before the victim leaves the hospital, provide a card with information about follow-up appointments and names and telephone numbers of local crisis and counseling centers.
- Plan a home visit or telephone call.
- Arrange for legal or pastoral counseling, if appropriate.
- Recommend and make referrals to a psychotherapist, mental health clinic, citizen action, or community group advocacy-related service.

Teach Management of Discomforts

- Gastrointestinal irritability: explain that the side effects of emergency contraceptive pills (ECP) are nausea and vomiting.
- Genitourinary discomfort: advise against scratching the area causing discomfort.
- Skeletal muscle tension:
  - Explain potential causes of discomfort.
  - Explain measures that may help release tension.
  - Teach relaxation methods.
- Follow-up counseling provides support over time and may lessen the intrapsychic effects of the rape (Carson & Smith-DiJulio, 2006).

POWERLESSNESS

Powerlessness

Risk for Powerlessness

NANDA-I Definition

The lived experience of lack of control over a situation, including a perception that one's actions do not significantly affect an outcome

Defining Characteristics

Major (Must Be Present)

Overt (anger, apathy) or covert expressions of dissatisfaction over inability to control a situation (e.g., work, illness, prognosis, care, recovery rate) that negatively affects outlook, goals, and lifestyle

Inability to access valued resources (food, shelter, income, education, employment)

Belief that one has little or no control over the cause or the solutions of one's problems

Minor (May Be Present)

Lack of information-seeking behaviors

Excessive dependence on others	Anger
	Feelings of alienation
Acting-out behavior	Low self-efficacy
Violent behavior	Resignation
Inability to effectively problem solve	Anxiety
	Depression
Passivity	Sense of vulnerability
Apathy	Feelings of helplessness

Related Factors

Pathophysiologic

Any disease process, acute or chronic, can cause or contribute to powerlessness. Some common sources are the following:

Related to inability to communicate secondary to:
Stroke   Intubation
Guillain–Barré syndrome

Related to inability to perform activities of daily living secondary to such conditions as:
Stroke   Myocardial infarction
Cervical trauma   Pain

Related to inability to perform role responsibilities secondary to surgery, trauma, or arthritis

Related to progressive debilitating disease secondary to such diseases as multiple sclerosis, terminal cancer, or AIDS

Related to substance abuse

Related to cognitive distortions secondary to:
Depression

Situational (Personal, Environmental)

Related to change from curative status to palliative status

Related to feeling of loss of control and lifestyle restrictions secondary to (specify)

Related to overeating patterns

Related to personal characteristics that highly value control (e.g., internal locus of control)

Related to effects of hospital or institutional limitations

Related to elevated fear of disapproval

Related to consistent negative feedback

Related to long-term abusive relationships

Related to oppressive patriarchal values with women

Related to the presence of an abusive relationships with a history of mental illness (Bengtsson-Tops, Saveman, & Tops, 2009)

Maturational

Older Adult
Related to multiple losses secondary to aging (e.g., retirement, sensory deficits, motor deficits, money, significant others)

Author's Note

Powerlessness is a feeling that all people experience to varying degrees in various situations. Stephenson (1979) described two types of pow-erlessness: (1) *situational powerlessness* occurs in a specific event and is probably short-lived; (2) *trait powerlessness* is more pervasive, affecting general outlook, goals, lifestyle, and relationships. The nursing diagnosis *Powerlessness* may be more useful clinically when describing a client experiencing trait rather than situational powerlessness.

   Hopelessness differs from powerlessness in that a hopeless client sees no solution to problems or no way to achieve what is desired, even if he or she feels in control. A powerless client may see an alternative or answer yet is unable to do anything about it because of perception of lack of control and resources. Prolonged powerlessness may lead to hopelessness.

NOC

Depression Control, Health Beliefs, Health Beliefs: Perceived Control, Participation: Health Care Decisions

Goal

The client will verbalize ability to control or influence situations and outcomes, as evidenced by the following indicators:

- Identify the factors that the client can control.
- The client will make decisions regarding his or her care, treat-ment, and future when possible.

NIC

Mood Management, Teaching: Individual, Decision-Making Support, Self-Responsibility Facilitation, Health System Guidance, Spiritual Support

Interventions

Assess for Causative and Contributing Factors

- Lack of knowledge
- Previous inadequate coping patterns (e.g., depression; for discussion, see *Ineffective Coping* related to depression)
- Insufficient decision-making opportunities

Eliminate or Reduce Contributing Factors, If Possible

Lack of Knowledge
- Increase effective communication between client and health care provider.
- Explain all procedures, rules, and options to the client; avoid medical jargon. Help the client anticipate situations that will occur during treatments (provides reality-oriented cognitive images that bolster a sense of control and coping strategies).
- Allow time to answer questions; ask the client to write questions down so that he or she does not forget them.
- Provide a specific time (10 to 15 minutes) per shift that the client knows can be used to ask questions or discuss subjects as desired.
- Anticipate questions/interest and offer information. Help the client to anticipate events and outcomes.
- While being realistic, point out positive changes in the client's condition, such as serum enzymes decreasing after myocardial infarction or surgical incision healing well.
- Be an active listener by allowing the client to verbalize concerns and feelings; assess for areas of concern.
- Designate one nurse to be responsible for a 24-hour plan of care, and provide opportunities for the client and family to identify with this nurse.
- If contributing factors are pain or anxiety, provide information about how to use behavioral control techniques (e.g., relaxation, imagery, deep breathing).

Provide Opportunities for the Client to Control Decisions and to Identify Personal Goals of Care

- Allow the client to manipulate surroundings, such as deciding what is to be kept where (shoes under bed, picture on window).
- If the client desires, and as hospital policy permits, encourage the client to bring personal effects from home (e.g., pillows, pictures).
- Keep needed items within reach (call bell, urinal, tissues).
- Do not offer options if there are none (e.g., a deep intramuscular [IM] Z-track injection must be rotated). Offer options that are personally relevant.
- Discuss daily plan of activities and allow the client to make as many decisions as possible about it.
- Increase decision-making opportunities as the client progresses.
- Respect and follow the client's decision if you have given options.
- Record the client's specific choices in care plan to ensure that others on staff acknowledge preferences ("dislikes orange juice," "takes showers," "plan dressing change at 7:30 AM before shower").
- Keep promises.
- Provide opportunity for the client and family to express feelings.
- Provide opportunities for the client and family to participate in care.

- Be alert for signs of paternalism/maternalism in health care providers (e.g., making decisions for clients).
- Plan a care conference to allow staff to discuss methods of individualizing care; encourage each nurse to share at least one action that he or she discovered a particular client likes.
- Shift emphasis from what one cannot do to what one can do.
- Set goals that are short term, behavioral, practical, and realistic (walk 5 more feet every day; then in 1 week, client can walk to the television room).
- Provide daily recognition of progress.
- Praise gains/achievements.
- Assist in identifying factors that are controllable and those that are not. Assist in accepting what cannot be changed and altering what can.
- Emphasize positive aspects when the client becomes focused on fears of the worst (reduces fear by shifting perspective and allowing the client to regain control).
- Allow the client to experience outcomes that result from his or her own actions.

Monitor a Client With External Locus of Control to Encourage Participation

- Have the client keep a record (e.g., food intake for 1 week; weight loss chart; exercise program; type and frequency of medications taken).
- Use telephone or e-mail contact to monitor the client, if feasible.
- Provide explicit written directions (e.g., meal plans; exercise regimen—type, frequency, duration; speech practice lessons for aphasia).
- Teach family methods to manipulate behaviors, if appropriate.
- Provide reward for each goal reached.

Assist the Client in Deriving Power From Other Sources

- Give permission to both client and family to use other power sources (e.g., prayer, stress reduction techniques).
- Suggest self-help groups focusing on empowerment. Learning, a component of the empowerment process, was found to occur in women with breast cancer who participated in self-help groups that focused on empowerment. Learning occurred by raising awareness, acquiring objective knowledge, learning form other's experiences, and discovering new perspectives about life and oneself (Stang and Mittelmark, 2008).
- Suggest support groups.
- Offer referral to religious leader.
- Provide privacy and support for other measures the client may request (e.g., meditation, imagery, special rituals).

Initiate Health Teaching and Referrals as Indicated (Social Worker, Psychiatric Nurse/Physician, Visiting Nurse, Religious Leader, Self-Help Groups)

Evaluate the Situation With the Client

- Once the outcome criteria have been accomplished or feelings of powerlessness are diminishing, discuss the process used to relieve powerlessness. Explain how factors contributed to the powerlessness, review why certain strategies were effective, and discuss how the client will manage feelings of powerlessness in the future.
- Advocate within the system to eliminate policies and routines that contribute to powerlessness.

Pediatric Interventions

- Provide opportunities for the child to make decisions (e.g., set time for bath, hold still for injection).
- Engage the child in play therapy before and after a traumatic situation (refer to *Delayed Growth and Development* for specific interventions for age-related development needs).

Risk for Powerlessness

NANDA-I Definition

At risk for the lived experience of lack of control over a situation, including a perception that one's actions do not significantly affect an outcome

Risk Factors

Refer to Related Factors in *Powerlessness*.

Goal

The client will continue to make decisions regarding his or her life, health care, and future, as evidenced by the following indicators:

- Engage in discussions of options.
- Raise questions regarding choices.

Interventions

Refer to *Powerlessness*.

INEFFECTIVE PROTECTION

Ineffective Protection

Risk for Dry Eye

Impaired Tissue Integrity

Impaired Skin Integrity

Risk for Impaired Skin Integrity

Impaired Oral Mucous Membrane

NANDA-I Definition

Decrease in the ability to guard self from internal or external threats, such as illness or injury

Defining Characteristics*

Deficient immunity	Fatigue
Impaired healing	Dyspnea
Altered clotting	Anorexia
Maladaptive stress response	Cough
Neurosensory alterations	Weakness
Pressure ulcers	Itching
Chilling	Immobility
Insomnia	Restlessness
Perspiring	Disorientation

 Author's Note

This broad diagnosis describes a client with compromised ability to defend against microorganisms, bleeding, or both because of immuno-suppression, myelosuppression, abnormal clotting factors, or all these. Use of this diagnosis entails several potential problems.

The nurse is cautioned against substituting *Ineffective Protection* for an immune system compromise, acquired immunodeficiency syndrome (AIDS), disseminated intravascular coagulation, diabetes mellitus, or other disorders. Rather, the nurse should focus on diagnoses describing the client's functional abilities that are or may be compromised by altered protection, such as *Fatigue, Risk for Infection*, and *Risk for Social Isolation*. The nurse also should address the physiologic complications of altered protection that require nursing and medical interventions for management, identifying appropriate collaborative problems.

For example, the nurse could use *Ineffective Protection* in each of these three cases: Mr. A, who has leukemia, leukopenia, and no evidence of infection; Mr. B, who is experiencing sickle cell crisis; and Mr. C, who has AIDS. The problem is that this diagnosis does not describe the specific focus of nursing but describes situations in which more specific responses can be diagnosed. For Mr. A, the nursing diagnosis of *Risk for Infection* related to compromised immune system would apply. For Mr. B., the collaborative problem *RC of Sickle Cell Crisis* best describes this situation, which the nurse monitors and manages using physician- and nurse-prescribed interventions. The nursing diagnosis *Risk for Infection* and the collaborative problem *RC of Opportunistic Infections* would apply for Mr. C. As these examples show, in most cases, the nursing diagnosis *Risk for Infection* and selected collaborative problems prove more clinically useful than *Ineffective Protection*.

Risk for Dry Eye

NANDA-I Definition

At risk for eye discomfort or damage to the cornea and conjunctiva due to reduced quantity or quality of tears to moisten the eye

Risk Factors

Pathophysiologic

Autoimmune diseases (rheumatoid arthritis, diabetes mellitus, thyroid disease, gout, osteoporosis, etc.)*
Collagen vascular disease
History of allergy*
Structural eyelid problems
Neurologic lesions with sensory or motor reflex loss (lagophthalmos, lack of spontaneous blink reflex due to decreased consciousness and other medical conditions)*
Ocular surface damage*
Vitamin A deficiency*
Deficient tear-producing glands
Tear gland damage from inflammation
Difficulty blinking due to eyelid problems (e.g., ectropion [turning out]; entropion [turning in])

Treatment Related

Pharmaceutical agents such as angiotensin-converting enzyme
inhibitors, antihistamines, diuretics, steroids, antidepressants,
tranquilizers, analgesics, sedatives, neuromuscular blockage
agents*
Surgical operations*
Anti-inflammatory agents (e.g., ibuprofen, naproxen, birth
control pills, decongestants)
After laser eye surgery
Tear gland damage from radiation
After cosmetic eyelid surgery
Oral contraceptives
Mechanical ventilation therapy*

Personal (Situational, Environmental)

Long hours looking at computer screen
Smoking
Heavy drinking
Contact lenses*
Environmental factors (air-conditioning, excessive wind,
sunlight exposure, air pollution, low humidity),* hot, dry,
windy climate
Place of living*
Female gender*
Lifestyle (e.g., smoking, caffeine use, prolonged reading)*
Air travel

Maturational

Aging   Postmenopause

 Author's Note

This new NANDA-I nursing diagnosis represents a common problem
experienced by most persons acutely or chronically. For some individuals, the problem is annoying, for others it causes a significant chronic
discomfort, and for a few individuals dry eye is a serious risk factor that
can cause corneal abrasions. Therefore, this diagnosis can be used to
prevent or reduce dry eyes.

For those individuals who are at risk for corneal abrasion, such as
those with chronic dry eyes or those so debilitated that the natural
lubrication system in the eye is compromised (e.g., comatose), *Risk for
Corneal Abrasion* would be more clinically useful.

NOC

Environmental, Health Promotion Behavior, Symptom Control

Goal

The client will report reduction of dry eye symptoms, as evidenced by the following indicators:

• Describe causes of dry eye.
• Identify strategies to prevent dry eyes.

NIC

Comfort Level, Hydration, Environmental Management, Nutritional Counseling

Interventions

Explain Factors That Contribute to Dry Eyes

Refer to Risk Factors.

Teach to Use Over-the-Counter Artificial Tears or Ocular Lubricants as Needed

• Before reading or other activities that increase eye movements
• Use preservative-free eye drops if they are used more than four times a day
• Avoid using drops that "get the red out," which are not effective in lubricating eyes

Increase Environmental Humidity, Especially in the Winter and Dry Climates

• Avoid hot rooms, high winds

Wear Wraparound Sunglasses or Other Type With Foam or Other Seals; When Swimming, Wear Goggles

Avoid Eye Irritants

• Hair sprays
• Tobacco smoke
• Air blowing in eyes (e.g., hair dryer, fans)

Use an Air Cleaner/Filter and a Humidifier, If Possible

• Advise client of medications that might increase dryness and discomfort. Advise them to discuss situation with their primary care provider.

For Contact Lens Wearers:
• If eye drops are used, be aware if lens must be removed before instillation of drops and not replaced for 15 minutes.
• Rewetting drops may be effective if eye dryness is mild.
• Wear lens for few hours daily if needed.

Advise of Nutritional and Hydration Effects on Eye Dryness
- Avoid dehydration. Advise to monitor hydration by keeping urine color pale.
- Advise that coffee and tea are diuretics and of the need to increase water intake, unless contraindicated.
- Discuss the relationship of nutritional intake of omega-3 fatty acids such as cold-water fish, sardines, tuna, salmon, cod, herring, flax seed oil, soybean oil, canola oil, fish oil supplements, and vitamin A (e.g., carrots, broccoli supplements).

When Reading or Using a Computer for Long Periods (Mayo Clinic, 2010):
- Take eye breaks, close eyes for a few minutes
- Blink repeatedly for a few seconds

Advise to See Primary Care Provider or an Eye Specialist If There Are Prolonged Signs and Symptoms of Dry Eyes

Impaired Tissue Integrity

NANDA-I Definition

Damage to mucous membranes, corneal integumentary, or subcutaneous tissues

Defining Characteristics

Damaged tissue or destroyed tissue (e.g., cornea, mucous membranes, integumentary, subcutaneous)

Related Factors

Pathophysiologic

Related to inflammation of dermal–epidermal junctions secondary to:

Autoimmune Alterations
Lupus erythematosus   Scleroderma

Metabolic and Endocrine Alterations
Diabetes mellitus   Cirrhosis
Jaundice   Thyroid dysfunction
Hepatitis   Renal failure
Cancer

Bacterial
Impetigo   Cellulitis
Folliculitis

Viral
Herpes zoster (shingles)	Gingivitis
Herpes simplex	AIDS

Fungal
Ringworm (dermatophytosis)	Vaginitis
Athlete's foot	

Related to decreased blood and nutrients to tissues secondary to:

Diabetes mellitus
Peripheral vascular alterations	Obesity
Anemia	Malnutrition
Venous stasis	Emaciation
Cardiopulmonary disorders	Edema*
Arteriosclerosis	Dehydration*

Treatment Related

Related to decreased blood and nutrients to tissues secondary to:
Therapeutic extremes in body temperature
NPO status
Surgery

Related to imposed immobility secondary to sedation

Related to mechanical trauma
Therapeutic fixation devices
  Wired jaw
  Casts
  Traction
Orthopedic devices/braces

Related to effects of radiation on epithelial and basal cells*

Related to effects of mechanical factors or pressure secondary to:*
Inflatable or foam donuts	Nasogastric (NG) tubes
Tourniquets	Shear
Footboards	Friction
Restraints	Endotracheal tubes
Dressings, tape, solutions	Oral prostheses/braces
External urinary catheters	Contact lenses

Related to the effects of medicines (specify) (e.g., steroids, antibiotics)

Situational (Personal, Environmental)

Related to chemical irritants secondary to:*
Excretions	Noxious agents/substances
Secretions	

Related to environmental irritants secondary to:

Radiation/sunburn   Temperature extremes*
Humidity   Parasites
Bites (insect, animal)   Inhalants
Poisonous plants

Related to the effects of pressure of impaired physical mobility*
secondary to:

Pain   Cognitive, sensory, or motor
Fatigue   deficits
Motivation

Related to inadequate personal habits (hygiene/dental/dietary/sleep)

Related to thin body frame

Maturational

Related to dry, thin skin and decreased dermal vascularity secondary to aging

 Author's Note

Impaired Tissue Integrity is the broad diagnosis under which fall the more specific diagnoses of *Impaired Skin Integrity* and *Impaired Oral Mucous Membranes*. Because tissue is composed of epithelium, connective tissue, muscle, and nervous tissue, *Impaired Tissue Integrity* correctly describes some pressure ulcers that are deeper than the dermis. *Impaired Skin Integrity* should be used to describe disruptions of epidermal and dermal tissue only.

When a pressure ulcer is stage IV, necrotic, or infected, it may be more appropriate to label the diagnosis a collaborative problem, such as *Risk for Complications of Stage IV Pressure Ulcer*. This would represent a situation in which a nurse manages with physician- and nurse-prescribed interventions. When a stage II or III pressure ulcer needs a dressing that requires a physician's order in an acute care setting, the nurse should continue to label the situation a nursing diagnosis because it would be appropriate and legal for a nurse to treat the ulcer independently in other settings (e.g., in the community).

If a client is immobile and multiple systems are threatened (respiratory, circulatory, musculoskeletal as well as integumentary), the nurse can use *Disuse Syndrome* to describe the entire situation. If a client is at risk for damage to corneal tissue, the nurse can use a diagnosis such as *Risk for Impaired Corneal Tissue Integrity* related to corneal drying and lower lacrimal production secondary to unconscious state.

 NOC

Tissue Integrity

Goal

The client will demonstrate progressive healing of tissue, as evidenced by the following indicators:

- Participate in risk assessment.
- Express willingness to participate in prevention of pressure ulcers.
- Describe etiology and prevention measures.
- Explain rationale for interventions.

NIC

Teaching: Individual, Surveillance

Interventions

Identify Causative/Contributing Factors

Refer to Related Factors.

Reduce Contributing Factors to Mechanical Irritants to Skin

- Encourage highest degree of mobility to avoid prolonged periods of pressure.

For neuromuscular impairment:

- Teach the client/family appropriate measures to prevent pressure, shear, friction, and maceration and to not use inflatable donuts or rings (Bergstrom et al., 1994; WOCN, 2003).
- Teach the client to recognize early signs of tissue damage.
- Change the client's position at least every 2 hours around the clock (Maklebust, 2005).
- Use a 30-degree lateral side-lying position.
- Frequently supplement full-body turns with minor shifts in body weight.
- Protect tissue from pressure (drains, tubes, dressings).
- Use pressure-dispersing devices as appropriate.
- Limit semi-Fowler's position in high-risk clients (limit elevation of head of bed to less than 30 degrees) (Bergstrom et al., 1994; Maklebust & Sieggreen, 1996; Reichel, 1958; WOCN, 2003).
- Avoid use of knee gatch on bed.
- Use lift sheet to reposition the client.
- Install an overhead trapeze to allow the clients increased mobility (Bergstrom et al., 1994; WOCN, 2003).

Reduce Causative Factors, If Possible

For casts:

- Monitor common pressure sites in relationship to cast application.
- Apply padding over bony prominence.
- Keep cast edges smooth and away from skin surfaces.
- Inspect for loose plaster and shifting of padding.

Protect Skin Around Feeding Tubes or Endotracheal Tubes With a Protective Barrier

- Change skin barrier when loose or leaking.
- Instruct to report discomforts.

Impaired Skin Integrity

NANDA-I Definition

Altered epidermis and/or dermis

Defining Characteristics*

Destruction of skin layers   Invasion of body structures
Disruption of skin surface

Related Factors

See *Impaired Tissue Integrity*.

Tissue Integrity: Skin and Mucous Membrane

Goals

The person will demonstrate progressive healing of tissue, as evidenced by the following indicators:

- Participate in risk assessment.
- Express willingness to participate in prevention of pressure ulcers.
- Describe etiology and prevention measures.

Pressure Management, Pressure Ulcer Care, Skin Surveillance, Positioning

Interventions

Identify the Stages of Pressure Ulcer Development

- Stage I: Nonblanchable erythema of intact skin
- Stage II: Ulceration of epidermis or dermis
- Stage III: Ulceration involving subcutaneous fat
- Stage IV: Extensive ulceration penetrating muscle, bone, or supporting structure

Assess Status of Ulcer

- Size, measuring longest and widest wound surface
- Depth:
  - No break in skin
  - Abrasion or shallow crater
  - Deep crater
  - Necrosis
- Edges:
  - Attached
  - Not attached
  - Fibrotic
- Undermining:
  - <2 cm
  - 2 to 4 cm
  - More than 4 cm
  - Tunneling
- Necrotic tissue type (color, consistency, adherence) and amount
- Exudate type, amount
- Surrounding skin color
- Presence of peripheral tissue edema, induration
- Granulation tissue
- Epithelialization

Wash Reddened Area Gently With a Mild Soap, Rinse Thoroughly to Remove Soap, and Pat Dry

Gently Massage Healthy Skin Around the Affected Area to Stimulate Circulation; Do Not Massage If Reddened

Protect the Healthy Skin Surface With One or a Combination of the Following

- Apply a thin coat of liquid copolymer skin sealant.
- Cover area with moisture-permeable film dressing.
- Cover area with a hydrocolloid wafer barrier, and secure with strips of 1-inch nonallergenic tape; leave in place for 2 to 3 days.

Increase Protein and Carbohydrate Intake to Maintain a Positive Nitrogen Balance; Weigh the Person Daily, and Determine Serum Albumin Level Weekly to Monitor Status

Devise Plan for Pressure Ulcer Management Using Principles of Moist Wound-Healing

- Débride necrotic tissue (collaborate with physician).
- Flush ulcer base with sterile saline solution.
- Protect granulating wound bed from trauma.
- Cover pressure ulcer with a sterile dressing that maintains a moist environment over the ulcer base (e.g., film dressing, hydrocolloid wafer dressing, moist gauze dressing).
- Avoid the use of drying agents (heat lamps, magnesium hydroxide [Maalox], milk of magnesia).
- Monitor for clinical signs of wound infection.

Consult With Nurse Specialist or Physician for Treatment of Stage IV Pressure Ulcers

Refer to Community Nursing Agency If Additional Assistance at Home Is Needed

Risk for Impaired Skin Integrity

NANDA-I Definition

At risk for alteration in epidermis and/or dermis

Risk Factors

Refer to related factors under *Impaired Skin Integrity*.

Tissue Integrity: Skin and Mucous Membrane

Goal

The client will demonstrate skin integrity free of pressure ulcers (if able), as evidenced by the following indicators:

- Participate in risk assessment.
- Express willingness to participate in prevention of pressure ulcers.
- Describe etiology and prevention measures.

Pressure Management, Pressure Ulcer Care, Skin Surveillance, Positioning

Interventions

Use a Formal Risk Assessment Scale to Identify Individual Risk Factors in Addition to Activity and Mobility Deficits (e.g., The Braden Scale, Worton Score [AHCPR, 1992]); Refer to Focus Assessment

Attempt to Modify Contributing Factors to Lessen the Possibility of a Pressure Ulcer Developing

Incontinence of Urine or Feces
• Determine the etiology of the incontinence.
• Maintain sufficient fluid intake for adequate hydration (approximately 2,500 milliliters daily, unless contraindicated); check oral mucous membranes for moisture and check urine specific gravity.
• Establish a schedule for emptying the bladder (begin with every 2 hours).
• If the client is confused, determine what his or her incontinence pattern is and intervene before incontinence occurs.
• Explain problem to the client; secure his or her cooperation with the plan.
• When incontinent, wash the perineum with a liquid soap that does not alter skin pH.
• Apply a protective barrier to the perineal region (incontinence film barrier spray or wipes).
• Check the client frequently for incontinence when indicated.
• For additional interventions, refer to *Impaired Urinary Elimination*.

Immobility
• Encourage range of motion exercises and weight-bearing mobility, when possible, to increase blood flow to all areas.
• Promote optimal circulation when in bed.
  • Use repositioning schedule that relieves vulnerable area most often (e.g., if the vulnerable area is the back, the turning schedule would be left side to back, back to right side, right side to left side, and left side to back); post "turn clock" at bedside.
  • Turn or instruct the client to turn or shift weight every 30 minutes to 2 hours, depending on other causative factors and the ability of the skin to recover from pressure.
  • Increase frequency of the turning schedule if any reddened areas that appear do not disappear within 1 hour after turning.

- Place the client in normal or neutral position with body weight evenly distributed. Use 30-degree laterally inclined position when possible.
- Keep the bed as flat as possible to reduce shearing forces; limit semi-Fowler's position to only 30 minutes at a time.
- Use foam blocks or pillows to provide a bridging effect to support the body above and below the high-risk or ulcerated area so the affected area does not touch the bed surface. Do not use foam donuts or inflatable rings because these increase the area of pressure.
- Alternate or reduce the pressure on the skin with an appropriate support surface.
- Suspend heels off bed surface.
- Use enough personnel to lift the client up in bed or a chair rather than pull or slide skin surfaces.
- Have the client wear a long-sleeved top and socks to reduce friction on elbows and heels.
- To reduce shearing forces, support the feet with a footboard to prevent sliding.
- Promote optimal circulation when the client is sitting.
  - Limit sitting time for the client at high risk for ulcer development.
  - Instruct the client to lift self using chair arms every 10 minutes, if possible, or assist the client in rising up off the chair at least every hour, depending on risk factors present.
  - Do not elevate the legs unless calves are supported to reduce the pressure over the ischial tuberosities.
  - Pad the chair with pressure-relieving cushion.
- Inspect areas at risk of developing ulcers with each position change.
  - Ears
  - Elbows
  - Occiput
  - Trochanter**
  - Heels
  - Ischia
  - Sacrum
  - Scapula
  - Scrotum
- Observe for erythema and blanching and palpate for warmth and tissue sponginess with each position change.
- Do not rub reddened areas. To avoid damaging the capillaries, do not perform massage.

** Areas with little soft tissue over a bony prominence are at greatest risk.

Malnourished State
- Consult a dietitian.
- Increase protein and carbohydrate intake to maintain a positive nitrogen balance; weigh the client daily and determine serum albumin level weekly to monitor status.
- Ascertain that daily intake of vitamins and minerals is maintained through diet or supplements.
- See *Imbalanced Nutrition: Less Than Body Requirements* for additional interventions.

Sensory Deficit
- Inspect the client's skin daily because he or she will not experience discomfort.
- Teach the client or family to inspect the skin with a mirror.

Initiate Health Teaching, as Indicated

- Instruct the client and family in specific techniques to use at home to prevent pressure ulcers.
- Consider the use of long-term pressure-relieving devices for clients with permanent disabilities.

Consult With Nurse Specialist or Physician for Treatment of Necrotic, Infected, or Deep Pressure Ulcers

Initiate Health Teaching and Referrals, as Indicated

- Instruct the client and family about care of ulcers.
- Teach the client the importance of good skin hygiene and optimal nutrition.
- Refer the client to a community nursing agency if additional assistance at home is needed.
- Humidity affects the rate of epithelialization and the amount of scar formation. A moist environment provides optimal conditions for rapid healing.

Impaired Oral Mucous Membrane

NANDA-I Definition

Disruption of the lips and/or soft tissue of the oral cavity

Defining Characteristics

Major (Must Be Present)

Disrupted oral mucous membranes

Minor (May Be Present)

Color changes—erythema, pallor, white patches, lesions, and ulcers
Moisture changes—increased or decreased saliva
Cleanliness changes—debris, malodor, discoloration of the teeth
Mucosal integrity changes—difficulty swallowing, decreased taste, difficulty weaning
Perception changes—difficulty swallowing, decreased taste, difficulty wearing dentures, burning, pain, and change in voice quality.

Related Factors

Pathophysiologic

Related to inflammation secondary to:

Diabetes mellitus	Oral cancer
Periodontal disease	Infection

Treatment Related

Related to drying effects of:
NPO more than 24 hours
Radiation to head or neck
Prolonged use of steroids or other immunosuppressive agents and other medications including opioids, antidepressants, phenothiazines, antihypertensives, antihistamines, diuretics, and sedatives.
Use of antineoplastic drugs
Oxygen therapy
Mouth breathing
Blood and marrow stem cell transplant

Related to mechanical irritation secondary to:

Endotracheal tube	NG tube

Situational (Personal, Environmental)

Related to chemical irritants* secondary to:

Acidic foods	Alcohol
Drugs	Tobacco
Noxious agents	High sugar intake

Related to mechanical trauma secondary to:

Broken or jagged teeth	Braces
Ill-fitting dentures	

Related to malnutrition*

Related to inadequate oral hygiene

Related to lack of knowledge of oral hygiene

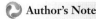 **Author's Note**

See *Impaired Tissue Integrity*.

NOC

Oral Tissue Integrity

Goal

The client will be free of oral mucosa irritation or exhibit signs of healing with decreased inflammation, as evidenced by the following indicators:

- Describe factors that cause oral injury.
- Demonstrate knowledge of optimal oral hygiene.

NIC

Oral Health Restoration, Chemotherapeutic Management, Oral Health Maintenance, Oral Health Promotion

Interventions

Assess for Causative or Contributing Factors

Refer to Related Factors.

Teach Preventive Oral Hygiene to Clients at Risk for Development of Mucositis

- Refer to *Impaired Oral Mucous Membrane Related to Inadequate Oral Hygiene* for specific instructions on brushing and flossing.
- Instruct client to:
  - Perform the regimen including brushing, flossing, rinsing, and moisturizing after meals and before sleep.
  - Avoid mouthwashes with alcohol content, lemon/glycerin swabs, or prolonged use of hydrogen peroxide.
  - Rinse mouth with saline or saline and bicarbonate solution.
  - Apply lubricant to lips every 2 hours and PRN (e.g., lanolin, A&D ointment).
  - Inspect mouth daily for lesions and inflammation and report alterations.
  - Avoid foods that are spicy, salty, hot, rough, or acidic.

- Report following symptoms: temperature greater than 101° F, new lesions or sores in mouth, bleeding from gums, difficulty swallowing or inability to take in fluids, and pain in the mouth.
- Keep mouth clean and moist.

Consult With Physician for Possible Need for Prophylactic Antifungal or Antibacterial Agent for Immunocompromised Clients at Risk for Mucositis (NCCN, 2008)

- Instruct client to see a dentist 2 to 3 weeks before therapy begins for diagnosis and treatment of infections and to ensure adequate time for healing.
- Consult with dentist for a regimen of daily fluoride treatments and oral hygiene.
- Instruct client to see a dentist during treatment as needed and 2 months after treatment.
- Refer any suspicious oral lesions to health care provider for culture to identify organism.
- Administer antibiotics, antifungals, or antivirals as prescribed.
- Monitor temperature every 4 hours and report abnormal readings to health care provider.
- Replace toothbrush after treatment of suspected or documented oral infection.

Promote Healing and Reduce Progression of Mucositis

- Inspect oral cavity three times daily with tongue blade and light; if mucositis is severe, inspect mouth every 4 hours.
- Ensure that oral hygiene regimen is done every 1 to 2 hours while awake and every 4 hours during the night.
- Use normal saline solution as a mouthwash.
- Floss teeth only once in 24 hours.
- Omit flossing if bleeding is excessive.

Reduce Oral Pain and Maintain Adequate Food and Fluid Intake

- Assess client's ability to chew and swallow.
- Administer mild analgesic every 3 to 4 hours as ordered by physician.
- Instruct client to:
  - Avoid commercial mouthwashes, citrus fruit juices, spicy foods, extremes in food temperature (hot, cold), crusty or rough foods, alcohol, mouthwashes with alcohol.
  - Eat bland, cool foods (e.g., sherbets).
  - Drink cool liquids every 2 hours and PRN.
- Consult with dietitian for specific interventions.
- Refer to *Impaired Nutrition: Less Than Body Requirements* related to anorexia for additional interventions.

- Consult with physician for an oral pain relief solution.
  - Xylocaine viscous 2% oral: swish and expectorate every 2 hours and before meals. (If throat is sore, the solution can be swallowed; if swallowed, Xylocaine produces local anesthesia and may affect the gag reflex.) The dose of the viscous Xylocaine is not to exceed 25 milliliters per day (NCCN, 2008).
  - Gelclair is a concentrated gel that provides a protective barrier and requires frequent applications because of limited duration. Prophylaxis is not recommended.
  - Topical morphine provides a reduction in pain severity and duration of pain. If the morphine is in an alcohol-based formula it may cause burning.

Initiate Health Teaching and Referrals, as Indicated

- Teach client and family the factors that contribute to stomatitis and its progression.
- Teach diet modifications to reduce oral pain and to maintain optimal nutrition.
- Have client describe or demonstrate home care regimen.

Pediatric Interventions

- If thrush (oral candidiasis) is present:
  - Rinse mouth with plain water after each feeding.
  - Boil nipples and bottles for at least 20 minutes.
  - Boil pacifiers once a day.
  - Apply topical medication as prescribed.
- Explain the need to teach 2-year-olds how to brush their teeth after meals and before bedtime.
- Encourage parent to have toddler accompany him or her to dentist office to meet personnel.
- Discuss the importance of routine dental examinations every 6 months beginning at 3 to 4 years old.

Maternal Interventions

- Stress the importance of good oral hygiene and dental examinations.
- Remind to advise dentist of pregnancy.
- Explain that gum hypertrophy and tenderness are normal during pregnancy.

Geriatric Interventions

- Explain high-risk age-related factors (Miller, 2009):
  - Degenerative bone disease
  - Diminished oral blood supply
  - Dry mouth
  - Vitamin deficiencies

- Explain that some medications cause dry mouth:
  - Laxatives
  - Antibiotics
  - Antidepressants
  - Analgesics
  - Iron sulfate
  - Cardiovascular
  - Anticholinergics
- Determine the presence of barriers to dental care:
  - Financial
  - Mobility
  - Dexterity
  - Lack of knowledge

INEFFECTIVE RELATIONSHIP

Ineffective Relationship

Risk for Ineffective Relationship

NANDA-I Definition

A pattern of mutual partnership that is insufficient to provide for each other's needs

Defining Characteristics*

No demonstration of mutual respect between partners
No demonstration of mutual support in daily activities between partners
No demonstration of understanding of partner's insufficient (physical, social, psychological) functioning
No demonstration of well-balanced autonomy between partners
No demonstration of well-balanced collaboration between partners
No identification of partner as a key person
Inability to communicate in a satisfying manner between partners
Report of dissatisfaction with complementary relation between partners
Report of dissatisfaction with fulfilling emotional needs by one's partner
Report of dissatisfaction with fulfilling physical needs by one's partner

Report of dissatisfaction with the sharing of ideas between partners

Report of dissatisfaction with the sharing of information between partners

Does not meet development goals appropriate for family life-cycle stage

Related Factors*

Cognitive changes in one partner	Poor communication skills
Developmental crises	Stressful life events
History of domestic violence	Substance abuse
	Unrealistic expectations

 Author's Note

This NANDA-I diagnosis represents problems or situations that can disrupt partner relationships. The list of related factors presents substantial different foci for interventions. For example, the interventions for relationship problems associated with substance abuse versus domestic violence and incarceration versus stressful life events are very different.

This book contains assessment and interventions for all of the Related Factors listed above, for example:

• Related to domestic violence, refer to *Dysfunctional Family Processes*.
• Related to substance abuse, refer to *Disturbed Self-Concept, Ineffective Denial*, and/or *Dysfunctional Family Processes*.
• Related to unrealistic expectations, refer to *Compromised Family Processes*.
• Related to poor communication skills, stressful life events, refer to *Compromised Family Processes, Readiness for Enhanced Relationships*.
• Related to cognitive changes, refer to *Chronic confusion, Altered Thought Processes*.

Thus, when *Ineffective or Risk for (Partner) Relationship* is validated, the nurse can find goals and interventions in sections listed above or can use one of the above diagnoses instead if found to be more descriptive.

Risk for Ineffective Relationship**

NANDA-I Definition

Risk for a pattern of mutual partnership that is insufficient to provide for each other's needs

---

** This diagnosis may be more clinically useful as *Risk for Ineffective Partner Relationships* because it is defined for partners.

Risk Factors

Cognitive changes in one's partner
Developmental crises
Domestic violence
Incarceration of one's partner

Poor communication skills
Stressful life events
Substance abuse
Unrealistic expectations

RELOCATION STRESS [SYNDROME]

Relocation Stress [Syndrome]

Risk for Relocation Stress [Syndrome]

NANDA-I Definition

Physiologic and/or psychological disturbance following transfer from one environment to another

Note: Other terms found in the literature that describe relocation stress include admission stress, postrelocation crisis, relocation crisis, relocation shock, relocation trauma, transfer stress, transfer trauma, translocation syndrome, and transplantation shock.

Defining Characteristics**

Major (80% to 100%)

Responds to transfer or relocation with:

Loneliness
Depression
Anger
Apprehension

Anxiety
Increased confusion
   (older adult population)

Minor (50% to 79%)

Change in former eating habits
Change in former sleep patterns

Increased verbalization of needs
Demonstration of dependency

** Harkulich, J. & Bruggler, C. (1988). *Nursing Diagnosis–translocation syndrome: Expert validation study.* Partial funding granted by the Peg Schlitz Fund, Delta Ix Chapter, Sigma Theta Tau International; Barnhouse, A. (1987). *Development of the nursing diagnosis of translocation syndrome with critical care patients.* Unpublished master's thesis, Kent State University, Kent, OH.

Demonstration of insecurity	Decrease in leisure activities
Demonstration of lack of trust	Gastrointestinal disturbances
Vigilance	Need for excessive reassurance
Weight change	Restlessness
Sad affect	Withdrawal
Decrease in self-care activities	Allergic symptoms

Unfavorable comparison of posttransfer to pretransfer staff
Verbalization of being concerned/upset about transfer
Verbalization of insecurity in new living situation

Related Factors

Pathophysiologic

Related to compromised ability to adapt to changes secondary to:

Decreased physical health status*	Increased/perceived stress before relocation
Physical difficulties	Depression
Decreased psychosocial health status	Decreased self-esteem

Situational (Personal, Environmental)

Related to insufficient finances, foreclosures

Related to high degree of changes secondary to:
Admission to a care facility

Related to:
Loss of social and familial ties
Abandonment
Change in relationship with family members

Related to little or no preparation for the impending move

Maturational

School-Aged Children and Adolescents
Related to losses associated with moving secondary to:
Fear of rejection, loss of peer group, or school-related problems
Decreased security in new adolescent peer group and school

Older Adult
Related to the need to be closer to family members for assistance
Related to admission to a care facility

Author's Note

NANDA-I has accepted *Relocation Stress* as a syndrome diagnosis. It does not fit the criterion for a syndrome diagnosis, which is a cluster of actual or risk nursing diagnoses as defining characteristics. The defining characteristics associated with *Relocation Stress* are observable or reportable cues consistent with *Relocation Stress*, not *Relocation Stress Syndrome*. The author recommends deleting "Syndrome" from the label.

Relocation represents a disruption for all parties involved. It can accompany a transfer from one unit to another or from one facility to another. It can involve a voluntary or forced permanent move to a long-term–care facility or new home. Since 2009, over 7 million housing units have been foreclosed on in the United States. This explosion of foreclosures in the United States and abroad has severely compromised individuals and families. The relocation disturbs all age groups involved. When physiologic and psychological disturbances compromise functioning, the nursing diagnosis *Relocation Stress Syndrome* is appropriate.

The optimal nursing approach to relocation stress is to initiate preventive measures, using *Risk for Relocation Stress* as the diagnosis.

NOC

Anxiety Self-Control, Coping, Loneliness, Psychosocial Adjustment: Life Change, Quality of Life

Goal

The client/family will report adjustment to the new environment with minimal disturbances, as evidenced by the following indicators:

* Share in decision-making activities regarding the new environment
* Express concerns regarding the move to a new environment
* Verbalize one positive aspect of the relocation
* Establish new bonds in the new environment
* Become involved in activities in the new environment

NIC

Anxiety Reduction, Coping Enhancement, Counseling, Family Involvement Promotion, Support System Enhancement, Anticipatory Guidance, Family Integrity Promotion, Transfer, Relocation Stress Reduction

Interventions

Encourage Each Family Member to Share Feelings About the Move

- Provide privacy for each client.
- Encourage family members to share feelings with one another.
- Discuss the possible and different effects of the move on each family member.
- Inform parents regarding potential changes in children's conduct with relocation, such as regression, withdrawal, acting out, and changes with eating (breast/bottle-feeding).
- Instruct parents to obtain all pertinent documents regarding children's medical/dental history (e.g., immunizations, communicable diseases, dental work).
- Allow for some ritual(s) when leaving the old environment. Encourage reminiscing, which will bring closure for many family members.

Teach Parents Techniques to Assist Their Children With the Move

- Remain positive about the move before, during, and after, accepting that the child may not be optimistic.
- Explore various options with children on how to communicate with friends/families in previous environment. Children's relationships with friends in the previous community are important, especially for "peer reassurance" after relocation.
- Keep regular routines in the new environment; establish them as soon as possible.
- Acknowledge the difficulty of peer losses with the adolescent.
- Join the organizations to which the child previously belonged (e.g., Scouts, sports).
- Assist children to focus on similarities between old and new environments (e.g., clubs, Scouts, church groups).
- Plan a trip to school during a class and lunch period to reduce fear of unknown.
- Allow children some choices regarding room arrangements, decorating, and the like.
- Ask teacher or counselor at the new school to introduce the adolescent to a student who recently relocated to that school.
- Allow children to mourn their losses as a result of the move.

Assess the Following Areas When Counseling a Relocated Adolescent

- Perceptions about the move
- Concurrent stressors
- Usual and present coping skills
- Support (family, peers, and community)

Initiate Health Teaching and Referrals, as Indicated

- Alert the family to the possible need for counseling before, during, or after the move.
- Furnish a written directory of relevant community organizations such as area churches, children's groups, Parents Without Partners, senior citizens' groups, and Welcome Wagon or other local new-neighbor groups.
- Instruct the family about appropriate community services.
- Consult the school nurse regarding school programs for new students.

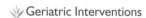 Geriatric Interventions

Promote Integration After Transfer Into a Long-Term Care Nursing Facility

- Allow as many choices as possible.
- Encourage person to bring familiar objects from home.
- Encourage person to interact with other individuals in new facility.
- Assist person to maintain previous interpersonal relationships.

Risk for Relocation Stress [Syndrome]

NANDA-I Definition

At risk for physiologic and/or psychological disturbance following transfer from one environment to another

Risk Factors

Refer to *Relocation Stress Syndrome*.

Goal

Refer to *Relocation Stress Syndrome*.

Interventions

Refer to *Relocation Stress Syndrome*.

RISK FOR COMPROMISED RESILIENCE

NANDA-I Definition

At risk for decreased ability to sustain a pattern of positive responses to an adverse situation or crisis

Risk Factors*

Chronicity of existing crises
Multiple coexisting adverse situations
Presence of additional new crisis (e.g., unplanned pregnancy,
    death of spouse, loss of job, illness, loss of housing, death of
    family member)

Author's Note

This NANDA-I diagnosis is not a response but an etiology of a coping problem. Resilience is a strength that can be taught to and nurtured in children. Resilient individuals and families can cope in adverse situations and crises. They problem solve and adapt their functioning to the situation. For example, when a mother of a family of five had to undergo chemotherapy, the family formulated a plan together to divide the responsibilities previously managed by the mother.

When a client or family is experiencing chronic, multiple adverse situations or a new crisis, refer to *Risk for Ineffective Coping*. In situations involving the loss of family member, significant other, or friend, refer to *Grieving* for Goals, and Interventions.

IMPAIRED INDIVIDUAL RESILIENCE

NANDA-I Definition

Decreased ability to sustain a pattern of positive responses to an adverse situation or crisis

Defining Characteristics*

Decreased interest in academic activities
Decreased interest in vocational activities
Depression, guilt, shame

Isolation
Low self-esteem
Lower perceived health status
Renewed elevation of distress

Social isolation
Using maladaptive coping skills
    (e.g., drug use, violence)

Related Factors*

Demographics that increase
    chance of maladjustment
Drug use
Inconsistent parenting
Low intelligence
Low maternal education
Large family size
Minority status

Parental mental illness
Poor impulse control
Poverty, violence
Psychological disorders
Vulnerability factors that
    encompass indices that
    exacerbate the negative
    effects of the risk condition

Author's Note

This NANDA-I diagnosis does not represent a nursing diagnosis. The defining characteristics are not defining resilience but in fact a variety of coping problems or mental disorders. Most of the related factors are prejudicial, pejorative, and cannot be changed by interventions. One related factor listed—poor impulse control—is a sign/symptom of hyperactivity disorders and some mental disorders. Resilience is a strength that can be taught to and nurtured in children. Resilient individuals and families can cope in adverse situations and crises. They problem solve and adapt their functioning to the situation. For example, when a mother of a family of five had to undergo chemotherapy, the family formulated a plan together to divide the responsibilities previously managed by the mother. When an individual or family has inadequate resilience, they are at risk for ineffective coping. Refer to *Ineffective Coping, Compromised or Disabled Family Coping* for Goals, and Interventions.

RISK FOR INEFFECTIVE RESPIRATORY FUNCTION**

Risk for Ineffective Respiratory Function

Dysfunctional Ventilatory Weaning Response

Risk for Dysfunctional Ventilatory Weaning Response

** This diagnosis is not currently on the NANDA list but has been included for clarity or usefulness.

Ineffective Airway Clearance

Ineffective Breathing Pattern

Impaired Gas Exchange

Impaired Spontaneous Ventilation

Definition

At risk for experiencing a threat to the passage of air through the respiratory tract and/or to the exchange of gases (O_2–CO_2) between the lungs and the vascular system

Risk Factors

Presence of risk factors that can change respiratory function (see Related Factors).

Related Factors

Pathophysiologic

Related to excessive or thick secretions secondary to:

Infection	Cardiac or pulmonary disease
Inflammation	Smoking
Allergy	Exposure to noxious chemical

Related to immobility, stasis of secretions, and ineffective cough secondary to:

Diseases of the nervous system (e.g., Guillain –Barré syndrome, multiple sclerosis, myasthenia gravis)

Central nervous system (CNS) depression/head trauma

Cerebrovascular accident (stroke)

Quadriplegia

Treatment Related

Related to immobility secondary to:

Sedating or paralytic effects of medications, drugs, or chemicals (specify)

Anesthesia, general or spinal

Related to suppressed cough reflex secondary to (specify)

Related to effects of tracheostomy (altered secretions)

Situational (Personal, Environmental)

Related to immobility secondary to:

Surgery or trauma	Fear
Fatigue	Anxiety
Pain	
Perception/cognitive impairment	

Related to extremely high or low humidity

For infants, related to placement on stomach for sleep

Exposure to cold, laughing, crying, allergens, smoke

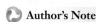 **Author's Note**

Nurses' many responsibilities associated with problems of respiratory function include identifying and reducing or eliminating risk (contributing) factors, anticipating potential complications, monitoring respiratory status, and managing acute respiratory dysfunction.

The author has added *Risk for Ineffective Respiratory Function* to describe a state that may affect the entire respiratory system, not just isolated areas, such as airway clearance or gas exchange. Allergy and immobility are examples of factors that affect the entire system; thus, it is incorrect to say *Impaired Gas Exchange* related to immobility, because immobility also affects airway clearance and breathing patterns. The nurse can use the diagnoses *Ineffective Airway Clearance* and *Ineffective Breathing Patterns* when nurses can definitely alleviate the contributing factors influencing respiratory function (e.g., ineffective cough, stress).

The nurse is cautioned not to use this diagnosis to describe acute respiratory disorders, which are the primary responsibility of medicine and nursing together (i.e., collaborative problems). Such problems can be labeled *RC of Acute Hypoxia* or *RC of Pulmonary Edema*. When a client's immobility is prolonged and threatens multiple systems—for example, integumentary, musculoskeletal, vascular, as well as respiratory—the nurse should use *Disuse Syndrome* to describe the entire situation.

NOC

Aspiration Control, Respiratory Status

Goal

The client will have a respiratory rate within normal limits compared with baseline, as evidenced by the following indicators:

- Express willingness to be actively involved in managing respiratory symptoms and maximizing respiratory function.
- Relate appropriate interventions to maximize respiratory status (varies depending on health status).
- Have satisfactory pulmonary function, as measured by PFTs.

Airway Management, Cough Enhancement, Respiratory Monitoring, Positioning

Interventions

Determine Causative Factors

Refer to Related Factors.

Eliminate or Reduce Causative Factors, If Possible

- Encourage ambulation as soon as consistent with the medical plan of care.
- If the client cannot walk, establish a regimen for being out of bed in a chair several times a day (e.g., 1 hour after meals and 1 hour before bedtime).
- Increase activity gradually. Explain that respiratory function will improve and dyspnea will decrease with practice.
- For neuromuscular impairment:
  - Vary the position of the bed, thereby gradually changing the horizontal and vertical position of the thorax, unless contraindicated.
  - Assist the client to reposition, turning frequently from side to side (hourly if possible).
  - In the hospital, especially if the client is on a ventilator, use beds with continuous lateral rotation (when available) (Swadener-Culpepper, 2010).
  - Encourage deep breathing and controlled coughing exercises five times every hour.
  - Teach the client to use a blow bottle or incentive spirometer every hour while awake. (With severe neuromuscular impairment, the client may have to be wakened during the night as well.)
  - For clients with quadriplegia, teach client and caregivers the "quad cough." (Caregiver places a hand on the client's diaphragm and thrusts upward and inward.)
  - For a child, use colored water in a blow bottle; have him or her blow up balloons.
  - Ensure optimal hydration status and nutritional intake.
- For the client with a decreased level of consciousness:
  - Position the client from side to side with a set schedule (e.g., left side on even hours, right side on odd hours); do not leave the client lying flat on his or her back.
  - Position the client on the right side after feedings (nasogastric tube feeding, gastrostomy) to prevent regurgitation and aspiration.

- Keep the head of the bed elevated 30 degrees unless contraindicated (Institute for Healthcare Improvement, 2008).
- See also *Risk for Aspiration*.

Prevent the Complications of Immobility

See *Disuse Syndrome*.

Dysfunctional Ventilatory Weaning Response

NANDA-I Definition

Inability to adjust to lowered levels of mechanical ventilator support that interrupts and prolongs the weaning process

Defining Characteristics

Dysfunctional ventilatory weaning response (DVWR) is a progressive state, and experienced nurses have identified three levels (Logan & Jenny, 1990): mild, moderate, and severe. The defining characteristics occur in response to weaning.

Mild

Restlessness
Slight increase of respiratory rate from baseline
Expressed feelings of increased oxygen need, breathing discomfort, fatigue, and warmth
Queries about possible machine dysfunction
Increased concentration on breathing

Moderate

Slight increase from baseline blood pressure (<20 mm Hg)*
Slight increase from baseline in heart rate (<20 beats/minute)*
Increase from baseline in respiratory rate (<5 breaths/minute)
Hypervigilance to activities
Inability to respond to coaching
Inability to cooperate
Apprehension
Diaphoresis
Wide-eyed look
Decreased air entry heard on auscultation
Color changes: pale, slight cyanosis
Slight respiratory accessory muscle use

Severe

Agitation*
Deterioration in arterial blood gases from current baseline
Increase from baseline blood pressure (≥20 mm Hg)
Increase from baseline heart rate (≥ 20 beats/min)
Shallow breaths
Cyanosis
Gasping breaths
Paradoxical abdominal breathing
Adventitious breath sounds
Full respiratory accessory muscle use
Profuse diaphoresis
Asynchronized breathing with the ventilator
Decreased level of consciousness
Paradoxical abdominal breathing

Related Factors

Pathophysiologic

Related to muscle weakness and fatigue secondary to:

Unstable hemodynamic status
Decreased level of
  consciousness
Chronic neuromuscular
  disability
Metabolic/acid–base
Abnormality
Severe disease process

Chronic respiratory disease
Multisystem disease
Fluid/electrolyte imbalance
Anemia
Infection
Chronic nutritional deficit
Debilitated condition
Pain

*Related to ineffective airway clearance**

Treatment Related

Related to obstructed airway

Related to muscle weakness and fatigue secondary to:

Excess sedation, analgesia   Uncontrolled pain

*Related to inadequate nutrition (deficit in calories, excess carbohydrates, inadequate fats and protein intake)**

Related to prolonged ventilator dependence (more than 1 week)

Related to previously unsuccessful ventilator weaning attempt(s)

Related to too-rapid pacing of the weaning process

Situational (Personal, Environmental)

*Related to insufficient knowledge of the weaning process**

Related to excessive energy demands (self-care activities, diagnostic and treatment procedures, visitors)

*Related to inadequate social support**

Related to insecure environment (noisy, upsetting events, busy room)

Related to fatigue secondary to interrupted sleep patterns

Related to inadequate self-efficacy

Related to moderate to high anxiety related to breathing efforts

Related to fear of separation from ventilator

*Related to feelings of powerlessness**

*Related to feelings of hopelessness**

 Author's Note

Dysfunctional Ventilatory Weaning Response is a specific diagnosis within the category of *Risk for Ineffective Respiratory Function. Ineffective Airway Clearance, Ineffective Breathing Patterns,* and *Impaired Gas Exchange* can also be encountered during weaning, either as indicators of lack of weaning readiness or as factors related to the onset of DVWR. DVWR is a separate client state. Its distinctive etiologies and treatments arise from the process of separating the client from the mechanical ventilator.

The process of weaning is an art and a science. Because weaning is a collaborative process, the nurse's ability to gain the client's trust and willingness to work is an important determinant of the weaning outcomes, especially with long-term clients. This trust is fostered by the knowledge and self-confidence nurses display and by their ability to deal with clients' specific concerns (Jenny & Logan, 1991).

NOC

Anxiety Control, Respiratory Status, Vital Signs Status, Knowledge: Weaning, Energy Conservation

Goal

The client will achieve progressive weaning goals, as evidenced by the following indicators:

- Spontaneous breathing for 24 hours without ventilatory support.

- Demonstrate a positive attitude toward the next weaning trial.
  - Collaborate willingly with the weaning plan.
  - Communicate comfort status during the weaning process.
  - Attempt to control the breathing pattern.
  - Try to control emotional responses.
- Be tired from the work of weaning, but not exhausted.

Anxiety Reduction, Preparatory Sensory Information, Respiratory Monitoring, Ventilation Assistance, Presence, Endurance

Interventions

If Applicable, Assess Causative Factors for Previous Unsuccessful Weaning Attempts

Refer to Related Factors.

Determine Readiness for Weaning (Morton et al., 2005)

- Respiratory rate less than 35 breaths per minute (but over-breathes the respiratory rate currently set on the ventilator)
- Oxygen concentration of 40% or less on the ventilator
- Negative inspiratory pressure less than -20 to -30 cm H_2O
- Positive expiratory pressure greater than -15 to -30 cm H_2O
- Spontaneous tidal volume 4 to 5 mL/kg
- Vital capacity greater than 10 to 15 mL/kg
- Rested, controlled discomfort
- Willingness to try weaning
- Absence of fever
- Normal hemoglobin levels

If Readiness for Weaning Is Present, Engage the Client in Establishing the Plan

- Explain the weaning process.
- Negotiate progressive weaning goals.
- Create a visual display of goals that uses symbols to indicate progression (e.g., bar or line graph to indicate increasing time off ventilator).
- Explain that these goals will be re-examined daily with the client.
- Refer to unit protocols for specific weaning procedures.

Explain the Client's Role in the Weaning Process

- From initial intubation, promote the understanding that mechanical ventilation is temporary.
- Share nurses' expectations of their collaborative work role when the client is judged ready to wean.

- Help the client to understand the importance of communicating comfort status and trying to reach the current weaning goals, and that rest will be allowed throughout the process.

Strengthen Feelings of Self-Esteem, Self-Efficacy, and Control

- Reinforce self-esteem, confidence, and control through normalizing strategies such as grooming, dressing, mobilizing, and conversing socially about things of interest to the client.
- Permit as much control as possible by informing the client of the situation and his or her progress, permitting shared decision-making about details of care, following the client's preferences as far as possible, and improving comfort status.
- Increase confidence by praising successful activities, encouraging a positive outlook, and reviewing positive progress to date. Explain that people usually succeed in weaning; reassure the client that you will be with him or her every step of the way.
- Demonstrate confidence in the client's ability to wean.
- Maintain the client's confidence by adopting a weaning pace that ensures success and minimizes setbacks.**
- Explain what you are doing and why to reduce the client's vigilance and feelings of uncertainty.
- Note concerns that hinder comfort and confidence (family members, topics of conversation, room events, previous weaning failures); discuss them openly and reduce them, if possible.

Reduce Negative Effects of Anxiety and Fatigue

- Monitor status frequently to avoid undue fatigue and anxiety. Use a systematic, comprehensive tool. A pulse oximeter is a noninvasive and unobtrusive way to monitor oxygen saturation levels.
- Provide regular periods of rest before fatigue advances.
  - Reduce activities.
  - Maintain or increase ventilator support and/or oxygen in consultation with a physician.
- During a rest period, dim lights, post "do not disturb" signs, and play instrumental music with 60 to 80 beats per minute. Allow the client to select type of music (Chan, 1998).
- Encourage calmness and breath control by reassuring the client that he or she can and will succeed.
- Consider use of alternative therapies such as music, hypnosis, and biofeedback.

** May require a primary professional's order.

- If the client is becoming agitated, calm him or her down while remaining at the bedside, and coach him or her to regain breathing control. Monitor oxygen saturation and vital signs closely during this intervention.
- If the weaning trial is discontinued, address the client's perceptions of weaning failure. Reassure the client that the trial was a good exercise and a useful form of training. Remind the client that the work is good for the respiratory muscles and will improve future performance.

Create a Positive Weaning Environment That Increases Feelings of Security

- Provide a room with a quiet atmosphere, low activity, soft music, and no chatter within the client's hearing.
- Delegate the most skilled staff to wean clients who have experienced moderate to severe responses or who are at high risk for doing so.
- Remain visible in the room to reinforce feelings of safety.
- Reassure the client that help is immediately available, if needed.
- Monitor visitors' effects on the client; help visitors understand how they can best assist.
- Encourage supportive visitors when possible during the weaning process. Visits from people who upset the client should be postponed.
- Ensure that clients are included in discussions that they are likely to overhear.

Promote Optimal Energy Resources

- Assist client to cough and deep-breathe regularly and use prescribed bronchodilators, humidification, and suctioning to improve air entry.
- Ensure that nutritional support falls within current guidelines for ventilated and weaning clients.
- Provide sufficient rest periods to prevent undue fatigue.
- Use ventilator support at night if necessary to increase sleep time, and try to avoid unnecessary awakening.
- Monitor the disease processes to determine the body systems' stability.

Control Activity Demands

- Coordinate necessary activities to promote adequate time for rest or relaxation.
- Ensure that all staff follow the individualized care plan.
- Coach the client in breath control by regular demonstrations of slow, deep, rhythmic patterns of breathing. Help the client to synchronize breathing with the ventilator.

- If the client's concentration creates tension and increases anxiety, provide distraction in the form of supportive visitors, radio, television, or conversation.

Follow the Institution's Multidiscipline Weaning Protocol (If Available)

- Document the specifics of the plan with a timetable.
- Establish predetermined criteria for terminating the weaning process.
- Outline each discipline's responsibilities.
- Review goals and progress at each shift. Document response.
- Collaborate if revisions are needed.

Risk for Dysfunctional Ventilatory Weaning Response

NANDA-I Definition

Inability to adjust to lowered levels of mechanical ventilator support during the weaning process, related to physical and/or psychological unreadiness to wean

Risk Factors

Pathophysiologic

Related to airway obstruction

Related to muscle weakness and fatigue secondary to:

Impaired respiratory functioning	Anemia
Metabolic abnormalities	Severe disease
Dysrhythmia	Unstable hemodynamic status
Fluid and/or electrolyte	Acid–base abnormalities
Decreased level of consciousness	Mental confusion
Fever	Infection
	Multisystem disease

Treatment Related

Related to ineffective airway clearance

Related to excess sedation, analgesia

Related to uncontrolled pain

Related to fatigue

Related to inadequate nutrition (deficit in calories, excess carbohydrates, inadequate fat and protein intake)

Related to prolonged ventilator dependence (more than 1 week)

Related to previous unsuccessful ventilator weaning attempt(s)

Related to too-rapid pacing of the weaning process

Situational (Personal, Environmental)

Related to muscle weakness and fatigue secondary to:
Chronic nutritional deficit   Ineffective sleep patterns
Obesity

Related to knowledge deficit related to the weaning process

Related to inadequate self-efficacy related to weaning

Related to moderate to high anxiety related to breathing efforts

Related to fear of separation from ventilator

Related to feelings of powerlessness

Related to depressed mood

Related to feelings of hopelessness

Related to uncontrolled energy demands (self-care activities, diagnostic and treatment procedures, visitors)

Related to inadequate social support

Related to insecure environment (noisy, upsetting events, busy room)

 Author's Note

See *Dysfunctional Ventilatory Weaning Response*.

NOC

Refer to *Dysfunctional Ventilatory Weaning Response*

Goals

The client will:

- Demonstrate a willingness to start weaning.
- Demonstrate a positive attitude about ability to succeed.
  - Maintain emotional control.
  - Collaborate with planning of the weaning.

NIC
Refer to *Dysfunctional Ventilatory Weaning Response.*

Interventions

Refer to *Dysfunctional Ventilatory Weaning Response.*

Ineffective Airway Clearance

NANDA-I Definition

State in which a client experiences inability to clear secretions or obstructions from the respiratory tract to maintain a clear airway

Defining Characteristics

Major (Must Be Present, One or More)

Ineffective or absent cough
Inability to remove airway secretions

Minor (May Be Present)

Abnormal breath sounds
Abnormal respiratory rate,
   rhythm, and depth

Related Factors
See *Risk for Ineffective
   Respiratory Function.*

NOC
Aspiration Control, Respiratory Status

Goal

The client will not experience aspiration, as evidenced by the following indicator:

• Demonstrate effective coughing.
• Demonstrate increased air exchange.

NIC
Cough Enhancement, Airway Suctioning, Positioning, Energy Management

Interventions

The nursing interventions for the diagnosis *Ineffective Airway Clearance* represent interventions for any client with this nursing diagnosis, regardless of the related factors.

Assess for Causative or Contributing Factors

Refer to Related Factors.

Assess and Evaluate

- Sputum (color, volume, odor).
- Respiratory status before and after coughing exercises (breath sounds, rate, rhythm).
- Provide oral care with a toothbrush at least every 4 hours.
- Use chlorhexidine gluconate rinse at least once per shift as prescribed.

Reduce or Eliminate Barriers to Airway Clearance

Inability to Maintain Proper Position
- Assist with positioning frequently; monitor for *Risk for Aspiration* (see *High Risk for Aspiration*).

Ineffective Cough
- Instruct the client on the proper method of controlled coughing.
  - Breathe deeply and slowly while sitting up as high as possible.
  - Use diaphragmatic breathing.
  - Hold the breath for 3 to 5 seconds, then slowly exhale as much of this breath as possible through the mouth (lower rib cage and abdomen should sink down).
  - Take a second breath; hold, slowly exhale, and cough forcefully from the chest (not from the back of the mouth or throat), using two short, forceful coughs.
  - Increase fluid intake if not contraindicated.

Pain or Fear of Pain Related to Surgery or Trauma
- Assess present analgesic regimen.
  - Administer pain medications as needed.
  - Coordinate analgesic doses with coughing sessions (e.g., give doses 30 to 60 minutes before coughing sessions).
  - Assess medication's effectiveness: Is the client too lethargic? Is he or she still in pain?
  - Note time when the client seems to have the best pain relief with optimal level of alertness and physical performance. This is the time for active breathing and coughing exercises.
- Provide emotional support.
  - Explain the importance of coughing after pain relief.
  - Reassure that suture lines are secure and that splinting by hand or pillow will minimize pain of movement.

- Use appropriate comfort measures for the site of pain.
  - Splint abdominal or chest incisions with hand, pillow, or both.
- For sore throat:
  - Provide humidity unless contraindicated.
  - Consider a warm saline gargle every 2 to 4 hours.
  - Consider use of an anesthetic lozenge or gargle, especially before coughing sessions.
  - Examine the throat for exudate, redness, and swelling; note if it is associated with fever.
  - Explain that a sore throat is common after anesthesia and should be a short-term problem.
- Maintain good body alignment to prevent muscular pain and strain.
  - Acquire and use extra pillows on both sides, especially the affected side, for support.
  - Position the client to prevent slouching and cramping positions of the thorax and abdomen; reassess positioning frequently.
- Assess understanding of the use of analgesia to enhance breathing and coughing effort.
  - Teach during periods of optimal level of consciousness.
  - Continually reinforce the rationale for the plan of nursing care. ("I will be back to help you cough when the pain medicine is working and you can be most effective.")

Viscous (Thick) Secretions
- Maintain adequate hydration (increase fluid intake to 2 to 3 quarts a day if not contraindicated by decreased cardiac output or renal insufficiency).
- Maintain adequate humidity of inspired air.

Fatigue, Weakness, and Drowsiness
- Plan and bargain for rest periods. ("Work to cough well now; then I can let you rest.")
- Vigorously coach and encourage coughing, using positive reinforcement. ("You worked hard; I know it's not easy, but it is important.")
- Be sure the coughing session occurs at the peak comfort period after analgesics, but not peak level of sleepiness.
- Allow for rest after coughing and before meals.
- For lethargy or decreased level of consciousness, stimulate the client to breathe deeply hourly. ("Take a deep breath.")

For Chronic, Unrelieved Coughing:
- Minimize irritants in the inspired air (e.g., dust, allergens).
- Provide periods of uninterrupted rest.
- Administer prescribed medications—cough suppressant, expectorant—as ordered by the physician/nurse practitioner (withhold food and drink immediately after administration of medications for best results).

Provide Health Teaching and Referrals, as Indicated

- Teach the client and family:
  - Hydration requirements
  - Mouth care
  - Effective coughing techniques
  - Signs of infection (change in sputum color, fever)
- Refer to home health nursing if needed.

Pediatric Interventions

- Instruct parents on the need for the child to cough, even if it is painful.
- Allow an adult and older child to listen to the lungs and describe if clear or if rales are present.
- Consult with a respiratory therapist for assistance, if needed.

Ineffective Breathing Pattern

NANDA-I Definition

Inspiration and/or expiration that does not provide adequate ventilation

Defining Characteristics*

Bradycardia	Dyspnea
Decreased expiratory pressure	Tachypnea, hyperpnea, hyperventilation
Decreased inspiratory pressure	
Alterations in depth of breathing	Increased anterior-posterior diameter
Orthopnea	Prolonged expiration phase
Dysrhythmic respirations	Use of accessory muscles to breathe
Altered chest excursion	
Assumption of three-point position	Splinted/guarded respirations
	Nasal flaring
Decreased minute ventilation	Pursed-lip breathing

Related Factors

See *Risk for Ineffective Respiratory Function*.

Author's Note

This diagnosis has limited clinical utility except to describe situations that nurses definitively treat, such as hyperventilation. For individuals with chronic pulmonary disease with *Ineffective Breathing Patterns,* refer to *Activity Intolerance.* Individuals with periodic apnea and hypoventilation have a collaborative problem that can be labeled *Risk for Complications of Hypoxemia* to indicate that they are to be monitored for various respiratory dysfunctions. If the person is more vulnerable to a specific respiratory complication, the nurse can write the collaborative problem as *Risk for Complications of Pneumonia* or *Risk for Complications of Pulmonary Embolism.* Hyperventilation is a manifestation of anxiety or fear. The nurse can use *Anxiety* or *Fear related to (specify event) as manifested by hyperventilation* as a more descriptive diagnosis.

 NOC

Respiratory Status, Vital Signs Status, Anxiety Control

Goals

The client will achieve improved respiratory function as evidenced by the following indicators:

- Demonstrate respiratory rate within normal limits, compared with baseline (8 to 24 breaths per minute).
- Express relief of or improvement in feelings of shortness of breath.
- Relate causative factors and ways of preventing or managing them.

NIC

Respiratory Monitoring, Progressive Muscle Relaxation, Teaching, Anxiety Reduction

Interventions

Assess History of Symptoms and Causative Factors

- Previous episodes—when, where, circumstances
- Causes:
  - Organic and physiologic
  - Emotional
- Faulty breathing habits

Remove or Control Causative Factors

- Explain the cause.
- Stay with the client.
- If fear or panic has precipitated the episode:
  - Remove the cause of the fear, if possible.
  - Reassure the client that measures are being taken to ensure safety.
  - Distract the client from thinking about the anxious state by having him or her maintain eye contact with you (or perhaps with someone else he or she trusts); say, "Now look at me and breathe slowly with me, like this."
  - Consider use of a paper bag as means of rebreathing expired air (expired CO_2 will be reinspired, thereby slowing respiratory rate).
  - Refer to *Fear*.
- Reassure the client that he or she can control breathing; tell him or her that you will help.
- Teach controlled breathing techniques (e.g., pursed-lip breathing) or consult with a respiratory therapist for training to overcome faulty breathing patterns.

Pediatric Interventions

- If child is prone to bronchospasm, medication may be indicated.

Impaired Gas Exchange

NANDA-I Definition

Excess or deficit in oxygenation and/or carbon dioxide elimination at the alveolar-capillary membrane

Defining Characteristics*

Abnormal arterial blood gases	Dyspnea
Abnormal arterial pH	Headache upon awakening
Abnormal breathing (e.g., rate, rhythm, depth)	Hypercapnia
	Hypoxemia
Abnormal skin color (e.g., pale, dusky)	Hypoxia
	Irritability
Confusion	Nasal flaring
Cyanosis (in neonates only)	Somnolence
Decreased carbon dioxide	Tachycardia
Diaphoresis	Visual disturbances

Related Factors

See Related Factors for *Risk for Ineffective Respiratory Function.*

 Author's Note

This diagnosis does not represent a situation for which nurses prescribe definitive treatment. Nurses do not treat *Impaired Gas Exchange,* but nurses can treat the functional health patterns that decreased oxygenation can affect, such as activity, sleep, nutrition, and sexual function. Thus, *Activity Intolerance related to insufficient oxygenation for activities of daily living* better describes the nursing focus. If an individual is at risk for or has experienced respiratory dysfunction, the nurse can describe the situation as *Risk for Complications of Ineffective Respiratory Function* or be even more specific with *Risk for Complications of Pulmonary Embolism.*

Impaired Spontaneous Ventilation

NANDA-I Definition

Decreased energy reserves resulting in an inability to maintain independent breathing that is adequate to support life

Defining Characteristics*

Major

Dyspnea   Increased metabolic rate

Minor

Increased restlessness   Increased PCO_2
Increased heart rate   Decreased tidal volume
Reports apprehension   Decreased cooperation
Decreased PO_2 Decreased SaO_2
Increased use of accessory
    muscles

 Author's Note

This diagnosis represents respiratory insufficiency with corresponding metabolic changes that are incompatible with life. This situation requires rapid nursing and medical management, specifically resuscitation and mechanical ventilation. *Inability to Sustain Spontaneous Ventilation* is not

appropriate as a nursing diagnosis; it is hypoxemia, a collaborative problem. *Hypoxemia* is insufficient plasma oxygen saturation from alveolar hypoventilation, pulmonary shunting, or ventilation-perfusion inequality. As a collaborative problem, physicians prescribe the definitive treatments; however, both nursing- and medical-prescribed interventions are required for management. The nursing accountability is to monitor status continuously and to manage changes in status with the appropriate interventions using protocols. For interventions, refer to *Risk for Complications of Hypoxemia* in Section 3 in Carpenito, L. J. (2013). *Nursing diagnosis: Application to clinical practice* [14th ed.]. Philadelphia: Lippincott Williams & Wilkins.

INEFFECTIVE ROLE PERFORMANCE

NANDA-I Definition

Patterns of behavior and self-expression that do not match environmental context, norms, and expectations

Defining Characteristics*

Altered role perceptions
    Anxiety
Inadequate adaptation to change
Role ambivalence

Role conflict, confusion, denial,
    dissatisfaction
Uncertainty
Role strain

Related Factors

Knowledge

Unrealistic role expectations
Inadequate role preparation
    (e.g., role transition, skill,
    rehearsal, validation)

Lack of education
Lack of role model

Physiologic

Body image alteration
Low self-esteem
Neurologic defects

Social

Conflict
Inadequate support system
Inappropriate linkage with
    the health care system
Job schedule demands
Young age
Cognitive deficits
Depression, mental illness

Pain
Developmental level
Domestic violence
Inadequate role socialization
Lack of resources
Lack of rewards
Low socioeconomic status
Stress

Author's Note

The nursing diagnosis *Ineffective Role Performance* has a defining characteristic of "conflict related to role perception or performance." All
people have multiple roles. Some are prescribed, such as gender and
age; some are acquired, such as parent and occupation; and some are
transitional, such as elected office or team member.

Various factors affect a client's role, including developmental stage,
societal norms, cultural beliefs, values, life events, illness, and disabilities. When a client has difficulty with role performance, it may be more
useful to describe the effect of the difficulty on functioning, rather than
to describe the problem as *Ineffective Role Performance*. For example,
a client who has experienced a cerebrovascular accident (CVA) may
undergo a change from being the primary breadwinner to becoming
unemployed. In this situation, the nursing diagnosis *Interrupted Family
Processes and/or Fear* related to loss of role as financial provider secondary to effects of CVA would be appropriate. In another example, if a
woman could not continue her household responsibilities because of
illness and other family members assumed these responsibilities, the
situations that may arise would better be described as *Risk for Disturbed
Self-Concept* related to recent loss of role responsibility secondary to
illness and *Risk for Impaired Home Maintenance Management* related to
lack of knowledge of family members.

A conflict in a family regarding others meeting role obligations or
expectations can represent related factors for the diagnosis *Ineffective
Family Processes* related to conflict regarding expectations of members
meeting role obligations.

Until clinical research defines this diagnosis and the associated nursing interventions, use *Ineffective Role Performance* as a related factor
for another nursing diagnosis (e.g., *Anxiety*, *Grieving*, *Stress Overload*,
or *Disturbed Self-Concept*).

SELF-CARE DEFICIT SYNDROME

Self-Care Deficit Syndrome**

Feeding Self-Care Deficit

Bathing Self-Care Deficit

Dressing Self-Care Deficit

Instrumental Self-Care Deficit**

Toileting Self-Care Deficit

Definition†

State in which a client experiences an impaired motor function or cognitive function, causing a decreased ability in performing each of the five self-care activities

Defining Characteristics

Major (One Deficit Must Be Present in Each Activity)

Feeding Self-Care Deficit
Inability (or unwilling) to†:
   Bring food from a receptacle to the mouth
   Complete a meal
   Place food onto utensils
   Handle utensils
   Ingest food in a socially acceptable manner
   Open containers
   Pick up cup or glass
   Prepare food for ingestion
   Use assistive device

Self-Bathing Deficits (Include Washing Entire Body, Combing Hair, Brushing Teeth, Attending to Skin and Nail Care, and Applying Makeup)†
Inability (or unwilling) to†:   Dry body
   Access bathroom   Obtain a water source
   Get bath supplies   Regulate bath water
   Wash body

** These diagnoses are not currently on the NANDA-I list but have been included by the author, for clarity or usefulness.
† This characteristic has been included by the author for clarity or usefulness.

Self-Dressing Deficits (Including Donning Regular or Special Clothing, Not Nightclothes)[†]

Inability or unwillingness to[†]:

Choose clothing or put clothing on lower body
Put clothing on upper body
Put on necessary items of clothing
Maintain appearance at a satisfactory level

Pick up clothing
Put on shoes/remove shoes
Put on/remove socks
Use assistive devices
Use zippers
Fasten, unfasten clothing
Obtain clothing

Self-Toileting Deficits

Unable or unwillingness to[†]:

Get to toilet or commode
Carry out proper hygiene
Manipulate clothing for toileting

Rise from toilet or commode
Sit on toilet or commode
Flush toilet or empty commode

Instrumental Self-Care Deficits[†]

Difficulty using telephone
Difficulty accessing transportation
Difficulty laundering, ironing
Difficulty managing money

Difficulty preparing meals
Difficulty with medication administration
Difficulty shopping

Related Factors

Pathophysiologic

Related to lack of coordination secondary to (specify)

Related to spasticity or flaccidity secondary to (specify)

Related to muscular weakness secondary to (specify)

Related to partial or total paralysis secondary to (specify)

Related to atrophy secondary to (specify)

Related to muscle contractures secondary to (specify)

Related to visual disorders secondary to (specify)

Related to nonfunctioning or missing limb(s)

Related to regression to an earlier level of development

Related to excessive ritualistic behaviors

Related to somatoform deficits (specify)

[†] This characteristic has been included by the author, for clarity or usefulness.

Treatment Related

Related to external devices (specify: casts, splints, braces, intravenous [IV] equipment)

Related to postoperative fatigue and pain

Situational (Personal, Environmental)

Related to cognitive deficits

Related to fatigue

Related to pain

Related to decreased motivation

Related to confusion

Related to disabling anxiety

Maturational

Older Adult

Related to decreased visual and motor ability, muscle weakness

---

🌀 Author's Note

Self-care encompasses the activities needed to meet daily needs, commonly known as activities of daily living (ADLs), which are learned over time and become lifelong habits. Self-care activities involve not only what is to be done (hygiene, bathing, dressing, toileting, feeding), but also how much, when, where, with whom, and how (Miller, 2009).

In every client, the threat or reality of a self-care deficit evokes panic. Many people report that they fear loss of independence more than death. A self-care deficit affects the core of self-concept and self-determination. For this reason, the nursing focus for self-care deficit should be not on providing the care measure, but on identifying adaptive techniques to allow the client the maximum degree of participation and independence possible.

The diagnosis *Total Self-Care Deficit* once was used to describe a client's inability to complete feeding, bathing, toileting, dressing, and grooming (Gordon, 1982). The intent of specifying "Total" was to describe a client with deficits in several ADLs. Unfortunately, sometimes its use invites, according to Magnan (1989, personal communication), "preconceived judgments about the state of an individual and the nursing interventions required." The client may be viewed as in a vegetative state, requiring only minimal custodial care. *Total Self-Care Deficit* has been eliminated because its language does not denote potential for growth or rehabilitation.

Currently not on the NANDA-I list, the diagnosis *Self-Care Deficit Syndrome* has been added here to describe a client with compromised ability in all five self-care activities. For this client, the nurse assesses functioning in each area and identifies the level of participation of which the client is capable. The goal is to maintain current functioning, to increase participation and independence, or both. The syndrome distinction clusters all five self-care deficits together to enable grouping of interventions when indicated, while also permitting specialized interventions for a specific deficit.

The danger of applying a *Self-Care Deficit* diagnosis lies in the possibility of prematurely labeling a client as unable to participate at any level, eliminating a rehabilitation focus. It is important that the nurse classify the client's functional level to promote independence. Use this scale with the nursing diagnosis (e.g., *Toileting Self-Care Deficit* 2 = minimal help). Continuous re-evaluation is also necessary to identify changes in the client's ability to participate in self-care.

NOC

See Bathing, Feeding, Dressing, Toileting, and/or Instrumental Self-Care Deficit

Goal

The client will participate in feeding, dressing, toileting, and bathing activities, as evidenced by the following indicators (specify what the client can perform with assistance and unassisted):

• Identify preferences in self-care activities (e.g., time, products, location).
• Demonstrate optimal hygiene after assistance with care.

NIC

See Feeding, Bathing, Dressing, Toileting, and/or Instrumental Self-Care Deficit

Interventions

Assess for Causative or Contributing Factors

Refer to Related Factors.

Use the Following Scale to Rate the Client's Ability to Perform

• 0 = Is completely independent
• 1 = Requires use of assistive device
• 2 = Needs minimal help
• 3 = Needs assistance and/or some supervision
• 4 = Needs total supervision
• 5 = Needs total assistance or unable to assist

Promote Optimal Participation

• Consult with a physical therapist to assess present level of participation and for a plan.
  • Determine areas for potentially increased participation in each self-care activity.
  • Explore the client's goals and determine what the client perceives as his or her own needs.
  • Compare what the nurse believes are the client's needs and goals, and then work to establish mutually acceptable goals.
  • Allow the client ample time to complete activities without help. Promote independence, but assist when the client cannot perform an activity.

Promote Self-Esteem and Self-Determination

• Determine preferences for:
  • Schedule
  • Products
  • Methods
  • Clothing selection
  • Hair styling
• During self-care activities, provide choices and request preferences.
• Do not focus on disability.
• Offer praise for independent accomplishments.

Evaluate the Client's Ability to Participate in Each Self-Care Activity (Feeding, Dressing, Bathing, Toileting)

• Reassess ability frequently and revise code as appropriate.

Refer to Interventions Under Each Diagnosis—Feeding, Bathing, Dressing, Toileting, and Instrumental Self-Care Deficit—as Indicated

Feeding Self-Care Deficit

NANDA-I Definition

Impaired ability to perform or complete self-feeding activities

Defining Characteristics*

Inability (or unwilling) to**:
  Bring food from a receptacle
    to the mouth
  Complete a meal
  Get food onto utensils
  Handle utensils

Ingest food in a socially
  acceptable manner
Open containers
Pick up cup or glass
Prepare food for ingestion
Use assistive device

Related Factors

Refer to *Self-Care Deficit Syndrome*.

 Author's Note

This diagnosis is appropriate for a client who has difficulty with the activities of self-feeding. Clients who have difficulty chewing and ingesting sufficient calories need an additional diagnosis of *Imbalanced Nutrition*.

NOC

Nutritional Status, Self-Care: Eating, Swallowing Status

Goal

The client will demonstrate increased ability to feed self or report that he or she needs assistance, as evidenced by the following indicators:

- Demonstrate ability to make use of adaptive devices, if indicated.
- Demonstrate increased interest and desire to eat.
- Describe rationale and procedure for treatment.
- Describe causative factors for feeding deficit.

NIC

Feeding, Self-Care Assistance: Feeding, Swallowing Therapy, Teaching, Aspiration Precautions

Interventions

Assess Causative Factors

Refer to Related Factors.

** These characteristics have been added by the author for clarity and usefulness.

Use the Following Scale to Rate the Client's Ability to Perform

- 0 = Is completely independent
- 1 = Requires use of assistive device
- 2 = Needs minimal help
- 3 = Needs assistance and/or some supervision
- 4 = Needs total supervision
- 5 = Needs total assistance or unable to assist

Provide Opportunities to Relearn or Adapt to Activity

Common Nursing Interventions for Feeding
- Ascertain from the client or the family members what foods the client likes or dislikes.
- Ensure the client eats meals in the same setting with pleasant surroundings that are not too distracting.
- Maintain correct food temperatures (hot foods hot, cold foods cold).
- Provide pain relief because pain can affect appetite and ability to feed self.
- Provide good oral hygiene before and after meals.
- Encourage the client to wear dentures and eyeglasses.
- Assist the client to the most normal eating position suited to his or her physical disability (best is sitting in a chair at a table).
- Provide social contact during eating.

Specific Interventions for People With Sensory/Perceptual Deficits
- Encourage the client to wear prescribed corrective lenses.
- Describe the location of utensils and food on the tray or table.
- Describe food items to stimulate appetite.
- For perceptual deficits, choose different colored dishes to help distinguish items (e.g., red tray, white plates).
- Ascertain usual eating patterns and provide food items according to preference (or arrange food items in clock-like pattern); record on the care plan the arrangement used (e.g., meat, 6 o'clock; potatoes, 9 o'clock; vegetables, 12 o'clock).
- Encourage eating of "finger foods" (e.g., bread, bacon, fruit, hot dogs) to promote independence.
- Avoid placing food to the blind side of the client with field cut until visually accommodated to surroundings; then encourage him or her to scan the entire visual field.

Specific Interventions for People With Missing Limbs
- Provide an eating environment that is not embarrassing to the client; allow sufficient time for eating.
- Provide only the supervision and assistance necessary for relearning or adaptation.

- To enhance independence, provide necessary adaptive devices:
  - Plate guard to avoid pushing food off the plate
  - Suction device under the plate or bowl for stabilization
  - Padded handles on utensils for a more secure grip
  - Wrist or hand splints with clamp to hold eating utensils
  - Special drinking cup
  - Rocker knife for cutting
- Assist with setup if needed, opening containers, napkins, condiment packages; cutting meat; and buttering bread.
- Arrange food so client has enough space to perform the task of eating.

Specific Interventions for People With Cognitive Deficits

- Provide an isolated, quiet atmosphere until the client can attend to eating and is not easily distracted from the task.
- Supervise the feeding program until there is no danger of choking or aspiration.
- Orient the client to location and purpose of feeding equipment.
- Avoid external distractions and unnecessary conversation.
- Place the client in the most normal eating position he or she can physically assume.
- Encourage the client to attend to the task, but be alert for fatigue, frustration, or agitation.
- Provide one food at a time in usual sequence of eating until the client can eat the entire meal in normal sequence.
- Encourage the client to be tidy, to eat in small amounts, and to put food in the unaffected side of the mouth if paresis or paralysis is present.
- Check for food in cheeks.
- Refer to *Impaired Swallowing* for additional interventions.

Initiate Health Teaching and Referrals, as Indicated

- Ensure that both client and family understand the reason and purpose of all interventions.
- Proceed with teaching as needed.
  - Maintain safe eating methods.
  - Prevent aspiration.
  - Use appropriate eating utensils (avoid sharp instruments).
  - Test the temperature of hot liquids and wear protective clothing (e.g., paper bib).
  - Teach the use of adaptive devices.

Bathing Self-Care Deficit

NANDA-I Definition

Impaired ability to perform or complete bathing activities for self

Defining Characteristics*

Self-bathing deficits (including washing the entire body, combing hair, brushing teeth, attending to skin and nail care, and applying makeup).**

Inability (or unwilling) to**:

Access bathroom	Wash and/or dry body
Get bath supplies	Obtain a water source
	Regulate bath water

Related Factors

Refer to *Self-Care Deficit Syndrome*.

 Author's Note

Refer to *Self-Care Deficit Syndrome*.

NOC

Self-Care: Activities of Daily Living, Self-Care: Bathing

Goal

The client will perform bathing activities at expected optimal level or report satisfaction with accomplishments despite limitations, as evidenced by the following indicators:

• Relate a feeling of comfort and satisfaction with body cleanliness.
• Demonstrate the ability to use adaptive devices.
• Describe causative factors of the bathing deficit.

NIC

Self-Care Assistance: Bathing Teaching: Individual

** These characteristics have been added by the author for clarity and usefulness.

Interventions

Assess Causative Factors

Refer to Related Factors.

Use the Following Scale to Rate the Client's Ability to Perform

0 = Is completely independent
1 = Requires use of assistive device
2 = Needs minimal help
3 = Needs assistance and/or some supervision
4 = Needs total supervision
5 = Needs total assistance or unable to assist

Provide Opportunities to Relearn or Adapt to Activity

General Nursing Interventions for Inability to Bathe
- Bathing time and routine should be consistent to encourage optimal independence.
- Encourage the client to wear prescribed corrective lenses or hearing aid.
- Keep the bathroom temperature warm; ascertain the client's preferred water temperature.
- Provide for privacy during bathing routine.
- Elicit from the client his or her usual bathing routine.
- Keep the environment simple and uncluttered.
- Observe skin condition during bathing.
- Provide all bathing equipment within easy reach.
- Provide for safety in the bathroom (nonslip mats, grab bars).
- When the client is physically able, encourage the use of either a tub or shower stall, depending on which he or she uses at home. (The client should practice in the hospital in preparation for going home).
- Provide for adaptive equipment as needed:
  - Chair or stool in bathtub or shower
  - Long-handled sponge to reach back or lower extremities
  - Grab bars on bathroom walls where needed to assist in mobility
  - Bath board for transferring to tub chair or stool
  - Safety treads or nonskid mat on floor of bathroom, tub, and shower
  - Washing mitts with pocket for soap
  - Adapted toothbrushes
  - Shaver holders
  - Handheld shower spray

- Provide for relief of pain that may affect the client's ability to bathe self.**
- Consider use of nondetergent, no-rinse, prepackaged bathing products.

Specific Bathing Interventions for People With Visual Deficits

- Place bathing equipment in a location most suitable to the client.
- Avoid placing bathing equipment to the blind side if the client has a field cut and is not visually accommodated to surroundings.
- Keep the call bell within reach if the client is to bathe alone.
- Give the client with visual impairment the same degree of privacy and dignity as any other client.
- Announce yourself before entering or leaving the bathing area.
- Observe the client's ability to locate all bathing utensils.
- Observe the client's ability to perform mouth care, hair combing, and shaving.
- Provide place for clean clothing within easy reach.

Specific Bathing Interventions for People With Affected or Missing Limbs

- Bathe early in the morning or before bed at night to avoid unnecessary dressing and undressing.
- Encourage client to use a mirror during bathing to inspect the skin of paralyzed areas.
- Encourage the client with amputation to inspect the remaining foot or stump for good skin integrity.
- For limb amputations, bathe the stump twice a day and be sure it is dry before wrapping it or applying the prosthesis.
- Provide only the supervision or assistance necessary for relearning the use of extremity or adaptation to the handicap.
- For lack of sensation, encourage the use of the affected area in the bathing process. (A client tends to forget the existence of body parts in which there is no sensation.)

Specific Bathing Interventions for People With Cognitive Deficits

- Provide a consistent time for bathing as part of a structured program to help decrease confusion.
- Keep instructions simple and avoid distractions; orient the client to the purpose of bathing equipment and put toothpaste on the toothbrush.
- If the client cannot bathe the entire body, have him or her bathe one part until he or she does it correctly; give positive reinforcement for success.
- Supervise activity until the client can safely perform the task unassisted.
- Encourage attention to the task, but be alert for fatigue that may increase confusion.

** May require a primary care professional's order.

- Preserve dignity and decrease agitation.
- Provide verbal warning prior to doing anything (e.g., touching, spraying with water).
- Apply firm pressure to the skin when bathing; it is less likely to be misinterpreted than a gentle touch.
- Use a warm shower or bath to help a confused or agitated client to relax.
- Add lavender oil to bath water (Morris, 2002).
- Determine the best method to bathe client (e.g., towel bath, shower, tub bath).

Initiate Health Teaching and Referrals, as Indicated

- Communicate to staff and family members the client's ability and willingness to learn.
- Teach the use of adaptive devices.
- Ascertain bathing facilities at home and assist in determining if there is any need for adaptations; refer to occupational therapy or social service for help in obtaining needed home equipment.
- Teach the client to use the tub or shower stall, depending on what is used at home.
- If the client is paralyzed, instruct the client or family to demonstrate complete skin check of key areas for redness (buttocks, bony prominences).
- Teach the family to maintain a safe bathing environment.
- Inability to care for oneself produces feelings of dependency and poor self-concept. With increased ability for self-care, self-esteem increases.

Dressing Self-Care Deficit

NANDA-I Definition

Impaired ability to perform or complete dressing activities for self

Defining Characteristics

Self-dressing deficits (including donning regular or special clothing, not nightclothes)**
Inability (or unwillingness) to**:

Choose clothing	Maintain appearance
Put clothing on lower or	at a satisfactory level
upper body	Pick up clothing
	Put on/remove shoes

** These characteristics have been added by the author for clarity and usefulness.

Put on/remove socks   Fasten, unfasten clothing
Use assistive devices   Obtain clothing
Use zippers

Related Factors

Refer to *Self-Care Deficit Syndrome.*

 Author's Note

Refer to *Self-Care Deficit Syndrome.*

NOC

Self-Care: Activities of Daily Living, Self-Care: Dressing

Goal

The client will demonstrate increased ability to dress self or report the need to have someone else assist him or her to perform
the task, as evidenced by the following indicators:

- Demonstrate ability to use adaptive devices to facilitate inde-
  pendence in dressing.
- Demonstrate increased interest in wearing street clothes.
- Describe causative factors for dressing deficits.
- Relate rationale and procedures for treatments.

NIC

Self-Care Assistance: Dressing/Grooming, Teaching: Individual, Dressing

Interventions

Assess for Causative Factors

Refer to Related Factors.

Use the Following Scale to Rate the Client's Ability to Perform

- 0 = Is completely independent
- 1 = Requires use of assistive device
- 2 = Needs minimal help
- 3 = Needs assistance and/or some supervision
- 4 = Needs total supervision
- 5 = Needs total assistance or unable to assist

General Nursing Interventions for Self-Dressing

- Obtain clothing that is larger-sized and easier to put on, including clothing with elastic waistbands, wide sleeves and pant legs, dresses that open down the back for women in wheelchairs and Velcro fasteners or larger buttons.
- Encourage the client to wear prescribed corrective lenses or hearing aid.
- Promote independence in dressing through continual and unaided practice.
- Allow sufficient time for dressing and undressing because the task may be tiring, painful, or difficult.
- Plan for the client to learn and demonstrate one part of an activity before progressing further.
- Lay clothes out in the order in which the client will need them to dress.
- Provide dressing aids as necessary (some commonly used aids include dressing stick, Swedish reacher, zipper pull, button-hook, long-handled shoehorn, and shoe fasteners adapted with elastic laces).
- Encourage the client to wear ordinary or special clothing as needed.
- If needed, increase participation in dressing by medicating for pain 30 minutes before it is time to dress or undress, if indicated.**
- Provide for privacy during dressing routine.
- Provide for safety by ensuring easy access to all clothing and by ascertaining the client's performance level.

Specific Dressing Interventions for People With Visual Deficits

- Allow the client to select the most convenient location for clothing and adapt the environment to accomplish the task best (e.g., remove unnecessary barriers).
- Announce yourself before entering or leaving the dressing area.
- If the client has a field cut, avoid placing clothing to the blind side until he or she is visually accommodated to the surroundings; then encourage him or her to turn the head to scan the entire visual field.

Specific Dressing Interventions for People With Cognitive Deficits (Miller, 2009)

- Keep verbal communication simple.
  - Ask yes/no questions.
  - Use one-step requests (e.g., "put your sock on").

** May require a primary care professional's order.

- Praise after each step.
- Be specific and concise.
- Call the client by name.
- Use the same word for the same thing (e.g., "shirt").
- Dress the bottom half, and then the top half.
- Prepare an uncluttered environment.
  - Ensure good lighting.
  - Make bed; minimize visual clutter.
  - Lay clothes face down.
  - Place clothes in the order that they will be used.
  - Allow the client a choice from only two pieces.
  - Place matching clothes together on hangers.
  - Remove dirty clothes from the dressing area.
- Provide nonverbal cues.
  - Hand one clothing item at a time in correct order.
  - Place shoes beside the correct foot.
  - Use gestures to explain.
  - Point or touch the body part to be used.
  - If the client cannot complete all the steps, always allow him or her to finish the dressing step, if possible—zipper pants, buckle belt.
  - Decrease assistance gradually.

Initiate Health Teaching and Referrals, as Indicated

- Access a home health nurse for an in-home evaluation.

Instrumental Self-Care Deficit **

Definition

Impaired ability to perform certain activities or access certain services essential for managing a household

Defining Characteristics

Observed or reported difficulty with one or more of the following:

Using a telephone	Shopping (food, clothes)
Accessing transportation	Managing money
Laundering and ironing	Administering medication
Preparing meals	

** This diagnosis is not currently on the NANDA-I list but has been included by the author for clarity or usefulness.

Related Factors

Refer to *Self-Care Deficit Syndrome*.

 Author's Note

Instrumental Self-Care Deficit is not currently on the NANDA-I list but has been added here for clarity and usefulness. This diagnosis describes problems with performing certain activities or accessing certain services needed to live in the community (e.g., phone use, shopping, money management). This diagnosis is important to consider when planning client discharge and during home visits by community nurses.

NOC

Self-Care: Instrumental Activities of Daily Living (IADL)

Goal

The client or family will report satisfaction with household management, as evidenced by the following indicators:

- Demonstrate use of adaptive devices (e.g., telephone, cooking aids).
- Describe a method to ensure adherence to medication schedule.
- Report ability to make calls and answer the telephone.
- Report regular laundering by self or others.
- Report daily intake of at least two nutritious meals.
- Identify transportation options to stores, physician, house of worship, and social activities.
- Demonstrate management of simple money transactions.
- Identify people who will assist with money matters.

NIC

Teaching: Individual, Referral, Family Involvement Promotion

Interventions

Assess for Causative and Contributing Factors

Refer to Related Factors.

Use the Following Scale to Rate the Client's Ability to Perform

- 0 = Is completely independent
- 1 = Requires use of assistive device
- 2 = Needs minimal help
- 3 = Needs assistance and/or some supervision
- 4 = Needs total supervision
- 5 = Needs total assistance or unable to assist

Assist the Client in Identifying Self-Help Devices

Grooming/Dressing Aids
Refer to *Impaired Physical Mobility*.

Kitchen/Eating Aids
• Dishes with one side built up
• Built-up handles on cutlery (use plastic foam curlers)
• Bulldog clip to secure a straw in a glass
• Built-up corner of a cutlery board to hold and anchor food or pot (e.g., to butter toast, mash potatoes)
• Mounted jar opener
• Nonskid material applied under dishes (same strips used to prevent slipping in bathtub)
• Two-sided suction holder to hold dishes in place

Communication/Security
• Motion-activated lights near walkway/entrance
• Nightlight for path to the bathroom
• Light next to the bed
• Specially adapted telephones (amplified, big buttons)
• Specially adapted safety devices (bracelet alarm)

Promote Self-Care and Safety for the Client With Cognitive Deficit

Evaluate Activities That Are Achievable
• Turn on lights before dark.
• Use nightlights.
• Keep the environment simple and uncluttered.
• Use clocks and calendars as cues.
• Mark on calendar (using picture symbols) reminders for shopping, laundry, cleaning, doctor's appointments, and the like.

For Laundry, Teach the Client to:
• Separate dark and light clothes.
• Use pictures to illustrate steps for washing clothes.
• Mark cup with line to indicate amount of soap needed.
• Minimize ironing.
• Use an iron with automatic shutoff mechanism.

Evaluate the Client's Ability to Select, Procure, and Prepare Nutritious Food Daily
• Prepare a permanent shopping list with cues for essential foods and products.
• Teach the client to review the list before shopping, check items needed, and, in the store, check off items selected. (Use a pencil that can be erased to reuse list.)
• Teach the client how to shop for single-person meals (refer to *Imbalanced Nutrition* for specific techniques).

- If possible, teach the client to use a microwave to reduce the risk of heat-related injuries or accidents.

Offer Hints to Improve Adherence to Medication Schedule
- Have someone place medications in a commercial pill holder divided into 7 days.
- Take out the exact amount of pills for the day. Divide them in small cups, each labeled with time of day.
- If needed, draw a picture of the pills and the quantity on each cup.
- Teach the client to transfer the pills from cup to small plastic bag when planning to be away from home.
- Tell the client whom to call for instructions if he or she misses a dose.

Initiate Health Teaching and Referrals, as Indicated

- Discuss the importance of identifying the need for assistance.
- Discuss the possibility of bartering for services (e.g., wash the neighbor's clothes in exchange for shopping help).
- Identify a person who can provide immediate help (e.g., neighbor, friend, hotline).
- Identify sources for help with laundry, shopping, and money matters.

Determine Available Sources of Transportation (Neighbors, Relatives, Community Centers)

- Church groups or social service agency
- Refer the client to community agencies for assistance (e.g., Department of Social Services, area agency on aging, senior neighbors, public health nursing, Meals on Wheels).

Toileting Self-Care Deficit

NANDA-I Definition

Impaired ability to perform or complete toileting activities for self

Defining Characteristics*

Unable (or unwilling) to**:
  Get to toilet or commode
  Carry out proper hygiene
  Manipulate clothing for
    toileting

Rise from toilet or commode
Sit on toilet or commode
Flush toilet or empty
  commode

** These characteristics have been added by the author for clarity and usefulness.

Related Factors

Refer to *Self-Care Deficit Syndrome*.

 Author's Note

Refer to *Self-Care Deficit Syndrome*.

NOC

Self-Care: Activities of Daily Living, Self-Care: Hygiene, Self-Care: Toileting

Goal

The client will demonstrate increased ability to toilet self or report the need to have someone assist him or her to perform the task, as evidenced by the following indicators (specify when assistance is needed):

- Demonstrate the ability to use adaptive devices to facilitate toileting.
- Describe causative factors for toileting deficit.
- Relate the rationale and procedures for treatment.

NIC

Self-Care Assistance: Toileting, Self-Care Assistance: Hygiene, Teaching Individual, Mutual Goal Setting

Interventions

Assess Causative Factors

Refer to Related Factors.

Use the Following Scale to Rate the Client's Ability to Perform

- 0 = Is completely independent
- 1 = Requires use of assistive device
- 2 = Needs minimal help
- 3 = Needs assistance and/or some supervision
- 4 = Needs total supervision
- 5 = Needs total assistance or unable to assist

Common Nursing Interventions for Toileting Difficulties
- Encourage the client to wear prescribed corrective lenses or hearing aid.
- Obtain bladder and bowel history from the client or family (see *Impaired Bowel Elimination* or *Impaired Urinary Elimination*).

- Ascertain the communication system the client uses to express the need to toilet.
- Maintain a bladder and bowel record to determine toileting patterns.
- Provide adequate fluid intake and a balanced diet to promote adequate urinary output and normal bowel evacuation.
- Promote normal elimination by encouraging activity and exercise within the client's capabilities.
- Avoid development of "bowel fixation" by less frequent discussion and inquiries about bowel movements.
- Be alert to the possibility of falls when toileting the client (be prepared to ease him or her to the floor without injuring either of you).
- Achieve independence in toileting by continual and unaided practice.
- Allow sufficient time for the task of toileting to avoid fatigue. (Lack of sufficient time to toilet may cause incontinence or constipation.)
- Avoid the use of indwelling and condom catheters to expedite bladder continence (if possible).

Specific Toileting Interventions for People With Visual Deficits
- Keep the call bell easily accessible so the client can quickly obtain help to toilet; answer the call bell promptly to decrease anxiety.
- If the bedpan or urinal is necessary for toileting, be sure it is within the client's reach.
- Avoid placing toileting equipment to the blind side of a client with field cut. (When he or she is visually accommodated to surroundings, you may suggest he or she search the entire visual field for equipment.)
- Announce yourself before entering or leaving the toileting area.
- Observe the client's ability to obtain equipment or get to the toilet unassisted.
- Provide for a safe and clear pathway to toilet area.

Specific Toileting Interventions for People With Affected or Missing Limbs
- Provide only the supervision and assistance necessary for relearning or adapting to the prosthesis.
- Encourage the client to look at the affected area or limb and use it during toileting tasks.
- Encourage useful transfer techniques taught by occupational or physical therapy. (The nurse becomes familiar with the planned mode of transfer.)
- Provide the necessary adaptive devices to enhance independence and safety (commode chairs, spill-proof urinals, fracture bedpans, raised toilet seats, side support rails for toilets).
- Provide for a safe and clear pathway to toilet area.

Specific Toileting Interventions for People With Cognitive Deficits

- Offer toileting reminders every 2 hours, after meals, and before bedtime.
- When the client can indicate the need to toilet, begin toileting at 2-hour intervals, after meals, and before bedtime.
- Answer the call bell immediately to avoid frustration and incontinence.
- Encourage wearing ordinary clothes. (Many confused people are continent while wearing regular clothing.)
- Avoid the use of bedpans and urinals; if physically possible, provide a normal atmosphere of elimination in bathroom. (The toilet used should remain constant to promote familiarity.)
- Give verbal cues as to what is expected of the client and positive reinforcement for success.
- Work to achieve daytime continence before expecting nighttime continence. (Nighttime incontinence may continue after daytime continence has returned.)
- Refer to *Impaired Urinary Elimination* for additional information on incontinence.

Initiate Health Teaching and Referrals, as Indicated

- Assess the understanding and knowledge of the client and family of foregoing interventions and rationales
- Ensure an in-home evaluation by a home health nurse

DISTURBED SELF-CONCEPT

Disturbed Self-Concept

Disturbed Body Image

Disturbed Personal Identity

Risk for Disturbed Personal Identity

Disturbed Self-Esteem

Chronic Low Self-Esteem

Risk for Chronic Low Self-Esteem

Situational Low Self-Esteem

Risk for Situational Low Self-Esteem

Definition**

A negative state of change about the way a person feels, thinks, or views him or herself. It may include a change in body image, self-esteem, or personal identity (Boyd, 2005).

Defining Characteristics

This diagnosis reflects a broad diagnostic category that can be
   used initially until more specific assessment data can support
   a more specific nursing diagnosis, such as *Disturbed Body Image*
   or *Disturbed Self-Esteem*.
Some examples of signs and symptoms (observed or reported) are:
   Verbal or nonverbal negative response to actual or perceived
      change in structure, function, or both (e.g., shame, embar-
      rassment, guilt, revulsion)
   Expression of shame or guilt
   Rationalization or rejection of positive feedback and exaggera-
      tion of negative feedback about self
   Hypersensitivity to slight criticism
   Episodic occurrence of negative self-appraisal in response to
      life events in a client with a previously positive self-evaluation
   Verbalization of negative feelings about self (helplessness,
      uselessness)

Related Factors

A disturbed self-concept can occur as a response to a variety of
   health problems, situations, and conflicts. Some common
   sources follow.

Pathophysiologic

*Related to change in appearance, lifestyle, role, response of others
secondary to:*
Chronic disease   Pain
Severe trauma   Loss of body functions
Loss of body parts

Situational (Personal, Environmental)

Related to feelings of abandonment or failure secondary to:
Divorce, separation from, or death of a significant other
Loss of job or ability to work

** This definition has been added by the author for clarity and usefulness.

Related to immobility or loss of function

Related to unsatisfactory relationships (parental, spousal)

Related to sexual preferences (homosexual, lesbian, bisexual, abstinent)

Related to teenage pregnancy

Related to gender differences in parental child-rearing

Related to experiences of parental violence

Related to change in usual patterns of responsibilities

Maturational

Middle Aged
Loss of role and responsibilities

Older Adult
Loss of role and responsibilities

Author's Note

Self-concept reflects self-view, encompassing body image, esteem, role performance, and personal identity. Self-concept develops over a life-time and is difficult to change. It is influenced by interactions with the environment and others and by the client's perceptions of how others view him or her.

Disturbed Self-Concept represents a broad diagnostic category under which fall more specific nursing diagnoses. Initially, the nurse may not have sufficient clinical data to validate a more specific diagnosis, such as Chronic Low Self-Esteem or Disturbed Body Image; thus, he or she can use Disturbed Self-Concept until data can support a more specific diagnosis.

Self-esteem is one of the four components of self-concept. Disturbed Self-Esteem is the general diagnostic category. Chronic Low Self-Esteem and Situational Low Self-Esteem represent specific types of Disturbed Self-Esteem and thus involve more specific interventions. Initially, the nurse may not have sufficient clinical data to validate a more specific diagnosis, such as Chronic Low Self-Esteem or Situational Low Self-Esteem; thus, Disturbed Self-Esteem may be appropriate to use. Refer to the major Defining Characteristics under these categories for validation.

Situational Low Self-Esteem is an episodic event; repeated occur-rence, continuous negative self-appraisals over time, or both can lead to Chronic Low Self-Esteem (Willard, 1990, personal communication).

NOC

Quality of Life, Depression Level, Depression, Self-Control, Self-Esteem, Coping

Goal

The client will demonstrate healthy adaptation and coping skills, as evidenced by the following indicators:

- Appraise self and situations realistically without distortions.
- Verbalize and demonstrate increased positive feelings.

NIC

Hope Instillation, Mood Management, Values Clarification, Counseling, Referral, Support Group, Coping Enhancement

Interventions

Nursing interventions for the various problems that might be associated with a diagnosis of *Disturbed Self-Concept* are similar.

Contact the Client Frequently and Treat Him or Her With Warm, Positive Regard

Encourage the Client to Express Feelings and Thoughts About the Following:

- Condition
- Progress
- Prognosis
- Effects on lifestyle
- Support system
- Treatment

Provide Reliable Information and Clarify Any Misconceptions

Explain the Process of Reimaging

- Explain that reimaging oneself after a loss of appearance or function is distinct and unique.
- Advise that the process takes at least 1 year.
- Assist client to examine societal homophobia and its results, so it is not internalized. Link him or her to appropriate groups and organizations.
- Provide maternal education and a sound supportive system, which includes alternatives for care of the infant when delivered.
- Provide education and refer to support groups that promote empowerment and change of focus to assist in evaluating and raising quality of life.

Help Client to Identify Positive Attributes and Possible New Opportunities

Assist With Hygiene and Grooming, as Needed

Encourage Visitors

Help Client Identify Strategies to Increase Independence and to Maintain Role Responsibilities

(continued)

- Prioritizing activities
- Using mobility aids and assistive devices, as needed

Discuss With Client's Family the Importance of Communicating the Client's Value and Importance to Them

Initiate Health Teaching, as Indicated

- Teach client what community resources are available, if needed (e.g., mental health centers, self-help groups such as Reach for Recovery, Make Today Count).
- Refer to specific health teaching issues under *Disturbed Body Image*, *Disturbed Self-Esteem* (*Chronic* and *Situational*).

✤ Pediatric Interventions

- Allow the child to bring his or her own experiences into the situation (e.g., "Some children say that an injection feels like an insect sting; some say they don't feel anything. After we do this, you can tell me how it feels"; Johnson, 1995).
- Avoid using "good" or "bad" to describe behavior. Be specific and descriptive (e.g., "You really helped me by holding still. Thank you for helping"; Johnson, 1995).
- Connect previous experiences with the present one (e.g., "The x-ray camera will look different from the last time. You will have to hold real still again. The table will move, too"; Johnson, 1995).
- Convey optimism with positive self-talk (e.g., "I am so busy today. I wonder if I will get all my work done? I bet I can." or "When you come back from surgery you will need to stay in bed. What would you like to do when you come back?").
- Help the child plan playtime with choices. Encourage crafts that produce an end product.
- Encourage interactions with peers and supportive adults.
- Encourage child to decorate room with crafts and personal items.

Disturbed Body Image

NANDA-I Definition

Confusion in mental picture of one's physical self

Defining Characteristics

Major (Must Be Present)

Verbal or nonverbal negative response to actual or perceived change in structure and/or function (e.g., shame, embarrassment, guilt, revulsion)

Minor (May Be Present)

Not looking at body part*
Not touching body part*
Intentional hiding or overexposing body part*
Change in social involvement*
Negative feelings about body; feelings of helplessness,
    hopelessness, powerlessness, vulnerability
Preoccupation with change or loss
Refusal to verify actual change
Depersonalization of part or loss
Self-destructive behaviors (e.g., mutilation, suicide attempts,
    overeating/undereating)

Related Factors

Pathophysiologic

Related to changes in appearance secondary to:

Chronic disease	Severe trauma
Loss of body part or body function	Illness*
	Aging

Related to unrealistic perceptions of appearance secondary to:

Psychosis	Bulimia
Anorexia nervosa	

Treatment Related

Related to changes in appearance secondary to:

Hospitalization	Radiation
Surgery*	Treatment regimen*
Chemotherapy	

Situational (Personal, Environmental)

Related to physical trauma* secondary to:
Sexual abuse
Accidents
Rape (perpetrator known or unknown)
Assault

Related to effects of (specify) on appearance:
Obesity
Related to cognitive/perceptual factors*
Related to morbid fear of obesity (Varcarolis, 2011)

Maturational

Related to developmental
  changes*

Immobility
Pregnancy

 Author's Note

See *Disturbed Self-Concept*.

NOC

Body Image, Child Development: (specify age), Grief Resolution, Psychosocial
Adjustment: Life Change, Self-Esteem

Goals

The person will implement new coping patterns and verbalize and
demonstrate acceptance of appearance (grooming, dress, posture,
eating patterns, presentation of self) as evidenced by the following
indicators:

• Demonstrate a willingness and ability to resume self-care/role
  responsibilities.
• Initiate new or re-establish contacts with existing support systems.

NIC

Self-Esteem Enhancement, Counseling, Presence, Active Listening, Body Image
Enhancement, Grief Work Facilitation, Support Group, Referral

Interventions

Establish a Trusting Nurse–Client Relationship

• Encourage person to express feelings, especially about the way
  he or she feels, thinks, or views self.
• Acknowledge feelings of hostility, grief, fear, and dependency;
  teach strategies for coping with emotions.
• Explore belief system (e.g., does pain, suffering, loss mean
  punishment?).
• Encourage client to ask questions about health problem, treat-
  ment, progress, and prognosis.
• Provide reliable information and reinforce information already
  given.
• Clarify any misconceptions about self, care, or caregivers.
• Avoid criticism.
• Provide privacy and a safe environment.

- Use therapeutic touch, with person's consent.
- Encourage client to connect with spiritual beliefs and values regarding a higher power.

Promote Social Interaction

- Assist client to accept help from others.
- Avoid overprotection, but limit the demands made.
- Encourage movement.
- Prepare significant others for physical and emotional changes.
- Support family as they adapt.
- Encourage visits from peers and significant others.
- Encourage contact (letters, telephone) with peers and family.
- Encourage involvement in unit activities.
- Provide opportunity to share with people going through similar experiences.
- Discuss the importance of communicating the client's value and importance to them with his or her support system.

Provide Specific Interventions in Selected Situations

Loss of Body Part or Function

- Assess the meaning of the loss for the client and significant others, as related to visibility of loss, function of loss, and emotional investment.
- Explore and clarify misconceptions and myths regarding loss or ability to function with loss.
- Expect the client to respond to the loss with denial, shock, anger, and depression.
- Be aware of the effect of the responses of others to the loss; encourage sharing of feelings between significant others.
- Validate feelings by allowing the client to express his or her feelings and to grieve.
- Use role playing to assist with sharing; if the client says, "I know my husband will not want to touch me with this colostomy," take the husband's role and discuss her colostomy, then switch roles so she can act out her feelings about her husband's response.
- Explore realistic alternatives and provide encouragement.
- Explore strengths and resources with person.
- Assist with the resolution of a surgically created alteration of body image:
  - Replace the lost body part with prosthesis as soon as possible.
  - Encourage viewing of site.
  - Encourage touching of site.
  - Encourage activities that encompass new body image (e.g., shopping for new clothes).

- Teach about the health problem and how to manage.
- Begin to incorporate person in care of operative site.
- Gradually allow client to assume full self-care responsibility, if feasible.
- Teach person to monitor own progress (Miller, 2009).
- Refer to *Sexual Dysfunction* for additional information, if indicated.
- Identifying personal attributes and strengths can help the client focus on the positive characteristics that contribute to the whole concept of self rather than only on the change in body image. The nurse should reinforce these positive aspects and encourage the client to reincorporate them into the new self-concept.

Changes Associated With Chemotherapy (Camp-Sorrell, 2007)

- Discuss the possibility of hair loss, absence of menses, temporary or permanent sterility, decreased estrogen levels, vaginal dryness, and mucositis.
- Encourage client to share concerns, fears, and perception of the effects of these changes on life.
- Explain where hair loss may occur (head, eyelashes, eyebrows; axillary, pubic, and leg hair).
- Explain that hair will grow back after treatment but may change in color and texture.
- Encourage client to select and wear a wig before hair loss. Suggest consulting a beautician for tips on how to vary the look (e.g., combs, clips).
- Encourage the wearing of scarves or turbans when wig is not on.
- Teach client to minimize the amount of hair loss by:
  - Cutting hair short.
  - Avoiding excessive shampooing, using a conditioner twice weekly.
  - Patting hair dry gently.
  - Avoiding electric curlers, dryers, and curling irons.
  - Avoiding pulling hair with bands, clips, or bobby pins.
  - Avoiding hair spray and hair dye.
  - Using wide-tooth comb, avoiding vigorous brushing.
- Refer client to American Cancer Society for information about new or used wigs. Inform the client that the wig is a tax-deductible item.
- Discuss the difficulty that others (spouse, friends, coworkers) may have with visible changes.
- Encourage client to initiate calls and contacts with others who may be having difficulty.
- Encourage client to ask for assistance of friends, relatives. Ask person if the situation were reversed, what he or she would want to do to help a friend.

- Allow significant others opportunities to share their feelings and fears.
- Assist significant others to identify positive aspects of the client and ways this can be shared.
- Provide information about support groups for couples.

Anorexia Nervosa, Bulimia Nervosa
- Differentiate between body image distortion and body image dissatisfaction.
- Provide factual feedback on low weight and determents to health. Do not argue or challenge their distorted perceptions (Varcarolis, 2011).
- Know that the person's distorted image is their reality (Varcarolis, 2011).
- Assist to identify their positive traits (Varcarolis, 2011).
- Refer individuals for psychiatric counseling.

Psychoses
- Refer to *Confusion* for specific information and interventions.

Sexual Abuse
- Refer to *Disabled Family Coping* for specific information and interventions.

Sexual Assault
- Refer to *Rape-Trauma Syndrome* for specific information and interventions.

Assault
- Refer to *Post-Trauma Response* for specific information and interventions.

Initiate Health Teaching, as Indicated

- Teach what community resources are available, if needed (e.g., mental health centers, self-help groups such as Reach for Recovery, Make Today Count).
- Teach wellness strategies.

Pediatric Interventions

For Hospitalized Child
- Prepare child for hospitalization, if possible, with an explanation and a visit to the hospital to meet personnel and examine the environment.
- Provide familiarities/routines of home as much as possible (e.g., favorite toy or blanket, story at bedtime).
- Provide nurturance (e.g., hug).
- Provide child with opportunities to share fears, concerns, and anger:
  - Provide play therapy.

- Correct misconceptions (e.g., that the child is being punished; that parents are angry).
- Encourage family to stay with or visit child, despite the child's crying when they leave; teach them to provide accurate information about when they will return to reduce fears of abandonment.
- Allow parents to help with care.
- Ask child to draw a picture of self, and then ask for a verbal description.
- Assist child to understand experiences:
  - Provide an explanation ahead of time, if possible.
  - Explain sensations and discomforts of condition, treatments, and medications.
  - Encourage crying.

Discuss With Parents How Body Image Develops and What Interactions Contribute to Their Child's Self-Perception

- Teach the names and functions of body parts.
- Acknowledge changes (e.g., height).
- Allow some choices for what to wear.

For Adolescents
- Discuss with parents the adolescent's need to "fit in":
  - Do not dismiss concerns too quickly.
  - Be flexible and compromise when possible (e.g., clothes are temporary, tattoos are not).
  - Negotiate a time period to think about options and alternatives (e.g., 4 to 5 weeks).
  - Provide with reasons for denying a request. Elicit adolescent's reasons. Compromise if possible (e.g., parents want curfew at 11:00; adolescent wants 12:00; compromise at 11:30).
  - Provide opportunities to discuss concerns when parents are not present.
  - Prepare for impending developmental changes.

Maternal Interventions

- Encourage the woman to share her concerns.
- Attend to each concern, if possible, or refer her to others for assistance.
- Discuss the challenges and changes that pregnancy and motherhood bring.
- Encourage her to share expectations: her own and those of her significant others.
- Assist her to identify sources for love and affection.
- Provide anticipatory guidance to both parents-to-be concerning:
  - Fatigue and irritability.
  - Appetite swings.

- Gastric disturbances (nausea, constipation).
- Back and leg aches.
- Changes in sexual desire and activity (e.g., sexual positions as pregnancy advances).
- Mood swings.
- Fear (for self, for unborn baby, of loss of attractiveness, of inadequacy as a parent).
- Encourage sharing of concerns between spouses.

Disturbed Personal Identity

NANDA-I Definition

Inability to maintain an integrated and complete perception of self

Defining Characteristics**

Appears unaware of or uninterested in others or their activities
Unable to identify parts of the body or body sensations
     (e.g., enuresis)
Excessively imitates other's activities or words
Fails to distinguish parent/caregiver as a whole person
Becomes distressed with bodily contact with others
Spends long periods of time in self-stimulating behaviors
     (self-touching, sucking, rocking)
Needs ritualistic behaviors and sameness to control anxiety
Cannot tolerate being separated from parent/caregiver

Related Factors**

Pathophysiologic

Related to biochemical imbalance

Related to impaired neurologic development or dysfunction

Maturational

Related to failure to develop attachment behaviors resulting in fixation at autistic phase of development

Related to interrupted or uncompleted separation/individualization process resulting in extreme separation anxiety

---

** Varcarolis, 2006.

Author's Note

Disturbed Personal Identity is a very complex diagnosis and should not be used to label autism. It may be more clinically useful in nursing to use *Anxiety* and/or *Impaired Social Interactions* for the nursing focus.

Risk for Disturbed Personal Identity

NANDA-I Definition

Risk for the inability to maintain an integrated and complete perception of self

Risk Factors*

Chronic low self-esteem
Psychiatric disorders
    (e.g., psychoses, depression,
    dissociative disorder)
Cult indoctrination
Situational crises
Situational low self-esteem
Cultural discontinuity
Social role change
Discrimination
Stages of development

Dysfunctional family processes
Stages of growth
Ingestion/inhalation of toxic
    chemicals
Use of psychoactive
    pharmaceutical agents
Manic states
Multiple personality disorder
Organic brain syndromes
Perceived prejudice

 Author's Note

Refer to *Disturbed Personal Identity*.

Disturbed Self-Esteem**

Definition

State in which a person experiences or is at risk of experiencing negative self-evaluation about self or capabilities

---

** This diagnosis is not presently on the NANDA-I list but has been added for clarity and usefulness.

Defining Characteristics**

Major (Must Be Present, One or More)

(Observed or reported)
Self-negating verbalization
Expressions of shame or guilt
Evaluates self as unable to deal with events
Rationalizes away or rejects positive feedback and exaggerates negative feedback about self

Lack of or poor problem-solving ability
Hesitant to try new things or situations
Rationalizes personal failures
Hypersensitivity to slight criticism

Minor (May Be Present)

Lack of assertion
Overly conforming
Indecisiveness
Passive
Seeks approval or reassurance excessively

Lack of culturally appropriate body presentation (posture, eye contact, movements)
Denial of problems obvious to others
Projection of blame or responsibility for problems

Related Factors

Disturbed Self-Esteem can be either episodic or chronic. Failure to resolve a problem or multiple sequential stresses can result in chronic low self-esteem (CLSE). Those factors that occur over time and are associated with CLSE are indicated by "CLSE" in parentheses.

Pathophysiologic

Related to change in appearance secondary to:
Loss of body parts
Loss of body functions

Disfigurement (trauma, surgery, birth defects)

Related to biochemical/neurophysiologic imbalance

Situational (Personal, Environmental)

Related to unmet dependency needs

** Leuner et al., 1994; Norris & Kunes-Connell, 1987.

Related to feelings of abandonment secondary to:
Death of significant other
Separation from significant other
Child abduction/murder

Related to feelings of failure secondary to:

Loss of job or ability to work	Relationship problems
Increase/decrease in weight	Marital discord
Unemployment	Separation
Financial problems	Stepparents
Premenstrual syndrome	In-laws

Related to assault (personal, or relating to the event of another's assault—e.g., same age, same community)

Related to failure in school

Related to history of ineffective relationship with parents (CLSE)

Related to history of abusive relationships (CLSE)

Related to unrealistic expectations of child by parent (CLSE)

Related to unrealistic expectations of self (CLSE)

Related to unrealistic expectations of parent by child (CLSE)

Related to parental rejection (CLSE)

Related to inconsistent punishment (CLSE)

Related to feelings of helplessness and/or failure secondary to institutionalization:

Mental health facility	Jail
Orphanage	Halfway house

Related to history of numerous failures (CLSE)

Maturational

Infant/Toddler/Preschool
Related to lack of stimulation or closeness (CLSE)

Related to separation from parents/significant others (CLSE)

Related to continual negative evaluation by parents

Related to inability to trust significant other (CLSE)

School-Aged
Related to failure to achieve grade-level objectives

Related to loss of peer group

Related to repeated negative feedback

Related to loss of independence and autonomy secondary to (specify)

Related to disruption of peer relationships

Related to scholastic problems

Related to loss of significant others

Middle-Aged
Related to changes associated with aging

Older Adult
Related to losses (people, function, financial, retirement)

 Author's Note

See *Disturbed Self-Concept.*

NOC

Refer to *Chronic Low Self-Esteem.*

Goals

The client will express a positive outlook for the future and resume previous level of functioning as evidenced by the following indicators:

- Identify source of threat to self-esteem and work through that issue.
- Identify positive aspects of self.
- Analyze own behavior and its consequences.
- Identify one positive aspect of change.

NIC

Refer to *Chronic Low Self-Esteem.*

Interventions

Establish a Trusting Nurse–Client Relationship

- Encourage client to express feelings, especially about the way he or she thinks or views self.
- Encourage client to ask questions about health problem, treatment, progress, prognosis.
- Provide reliable information and reinforce information already given.
- Clarify any misconceptions the client has about self, care, or caregivers. Avoid criticism.

Promote Social Interaction

- Assist client to accept help from others.
- Avoid overprotection while still limiting the demands made on the individual.
- Encourage movement.

Explore Strengths, Resources, and Expectations With Client

- Explore realistic alternatives.

Refer to Community Resources as Indicated (e.g., Counseling, Assertiveness Courses)

Chronic Low Self-Esteem

NANDA-I Definition

Long-standing negative self-evaluating/feelings about self or self-capabilities

Defining Characteristics†

Major (80% to 100%)

Long-Standing or Chronic
Self-negating verbalization
Reports feelings of shame/guilt*
Evaluates self as unable to deal with events*
Rationalizes away/rejects positive feedback and exaggerates
    negative feedback about self*
Hesitant to try new things/situations*
Exaggerating negative feedback about self*

Minor (50% to 79%)

Frequent lack of success in work or other life events*
Overly conforming, dependent on others' opinions*
Lack of culturally appropriate body presentation (eye contact,
    posture, movements)
Nonassertive/passive*
Indecisive
Excessively seeks reassurance*

---

† Leuner et al., 1994; Norris & Kunes-Connell, 1987.

Related Factors

See *Disturbed Self-Esteem*.

 Author's Note

See *Disturbed Self-Concept*.

NOC

Depression Level, Depression Self-Control, Anxiety Level, Quality of Life, Self-Esteem

Goals

The client will identify positive aspects of self and a realistic appraisal of limitations as evidenced by the following indicators (Varcarolis, 2011):

* Identify two strengths.
* Identify two unrealistic expectations and modify more realistic life goals.
* Verbalize acceptance of limitations.
* Cease self-abusive descriptions of self (e.g., I am stupid).

NIC

Hope Instillation, Anxiety Reduction, Self-Esteem Enhancement, Coping Enhancement, Socialization Enhancement, Referral

Interventions

Assist the Person to Reduce Present Anxiety Level

* Be supportive, nonjudgmental.
* Accept silence, but let him or her know you are there.
* Orient as necessary.
* Clarify distortions; do not use confrontation.
* Be aware of your own anxiety and avoid communicating it to the person.
* Refer to *Anxiety* for further interventions.

Enhance the Person's Sense of Self

* Be attentive.
* Respect personal space.
* Validate your interpretation of what he or she is saying or experiencing ("Is this what you mean?").
* Help him or her to verbalize what he or she is expressing nonverbally.

- Assist client to reframe and redefine negative expressions (e.g., not "failure," but "setback").
- Use communication that helps to maintain his or her individuality ("I" instead of "we").
- Pay attention to person, especially new behavior.
- Encourage good physical habits (healthy food and eating patterns, exercise, proper sleep).
- Provide encouragement as he or she attempts a task or skill.
- Provide realistic positive feedback on accomplishments.
- Teach person to validate consensually with others.
- Teach and encourage esteem-building exercises (self-affirmations, imagery, mirror work, use of humor, meditation/prayer, relaxation).

Promote Use of Coping Resources

- Identify the client's areas of personal strength:
  - Sports, hobbies, crafts
  - Health, self-care
  - Work, training, education
  - Imagination, creativity
  - Writing skills, math
  - Interpersonal relationships
- Share your observations with the client.
- Provide opportunities for client to engage in the activities.

Assist to Identify Cognitive Distortions That Increase Negative Self-Appraisal (Varcarolis, 2011)

- Overgeneralization: Teach to focus on each event as separate.
- Self-Blame: Teach to evaluate if she/he is really responsible and why.
- Mind-Reading: Advise to clarify verbally what he/she thinks is happening.
- Discounting positive responses of others: Teach to respond with only "thank you."

Provide Opportunities for Positive Socialization

- Encourage visits/contact with peers and significant others (letters, telephone).
- Be a role model in one-to-one interactions.
- Involve in activities, especially when strengths can be used.
- Do not allow person to isolate self (refer to *Social Isolation* for further interventions).
- Involve the client in supportive group therapy.
- Teach social skills as required (refer to *Impaired Social Interaction* for further interventions).
- Encourage participation with others sharing similar experiences.

Set Limits on Problematic Behavior Such as Aggression, Poor Hygiene, Ruminations, and Suicidal Preoccupation

Refer to *Risk for Suicide* and/or *Risk for Violence* if these are assessed as problems.

Provide for Development of Social and Vocational Skills

- Refer for vocational counseling.
- Involve the client in volunteer organizations.
- Encourage participation in activities with others of same age.
- Arrange for continuation of education (e.g., literacy class, vocational training, art/music classes).

Risk for Chronic Low Self-Esteem

NANDA-I Definition

At risk for longstanding negative self-evaluating/feelings about self or self-capabilities

Risk Factors*

Ineffective adaptation to loss
Lack of affection
Lack of membership in group
Perceived discrepancy between self and cultural norms
Perceived discrepancy between self and spiritual norms
Perceived lack of belonging
Perceived lack of respect from others
Psychiatric disorder
Repeated failures
Repeated negative reinforcement
Traumatic event
Traumatic situation

NOC
Depression Level, Depression Self-Control, Anxiety Level, Quality of Life, Self-Esteem

Goal

The person will identify positive aspects of self and a realistic appraisal of limitations as evidenced by the following indicators (Varcarolis, 2011):

- Identify two strengths.
- Identify two unrealistic expectations and modify more realistic life goals.
- Verbalize acceptance of limitations.
- Cease self-abusive descriptions of self (e.g., I am stupid, etc.).

Hope Instillation, Anxiety Reduction, Self-Esteem Enhancement, Coping
Enhancement, Socialization Enhancement, Referral

Interventions

Refer to *Chronic Low Self-Esteem*.

Situational Low Self-Esteem

NANDA-I Definition

Development of a negative perception of self-worth in response
to a current situation

Defining Characteristics**

Major (80% to 100%)

Episodic occurrence of negative self-appraisal in response to life
   events in a person with a previously positive self-evaluation
Verbally reports current situational challenge to self-worth*
Verbalization of negative feelings about self (helplessness,
   uselessness)*

Minor (50% to 79%)

Self-negating verbalizations*
Expressions of shame/guilt
Evaluates self as unable to handle situations/events*
Difficulty making decisions

Related Factors

See *Disturbed Self-Esteem*.

 Author's Note

See *Disturbed Self-Concept*.

** Leuner et al., 1994; Norris & Kunes-Connell, 1987.

NOC

Decision-Making, Grief Resolution, Psychosocial Adjustment: Life Change, Self-Esteem

Goal

The client will express a positive outlook for the future and resume previous level of functioning as evidenced by the following indicators:

- Identify source of threat to self-esteem and work through that issue.
- Identify positive aspects of self.
- Analyze his or her own behavior and its consequences.
- Identify one positive aspect of change.

NIC

Active Listening, Presence, Counseling, Cognitive Restructuring, Family Support, Support Group, Coping Enhancement

Interventions

Assist the Client to Identify and to Express Feelings

- Be empathic, nonjudgmental.
- Listen. Do not discourage expressions of anger, crying, and so forth.
- Ask what was happening when he or she began feeling this way.
- Clarify relationships between life events.

Assist the Client to Identify Positive Self-Evaluations

- How has he or she handled other crises?
- How does he or she manage anxiety—through exercise, withdrawal, drinking/drugs, talking?
- Reinforce adaptive coping mechanisms.
- Examine and reinforce positive abilities and traits (e.g., hobbies, skills, school, relationships, appearance, loyalty, industriousness).
- Help client accept both positive and negative feelings.
- Do not confront defenses.
- Communicate confidence in the client's ability.
- Involve client in mutual goal setting.
- Have client write positive true statements about self (for his or her eyes only); have client read the list daily as a part of normal routine.
- Reinforce use of esteem-building exercises (self-affirmations, imagery, meditation/prayer, relaxation, use of humor).

Assist to Identify Cognitive Distortions That Increase Negative Self-Appraisal (Varcarolis, 2011)

- Overgeneralization.
- Teach to focus on each event as separate.
- Self-blame.
- Teach to evaluate if she/he is really responsible and why.
- Mind-reading.
- Advise to clarify verbally what he/she thinks is happening.
- Discounting positive responses of others.
- Teach to respond with only "thank you."

Assess and Mobilize Current Support System

- Does he or she live alone? Is he or she employed?
- Does he or she have available friends and relatives?
- Is religion a support?
- Has he or she previously used community resources?
- Refer client to vocational rehabilitation for retraining.
- Support returning to school for further training.
- Assist client to involve local volunteer organizations (senior citizens employment, foster grandparents, local support groups).
- Arrange continuation of school studies for students.

Assist the Client to Learn New Coping Skills

- Practice self-talk (Murray, 2000):
  - Write a brief description of the change and its consequence (e.g., My spouse had an affair. I am betrayed.).
  - Write three things that may be useful about this situation.
- Communicate that the client can handle the change.
- Challenge the client to imagine positive futures and outcomes.
- Encourage a trial of new behavior.
- Reinforce the belief that the client does have control over the situation.
- Obtain a commitment to action.

Assist the Client to Manage Specific Problems

- Rape—refer to *Rape-Trauma Syndrome*.
- Loss—refer to *Grieving*.
- Hospitalization—refer to *Powerlessness* and *Parental Role Conflict*.
- Ill family member—refer to *Interrupted Family Processes*.
- Change or loss of body part—refer to *Disturbed Body Image*.
- Depression—refer to *Ineffective Coping* and *Hopelessness*.
- Domestic violence—refer to *Disabled Family Coping*.

Pediatric Interventions

- Provide opportunities for child to be successful and needed.
- Personalize the child's environment with pictures, possessions, and crafts he or she made.
- Provide structured and unstructured playtime.
- Ensure continuation of academic experiences in the hospital and home. Provide uninterrupted time for schoolwork.

Geriatric Interventions

- Acknowledge the client by name.
- Use a tone of voice that you use for your peer group.
- Avoid words associated with infants (e.g., "diapers").
- Ask about family pictures, personal items, and past experiences.
- Avoid attributing disabilities to "old age."
- Knock on door of bedrooms and bathrooms.
- Allow enough time to accomplish tasks at own pace.

Risk for Situational Low Self-Esteem

NANDA-I Definition

At risk for developing a negative perception of self-worth in response to a current situation

Risk Factors

See *Situational Low Self-Esteem.*

Author's Note

See *Situational Low Self-Esteem.*

Goal

The client will continue to express a positive outlook for the future to identify positive aspects of self as evidenced by the following indicators:

- Identify threats to self-esteem.
- Identify one positive aspect of change.

Interventions

See *Situational Low Self-Esteem.*

RISK FOR SELF-HARM**

Risk for Self-Harm

Self-Mutilation

Risk for Self-Mutilation

Risk for Suicide

Definition

State in which a client is at risk for inflicting direct harm on him or herself. This may include one or more of the following: self-abuse, self-mutilation, and suicide.

Defining Characteristics

Major (Must Be Present, One or More)

Expresses desire or intent to harm self
Expresses desire to die or commit suicide
History of attempts to harm self

Minor (May Be Present)

Reported or Observed:

Depression	Hallucinations/	Lack of support
Helplessness	delusions	system
Substance abuse	Emotional pain	Poor impulse
Hostility	Agitation	control
Hopelessness	Poor self-concept	

Related Factors

Risk for Self-Harm can occur as a response to a variety of health problems, situations, and conflicts. Some sources are listed next.

** This diagnosis is not currently on the NANDA-I list but has been added for clarity or usefulness.

Pathophysiologic

Related to feelings of helplessness, loneliness, or hopelessness secondary to:

Disabilities
Terminal illness
Chronic illness
Chronic pain
Chemical dependency
Substance abuse
New diagnosis of positive
   human immunodeficiency
   virus (HIV) status
Mental impairment
   (organic or traumatic)

Psychiatric disorder
   Schizophrenia
   Personality disorder
   Bipolar disorder
   Adolescent adjustment
      disorder
   Post-trauma syndrome
   Somatoform disorders

Treatment Related

Related to unsatisfactory outcome of treatment (medical, surgical, psychological)

Related to prolonged dependence on:

Dialysis
Chemotherapy/radiation

Insulin injections
Ventilator

Situational (Personal, Environmental)

Related to:

Incarceration
Depression
Ineffective coping skills

Parental/marital conflict
Substance abuse in family
Child abuse

Real or perceived loss secondary to:

Finances/job
Death of significant others
Separation/divorce
Threat of abandonment

Status/prestige
Someone leaving home
Natural disaster

Related to wish for revenge on real or perceived injury (body or self-esteem)

Maturational

Related to indifference to pain secondary to autism

Adolescent
Related to feelings of abandonment

Related to peer pressure

Related to unrealistic expectations of child by parents

Related to depression

Related to relocation

Related to significant loss

Older Adult
Related to multiple losses secondary to:

Retirement	Significant loss
Social isolation	Illness

 Author's Note

Risk for Self-Harm represents a broad diagnosis that can encompass self-abuse, self-mutilation, and/or risk for suicide. Although initially they may appear the same, the distinction lies in the intent. Self-mutilation and self-abuse are pathologic attempts to relieve stress temporarily, whereas suicide is an attempt to die to relieve stress permanently (Carscadden, 1992, personal communication).

   Risk for Self-Harm also can be a useful early diagnosis when insufficient data are present to differentiate one from the other. In some clinical situations the person may have delirium or dementia. This person is at risk of harming themselves (e.g., pulling out a Foley catheter or IV). *Risk for Self-Harm* would be clinically useful.

   Risk for Suicide has been in this author's work for more than 20 years. *Risk for Suicide* was added to the NANDA list in 2006. Previously, *Risk for Violence to Self* was included under *Risk for Violence*. The term *violence* is defined as a swift and intense force or a rough or injurious physical force. As the reader knows, suicide can be either violent or nonviolent (e.g., overdose of barbiturates). Using the term "violence" in this diagnostic context, unfortunately, can lead to non detection of a client at risk for suicide because of the perception that the client is not capable of violence.

   Risk for Suicide clearly denotes a client at high risk for suicide and in need of protection. Treatment of this diagnosis involves validating the risk, contracting with the client, and providing protection. Treatment of the client's underlying depression and hopelessness should be addressed with other applicable nursing diagnoses (e.g., *Ineffective Coping, Hopelessness*).

NOC

Aggression Self-Control, Impulse Self-Control

Goal

The client will choose alternatives that are not harmful as evidenced by the following indicators:

- Acknowledge self-harm thoughts.
- Admit to use of self-harm behavior if it occurs.
- Be able to identify personal triggers.
- Learn to identify and tolerate uncomfortable feelings.

Presence, Anger Control, Environmental Management: Violence Prevention, Behavior Modification, Security Enhancement, Therapy Group, Coping Enhancement, Impulse Control Training, Crisis Intervention

Interventions

Establish a Trusting Nurse–Client Relationship

- Demonstrate acceptance of the client as a worthwhile person through nonjudgmental statements and behavior.
- Ask questions in a caring, concerned manner.
- Encourage expression of thoughts and feelings.
- Actively listen or provide support by just being there if the client is silent.
- Be aware of the client's supersensitivity.
- Label the behavior, not the client.
- Be honest in your interactions.
- Assist the client in recognizing hope and alternatives.
- Provide reasons for necessary procedures or interventions.
- Maintain the client's dignity throughout your therapeutic relationship.

Validate Reality

Schizophrenia or Drug-Induced Psychosis

- Tell the client, "You are safe."
- Use a quiet, calming voice.
- Use "talk downs" when the client has taken a hallucinogenic drug. If agitation increases, stop immediately.
- Orient the client as required. Point out sensory/environmental misperceptions without belittling his or her fears or indicating disapproval of verbal expressions.
- Reassure the client that this will pass.
- Watch for signs of increased delusional thinking and/or frightening hallucinations (increased anxiety, agitation, irritability, pacing, hypervigilance).

Post-Trauma or Dysfunctional
- Tell the client, "You are not bad, crazy, or hopeless."
- Say you believe the client when he or she tells you personal history; many grew up in denial or minimization.
- Let the client know he or she is not the only one.

Help Reframe Old Thinking/Feeling Patterns (Carscadden, 1993)

- Encourage the belief that change is possible.
- Assist the client to identify thought–feeling–behavior concept.
- Help the client assess payoffs and drawbacks to self-harm.
- Rename words that have a negative connotation (e.g., "setback," not "failure").
- Encourage identification of personal triggers.
- Assist the client in exploring viable alternatives.
- Help the client to examine feelings of ambivalence about recovery.
- Encourage the client to become comfortable with and to use feelings.

Facilitate the Development of New Behavior

- Validate good coping skills already in existence.
- Serve as a role model in your own behavior and interactions.
- Encourage the use of positive affirmations, meditation and relaxation techniques, and other esteem-building exercises.
- Promote the concept of being helpful instead of helpless.
- Encourage journaling: keeping a diary of triggers, thoughts, feelings, and alternatives that work or do not work.
- Assist the client to develop body awareness as a method of ascertaining triggers and determining levels of impending self-harm.
- Assist with role playing to work on situations/relationships.
- Promote the development of healthy self-boundaries for the client.

Endorse an Environment That Demotes Self-Harm

- How much control or influence a professional exerts in this area will depend on the diagnosis, the environmental setting, and the policies of that setting (e.g., a client's home, residential setting, treatment facility, or institution).
- If mandated by the setting's policies to intervene in self-harm attempts, the following interventions should take place.

Structure the Client's Time and Activities
- Provide a scheduled day that meets the client's need for activity and rest.
- Encourage activities with others without competitiveness.
- Relieve pent-up tension and purposeless hyperactivity with physical activity (e.g., brisk walk, dance therapy, aerobics).

Reduce Excessive Stimuli
- Provide a quiet, serene atmosphere.
- Establish firm, consistent limits while giving the client as much control/choice as possible within those boundaries.
- Intervene at the earliest stages to assist the client in regaining control, prevent escalation, and allow treatment in the least restrictive manner.
- Keep communication simple. Agitated people cannot process complicated communication.
- Provide an area where the client can retreat to decrease stimuli (e.g., time-out room, quiet room; clients on hallucinogens need a darkened, quiet room with a nonintrusive observer).
- Remove potentially dangerous objects from the environment (if the client is in crisis stage).

Promote the Use of Alternatives
- Stress that there are always alternatives.
- Stress that self-harm is a choice, not something uncontrollable.
- Allow opportunities for verbal expression of thoughts and feelings (e.g., anger, depression).
- Provide acceptable physical outlets (e.g., yelling, pounding pillow, tearing up newspapers, using clay or Play-Doh, taking a brisk walk).
- Provide for less physical alternatives (e.g., relaxation tapes, soft music, warm bath, diversional activities).

Determine Present Level of Impending Self-Harm, If Indicated

Beginning Stage (Thought Stage)
- Provide soothing touch if permitted by the client (predetermined).
- Remind the client that this is an "old tape" and to replace it with new thinking and belief patterns.
- Provide nonintrusive, calming alternatives.

Climbing Stage (Feeling Stage)
- Remind the client to consider alternatives.
- Give as much control to the client as possible to support his or her accountability.
- Are you in control? How can I help? Would you like me to assist?
- Provide more intense interventions at this stage.
- Encourage the client to turn over any potential items of self-harm.

Crisis Stage (Behavior Stage)
- Give positive feedback if the client chooses an alternative and does not harm himself or herself.
- Ask the client to put down any object of harm if he or she possesses one.

- Continue to emphasize there are always alternatives.
- Restrain the client only if he or she becomes out of control.
- Release the client from restraints as soon as possible to give responsibility back to him or her. "Are you in control now?" "Are you feeling safe?"
- Remain calm and caring throughout the crisis period.
- Attend to practical issues in a nonpunitive, nonjudgmental manner.

Post Crisis Stage
- Give positive reinforcements if the client did not harm himself or herself.
- Assist the client in problem solving on how to divert himself before the crisis stage.
- Assess the degree of injury/harm if the client did not choose the alternative.
- Provide assistance or medical care, as necessary.
- Pay as little attention as possible to the act of self-harm and focus on prior stages (e.g., "Can you remember what triggered you?" "What kinds of things were going through your mind?" "What do you think you might have done instead?").
- Return the client to normal activities/routine as soon as possible.

Initiate Support Systems to Community, When/Where Indicated

Teach Family
- Constructive expression of feelings.
- How to recognize levels of impending self-harm.
- How to assist with appropriate interventions.
- How to deal with self-harm behavior/results.

Supply Phone Number of 24-Hour Emergency Hotlines

Provide Referral to:
- Individual therapist
- Family counseling
- Peer support group
- Leisure/vocational counseling
- Halfway houses
- Other community resources

Self-Mutilation

NANDA-I Definition

Deliberate self-injurious behavior causing tissue damage with the intent of causing nonfatal injury to attain relief of tension

Defining Characteristics*

Expresses desire or intent to harm self**
Past history of attempts to harm self, including:
Cuts on body
Scratches on body
Picking at wounds
Abrading
Constricting a body part
Biting

Self-inflicted burns
Severing
Inhalation of harmful substances
Insertion of object into body orifice
Hitting
Ingestion of harmful substances

Related Factors

See *Risk for Self-Harm*.

 Author's Note

See *Risk for Self-Harm*.

Goal

See *Risk for Self-Harm*.

Interventions

See *Risk for Self-Harm*.
    Frequency changing with progress or relapse.

Risk for Self-Mutilation

NANDA-I Definition

At risk for deliberate self-injurious behavior causing tissue damage with the intent of causing nonfatal injury to attain relief of tension

---

** This has been added by the author for clarity and usefulness.

Related Factors†

Pathophysiologic

Related to biochemical/neurophysiologic imbalance secondary to:

Bipolar disorder	Autism
Psychotic states	Mentally impaired

Personal

Related to:

History of self-injury	Impulsive behavior
Desperate need for attention	Feelings of depression,
History of physical, emotional,	rejection, self-hatred,
or sexual abuse	separation anxiety, guilt,
Ineffective coping skills	and/or depersonalization
Eating disorders	
Inability to verbally express	
tensions	

Maturational

Children/Adolescents

Related to emotional disturbed or battered children

 Author's Note

See *Risk for Self-Harm.*

 NOC

Impulse-Self Control, Self-Mutilation Restraint

Goal

The client will identify persons to contact if thoughts of self-harm occur as evidenced by the following indicators:

Long term (Varcarolis, 2011):
- Demonstrate a decrease in frequency and intensity of self-inflicted injury by (date).
- Participate in therapeutic regimen.
- Demonstrate two new coping skills that work for the client. when tension mounts and impulse is present instead of acting-out behaviors by (date).

---

† Varcarolis, 2011.

Short term:
- Respond to external limits.
- Express feelings related to stress and tension instead of acting out behaviors by (date).
- Discuss alternative ways the client can meet demands of current situation by (date).

NIC

Active Listening, Coping Enhancement, Impulse Control Training, Behavior Management: Self-Harm, Hope Instillation, Contracting, Surveillance: Safety

Interventions[†]

- Assess client's history of self-mutilation (Varcarolis, 2011).
  - Types of mutilating behaviors.
  - Frequency of behaviors.
  - Stressors preceding events.
- Explore for feeling before the act of mutilation and what they mean (e.g., gain control over others, attention, method to feel alive, expression of guilt or self-hate).
- Establish a written no harm contract with specific steps to initiate when feeling of self-mutilation occurs and identify persons to contact.
- Respond to self-mutilation episodes matter-of-fact.
- Provide treatment for injuries and what provoked the act.
- Collaborate on alternative behaviors to self-mutilation.
  - Avoidance of certain activities that trigger behavior.
  - Discussion of intense feelings with designated person before self-mutilation.
- Clearly establish limits on behavior.
- Initiate referrals as needed.
  - Connect with community resources (therapist, support groups).

Risk for Suicide

NANDA-I Definition

At risk for self-inflicted, life-threatening injury

[†] Varcarolis, 2006.

Risk Factors

Suicidal behavior (ideation, talk, plan, available means)
    (Varcarolis, 2011)
Persons high risk for suicide
Poor support system*
Family history of suicide *
Hopelessness/helplessness*
Poor support system
History of prior suicidal attempts*
Alcohol and substance abuse*
Legal or disciplinary problems*
Grief/bereavement (loss of person, job, home)
Suicidal cues (Varcarolis, 2011)
Overt ("No one will miss me," "I am better off dead," "I have
    nothing to live for")
Covert (making out a will, giving valuables away, writing forlorn
    love notes, acquiring life insurance)

NOC

Impulse-Self Control, Suicide Self-Restraint

Goal

The client will identify persons to contact if suicidal thoughts occur, and he or she will not commit suicide as evidenced by the
following indicators:

Long term (Varcarolis, 2011):
• State the desire to live.
• Name two people he/she can call if thoughts of suicide recur
  before discharge.
• Name at least one acceptable alternative to his or her situation.
• Identify at least one realistic goal for the future.

Short term:
• Remain safe while in the hospital.
• Stay with a friend or family if person has a potential for suicide
  (if in the community).
• Keep an appointment for the next day with a crisis counselor
  (if in the community).
• Join family in crisis family counseling.
• Have links to self-help groups in the community.

NIC
Active Listening, Coping Enhancement, Suicide Prevention, Impulse Control Training, Behavior Management: Self-Harm, Hope Instillation, Contracting, Surveillance: Safety

Interventions

Assist the Client in Reducing His or Her Present Risk for Self-Destruction

- Assess level of present risk.
- See Table II.5.
  - High
  - Moderate
  - Low
- Assess level of long-term risk:
  - Lifestyle
  - Lethality of plan
  - Usual coping mechanisms
  - Support available

Provide a Safe Environment Based on Level of Risk; Notify All Staff That the Client Is at Risk for Self-Harm; Use Both Written and Oral Communication (Varcarolis, 2011)

- Initiate suicide precaution for immediate management for the high-risk client.
  - When the client is being constantly observed, he or she is not to be allowed out of sight, even though privacy is lost.
  - Arm's length is the most appropriate space for a high-risk client.
- Initiate suicide observation for risk persons.
  - Provide 15 minute visual check of mood, behaviors, and verbatim statements.
- Restrict glass, nail files, scissors, nail polish remover, mirrors, needles, razors, soda cans, plastic bags, lighters, electric equipment, belts, hangers, knives, tweezers, alcohol, and guns.
- Provide meals in a closely supervised area, usually on the unit or in client's room:
  - Ensure adequate food and fluid intake.
  - Use paper/plastic plates and utensils.
  - Check to be sure all items are returned on the tray.
- When administering oral medications, check to ensure that all medications are swallowed.
- Designate a staff member to provide checks on the client as designated by the institution's policy. Provide relief for the staff member.

Table II.5   ASSESSING THE DEGREE OF SUICIDAL RISK

Behavior or Symptom	Intensity of Risk		
	Low	Moderate	High
Anxiety	Mild	Moderate	High, or panic state
Depression	Mild	Moderate	Severe or a sudden change to a happy or peaceful state**
Isolation/withdrawal	Some feelings of isolation, no withdrawal	Some feelings of hopelessness, and withdrawal	Hopeless, withdrawn, and self-deprecating, isolation
Daily functioning	Effective	Moody	Depressed
	Good grades in school*	Some friends	Poor grades*
	Close friends	Prior suicidal thoughts	Few or no close friends
	No prior suicide attempt		Prior suicide attempts
	Stable job		Erratic or poor work history
Lifestyle	Stable	Moderately stable	Unstable
Alcohol/drug use	Infrequently to excess	Frequently to excess	Continual abuse
Previous suicide attempts	None or of low lethality (few pills)	One or more (pills, superficial wrist slash)	One or more (entire bottle of pills, gun, hanging)
Associated events	None or an argument	Disciplinary action*	Relationship breakup
		Failing grades*	Death of a loved one
		Work problems	Loss of job
		Family illness	Pregnancy*
Purpose of act	None or not clear	Relief of shame or guilt	Wants to die
		To punish others	Escape to join deceased
		To get attention	Debilitating disease

Family's reaction and structure	Supportive Intact family Good coping and mental health No history of suicide	Mixed reaction Divorced/separated Usually copes and understands	Angry and unsupportive Disorganized Rigid/abusive Prior history of suicide in family
Suicide plan (method, location, time)	No plan	Frequent thoughts, occasional ideas about a plan	Specific plan Firearms Hanging Jumping Carbon monoxide Overdose of antidepressants, barbiturates, aspirin, acetaminophen
Lethality of suicide attempts		Wrist slashing Overdose of nonprescription drugs except aspirin and acetaminophen.	

*Applies only to children and adolescents.

**Added by Lynda Juall Carpenito.

Adapted from Hatton, C. L. & McBride, S. (1984). *Suicide: Assessment and intervention.* Norwalk, CT: Appleton-Century-Crofts; Jackson, D. B. & Saunders, R. B. (1993). *Child health nursing.* Philadelphia, PA: J. B. Lippincott; and Mohr, W. (2009). *Psychiatric-Mental Health Nursing* (7th ed.). Philadelphia, PA: J. B. Lippincott.

- Restrict the client to the unit unless specifically ordered by physician. When the client is off unit, provide a staff member to accompany him or her.
- Instruct visitors on restricted items (e.g., ensure they do not give the client food in a plastic bag).
- The client may use restricted items in the presence of staff, depending on level of risk.
- For acutely suicidal clients, provide a hospital gown to deter the client from leaving the facility. As risk decreases, the client may be allowed own clothing.
- Conduct room searches periodically according to institution policy.
- Use seclusion and restraint if necessary (refer to *Risk for Violence* for discussion).
- Notify the police if the client leaves the facility and is at risk for suicide.
- Keep accurate and thorough records of the client's behaviors and all nursing assessments and interventions.

Emphasize the Following (Varcarolis, 2011)

- The crisis is temporary.
- Unbearable pain can be survived.
- Help is available.
- You are not alone.

Observe for a Sudden Change in Emotions from Sad, Depressed to Elated, Happy, or Peaceful

Help Build Self-Esteem and Discourage Isolating Behaviors

- Be nonjudgmental and empathic.
- Be aware of own reactions to the situation.
- Provide genuine praise.
- Encourage interactions with others.
- Divert attention to the external world (e.g., odd jobs).
- Convey a sense that the client is not alone (use group or peer therapy).
- Seek out the client for interactions.
- Set limits by informing the client of the rules.
- Use a firm, consistent approach.
- Provide planned daily schedules for people with low impulse control.

Assist the Client to Identify and Contact Support System

- Inform family and significant others.
- Enlist support.
- Do not provide false reassurance that behavior will not recur.
- Encourage an increase in social activity.
- Refer the client to read "If You Are Thinking About Suicide..... Read This First" found at www.metanoia.org/suicide.

Assist the Client in Developing Positive Coping Mechanisms

* Encourage appropriate expression of anger and hostility.
* Set limits on ruminations about suicide or previous attempts.
* Assist the client in recognizing predisposing factors: "What was happening before you started having these thoughts?"
* Facilitate examination of life stresses and past coping mechanisms.
* Explore alternative behaviors.
* Anticipate future stresses and assist in planning alternatives.
* Use appropriate behavior modification techniques for non-compliant, resistive people.
* Help the client to identify negative thinking patterns and direct the client to practice altering them.
* Involve the client in planning the treatment goals and evaluating progress.
* Refer to *Anxiety*, *Ineffective Coping*, and *Hopelessness* for further interventions.

Initiate Health Teaching and Referrals, When Indicated

* Provide teaching that prepares the client to deal with life stresses (relaxation, problem-solving skills, how to express feelings constructively).
* Refer for peer or group therapy.
* Refer for family therapy, especially when a child or adolescent is involved.
* Teach the family limit-setting techniques.
* Teach the family constructive expression of feelings.
* Instruct significant others in how to recognize an increase in risk: change in behavior, verbal or nonverbal communication, withdrawal, or signs of depression.
* Supply the phone number of 24-hour emergency hotline.
* Refer to vocational training if appropriate.
* Refer to halfway house or other agencies, as appropriate.
* Refer for ongoing psychiatric follow-up.
* Refer to senior citizen centers or other agencies to increase leisure activities.
* Initiate referral for family intervention after a completed suicide.

Pediatric Interventions

* Take all suicide threats seriously. Listen carefully.
* Determine whether the child understands the finality of death (e.g., "What does it mean to die?").
* "Have you ever seen a dead animal on the road? Can it get up and run?"

- Engage parents, friends, school personnel, and the client in behavior contracts to "keep safe."
- Explore feelings and reason for suicidal feelings.
- Consult with a psychiatric expert regarding the most appropriate environment for treatment.
- Participate in programs in school to teach about the symptoms of depression and signs of suicidal behavior.
- With adolescents, explore (Mohr, 2009; Hockenberry et al., 2009):
  - Family problems.
  - Mental status.
  - Strength of support systems.
  - Disruption of friendship or romantic relationship.
  - Seriousness of the attempt.
  - Presence of performance failure (e.g., examination, course).
  - Recent or upcoming change (change of school, relocation).
  - Sexual orientation.
- Convey empathy regarding problems and/or losses.
- Be alert for symptoms of a masked depression (e.g., boredom, restlessness, irritability, difficulty concentrating, somatic preoccupation, excessive dependence on or isolation from others, especially adults; Mohr, 2007).

INEFFECTIVE SELF-HEALTH MANAGEMENT

NANDA-I Definition

Pattern of regulating and integrating into daily living a therapeutic regimen for treatment of illness and its sequelae that is unsatisfactory for meeting specific health goals

Defining Characteristics

Verbalized desire to manage the treatment of illness* and prevention of complications
Verbalized difficulty with one or more prescribed regimens* for treatment of illness and its effects or prevention of complications
Acceleration (expected or unexpected) of illness symptoms
Failure to include treatment regimens in daily routines*

Verbalized to reduce risk factors for progression of illness and
    sequelae
Makes choices in daily living ineffective for meeting health goals*

Related Factors

Treatment Related

Related to:
Complexity of therapeutic regimen*
Complexity of health care system*
Financial cost of regimen
Side effects of therapy*

Situational (Personal, Environmental)

Related to:

Previous unsuccessful   Excessive demands (individual,
    experiences   family)*
Family patterns of health care*   Deficient knowledge*
Mistrust of health care   Family conflict*
    personnel   Powerlessness*
Perceived barriers*   Mistrust of regimen
Health belief conflicts   Insufficient confidence
Perceived susceptibility   Economic difficulties*
Questions seriousness of   Questions benefits of regimen
    problem   Decisional conflicts*

Related to insufficient or unavailable family support

Related to barriers to comprehension secondary to:
Cognitive deficits   Motivation
Fatigue   Anxiety
Hearing impairments   Memory problems

🔄 Author's Note

Ineffective Self-Help Management is a very useful diagnosis for nurses in
most settings. Individuals and families experiencing various health problems,
acute or chronic, usually face treatment programs that require changes
in previous functioning or lifestyle. These changes or adaptations can be
instrumental in influencing positive outcomes.

This diagnosis describes individuals or families experiencing difficulty
achieving positive outcomes. The nurse is the primary professional who,
with the client, determines available choices and how to achieve success.
The primary nursing interventions are exploring the options available
and teaching the client how to implement a treatment plan

When a person faces a complex regimen or has compromised functioning that impedes successful management, the diagnosis *Risk for Ineffective Self-Health Management* would be appropriate. In addition to teaching how to manage the regimen, the nurse also must assist the client to identify the adjustments needed because of a functional deficit.

Ineffective Self-Health Management focuses on assisting the person and family to identify barriers in management of the condition and to prevention complications at home. A new nursing diagnosis, *Risk–Prone Health Behavior*, approved in 2006, is different. This diagnosis focuses on habits or lifestyles which are unhealthy and can aggravate an existing condition or contribute to developing a disorder.

NOC

Compliance Behavior, Knowledge: Treatment Regimen/Procedure, Participation in Health Care Decisions, Treatment Behavior: Illness or Injury

Goal

The person/family will relate the intent to implement a treatment plan needed or desired for recovery from illness and prevention of recurrence or complications as evidenced by the following indicators:

• Relate less anxiety regarding home management of the condition.
• Describe disease process, causes of and factors contributing to symptoms.
• Demonstrate or describe the treatment regimen for disease or symptom control.

NIC

Teaching: Disease process, Referral, Family Support, Health System Guidance

Interventions

Identify Causative or Contributing Factors That Impede Effective Management

• Refer to Related Factors.

Implement Symptom-Focused Self-Care (Skelly et al., 2008)

• Elicit from person their present symptoms.
• Explain the causes of symptoms (e.g., headache with high blood pressure, blurred vision with elevated glucose levels, leg cramps when walking with tobacco use, intermittent leg swelling with obesity, and decreased sensation in feet with nerve damage from elevated glucose levels).

- If possible, emphasize early symptoms that can be reversed or not worsen.
- Discuss symptom management:
  - *Medical*: medication compliance, how it works.
  - *Behavioral* (self-care practices): e.g., exercise, food portion management, low salt diet, foot care.
  - *Socio-psychological* (coping, stress reduction): e.g., meditation, yoga, walking, assertiveness training.
  - *Focus of health outcomes* (metabolic control indicators): e.g., blood pressure, weight loss, glucose readings.
- Parent–child relationship.
- Family caregiving abilities.

Consider Cultural Preferences or Practices

- What does family do to maintain health?
- What does family do to prevent illness?
- What home remedies do you or your family use?

Promote Confidence and Positive Self-Efficacy (Bandura, 1982)

- Explore past successful management of problems.
- Emphasize past successful coping.
- Tell stories of other "successes."
- If appropriate, encourage opportunities to witness others successfully coping in a similar situation.
- Encourage participation in self-help groups.

Reduce or Eliminate Barriers to Learning

- Adapt teaching to person's physical and psychological status.
  - Comfort levels.
  - Fatigue levels.
  - Not concurrent with peaks of medications that alter perception or cognition.
- Allow person to work through and express intense emotions before beginning to teach.
- Examine person's health beliefs and past experiences related to illness; Assess their effects on desire to learn.
  - Delay teaching until person is ready.

Reduce Anxiety

- Encourage verbalization.
- Listen attentively.
- Meet the client's expressed needs before giving other information.
- Develop trust with frequent, consistent interactions.
- Give correct, relevant information.
- Give nonthreatening information before delivering more anxiety-producing information.

- Explain reason for and intended effect of treatment; emphasize the positive.
- Explore with the client the effects of a new diagnosis, treatment, or surgery on significant others.
- Do not overwhelm the client with too much information if anxiety is high or physical condition is unstable.
- Allow the client to maintain some control over self and routines by involving him or her in care.

Initiate Teaching Home Care

- Determine if the client is inexperienced in the situation.
- When providing care explain the procedure to the client.
- Emphasize important points (safety, infection prevention).
- Allow the person to participate if possible.
- Present information at a level consistent with the client's ability.
- Adjust the explanation according to the client's physical ability.
- Use terminology that is commonly known:
  - Avoid too much information at the first session.
  - Repeat important points of information.
  - Ask client to share what he or she learned and what additional information is desired.
  - Write down step by step procedures and what signs of complications should be reported.

Ensure Family are Included in Teaching Sessions

Clearly Explain That the Person Responsible for Their Health Outcomes Is the Individual Unless the Person Is Dependent on Others for Assistance (E.g., Self-Care, Meals, Blood Glucose Monitoring)

- Explain and discuss:
  - Disease process.
  - Treatment regimen (medications, diet, procedures, exercises, equipment).
  - Rationale for regimen.
  - Expectations (client, family) of regimen.
  - Side effects of regimen.
  - Lifestyle changes needed.
  - Methods to monitor condition.
  - Follow-up care needed.
  - Signs/symptoms of complications.
  - Resources, support available.
  - Home environment alterations needed.

Initiate Health Teaching and Referral as Indicated

- Consult with discharge planner or social services to determine what resources are needed at home.
- Ensure a home health nurse assessment at discharge.
- Ensure sufficient supplies at discharge.

INEFFECTIVE FAMILY SELF-HEALTH MANAGEMENT**

Definition

Pattern in which the family experiences or is at risk to experience difficulty integrating into daily living a program for treatment of illness and the sequelae of illness that meets specific health goals

Defining Characteristics

Major (Must Be Present)

Inappropriate family activities for meeting the goals of a treatment or prevention program

Minor (May Be Present)

Acceleration (expected or unexpected) of illness symptoms of a family member

Lack of attention to illness and its sequelae

Verbalized desire to manage the treatment of illness and prevention of sequelae

Verbalized difficulty with regulation/integration of one or more prescribed regimens for treatment of illness and its effects or prevention of complications

Verbalized that family did not take action to reduce risk factors for progression of illness and sequelae

Related Factors

Refer to *Ineffective Self-Health Management.*

Author's Note

Refer to *Ineffective Self-Health Management.*

Interventions

Refer to *Ineffective Self-Health Management.*

** This diagnosis is not presently on the NANDA-I list but has been added for clarity and usefulness.

INEFFECTIVE COMMUNITY SELF-HEALTH MANAGEMENT**

Definition

Pattern of regulating and integrating into community processes programs for treatment of illness and the sequelae of illness that are unsatisfactory for meeting health-related goals

Defining Characteristics

Verbalized difficulty meeting health needs in communities
Acceleration (expected or unexpected) of illness(es)
Morbidity, mortality rates above norm

Related Factors

Situational (Environmental)

Related to unavailability of community programs for (specify):

Prevention of diseases	Fire safety
Screening for diseases	Smoking cessation
Immunizations	Substance abuse
Dental care	Alcohol abuse
Accident prevention	Child abuse

Related to problem accessing program secondary to:

Inadequate communication	Lack of transportation
Limited hours	Insufficient funds

Related to complexity of population's needs

Related to lack of awareness of availability

Related to multiple needs of vulnerable groups (specify):

Homeless	Below poverty level
Pregnant teenagers	Home-bound individuals

Related to unavailable or insufficient health care agencies

 Author's Note

This diagnosis describes a community that is experiencing unsatisfactory management of its health problems. This diagnosis can also describe a

---

** This diagnosis is not presently on the NANDA-I list but has been added for clarity and usefulness.

community with evidence that a population is underserved because of the lack of availability of, access to, or knowledge of health care resources. Using the results of community assessments, community nurses can identify at-risk groups and overall community needs. In addition, they assess health systems, transportation, social services, and access.

NOC

Participation: Health Care Decisions, Risk Control, Risk Detection

Goal

This community will achieve the following goals:

- Identify needed community resources.
- Promote the use of community resources for health problems.

NIC

Decision-Making Support, Health System Guidance, Risk Identification, Community Health Development, Risk Identification

Interventions

Use Health Department Data (Local, County, State, National) to Identify Major Health Problems and Associated Risks; for Example:

- Obesity
- Heart disease
- Asthma
- Automobile accidents

Organize Focus Groups to Assess Health Needs and Assets; Include Different Age Groups, Ethnic/Racial Groups, and Residents With Varied Lengths of Residence (Clarke et al., 2003)

- Initiate discussion with questions such as (Clarke et al., 2003):
  - What is it like to live in this community?
  - What could make life in this community better?
  - What kinds of things could improve the health of people who live in this community?
  - What could the health department do to improve the health of people who live in this community?
  - What could you, or people you know, do to improve life in this community?

Meet With Community Groups (Health Centers, Faith-Based Groups, Government Agencies) to Review Findings of Focus Groups and to Discuss Collaborative Planning

Organize Response Data

- Rank-order entire sample.
- Group responses of selected groups (e.g., age, gender, income level, disabled).

Analyze the Findings

- What overall health problems are reported?
- What are the health concerns of:
  - Older population
  - Households with children up to 20 years of age
  - Single-parent households
  - Respondents younger than 45 years
  - People living below poverty level
  - Uninsured
  - Adolescents
  - New immigrants

Evaluate Community Resources

- What resources are available for the health problems identified?
- Are there utilization or access problems with the services?
- How does the population learn about services?
- Identify problems that do not have community services available.

If Services Are Unavailable, Pursue Program Development

Examine and Evaluate Similar Programs in Other Communities

- Basic information
- Purpose, goals
- Services available
- Funding
- Cost to participants
- Accessibility of services

Meet With Appropriate People to Discuss Findings (Survey, On-Site Visits); Address the Following:

- Presence of community support
- Available expertise and technology in community
- Financial support

Identify Appropriate Community Sources of Assistance

- Hospital departments
- Health departments
- Faith-based organizations

- Chamber of Commerce
- Health care professionals
- Industry
- Private foundations
- Public assistance agencies
- Professional societies

Collaborate With University Faculty for Collaborative Grant Writing

Plan the Program (Refer to *Readiness for Enhanced Community Coping* for Interventions for Community Planning)

If Services Are Available But Are Underutilized, Assess for (Bamberger et al., 2000):

System Barriers
- Hours of operation (inconvenient)
- Location of services (access, aesthetics, distance)
- Efficiency and atmosphere
- Cost
- Complicated appointment system
- Unfriendly

Personal Barriers
- Mistrust
- Competing life priorities
- Powerlessness
- Illiteracy
- Lacking resources (e.g., telephone, transportation, child care, finances)
- Unpredictable work schedule
- Language other than English

Evaluate Vulnerable Population's Access to Health Care and Knowledge of Risk Factors

- Rural families, elderly
- Migrant workers
- New immigrants
- Homeless
- Those living below poverty level

Make a Priority of Ensuring That Basic Needs (Food, Shelter, Clothing, and Safety) Are Met Before Attempting to Address Higher Health Needs

Provide Information Regarding Illness Prevention, Health Promotion, and Health Services to Vulnerable Populations (e.g., Federally Funded Community Health Centers)

- Be sure reading material is appropriate for targeted group (e.g., reading level, language, pictures).
- Use posters, flyers.
- Select locations that the targeted populating uses regularly:
  - Grocery, convenience stores
  - Day care centers
  - School activities
  - Religious services
  - Laundromats
  - Community fairs
  - Meetings
  - Sporting events

INEFFECTIVE SEXUALITY PATTERN

Ineffective Sexuality Pattern

Sexual Dysfunction

NANDA-I Definition

Expressions of concern regarding own sexuality

Defining Characteristics

Actual concerns regarding sexual behaviors, sexual health, sexual functioning, or sexual identity.

Expression of concern about impact a medical diagnosis or treatment for a medical condition may have on sexual functioning or sexual desirability.

Related Factors

Ineffective sexual patterns can occur as a response to various health problems, situations, and conflicts. Some common sources are listed next.

Pathophysiologic

Related to biochemical effects on energy and libido secondary to:

Endocrine
Diabetes mellitus
Hyperthyroidism
Addison's disease

Decreased hormone
  production
Myxedema
Acromegaly

Genitourinary
Chronic renal failure

Neuromuscular and Skeletal
Arthritis
Amyotrophic lateral sclerosis
Multiple sclerosis
Disturbances of nerve supply to brain, spinal cord, sensory
  nerves, or autonomic nerves

Cardiorespiratory
Peripheral vascular disorders
Cancer
Myocardial infarction

Congestive heart failure
Chronic respiratory disorders

Related to fears associated with (sexually transmitted diseases [STDs])*
(specify):
Human immunodeficiency virus (HIV)/Acquired immunodeficiency
  syndrome (AIDS)
Human papilloma virus
Herpes
Gonorrhea
Chlamydia
Syphilis

Related to effects of alcohol on performance

Related to decreased vaginal lubrication secondary to (specify)

Related to fear of premature ejaculation

Related to pain during intercourse

Treatment Related

Related to effects of:
Medications   Radiation therapy

Related to altered self-concept from change in appearance (trauma,
radical surgery)

Related to knowledge/skill deficit about alternative responses to health related transitions, altered body function or structure, illness or medical treatment*

Situational (Personal, Environmental)

Related to fear of pregnancy*

Related to lack of significant other*

Related to conflicts with sexual orientation preferences*

Related to conflicts with variant preferences

Related to partner problem (specify):

Unwilling	Conflicts
Not available	Abusive
Uninformed	Separated, divorced

Related to lack of privacy*

Related to ineffective role model*

Related to stressors secondary to:

Job problems	Financial worries
Value conflicts	Relationship conflicts

Related to misinformation or lack of knowledge

Related to fatigue

Related to fear of rejection secondary to obesity

Related to pain

Related to fear of sexual failure

Related to fear of pregnancy

Related to depression

Related to anxiety

Related to guilt

Related to history of unsatisfactory sexual experiences

Maturational

Adolescent
Related to ineffective/absent role models*

Related to negative sexual teaching

Related to absence of sexual teaching

Adult

Related to adjustment to parenthood

Related to effects of menopause on libido and vaginal tissue atrophy

Related to values conflict

Related to effects of pregnancy on energy levels and body image

Related to effects of aging on energy levels and body image

 Author's Note

The diagnoses *Ineffective Sexuality Pattern* and *Sexual Dysfunction* are difficult to differentiate. *Ineffective Sexuality Pattern* represents a broad diagnosis, of which sexual dysfunction can be one part. *Sexual Dysfunction* may be used most appropriately by a nurse with advanced preparation in sex therapy. Until *Sexual Dysfunction* is well differentiated from *Ineffective Sexuality Pattern*, most nurses should not use it.

NOC

Body Image, Self-Esteem, Role Performance, Sexual Identity

Goal

The client will resume previous sexual activity or engage in alternative satisfying sexual activity as evidenced by the following indicators:

- Identify effects of stressors, loss, or change on sexual functioning.
- Modify behavior to reduce stressors.
- Identify limitations on sexual activity caused by a health problem.
- Identify appropriate modifications in sexual practices in response to these limitations.
- Report satisfying sexual activity.

NIC

Behavioral Management, Sexual Counseling, Emotional Support, Active Listening, Teaching: Sexuality

Interventions

Assess for Causative or Contributing Factors (See Related Factors)

Explore the Client's Patterns of Sexual Functioning

* Encourage him or her to share concerns; assume that clients of all ages have had some sexual experience, and convey a willingness to discuss feelings and concerns.

Discuss the Relationship Between Sexual Functioning and Life Stressors

* Clarify the relation between stressors and problem in sexual functioning.
* Explore options available for reducing the effects of the stressor on sexual functioning (e.g., increase sleep, increase exercise, modify diet, explore stress reduction methods).

Reaffirm the Need for Frank Discussion Between Sexual Partners

* Explain how the client and partner can use role playing to discuss concerns about sex.
* Reaffirm the need for closeness and expressions of caring through touching, massage, and other means.
* Suggest that sexual activity need not always culminate in vaginal intercourse, but that the partner can reach orgasm through noncoital manual or oral stimulation.

Address Factors for Clients With Acute or Chronic Illness

* Eliminate or reduce causative or contributing factors, if possible, and teach the importance of adhering to medical regimen designed to reduce or control disease symptoms.
* Provide limited information and specific suggestions.
  * Provide appropriate information to client and partner concerning actual limitations on sexual functioning caused by the illness (limited information).
  * Teach possible modifications in sexual practices to assist in dealing with limitations caused by illness.

Facilitate Adaptation to Change in or Loss of Body Part

* Assess the stage of adaptation of the client and partner to the loss (denial, depression, anger, resolution; see *Grieving*).
* Encourage adherence to the medical regimen to promote maximum recovery.
* Encourage the couple to discuss the strengths of their relationship and to assess the influence of the loss on these strengths.

- Clarify the relationship between loss or change and the problem in sexual functioning.

Provide Referrals as Indicated:

- Enterostomal therapist
- Physician
- Nurse specialist
- Sex therapist

Pediatric Interventions

- Clarify the confidentiality of the discussion.
- Strive to be open, warm, objective, unembarrassed, and reassuring.
- Explore feelings and sexual experiences. Encourage questions. Dispel myths.
- Discuss how bacteria are transferred (vaginally, anally, orally).
- For young women, explain the relationship of STDs and pelvic inflammatory disease, infertility, and ectopic pregnancies.
- Show a diagram of reproductive structures.
- Emphasize that most STDs have no symptoms initially.
- Discuss abstinence from sexual perspective (e.g., right to say no, commitment, unwanted pregnancies, STDs).
- Discuss contraceptive methods available (e.g., pill, depo-provera, intrauterine device, condoms, foam, diaphragm, spermicides):
  - How it works
  - Effectiveness
  - Cost
  - Prevention of STDs
- Explain and provide written instructions for method chosen.
- Maternal interventions.
- Discuss body changes during pregnancy.
- Encourage couple to share their feelings.
- Reassure that unless problems exist (preterm labor, previous early loss, bleeding or rupture of membranes) intercourse is allowed until labor begins.
- Suggest alternative sexual positions for later pregnancy to prevent abdominal pressure (e.g., side-lying, woman kneeling, woman on top).
- Give reassurance about postpartum changes. Reassure that this is a temporary state and will resolve in 2 to 3 months.
- Reassure that sexual attitudes change throughout pregnancy from feeling very desirous of sex to wanting only to be cuddled.
- Discuss techniques to enhance the couple's relationship (Polomeno, 1999).
- Explore fears and anxieties (separately).

- Discuss barriers to disclosing fears and anxieties.
- Role-play disclosure.
- Encourage client to share the "little things" that represent caring.
- Instruct on "heart talks." One partner talks for 5 minutes with no interruption or argument. The other partner then has a chance to talk. At the end the couple hugs and says, "I love you" (Polomeno, 1999).
- Instruct on "sexual conversation" (Gray, 1995). Useful questions are:
  - What do you like about having sex with me?
  - Would you like more sex?
  - Would you like more or less foreplay?
  - Is there a way that you would like me to touch you?
- Discuss methods to keep romance alive (Gray, 1995):
  - Set aside regular time with each other.
  - Hold hands.
  - Send messages that partner is appreciated.
- Acknowledge fatigue, especially during first trimester, last month, and postpartum.
- Encourage person to make time for her relationship in sexual and other contexts.
- Teach couples to abstain from any sex play or intercourse and seek the advice of their health care provider if any of the following situations are present (Pillitteri, 2010):
  - Vaginal bleeding
  - Premature dilation
  - Multiple pregnancy
  - Engaged fetal head or lightening
  - Placenta previa
  - Rupture of membranes
  - History of premature delivery
  - History of miscarriage

✹ Geriatric Interventions

- Explain that normal aging affects reproductive abilities but has little effect on sexual functioning.
- Explore interest, activity, attitude, and knowledge regarding sexual functioning.
- If pertinent, discuss the effects of chronic diseases on functioning.
- Explain the effects of certain medications on sexual functioning (e.g., cardiovascular, antidepressants, antihistamine, gastrointestinal, sedatives, alcohol).
- If sexual dysfunction is related to medications, explore alternatives (e.g., medication change, dose reduction).

- With women, discuss the quality of vaginal lubrication and available water-soluble lubricants.
- Encourage questions. If needed, refer to urologist or other specialist.

Sexual Dysfunction

NANDA-I Definition

The state in which an individual experiences a change in sexual function during the sexual response phases of desire, excitation and/or orgasm, which is viewed as unsatisfying, unrewarding, or inadequate

Defining Characteristics*

Alterations in achieving sexual satisfaction and/or perceived sex role
Actual or perceived limitations imposed by disease and/or therapy
Change in interest in others and/or in self
Inability to achieve desired satisfaction
Perceived alteration in sexual excitement
Perceived deficiency of sexual desire
Seeking confirmation of desirability
Verbalization of problem

Related Factors

See *Ineffective Sexuality Pattern*

 Author's Note

See *Ineffective Sexuality Pattern*

RISK FOR SHOCK

See also *Risk for Complications of Hypovolemia* that can be found on http://thePoint.lww.com/CarpenitoHB14e.

NANDA-I Definition

At risk for inadequate blood flow to the body's tissues, which may lead to life-threatening cellular dysfunction

Risk Factors*

Hypertension	Infection
Hypovolemia	Sepsis
Hypoxemia	Systemic inflammatory
Hypoxia	response syndrome

Author's Note

This NANDA-I diagnosis represents several collaborative problems. In order to decide which of the following collaborative problems is appropriate for an individual client, determine what you are monitoring for. Which of the following describes the focus of nursing for this client?

- *Risk for Complications of Hypertension*
- *Risk for Complications of Hypovolemia*
- *Risk for Complications of Sepsis*
- *Risk for Complications of Decrease Cardiac Output*
- *Risk for Complications of Hypoxemia*
- *Risk for Complications of Allergic Reaction*

Refer to http://thePoint.lww.com/CarpenitoHB14e for related Goals and Interventions.

DISTURBED SLEEP PATTERN

Disturbed Sleep Pattern

Insomnia

Sleep Deprivation

NANDA-I Definition

Time-limited interruptions of sleep amount and quality due to external factors

Defining Characteristics

Major (Must Be Present)

Adults
Difficulty falling or remaining asleep

Minor (May Be Present)

Adults
Fatigue on awakening or
  during the day
Dozing during the day

Agitation
Mood alterations

Children
Reluctance to retire
Persists in sleeping with
  parents

Frequent awakening during
  the night

Related Factors

Many factors can contribute to disturbed sleep patterns. Some
common factors follow.

Pathophysiologic

Related to frequent awakenings secondary to:
Impaired oxygen transport
  Angina
  Respiratory disorders
  Peripheral arteriosclerosis
  Circulatory disorders
Impaired elimination;
  bowel or bladder
  Diarrhea
  Retention

Constipation
Dysuria
Incontinence
Frequency
Impaired metabolism
  Hyperthyroidism
  Hepatic disorders
  Gastric ulcers

Treatment Related

*Related to Interruptions (e.g., for therapeutic monitoring, laboratory
tests)**

Related to physical restraints*

Related to difficulty assuming usual position secondary to (specify)

*Related to excessive daytime sleeping or hyperactivity secondary to
(specify medication):*
Tranquilizers
Sedatives
Amphetamines
Monoamine oxidase inhibitors
Hypnotics

Barbiturates
Antidepressants
Corticosteroids
Antihypertensives

Situational (Personal, Environmental)

*Related to lack of sleep privacy/control**

*Related to lighting, noise, noxious odors**

*Related to sleep partner (e.g., snoring)**

*Related to unfamiliar sleep furnishings**

*Related to ambient temperature, humidity**

*Related to caregiving responsibilities**

*Related to change in daylight/darkness exposure**

Related to excessive hyperactivity secondary to:
Bipolar disorder   Panic anxiety
Attention-deficit disorder   Illicit drug use

Related to excessive daytime sleeping

Related to depression

Related to inadequate daytime activity

Related to pain

Related to anxiety response

Related to discomfort secondary to pregnancy

Related to lifestyle disruptions
Occupational   Sexual
Emotional   Financial
Social

Related to environmental changes (specify)
Hospitalization (noise, disturbing roommate, fear)
Travel

Related to fears

Related to circadian rhythm changes

Maturational

Children
Related to fear of dark

Related to fear

Related to enuresis

Related to inconsistent parenteral responses

Related to inconsistent sleep rituals

Adult Women
Related to hormonal changes (e.g., perimenopausal)

 Author's Note

Sleep disturbances can have many causes or contributing factors. Some examples are asthma, tobacco use, stress, marital problems, and traveling. *Disturbed Sleep Pattern* describes a situation that is probably transient due to a change in the client or environment (e.g., acute pain, travel, hospitalization). *Risk for Disturbed Sleep Pattern* can be used when a client is at risk due to travel or shift work. *Insomnia* describes a client with a persistent problem falling asleep or staying asleep because of chronic pain and multiple chronic stressors. It may be clinically useful to view sleep problems as a sign or symptom of another nursing diagnosis such as *Stress Overload, Pain, Ineffective Coping, Dysfunctional Family Coping,* or *Risk-Prone Health Behavior.*

NOC

Rest, Sleep, Well-Being, Parenting Performance

Goal

The client will report an optimal balance of rest and activity, as evidenced by the following indicators:

- Describe factors that prevent or inhibit sleep.
- Identify techniques to induce sleep.

NIC

Energy Management, Sleep Enhancement, Relaxation Therapy, Exercise Promotion, Environmental Management, Parent Education: Childrearing Family

Interventions

Because various factors can disrupt sleep patterns, the nurse should consult the index for specific interventions to reduce certain factors (e.g., pain, anxiety, fear). The following suggests general interventions for promoting sleep and specific interventions for selected clinical situations.

Identify Causative Contributing Factors

- Refer to Related Factors.
- Explain that sleep cycles include REM, NREM, and wakefulness, and explain sleep requirements.

Reduce or Eliminate Environmental Distractions and Sleep Interruptions

* Assess with client and family their usual bedtime routine—time, hygiene practices, rituals such as reading—and adhere to it as closely as possible.
* Encourage or provide evening care:
  * Bathroom or bedpan
  * Personal hygiene (mouth care, bath, shower, partial bath)
  * Clean linen and bedclothes (freshly made bed, sufficient blankets)

Noise
* Close the door to the room.
* Pull the curtains.
* Unplug the telephone.
* Use "white noise" (e.g., fan, quiet music, tape of rain, waves).
* Eliminate 24-hour lighting.
* Provide night lights.
* Decrease the amount and kind of incoming stimuli (e.g., staff conversations).
* Cover blinking lights with tape.
* Reduce the volume of alarms and televisions.
* Place the client with a compatible roommate, if possible.

Interruptions
* Organize procedures to minimize disturbances during sleep period (e.g., when the client awakens for medication, also administer treatments and obtain vital signs).
* Avoid unnecessary procedures during sleep period.
* Limit visitors during optimal rest periods (e.g., after meals).
* If voiding during the night is disruptive, have the client limit nighttime fluids and void before retiring.

Increase Daytime Activities, as Indicated

* Establish with the client a schedule for a daytime program of activity (walking, physical therapy).
* Discourage naps longer than 90 minutes.
* Encourage naps in the morning.
* Limit the amount and length of daytime sleeping if excessive (i.e., more than 1 hour).
* Encourage others to communicate with the client and stimulate wakefulness.

Promote a Sleep Ritual or Routine

* Maintain a consistent daily schedule for waking, sleeping, and resting (weekdays, weekends).

- Arise at the usual time even after not sleeping well; avoid staying in bed when awake.
- Use the bed only for activities associated with sleeping; avoid TV watching.
- If the client is awakened and cannot return to sleep, tell him or her to get out of bed and read in another room for 30 minutes.
- Take a warm bath.
- Consume a desired bedtime snack (avoid highly seasoned and high-roughage foods) and warm milk.
- Use herbs that promote sleep (e.g., lavender, ginseng, chamomile, valerian, rose hips, lemon balm, passion flower [Miller, 2009]). Consult with the primary care provider prior to use.
- Avoid alcohol, caffeine, and tobacco at least 4 hours before retiring.
- Go to bed with reading material.
- Get a back rub or massage.
- Listen to soft music or a recorded story.
- Practice relaxation/breathing exercises.
- Ensure that the client has at least four or five periods of at least 90 minutes each of uninterrupted sleep every 24 hours.
- Document the amount of the client's uninterrupted sleep each shift.

Provide Health Teaching and Referrals, as Indicated

- Teach an at-home sleep routine (Miller, 2009). See above for specifics.
- Teach the importance of regular exercise (walking, running, aerobic dance) for at least 30 minutes three times a week (if not contraindicated). Avoid exercise in the evening.
- Explain risks of hypnotic medications with long-term use.
- Refer a client with a chronic sleep problem to a sleep disorders center.
- For peri- and postmenopausal women, explain the following:
  - Sedative and hypnotic drugs begin to lose their effectiveness after 1 week of use, requiring increasing dosages and leading to the risk of dependence.
  - Warm milk contains L-tryptophan, which is a sleep inducer.
  - Caffeine and nicotine are CNS stimulants that lengthen sleep latency and increase nighttime wakening (Miller, 2009).
- Alcohol induces drowsiness but suppresses REM sleep and increases the number of awakenings (Miller, 2009).
- Early-morning naps produce more REM sleep than do afternoon naps. Naps longer than 90 minutes decrease the stimulus for longer sleep cycles in which REM sleep is obtained.

🎏 Pediatric Interventions

Explain the Sleep Differences of Infants and Toddlers (Murray, Zentner, & Yakimo, 2009)

15 months	Shorter morning nap, needs afternoon nap
17 to 24 months	Has trouble falling asleep
18 months	Has a favorite sleep toy, pillow, or blanket
19 months	Tries to climb out of bed
20 months	May awake with nightmares
21 months	Sleeps better, shorter afternoon naps
24 months	Wants to delay bedtime, needs afternoon nap, sleeps less time
2 to 3 years	Can change to bed from crib, needs closely spaced side rails

- Explain night to the child (stars and moon).
- Discuss how some people (nurses, factory workers) work at night.
- Explain that when night comes for them, day is coming for other people elsewhere in the world.
- If a nightmare occurs, encourage the child to talk about it, if possible. Reassure the child that it is a dream, even though it seems very real. Share with the child that you have dreams too.

Stress the Importance of Establishing a Sleep Routine (Murray, Zentner, & Yakimo, 2009)

- Set a definite time and bedtime routine. Begin 30 minutes before bedtime. Try to prevent the child from becoming overtired and agitated.
- Establish a bedtime ritual with bath, reading a story, and soft music.
- Ensure that the child has his or her favorite bedtime object/toy, pillow, blanket, etc.
- Quietly talk and hold the child.
- Avoid TV and videos.
- If the child cries, go back in for a few minutes and reassure for less than a minute. Do not pick up the child. If crying continues, return in 5 minutes and repeat the procedure.
- "If extended crying continues, lengthen the time to return to the child to 10 minutes" (Murray, Zentner, & Yakimo, 2009) Eventually the child will fatigue and fall asleep.
- "The child should remain in his or her bed rather than co-sleep for part or all of the night with parents" (Murray, Zentner, & Yakimo, 2009). Occasional exceptions can be made for family crises, trauma, and illness.

- Provide a night light or a flashlight to give the child control over the dark.
- Reassure the child that you will be nearby all night.

Maternal Interventions

- Discuss reasons for sleeping difficulties during pregnancy (e.g., leg cramps, backache, fetal movements).
- Teach the client how to position pillows in side-lying position (one between legs, one under abdomen, one under top arm, one under head).
- Refer to Interventions for *Sleep Promotion Strategies.*

Geriatric Interventions

Explain the Age-Related Effects on Sleep

Explain That Medications (Prescribed, Over the Counter) Should Be Avoided Because of Their Risk for Dependence and the Risks of Drowsiness

- If the client needs sleeping pills occasionally, advise him or her to consult primary care provider for a type with a short half-life.

Insomnia

NANDA-I Definition

A disruption in amount and quality of sleep that impairs functioning

Defining Characteristics*

Observed changes in affect
Increased absenteeism (e.g., school, work)
Reports:

Changes in mood	Observed lack of energy
Decreased health status	Decreased quality of life
Dissatisfaction with sleep (current)	Difficulty concentrating
Increased accidents	Difficulty falling or staying asleep
Lack of energy	Nonrestorative sleep
Waking up too early	Sleep disturbances that produce next-day consequences

Related Factors

Refer to *Disturbed Sleep Pattern.*

Refer to *Disturbed Sleep Pattern*.

Goal

Refer to *Disturbed Sleep Pattern*.

Refer to *Disturbed Sleep Pattern*.

Interventions

- Have the client keep a sleep–awake diary for one month to include bedtime, arising time, difficulty getting sleep, number of awakenings (reason), and naps.
- Evaluate if there is a physiologic condition or medication that is interfering with sleep. Refer to Related Factors under Pathophysiologic and Treatment Related Factors under *Disturbed Sleep Pattern*. Refer to the primary care provider for management.
- Evaluate if a psychological state is interfering with sleep. Refer to Situational Related Factors. Refer to mental health professions.
- Determine if the lifestyle or life events are interfering with sleep. Refer to other nursing diagnoses if appropriate: *Grieving*, *Stress Overload*, *Ineffective Coping*, or *Risk-Prone Health Behavior*.

Refer to *Disturbed Sleep Pattern* for Interventions to Establish a Sleep Ritual or Routine

Sleep Deprivation

NANDA-I Definition

Prolonged periods without sleep (sustained natural, periodic suspension of relative unconsciousness)

Defining Characteristics

Refer to *Disturbed Sleep Pattern*.

Related Factors

Refer to *Disturbed Sleep Pattern*.

 Author's Note

This diagnostic label represents a situation in which the client's sleep is insufficient. It is difficult to differentiate this diagnosis from the others. Refer to *Disturbed Sleep Pattern* for interventions.

Goal/Interventions

Refer to *Disturbed Sleep Pattern*.

IMPAIRED SOCIAL INTERACTION

NANDA-I Definition

Insufficient or excessive quantity or ineffective quality of social exchange

Defining Characteristics*

Social isolation is a subjective state. Thus, the nurse must validate all inferences about a client's feelings of aloneness because the causes vary and people show their aloneness in different ways.

Discomfort in social situations

Dysfunctional interaction with others

Family report of changes in interaction (e.g., style, pattern)

Inability to communicate a satisfying sense of social engagement (e.g., belonging, caring, interest, shared history)

Inability to receive a satisfying sense of social engagement (e.g., belonging, caring, interest, shared history)

Use of unsuccessful social interaction behaviors

Related Factors

Impaired social interactions can result from a variety of situations and health problems related to the inability to establish and maintain rewarding relationships. Some common sources follow.

612   SECTION 1 • Nursing Diagnoses

Pathophysiologic

Related to embarrassment, limited physical mobility, or energy*
secondary to:

Loss of body function   Terminal illness
Loss of body part

Related to communication barriers secondary to:*

Hearing deficits   Chronic mental illness
Speech impediments   Visual deficits
Mental retardation

Treatment Related

Related to surgical disfigurement

*Related to therapeutic isolation**

Situational (Personal, Environmental)

Related to alienation from others secondary to:

Constant complaining   Disorganized thinking
High anxiety   Illogical ideas
Rumination   Dependent behavior
Impulsive behavior   Egocentric behavior
Overt hostility   Strong unpopular beliefs
Delusions   Emotional immaturity
Manipulative behaviors   Depressive behavior
Hallucinations   Aggressive responses
Mistrust or suspicion

Related to language/cultural barriers

Related to lack of social skills

Related to change in usual social patterns secondary to:

Divorce   Death
Relocation

Maturational

Child/Adolescent
Related to inadequate sensory stimulation

Related to altered appearance

Related to speech impediments

Adult
Related to loss of ability to practice vocation

Older Adult
Related to change in usual social patterns secondary to:
Death of spouse   Retirement
Functional deficits

 Author's Note

Social competence refers to a client's ability to interact effectively with others. Interpersonal relationships assist a client through life experiences, both positive and negative. Positive relationships with others require positive self-concept, social skills, social sensitivity, and acceptance of the need for independence. To interact satisfactorily with others, a client must acknowledge and accept his or her limitations and strengths (Maroni, 1989).

A client without positive mental health usually does not have social sensitivity and thus is uncomfortable with the interdependence necessary for effective social interactions. A client with poor self-concept may constantly sacrifice his or her needs for those of others or may always put personal needs before the needs of others.

The diagnosis *Impaired Social Interaction* describes a client who exhibits ineffective interactions with others. If extreme, prolonged, or both, this problem can lead to a diagnosis of *Social Isolation*. The nursing focus for *Impaired Social Interaction* is increasing the client's sensitivity to the needs of others and teaching reciprocity.

NOC

Family Functioning, Social Interaction Skills, Social Involvement

Goal

The client/family will report increased satisfaction in socialization, as evidenced by the following indicators:

- Identify problematic behavior that deters socialization.
- Substitute constructive behavior for disruptive social behavior (specify).
- Describe strategies to promote effective socialization.

NIC

Anticipatory Guidance, Behavior Modification, Family Integrity Promotion, Counseling, Behavior Management, Family Support, Self-Responsibility Facilitation

Interventions

Provide Support to Maintain Basic Social Skills and Reduce Social Isolation (See *Risk for Loneliness* or Further Interventions)

Provide an Individual, Supportive Relationship

- Assist the client to manage life stresses.
- Focus on present and reality.
- Help the client to identify how stress precipitates problems.
- Support healthy defenses.
- Help the client to identify alternative courses of action.
- Assist the client to analyze approaches that work best.

Provide Supportive Group Therapy

- Focus on the here and now.
- Establish group norms that discourage inappropriate behavior.
- Encourage testing of new social behavior.
- Use snacks or coffee to decrease anxiety during sessions.
- Model certain accepted social behaviors (e.g., respond to a friendly greeting instead of ignoring it).
- Foster development of relationships among members through self-disclosure and genuineness.
- Use questions and observations to encourage people with limited interaction skills.
- Encourage members to validate their perception with others.
- Identify strengths among members and ignore selected weaknesses.
- Activity groups and drop-in socialization centers can be used for some clients.
- Contact the client when he or she fails to attend a scheduled appointment, job interview, and so forth.
- Do not wait for the client to initiate participation.

Hold People Accountable for Their Own Actions

- Contact the client when he or she fails to attend a scheduled appointment, job interview, and so forth.
- Do not wait for the client to initiate participation.
- Treat clients as responsible citizens.
- Allow decision making, but outline limits as necessary.
- Do not allow clients to use their illness as an excuse for their behavior.
- Set consequences and enforce when necessary, including encounters with the law.
- Help client to see how his or her behaviors or attitudes contribute to their frequent interpersonal conflicts.

Provide for Development of Social Skills

- Identify the environment in which social interactions are impaired: living, learning, and working.
- Provide instruction in the environment where the client is expected to function, when possible (e.g., accompany to a job site, work with the client in his or her own residence).
- Develop an individualized social skill program. Examples of some social skills are grooming and personal hygiene, posture, gait, eye contact, beginning a conversation, listening, and ending a conversation. Include modeling, behavior rehearsal, and homework.
- Combine verbal instructions with demonstration and practice.
- Be firm in setting parameters of appropriate social behaviors, such as punctuality, attendance, managing illnesses with employers, and dress.
- Use the group as a method of discussing work-related problems.
- Use sheltered workshops and part-time employment depending on level at which success can best be achieved.
- Give positive feedback; make sure it is specific and detailed. Focus on no more than three behavioral connections at a time; too-lengthy feedback adds confusion and increases anxiety.
- Convey a "can-do" attitude.
- Role play aspects of social interactions (McFarland et al., 1996):
  - How to initiate a conversation
  - How to continue a conversation
  - How to terminate a conversation
  - How to refuse a request
  - How to ask for something
  - How to interview for a job
  - How to ask someone to participate in an activity (e.g., going to the movies)

Assist Family and Community Members in Understanding and Providing Support

- Provide facts concerning mental illness, treatment, and progress to family members. Gently help family accept the illness.
- Validate family members' feelings of frustration in dealing with daily problems.
- Provide guidance on overstimulating or understimulating environments.
- Allow families to discuss their feelings of guilt and how their behavior affects the client. Refer to a family support group, if available.

- Develop an alliance with family.
- Arrange for periodic respite care.

Explore Strategies for Handling Difficult Situations (e.g., Disrupted Communications, Altered Thoughts, Alcohol and Drug Use) (Stuart & Sundeen, 2002)

Refer to *Disabled Family Coping* or *Confusion* for Additional Interventions

Initiate Health Teaching and Referrals, as Indicated

- Teach the client (McFarland et al., 1996):
  - Responsibilities of role as client (making requests clearly known, participating in therapies)
  - To outline activities of the day and to focus on accomplishing them
  - How to approach others to communicate
  - To identify which interactions encourage others to give him or her consideration and respect
  - To identify how he or she can participate in formulating family roles and responsibility to comply
  - To recognize signs of anxiety and methods to relieve them
  - To identify positive behavior and to experience self-satisfaction in selecting constructive choices
- Refer to a variety of social agencies; however, one agency should maintain coordination and continuity (e.g., job training, anger management).
- Refer for supportive family therapy as indicated.
- Refer families to local self-help groups.
- Provide numbers for crisis intervention services.

Pediatric Interventions

If Impulse Control Is a Problem:

- Set firm, responsible limits.
- Do not lecture.
- State limits simply and back them up.
- Maintain routines.
- Limit play to one playmate to learn appropriate play skills (e.g., relative, adult, quiet child).
- Gradually increase number of playmates.
- Provide immediate and constant feedback.

Discuss Selective Parenting Skills

- Reward small increments of desired behavior.
- Contract appropriate age-related consequences (e.g., time out, loss of activity [use of car, bicycle]).

- Avoid harsh criticism.
- *Do not* disagree in front of child.
- Establish eye contact before giving instructions and ask child to repeat back what was said.
- Teach older child to self-monitor target behaviors and to develop self-reliance.

If Antisocial Behavior Is Present, Help to:

- Describe behaviors that interfere with socialization.
- Role play alternative responses.
- Limit social circle to a manageable size.
- Elicit peer feedback for positive and negative behavior.

Assist the Adolescent to Decrease Social Deficits

- Assertiveness
- Anger management
- Problem solving
- Refusal skills
- Stress management
- Clarification of values

SOCIAL ISOLATION

NANDA-I Definition

Aloneness experienced by the individual and perceived as imposed by others and as a negative or threatening state

Defining Characteristics

Social isolation is a subjective state. Thus, the nurse must validate all inferences concerning a client's feelings of aloneness because the causes vary and people show their aloneness in different ways.**

Absence of supportive family*

Seeks to be alone*

Shows behavior unaccepted by dominant culture*

Expressed feelings of aloneness imposed by others and/or rejection*

Inability to meet expectations of others*

Insecurity in public*

** This statement has been added by the author, Lynda Juall Carpenito, for clarity and usefulness.

Desire for more contact with people
Describes a lack of meaningful relationships
Uncommunicative*
Feeling of rejection
Projects hostility*
Withdrawn*
Sad, dull affect*
Poor eye contact
Preoccupied with own thoughts* and memories

Related Factors

A state of social isolation can result from a variety of situations and health problems that are related to a loss of established relationships or to a failure to generate these relationships. Some common sources include the following.

Pathophysiologic

Related to fear of rejection secondary to:
Obesity
Cancer (disfiguring surgery of head or neck, superstitions of others)
Physical handicaps (paraplegia, amputation, arthritis, hemiplegia)
Emotional handicaps (extreme anxiety, depression, paranoia, phobias)
Incontinence (embarrassment, odor)
Communicable diseases (AIDS, hepatitis)
Psychiatric illness (schizophrenia, bipolar affective disorder, personality disorders)

Situational (Personal, Environmental)

Related to death of a significant other

Related to divorce

Related to disfiguring appearance

Related to fear of rejection secondary to:
Obesity   Extreme poverty
Hospitalization or terminal   Unemployment
   illness (dying process)

Related to moving to another culture (e.g., unfamiliar language)

Related to loss of usual means of transportation

Related to history of unsatisfactory relationships secondary to:
Unacceptable social behavior   Delusional thinking
Drug abuse   Immature behavior
Alcohol abuse

Maturational

Child
Related to protective isolation or a communicable disease

Older Adult
Related to loss of usual social contacts

 Author's Note

In 1994, NANDA added a new diagnosis: *Risk for Loneliness*. Although this diagnosis is only in stage I of a four-stage developmental process, it more accurately adheres to the NANDA definition of "response to." Social isolation is not a response but a cause or be a contributing factor to loneliness. In addition, a client can experience loneliness even with many people around. This author recommends deleting *Social Isolation* from clinical use and using *Loneliness* or *Risk for Loneliness* instead.

CHRONIC SORROW

Definition

Cyclical, recurring, and potentially progressive pattern of pervasive sadness experienced (by parent, caregiver, individual with chronic illness or disability) in response to continual loss throughout the trajectory of an illness or disability (NANDA-I)

State in which a client experiences, or is at risk to experience, permanent pervasive psychic pain and sadness, variable in intensity, in response to a loved one forever changed by an event or condition and the ongoing loss of normalcy (Teel, 1991)

Defining Characteristics

Major (Must Be Present, One or More)

Lifelong episodic sadness to loss of a loved one or loss of normalcy in a loved one who is has been changed by an event or disability
Variable intensity

Expresses feelings that interfere with ability to reach highest
    level of personal and/or social well-being*
Negative feelings of variable intensity, periodic, recurrent*
Anger
Loneliness
Sadness
Frustration
Guilt
Self-blame
Fear
Overwhelmed
Emptiness
Helplessness
Confusion
Disappointment

Related Factors

Situational (Personal, Environmental)

*Related to the chronic loss of normalcy secondary to a child's or adult
child's condition*

Autism	Spina bifida
Severe scoliosis	Sickle cell disease
Chronic psychiatric condition	Type I diabetes mellitus
Down syndrome	Human immunodeficiency
Mental retardation	virus

Related to lifetime losses associated with infertility

*Related to ongoing losses associated with a degenerative condition
(e.g., multiple sclerosis, Alzheimer's disease)*

Related to loss of loved one

Related to losses associated with caring for a child with fatal illness

⟳ Author's Note

Olchansky identified *Chronic Sorrow* in 1962. Chronic sorrow differs
from grieving, which is time-limited and results in adaptation to the loss.
Chronic sorrow varies in intensity but persists as long as the client with
the disability or chronic condition lives (Burke et al., 1992). Chronic sorrow can also accompany the loss of a child and can occur in an individual
who suffers from a chronic disease that regularly impairs his or her ability to live a "normal life" (e.g., paraplegic, AIDS, sickle cell disease).
    Chronic sorrow can be described as an "ongoing funeral" because
there is no psychological closure or opportunity for resolution (Lindgren
et al., 1992; Northington, 2000).

Depression Level, Coping, Mood Equilibrium Acceptance: Health Status

Goal

The client will be assisted in anticipating events that can trigger heightened sadness, as evidenced by the following indicators:

- Express sadness.
- Discuss the loss(es) periodically.

NIC

Anticipatory Guidance, Coping Enhancement, Referral, Active Listening, Presence, Resiliency Promotion

Interventions

Explain Chronic Sorrow

- Normal response
- Focus on loss of normalcy
- Not time limited
- Episodic
- Persists throughout life

Encourage the Client to Share Feelings Since the Change (e.g., Birth of Child, Accident)

Promote Hopefulness (Hockenberry & Wilson, 2009)

- Advise of age-related health promotion needs.
- Provide anticipatory guidance for maturational stages (e.g., puberty).
- Discuss possible age-related self-care responsibilities.
- Advise how to negotiate self-care activities between parent and child.

Prepare the Client for Subsequent Crises Over the Life Span

- Gently encourage the client to share lost dreams or hopes.
- Assist the client to identify developmental milestones that will exacerbate the loss of normalcy (e.g., school play, sports, prom, dating).
- Clarify that feelings will fluctuate (intense, diminished) over the years, but the sorrow will not disappear.
- Advise client that these crises may feel like the first response to the "news."

Encourage Participation in Support Groups With Others Experiencing Chronic Sorrow and Expression of Grief

- Stress the importance of maintaining support systems and friendships.
- Share the difficulties of the following (Monsen, 1999):
  - Living worried
  - Treating the child like other children
  - Staying in the struggle

Acknowledge That Parent(s) Is the Child's Expert Caregiver (Melnyk et al., 2001)

- Elicit routines from the parents.
- Prepare the family for transition to another health care provider (e.g., child to adult providers).
- Educate the parents about specific procedures.

Link the Family With Appropriate Services (e.g., Home Health, Respite Counselor)

Refer to *Caregiver Role Strain* for Additional Interventions

SPIRITUAL DISTRESS

Spiritual Distress
Risk for Spiritual Distress
Impaired Religiosity
Risk for Impaired Religiosity

NANDA-I Definition

Impaired ability to experience and integrate meaning and purpose in life through connectedness with self, others, art, music, literature, nature, and/or a power greater than oneself

Defining Characteristics

Questions meaning of life, death, and suffering
Reports no sense of meaning and purpose in life
Lacks enthusiasm for life, feelings of joy, inner peace, or love
Demonstrates discouragement or despair
Feels a sense of emptiness
Experiences alienation from spiritual or religious community

Expresses need to reconcile with self, others, God, or creator

Presents with sudden interest in spiritual matters (reading spiritual or religious books, watching spiritual or religious programs on television)

Displays sudden changes in spiritual practices (rejection, neglect, doubt, fanatical devotion)

Verbalizes that family, loved ones, peers, or health care providers opposed spiritual beliefs or practices

Questions credibility of religion or spiritual belief system

Requests assistance for a disturbance in spiritual beliefs or religious practice

Related Factors

Pathophysiologic

Related to challenge in spiritual health or separation from spiritual ties secondary to:

Hospitalization	Trauma
Pain	Debilitating disease
Terminal illness	Miscarriage, stillbirth
Loss of body part or function	

Treatment Related

Related to conflict between (specify prescribed regimen) and beliefs:

Abortion	Medications
Isolation	Dietary restrictions
Surgery	Medical procedures
Blood transfusion	Dialysis

Situational (Personal, Environmental)

Related to death* or illness of significant other

Related to embarrassment of expressions of spirituality or religion, such as prayers, meditation, or other rituals

Related to barriers to practicing spiritual rituals:
Restrictions of intensive care
Lack of privacy
Unavailability of special foods/diet or ritual objects
Confinement to bed or room

Related to spiritual or religious beliefs opposed by family, peers, health care providers

Related to divorce, separation from loved one, or other perceived loss

Author's Note

Wellness represents a response to a client's potential for personal growth, involving use of all of a client's resources (social, psychological, cultural, environmental, spiritual, and physiologic). Nurses profess to care for the whole client, but several studies report that they commonly avoid addressing the spiritual dimension of clients, families, and communities (Kendrick & Robinson, 2000; Puchalski & Ferrell, 2010; Swift, Calcutawalla, & Elliott, 2007).

To promote positive spirituality with clients and families, the nurse must possess spiritual self-knowledge. For the nurse, self-evaluation must precede assessment of spiritual concerns, and assessment of spiritual health should be confined to the context of nursing. The nurse can assist people with spiritual concerns or distress by providing resources for spiritual help, by listening nonjudgmentally, and by providing opportunities to meet spiritual needs (O'Brien, 2010; Wright, 2004).

Spirituality and religiousness are two different concepts. Burkhart and Solari-Twadell (2001) define spirituality as the "ability to experience and integrate meaning and self; others, art, music, literature, nature, or a power greater than oneself." Religiousness is "the ability to exercise participation in the beliefs of a particular denomination of faith community and related rituals" (Burkhart & Solari-Twadell, 2001). Although the spiritual dimension of human wholeness is always present, it may or may not exist within the context of religious traditions or practices.

Impaired Religiousness was approved by NANDA in 2004. This diagnosis can be used for *Spiritual Distress* when a client has a barrier to practicing his or her religious rituals that the nurse can assist by decreasing or removing. *Impaired Religiosity* would be appropriate.

NOC
Hope, Spiritual Well-Being

Goal

The client will find meaning and purpose in life, even during illness, as evidenced by the following indicators:

- The client expresses his or her feelings related to beliefs and spirituality.
- The client describes his or her spiritual belief system as it relates to illness.
- The client finds meaning and comfort in religious or spiritual practice.

Spiritual Growth Facilitation, Hope Instillation, Active Listening, Presence, Emotional Support, Spiritual Support

Interventions

Assess for Causative and Contributing Factors

- Failure of spiritual beliefs to provide an explanation or comfort during a crisis of illness/suffering/impending death
- Doubting quality or strength of own faith to deal with current crisis
- Anger toward God or spiritual beliefs for allowing or causing illness/suffering/death

Eliminate or Reduce Causative and Contributing Factors, If Possible

Feeling Threatened and Vulnerable Because of Symptoms or Possible Death

- Inform clients and families about the importance of finding meaning in illness.
- Suggest using prayer, imagery, and meditation to reduce anxiety and provide hope and a sense of control.

Failure of Spiritual Beliefs to Provide Explanation or Comfort During Crisis of Illness/Suffering/Impending Death

- Communicate your concern seriously by being available to listen to feelings, questions, and so forth.
- Give "permission" to discuss spiritual matters with the nurse by bringing up the subject of spiritual welfare, if necessary.
- Use questions about past beliefs and spiritual experiences to assist the client in putting this life event into wider perspective.
- Assist the client in beginning the problem-solving process and moving toward new spiritual understandings, if necessary.
- Offer to contact the usual or a new spiritual leader.
- Offer to pray/meditate/read with the client if you are comfortable with this, or arrange for another member of the health care team if more appropriate.
- Provide uninterrupted quiet time for prayer/reading/meditation on spiritual concerns.

Doubting Quality of Own Faith to Deal With Current Illness/Suffering/Death

- Be available and willing to listen when client expresses self-doubt, guilt, or other negative feelings.
- Silence, touch, or both may be useful in communicating the nurse's presence and support during times of doubt or despair.

- Suggest the process of "life review" to identify past sources of strength or spiritual support.
- Suggest guided imagery or meditation to reinforce faith/beliefs.
- Offer to contact usual or new spiritual leader.

Anger Toward God or Spiritual Beliefs for Allowing or Causing Illness/Suffering/Death

- Express to the client that anger toward God is a common reaction to illness/suffering/death.
- Help the client recognize and discuss feelings of anger.
- Allow client to problem solve to find ways to express and relieve anger.
- Offer to contact the usual spiritual leader.
- Offer to contact another spiritual support person (e.g., pastoral care, hospital chaplain) if the client cannot share feelings with the usual spiritual leader.

Listening Skills (Puchalski & Ferrill, 2010)

- Create an environment of trust.
- Be open to listening to the client's story, not just the medical facts.
- Listen for the content, emotion and manner, and spiritual meanings.
- Be fully present.
- Communicate acceptance of various spiritual beliefs and practices.
- Convey nonjudgmental attitude.
- Acknowledge importance of spiritual needs.
- Express willingness of health care team to help in meeting spiritual needs.
  - Maintain diet with religious restrictions when not detrimental to health.
  - Encourage spiritual rituals not detrimental to health.
  - Provide opportunity for individual to pray with others or be read to by members of own religious group or a member of the health care team who feels comfortable with these activities.

Pediatric Interventions

- Encourage children to maintain bedtime or before-meal prayer rituals.
- If compatible with the child's religious beliefs:
  - Share religious picture books and other religious articles.
  - Consult with the family for appropriate books or objects (e.g., medals, statues).

- Explore the child's feelings regarding illness as punishment for wrongdoing (Hockenberry & Wilson, 2009).
- Discuss if being sick has changed his or her beliefs (e.g., prayer requests).
- Support an adolescent who may be struggling for understanding of spiritual teachings.
- For parental conflict about treatment of child:
  - If parents refuse treatment of child, encourage consideration of alternative methods of therapy (e.g., use of Christian Science nurses and practitioners; special surgeons and techniques for surgery without blood transfusions); support individual making informed decision even if decision conflicts with own values.
  - If treatment is still refused, physician or hospital administrator may obtain court order appointing temporary guardian to consent to treatment.
  - Call spiritual leader to support parents (and possibly child).
  - Encourage expression of negative feelings.

Risk for Spiritual Distress

NANDA-I Definition

At risk for an impaired ability to experience and integrate meaning and purpose in life through connectedness with self, others, art, music, literature, nature, and/or a power greater than oneself

Risk Factors

Refer to *Spiritual Distress*.

Author's Note

Refer to *Spiritual Distress*.

NOC

Refer to *Spiritual Distress*.

Goal

The client will find meaning and purpose in life, including during illness, as evidenced by the following indicators:

- Practice spiritual rituals.
- Express comfort with beliefs.

Refer to *Spiritual Distress*.

Interventions

Refer to *Spiritual Distress*.

Impaired Religiosity

NANDA-I Definition

Impaired ability to exercise reliance on beliefs and/or participate in rituals of a particular faith tradition

Defining Characteristics

Individuals experience distress because of difficulty with adhering to prescribed religious rituals such as:
  Religious ceremonies
  Dietary regulations
  Certain clothing
  Prayer
  Request to worship
  Holiday observances
  Separation from faith community*
  Emotional distress regarding religious beliefs, religious social network, or both
  Need to reconnect with previous belief patterns and customs
  Questioning of religious belief patterns and customs*

Related Factors

Pathophysiologic

*Related to sickness/illness**

Related to suffering

*Related to pain**

Situational (Personal, Environmental)

Related to personal crisis secondary to activity*

*Related to fear of death**

Related to embarrassment at practicing spiritual rituals

Related to barriers to practicing spiritual rituals

Intensive care restrictions	Lack of availability of special
Confinement to bed or the	foods/diets
room	Hospitalization
Lack of privacy	

Related to crisis within the faith community, which causes distress in the believer

 Author's Note

Refer to *Spiritual Distress.*

 NOC

Spiritual Well-Being

Goal

The client will express satisfaction with ability to practice or exercise beliefs and practices, as evidenced by the following indicators:

- Continue spiritual practices not detrimental to health.
- Express decreasing feelings of guilt and anxiety.

NIC

Spiritual Support

Interventions

Explore Whether the Client Desires to Engage in an Allowable Religious or Spiritual Practice or Ritual; If So, Provide Opportunities To Do So

Express Your Understanding and Acceptance of the Importance of the Client's Religious or Spiritual Beliefs and Practices

Assess for Causative and Contributing Factors

- Hospital or nursing home environment
- Limitations related to disease process or treatment regimen (e.g., cannot kneel to pray because of traction; prescribed diet differs from usual religious diet)
- Fear of imposing on or antagonizing medical and nursing staff with requests for spiritual rituals

- Embarrassment over spiritual beliefs or customs (especially common in adolescents)
- Separation from articles, texts, or environment of spiritual significance
- Lack of transportation to spiritual place or service
- Spiritual leader unavailable because of emergency or lack of time

Eliminate or Reduce Causative and Contributing Factors, If Possible

Limitations Imposed by the Hospital or Nursing Home Environment

- Provide privacy and quiet as needed for daily prayer, visit by spiritual leader, and spiritual reading and contemplation.
  - Pull the curtains or close the door.
  - Turn off the television and radio.
  - Ask the desk to hold calls, if possible.
  - Note the spiritual interventions on Kardex and include in the care plan.
- Contact the spiritual leader to clarify practices and perform religious rites or services, if desired.
  - Communicate with the spiritual leader concerning the client's condition.
  - Address Roman Catholic, Orthodox, and Episcopal priests as "Father," other Christian ministers as "Pastor," and Jewish rabbis as "Rabbi."
- Prevent interruption during the visit, if possible.
- Offer to provide a table or stand covered with a clean white cloth.
- Inform the client about religious services and materials available within the institution.

Limitations Related to Disease Process or Treatment Regimen

- Encourage spiritual rituals not detrimental to health (see Box II.4):
  - Assist clients with physical limitations in prayer and spiritual observances (e.g., help to hold rosary; help to kneeling position, if appropriate).
  - Assist in habits of personal cleanliness.
  - Avoid shaving if beard is of spiritual significance.
  - Allow the client to wear religious clothing or jewelry whenever possible.
  - Make special arrangements for burial of respected limbs or body organs.
  - Allow the family or spiritual leader to perform ritual care of the body.
  - Make arrangements as needed for other important spiritual rituals (e.g., circumcisions).

- Maintain diet with spiritual restrictions when not detrimental to health (see Box II.4):
  - Consult with a dietitian.
  - Allow fasting for short periods, if possible.
  - Change the therapeutic diet as necessary.
  - Have family or friends bring in special food, if possible.
  - Have members of the spiritual group supply meals to the client at home.
  - Be as flexible as possible in serving methods, times of meals, and so forth.

Fear of Imposing or Embarrassment
- Communicate acceptance of various spiritual beliefs and practices.
- Convey a nonjudgmental, respectful attitude.
- Acknowledge the importance of spiritual needs.
- Express the willingness of the health care team to help the client meet spiritual needs.
- Provide privacy and ensure confidentiality.

Separation from Articles, Texts, or Environment of Spiritual Significance
- Question the client about missing religious or spiritual articles or reading material.
- Obtain missing items from the clergy in the hospital, spiritual leader, family, or members of the spiritual group.
- Treat these articles and books with respect.
- Allow the client to keep spiritual articles and books within reach as much as possible or where they can be easily seen.
- Protect articles from loss or damage (e.g., a medal pinned to a gown can be lost in the laundry).
- Recognize that articles without overt religious meaning may have spiritual significance for the client (e.g., wedding band).
- Use spiritual texts in large print, in Braille, or on tape when appropriate and available.
- Provide an opportunity for the client to pray with others or be read to by members of his or her own religious group or a member of the health care team who feels comfortable with these activities.

Suggested Readings
1. Jews and Seventh-Day Adventists would find Psalms 23, 34, 42, 63, 71, 103, 121, and 127 appropriate.
2. Christians would also appreciate I Corinthians 13, Matthew 5:3–11, Romans 12, and the Lord's Prayer.

Lack of Transportation
- Take the client to the chapel or quiet environment on hospital grounds.
- Arrange transportation to the church or synagogue for the client at home.
- Provide access to spiritual programming on radio and television when appropriate.

Spiritual Leader Unavailable Because of Emergency or Lack of Time
- Baptize the critically ill newborn of Greek Orthodox, Episcopal, or Roman Catholic parents.
- Perform other mandatory spiritual rituals, if possible.
- Offer a visit from the hospital spiritual care professional.

Risk for Impaired Religiosity

NANDA-I Definition

At risk for an impaired ability to exercise reliance on religious beliefs and/or participate in rituals of a particular faith tradition

Related Factors

Refer to *Impaired Religiosity*.

Spiritual Well-Being

Goal

The client will express continued satisfaction with religious activities, as evidenced by the following indicators:

- Continue to practice religious rituals.
- Described increased comfort after assessment.

Spiritual Support

Interventions

Refer to *Impaired Religiosity* for interventions.

STRESS OVERLOAD

NANDA-I Definition

Excessive amounts and types of demands that require action

Defining Characteristics

Reports excessive situational stress (e.g., rates stress level as 7 or above on a 10-point scale)*

Reports negative impact from stress (e.g., physical symptoms, psychological distress, feeling of being sick or of going to get sick)*

Physiologic

Headaches
Indigestion
Sleep difficulties

Restlessness
Fatigue

Emotional

Crying
Increased anger*
Edginess
Increased impatience*
Nervousness

Easily upset
Overwhelmed
Feeling sick
Feeling of pressure*
Feeling of tension*

Cognitive

Memory loss
Constant worry
Forgetfulness

Loss of humor
Problems with decision making*
Trouble thinking clearly

Behavioral

Isolation
Intolerance
Lack of intimacy
Compulsive eating

Excessive smoking
Resentment
Difficulty functioning*

Related Factors

The Related Factors of *Stress Overload*; one person can be influenced by multiple coexisting stressors that can be pathophysiologic, maturational, treatment related, situational, environmental, personal, or all of these.

Pathophysiologic

Related to coping with:
Acute illness (myocardial infarction, fractured hip)
Chronic illness* (arthritis, depression, chronic obstructive
    pulmonary disorder)
Terminal illness*
New diagnosis (cancer, genital herpes, HIV, multiple sclerosis,
    diabetes mellitus)
Disfiguring condition

Situational (Personal, Environmental)

Related to actual or anticipated loss of a significant other secondary to:

Death, dying	Divorce
Moving	Military duty

Related to coping with:

Dying	Assault
War	

Related to actual or perceived change in socioeconomic status secondary to:

Unemployment	Foreclosure
New job	Destruction of personal
Promotion	property
Illness	

Related to coping with:

Family violence*	Substance abuse
New family member	Relationship problems

Maturation

Related to coping with:

Retirement	Loss of residence
Financial changes	Functional losses

Author's Note

This diagnosis represents a client in an overwhelming situation influenced by multiple varied stressors. If stress overload is not reduced, the client will deteriorate and may be in danger of injury and illness.

NOC

Well–Being: Health Beliefs, Anxiety Reduction, Coping, Knowledge: Health Promotion, Knowledge: Health Resources

Goal

The client will verbalize intent to change two behaviors to decrease or manage stressors, as evidenced by the following indicators:

- Identify stressors that can be controlled and those that cannot.
- Identify one successful behavior change to increase stress management.
- Identify one behavior to reduce or eliminate that will increase successful stress management.

Anxiety Reduction, Behavioral Modification, Exercise Promotion

Interventions

Assist the Client to Recognize His or Her Thoughts, Feelings, Actions, and Physiologic Responses

Teach the Client How to Break the Stress Cycle in a Traffic Jam and How to Decrease Heart Rate, Respirations, and Strong Feelings of Anger (Edelman & Mandle, 2010)

- Purposefully distract yourself by thinking of something pleasant.
- Engage in a diversional activity.
- Initiate relaxation breaking: inhale through nose for 4 seconds.
- Refer to resources to learn relaxation techniques such as audiotapes, printed material, and yoga.

Ask the Client to List One or Two Changes They Would Like to Make in the Next Week

- Diet (eat one vegetable a day)
- Exercise (walk one to two blocks each day)

If Sleep Disturbances Are Present, Refer to *Insomnia*

- Ask what activity brings the client feelings of peace, joy, and happiness. Ask them to incorporate one of these activities each week.

If Spiritual Needs Are Identified as Deficient, Refer to *Spiritual Distress*

- Ask the client what is important, and if change is needed in their life.

Assist the Client to Set Realistic Goals to Achieve a More Balanced Health-Promoting Lifestyle (Wells-Federman, 2000)

- What is most important?
- What aspects of your life would you like to change most?

- What is the first step?
- When?

Initiate Health Teaching and Referrals, as Necessary

- If client is engaged in substance or alcohol abuse, refer for drug and alcohol abuse.
- If client has severe depression or anxiety, refer for professional counseling.
- If family functioning is disabled, refer for family counseling.

RISK FOR SUDDEN INFANT DEATH SYNDROME

NANDA-I Definition

At risk for sudden death of an infant under 1 year of age

Risk Factors

There is no single risk factor. Several risk factors combined may be contributory (refer to Related Factors).

Related Factors[†]

Pathophysiologic

Related to increased vulnerability secondary to:

Cyanosis	Low birth weight*
Hypothermia	Small for gestational age*
Fever	Prematurity *
Poor feeding	Low Apgar score (less than 7)
Irritability	History of diarrhea, vomiting,
Respiratory distress	or listlessness 2 weeks before
Tachycardia	death
Tachypnea	

Related to increased vulnerability secondary to prenatal maternal:

Anemia*	Poor weight gain
Urinary tract infection	Sexually transmitted infections

[†] McMillan et al., 1999.

Situational (Personal, Environmental)

Related to increased vulnerability secondary to maternal:

Cigarette smoking*
Drug use during pregnancy
Lack of breastfeeding*
Inadequate prenatal care*
Low educational levels*

Single mother*
Multiparity with first
Young age (younger than 20)*
Young age during pregnancy*

Related to increased vulnerability secondary to:

Crowded living conditions*
Sleeping on stomach*
Poor family financial status

Cold environment
Low socioeconomic status

Related to increased vulnerability secondary to:

Male gender*
Native Americans*
Multiple births
African descent*

Previous sudden infant death syndrome (SIDS) death in family

NOC

Knowledge: Maternal–Child Health, Risk Control: Tobacco Use, Risk Control, Knowledge: Infant Safety

Goal

The caregiver will reduce or eliminate risk factors that are modifiable, as evidenced by the following indicators:

- Position the infant on the back or lying on the side.
- Eliminate smoking in the home, near the infant, and during pregnancy.
- Participate in prenatal and newborn medical care.
- Improve maternal health (e.g., treat anemia, promote optimal nutrition).
- Enroll in drug and alcohol programs, if indicated.

NIC

Teaching: Infant Safety, Risk Identification

Interventions

Explain SIDS to Caregivers and Identify Risk Factors Present

Reduce or Eliminate Risk Factors That Can Be Modified

Determine If Home Cardiorespiratory Monitoring Is Indicated; Consult With Pediatrician or Neonatal/Pediatric Nurse Practitioner (Hockenberry & Wilson, 2009)

- Teach parents to focus on the infant when the alarm sounds, not on the machine.
- Teach parents to assess:
  - Infant's color (pink?)
  - Infant's breathing

Teach Environmental Practices to Reduce SIDS

- Position infant on his or her back.
- Avoid overheating the infant during sleep.
- Avoid soft bedding (e.g., mattresses).
- Avoid pillows.
- Avoid sleeping with the infant (Anderson, 2000).
- Avoid tobacco smoke.

Initiate Health Teaching and Referrals, as Indicated

- Provide instructions on use of the home monitor and cardio-pulmonary resuscitation if appropriate.
- Refer the client to drug and alcohol treatment programs, as indicated.
- Discuss strategies to stop smoking (refer to index—*smoking*).
- Provide emergency numbers, as indicated.
- Refer to social agencies, as indicated.

DELAYED SURGICAL RECOVERY

NANDA-I Definition

Extension of the number of postoperative days required to initiate and perform activities that maintain, life, health, and well-being

Defining Characteristics

Postpones resumption of work/employment activities*
Requires help to complete self-care*
Loss of appetite with or without nausea*
Fatigue*
Perceives that more time is needed to recover*
Evidence of interrupted healing of surgical area
    (e.g., red, indurated, draining, immobilized)*

Difficulty moving about*
Venous obstruction/pooling

 Author's Note

This diagnosis represents a client who has not achieved recovery from a surgical procedure within the expected time. Based on the defining characteristics from NANDA-I, some confusion exists regarding the difference between defining characteristics (signs and symptoms) and related factors. A possible use of this diagnosis is as a risk diagnosis. Persons who are high risk for *Delayed Surgical Recovery*, for example, the obese, those with diabetes mellitus, or cancer, could by identified. Interventions to prevent this state could be implemented. The diagnosis has not been developed sufficiently for clinical use. This author recommends using other nursing diagnoses, such as *Self-Care Deficit*, *Acute Pain*, or *Imbalanced Nutrition*.

INEFFECTIVE TISSUE PERFUSION**

Ineffective Tissue Perfusion

Risk for Decreased Cardiac Tissue Perfusion

Risk for Ineffective Cerebral Tissue Perfusion

Risk for Ineffective Gastrointestinal Tissue Perfusion

Ineffective Peripheral Tissue Perfusion

Risk for Ineffective Peripheral Tissue Perfusion

Risk for Peripheral Neurovascular Dysfunction

Risk for Ineffective Renal Perfusion

Definition

Decrease in oxygen resulting in failure to nourish tissues at capillary level

 Author's Note

The use of any *Ineffective Tissue Perfusion* diagnosis other than *Peripheral* merely provides new labels for medical diagnoses, labels that do not describe the nursing focus or accountability.

** This diagnosis presently not on the NANDA-I list has been added by this author for clarity and usefulness.

NANDA-I approved the diagnosis *Ineffective Tissue Perfusion* in 1980. It does not conform to the NANDA-I definition approved in 1990. When using these diagnoses, nurses cannot be accountable for prescribing the interventions for outcome achievement. Instead of using *Ineffective Tissue Perfusion*, the nurse should focus on the nursing diagnoses and collaborative problems applicable because of altered renal, cardiac, cerebral, pulmonary, or gastrointestinal (GI) tissue perfusion. Refer to http://thePoint.lww.com/CarpenitoHB14e for specific collaborative problems for example: *RC of Increased Intracranial Pressure, RC of GI Bleeding.*

Ineffective Peripheral Tissue Perfusion can be a clinically useful nursing diagnosis if used to describe chronic arterial or venous insufficiency or potential thrombophlebitis. (In contrast, acute embolism and thrombophlebitis represent collaborative problems.) A nurse focusing on preventing thrombophlebitis in a postoperative client would write the diagnosis *Risk for Ineffective Peripheral Tissue Perfusion related to postoperative immobility and dehydration.*

Risk for Decreased Cardiac Tissue Perfusion

NANDA-I Definition

Risk for a decrease in cardiac (coronary) circulation

Risk Factors*

Birth control pills* (medication side effect of combination pills)**
Cardiac surgery* (treatment)
Cardiac tamponade* (clinical emergency)
Coronary artery spasm* (clinical emergency)
Diabetes mellitus* (medical diagnosis with multiple complications with associated modifiable risk lifestyles)
Drug abuse* (clinical situations with multiple complications)
Elevated C-reactive protein* (positive laboratory test)
Family history of coronary artery disease* (factor with associated modifiable risk lifestyles)
Hyperlipidemia* (medical diagnosis with associated modifiable risk lifestyles)

** Text in parentheses has been added by author.

Hypertension* (medical diagnosis with multiple complications with associated modifiable risk lifestyles)

Hypoxemia* (complication)

Hypovolemia* (complication)

Hypoxia* (complication)

Lack of knowledge of modifiable risk factors (e.g., smoking, sedentary lifestyle, obesity)

(These relate to nursing diagnoses of *Risk Prone Health Behavior* and/or *Ineffective Self-Health Management*)

 Author's Note

This NANDA-I nursing diagnosis represents a collection of risk factors that have different clinical implications. Some include a collection of physiological complications that relate to the situation and can be labeled as *Risk for Complications of Cardiac Surgery*, *RC of Acute Coronary Syndrome*, and *RC of Diabetes Mellitus*. Some are single complications such as *RC of Hypovolemia* and *RC of Hypoxia*.

For example, *Risk for Complications of Cocaine Abuse* would describe monitoring and management of complications such as cardiac/vascular shock, seizures, coma, respiratory insufficiency, stroke, and hyperpyrexia. These complications are different than *Risk for Complications of Alcohol Abuse* which describes the monitoring and management of complications of delirium tremens, seizures, autonomic hyperactivity, hypovolemia, hypoglycemia, alcohol hallucinosis, and cardio/vascular shock.

Some complications are medical emergencies such as cardiac tamponade, coronary artery spasm or occlusion, all of which have protocols for medical interventions.

If a diagnosis is needed for this clinical situation, use *Risk for Complications of Medication Therapy Adverse Effects*, specifically, *Risk for Complications of Oral Combination Contraception Therapy*.

Outcomes/Interventions

Refer to *Risk for Complications of Cardiovascular Dysfunction* on http://thePoint.lww.com/CarpenitoHB14e for specific interventions for cardiovascular complications. If the focus is on modifying one's lifestyle, refer to *Sedentary Lifestyle*, *Risk-Prone Health Behavior*, or *Ineffective Self-Health Management* in Section 1.

Risk for Ineffective Cerebral Tissue Perfusion

NANDA-I Definition

At risk for a decrease in cerebral tissue circulation that may compromise health

Risk Factors*

Abnormal partial thromboplastin time
Abnormal prothrombin time
Akinetic left ventricular segment
Aortic atherosclerosis
Arterial dissection
Atrial fibrillation
Atrial myxoma
Brain Tumor
Carotid stenosis
Cerebral aneurysm
Coagulopathies (e.g., sickle cell anemia)
Dilated cardiomyopathy
Disseminated intravascular coagulation
Embolism
Head trauma
Hypercholesterolemia
Hypertension
Endocarditis
Left atrial appendage thrombosis
Mechanical prosthetic valve
Mitral stenosis
Neoplasm of the brain
Recent myocardial infarction
Sick sinus syndrome
Substance abuse
Thrombolytic therapy
Treatment-related side effects (cardiopulmonary bypass, pharmaceutical agents)

 Author's Note

This NANDA-I nursing diagnosis represents a collection of risk factors that have very different clinical implications. Some are physiologic complications that are related to a medical diagnosis or treatment and can be labeled as *Risk for Complications of Head Trauma*, *RC of Brain Tumor*, or *RC of Thrombolytic Therapy*. These clinical situations have both nursing diagnoses and collaborative problems that require interventions.

For example, *Risk for Complications of Cranial Surgery* would have the following collaborative problems:

• *RC of Increase Intracranial Pressure*
• *RC of Hemorrhage, Hypovolemia/Shock*
• *RC of Thromboembolism*
• *RC of Cranial Nerve Dysfunction*
• *RC of Cardiac Dysrhythmias*

- *RC of Seizures*
- *RC of Sensory/Motor Alterations*

Nursing diagnoses associated with this clinical situation:**

- *Anxiety to impending surgery and fear of outcomes*
- *Acute Pain related to compression/displacement of brain tissue and increased intracranial pressure*
- *Risk for Ineffective Self Heath Management related to insufficient knowledge of wound care signs and symptoms of complications, restrictions and follow-up care*

Goals/Interventions

Refer to http://thePoint.lww.com/CarpenitoHB14e for specific collaborative problems under *Risk for Complications of Neurologic Dysfunction*.

Risk for Ineffective Gastrointestinal Tissue Perfusion

NANDA-I Definition

At risk for decrease in gastrointestinal circulation

Risk Factors*

Abdominal aortic aneurysm
Abdominal compartment syndrome
Abnormal partial thromboplastin time
Abnormal prothrombin time
Acute gastrointestinal bleed
Acute gastrointestinal hemorrhage
Age >60 years
Anemia
Coagulopathies (e.g., sickle cell anemia)
Diabetes mellitus
Disseminated intravascular coagulation
Female gender

** For more specific care plans with nursing interventions/rationales and outcomes for clinical situations, such as medical diagnoses (e.g., acute coronary syndrome, hypertension, stroke), surgical procedures (e.g., coronary bypass surgery), therapy treatments (e.g., anticoagulant therapy), pacemaker insertion, and 70 other situations refer to Carpenito-Moyet, L. J. (2009). *Nursing Care Plans and Documentation* (5th ed.). Philadelphia, PA: Lippincott, Williams & Wilkins.

Gastric paresis (e.g., diabetes mellitus)
Gastrointestinal disease (e.g., duodenal or gastric ulcer, ischemic colitis, ischemic pancreatitis)
Hemodynamic instability
Liver dysfunction
Myocardial infarction
Poor left ventricular performance
Renal failure
Stroke
Treatment-related side effects (e.g., cardiopulmonary bypass, medications, anesthesia, gastric surgery)
Vascular disease (e.g., peripheral vascular disease, aortoiliac occlusive disease)

 Author's Note

This diagnosis is too general for clinical use because it represents a variety of physiologic complications related to GI perfusion. These complications are collaborative problems and should be separated to more specific complications as:

• *RC of GI Bleeding*
• *RC of Paralytic Ileus*
• *RC of Hypovolemia/Shock*

Goals/Interventions

Refer to http://thePoint.lww.com/CarpenitoHB14e for goals and interventions for Risk *for Complications of GI Bleeding or Paralytic Ileus or Hypovolemia/Shock.*

Ineffective Peripheral Tissue Perfusion

NANDA-I Definition

Decrease in blood circulation to the periphery that may compromise health

Defining Characteristics

Major (Must Be Present, One or More)

Presence of one of the following types:

Claudication (arterial)*
Aching pain (arterial or venous)

Rest pain (arterial)
Diminished or absent arterial pulses* (arterial)
Skin color changes*
Pallor (arterial)
Reactive hyperemia (arterial)
Cyanosis (venous)
Skin temperature changes
   Cooler (arterial)
   Warmer (venous)
Decreased blood pressure (arterial)
Capillary refill longer than 3 seconds (arterial)*

Minor (May Be Present)

Edema* (venous)
Change in sensory function
   (arterial)
Change in motor function
   (arterial)

Trophic tissue changes
   (arterial)
Hard, thick nails
Loss of hair
Nonhealing wound

Related Factors

Pathophysiologic

Related to compromised blood flow secondary to:
Vascular disorders
   Arteriosclerosis
   Raynaud's disease/syndrome
   Arterial thrombosis
   Sickle cell crisis
   Rheumatoid arthritis
   Leriche's syndrome
   Aneurysm
Diabetes mellitus
Hypotension
Blood dyscrasias
Renal failure
Cancer/tumor

   Buerger's disease
   Collagen vascular disease
   Alcoholism
   Venous hypertension
   Varicosities
   Deep vein thrombosis
   Cirrhosis

Treatment Related

Related to immobilization

Related to presence of invasive lines

Related to pressure sites/constriction (elastic compression bandages, stockings, restraints)

Related to blood vessel trauma or compression

Situational (Personal, Environmental)

Related to pressure of enlarging uterus on pelvic vessels

Related to pressure of enlarged abdomen on pelvic vessels

Related to vasoconstricting effects of tobacco

Related to decreased circulating volume secondary to dehydration

Related to dependent venous pooling

Related to hypothermia

Related to pressure of muscle mass secondary to weight lifting

 Author's Note

See *Ineffective Peripheral Tissue Perfusion.*

NOC

Sensory Functions; Cutaneous, Tissue Integrity, Tissue perfusion: Peripheral

Goal

The individual will report a decrease in pain as evidenced by the following indicators:

- Define peripheral vascular problem in own words.
- Identify factors that improve peripheral circulation.
- Identify necessary lifestyle changes.
- Identify medical regimen, diet, medications, activities that promote vasodilation.
- Identify factors that inhibit peripheral circulation.
- State when to contact physician or health care professional.

NIC

Peripheral Sensation Management, Circulatory Care: Venous Insufficiency, Circulatory Care: Arterial Insufficiency, Positioning, Exercise Promotion

Interventions

Assess Causative and Contributing Factors

- Underlying disease.
- Inhibited arterial blood flow.
- Inhibited venous blood flow.
- Fluid volume excess or deficit.

- Hypothermia or vasoconstriction.
- Activities related to symptom/sign onset.

Promote Factors That Improve Arterial Blood Flow

- Keep extremity in a dependent position.
- Reduce risk for trauma:
  - Change positions at least every hour.
  - Avoid leg crossing.
  - Reduce external pressure points (inspect shoes daily for rough lining).
  - Avoid sheepskin heel protectors (they increase heel pressure and pressure across dorsum of foot).
  - Encourage range-of-motion exercises.
  - Discuss smoking cessation (see *Ineffective Health Maintenance related to tobacco use*).

Promote Factors That Improve Venous Blood Flow

- Elevate extremity above the level of the heart (may be contraindicated if severe cardiac or respiratory disease is present).
- Avoid standing or sitting with legs dependent for long periods.
- Consider the use of elastic compression stockings.
- Teach client to:
  - Avoid pillows behind the knees or Gatch bed, which is elevated at the knees.
  - Avoid leg crossing.
  - Change positions, move extremities, or wiggle fingers and toes every hour.
  - Avoid garters and tight elastic stockings above the knees.
  - Measure baseline circumference of calves and thighs if the client is at risk for deep venous thrombosis, or if it is suspected.

Plan a Daily Walking Program

- Refer to *Sedentary Lifestyle* for specific interventions.

Initiate Health Teaching, as Indicated

- Teach client to
  - Avoid long car or plane rides (get up and walk around at least every hour).
  - Keep dry skin lubricated (cracked skin eliminates the physical barrier to infection).
  - Wear warm clothing during cold weather.
  - Wear cotton or wool socks.
  - Use gloves or mittens if hands are exposed to cold (including home freezers).
  - Avoid dehydration in warm weather.

- Give special attention to feet and toes:
  - Wash feet and dry well daily.
  - Do not soak feet.
  - Avoid harsh soaps or chemicals (including iodine) on feet.
  - Keep nails trimmed and filed smooth.
- Inspect feet and legs daily for injuries and pressure points.
- Wear clean socks.
- Wear shoes that offer support and fit comfortably.
- Inspect the inside of shoes daily for rough lining.

Explain the Relation of Certain Risk Factors to the Development of Atherosclerosis

- Smoking
  - Vasoconstriction
  - Elevated blood pressure
  - Decreased oxygenation of the blood
  - Increased lipidemia
  - Increased platelet aggregation
- Hypertension/hyperlipidemia
- Sedentary lifestyle
- Excess weight (greater than 10% of ideal)
- Refer to community resources for lifestyle changes.

Maternal Interventions

- Explain that uterine pressure can cause pooling of venous blood in lower extremities.
- Teach to report immediately signs and symptoms of thrombosis:
  - Pain in leg, groin
  - Unilateral leg swelling
  - Pale skin
- Refer to Interventions for specific techniques to reduce edema.

Risk for Ineffective Peripheral Tissue Perfusion

NANDA-I Definition

At risk for a decrease in blood circulation to the periphery that may compromise health

Risk Factors*

Age >60 years

Deficient knowledge of aggravating factors (e.g., smoking,
   sedentary lifestyle, trauma, obesity, salt intake, immobility)
Deficient knowledge of disease process (e.g., diabetes mellitus,
   hyperlipidemia)
Diabetes mellitus
Endovascular procedures
Hypertension
Sedentary lifestyle
Smoking

Goal

Refer to *Ineffective Peripheral Tissue Perfusion.*

Interventions

Refer to *Ineffective Peripheral Tissue Perfusion.*

Risk for Peripheral Neurovascular Dysfunction

NANDA-I Definition

At risk for disruption in the circulation, sensation, or motion of
an extremity

Risk Factors*

Burns
Fractures
Immobilization
Mechanical compression (e.g., tourniquet, cane, cast, brace,
   dressing, restraint)
Orthopedic surgery
Trauma
Vascular obstruction

Pathophysiologic

Related to increased volume of (specify extremity) secondary to:
Arterial obstruction
Bleeding (e.g., trauma*, fractures*)

Coagulation disorder
Venous obstruction*/pooling

Related to increased capillary filtration secondary to:
Allergic response (e.g., insect   Severe burns (thermal,
    bites)   electrical)
Frostbite   Trauma
Hypothermia   Venomous bites (e.g., snake)
Nephrotic syndrome

Related to restrictive envelope secondary to circumferential burns

Treatment Related

Related to increased capillary filtration secondary to:
Total knee replacement
Total hip replacement

Related to restrictive envelope secondary to:
Tourniquet   Brace
Antishock trousers   Air splints
Circumferential dressings   Premature or tight closure of
Ace wraps   fascial defects
Excessive traction   Restraints
Cast

🌀 Author's Note

This diagnosis represents a situation that nurses can prevent complications by identifying who is at risk and implementing measures to reduce or eliminate causative or contributing factors. *Risk for Peripheral Neurovascular Dysfunction* can change to compartment syndrome. *RC of Compartment Syndrome* is inadequate tissue perfusion in a muscle, usually an arm or leg, caused by edema, which obstructs venous and arterial flow and compresses nerves. The nursing focus for compartment syndrome is diagnosing early signs and symptoms and notifying the physician. The medical interventions required to abate the problem are surgical, such as evacuation of hematoma, repair of damaged vessels, or fasciotomy. Refer to *RC of Compartment Syndrome* on http://thePoint.lww.com/CarpenitoHB14e for specific interventions for either diagnosis. Students should consult with their faculty for direction to use either *Risk for Peripheral Vascular Dysfunction* or *RC of Compartment Syndrome*.

NOC
Neurologic Status

Goal

The individual will report changes in peripheral sensation or movement as evidenced by the following indicators:

• Have palpable peripheral pulses.
• Have warm extremities.
• Have capillary refill less than 3 seconds.

 NIC

Peripheral Sensation Management, Positioning, Embolus Precautions

Interventions

Assess and Evaluate Neurovascular Status at Least Every Hour for First 24 Hours, and Compare with Unaffected Limb if Possible

• Peripheral pulses
• Skin color, temperature
• Capillary refill time

For Injured Arms
• Assess for ability to:
  • Hyperextend thumbs, wrist, and four fingers
  • Abduct (fan out) all fingers
  • Touch thumb to small finger
• Assess sensation with pressure from a sharp point.
  • Web space between thumb and index finger
  • Distal fat pad of small finger
  • Distal surface of the index finger

For Injured Legs
• Assess for ability to:
  • Dorsiflex (upward movement) ankle and extend toes at metatarsal phalangeal joints
  • Plantarflex (downward movement) ankle and toes
• Assess sensation with pressure from a sharp point:
  • Web space between great toe and second toe
  • Medial and lateral surfaces of the sole (upper third)

Instruct to Report Unusual, New, or Different Sensations (e.g., Tingling, Numbness, or Decreased Ability to Move Toes or Fingers; Pain with Passive Stretch; Unrelieved Pain)

Reduce Edema or Its Effects on Function

• Remove jewelry from affected limb.
• Elevate limbs unless contraindicated.

- Advise to move fingers or toes of affected limb two to four times per hour.
- Apply ice bags around injured site. Place a cloth between ice bag and skin.
- Monitor drainage (characteristics, amount) from wounds or incisional site.
- Maintain patency of the wound drainage system.

Notify the Physician If the Following Occur:

- Change in sensation
- Change in movement ability
- Pale, mottled, or cyanotic skin
- Slowed capillary refill more than 3 seconds
- Diminished or absent pulse
- Increasing pain or pain not controlled by medication
- Pain with passive stretching of muscle
- Pain increased with elevation

Discontinue Elevation and Ice Application If Previous Signs or Symptoms Occur

- Promote circulation in affected limb.
- Ensure hydration is optimal to maximize circulation.
- Monitor traction apparatus and splints for pressure on vessels or nerves.
- If wrist or ankle restraints are used, monitor for pressure on vessels or nerves. Remove at least every hour, and perform range-of-motion (ROM) exercises.
- Encourage active ROM exercises of unaffected body parts and ambulation if permissible.

Maintain Correct Positioning to Prevent Prosthetic Dislocation After Hip or Knee Joint Replacement

Initiate Health Teaching As Indicated

- Teach client and family to watch for and report the following symptoms:
  - Severe pain
  - Numbness or tingling
  - Swelling
  - Skin discoloration
  - Paralysis or reduced movement
  - Cool, white toes or fingertips
  - Foul odor, warm spots, soft areas, or cracks in the cast
- Emphasize the importance of follow-up evaluations.

Risk for Ineffective Renal Perfusion

NANDA-I Definition

At risk for a decrease in blood circulation to the kidney that may compromise health

Risk Factors*

Abdominal compartment syndrome
Advance age
Bilateral cortical necrosis
Burns
Cardiac surgery
Cardiopulmonary bypass
Diabetes mellitus
Exposure to toxins
Female glomerulonephritis
Hyperlipidemia
Hypertension
Hypovolemia
Hypoxemia
Hypoxia
Infection (e.g., sepsis, localized infection)
Malignancy
Malignant hypertension
Metabolic acidosis
Multitrauma
Polynephritis
Renal artery stenosis
Renal disease (polycystic kidney)
Smoking
Systemic inflammatory response syndrome
Treatment-related side effects (e.g., pharmaceutical agents, surgery)
Vascular embolism vasculitis

🌀 Author's Note

This NANDA-I diagnosis represents a potential complication which is a collaborative problem, *Risk for Complications of Renal Insufficiency*.

If the situation is a medical diagnosis of Acute Kidney Failure or Chronic Renal Disease, using *Risk for Complications of Acute Kidney Failure* would include the following collaborative problems:[†]

- *RC of Fluid Overload*
- *RC of Metabolic Acidosis*
- *RC of Acute Albuminemia*
- *RC of Hypertension*
- *RC of Pulmonary Edema*
- *RC of Dysrhythmias*
- *RC of Gastrointestinal Bleeding*

Nursing diagnoses associated with this clinical situation:

- *Risk for Infection related to invasive procedures*
- *Imbalanced Nutrition: Less that Body Requirements related to anorexia, nausea, vomiting, loss of taste, loss of smell, stomatitis, and dietary restrictions*
- *Risk for Impaired Tissue Integrity related to retention of metabolic wastes, increased capillary fragility and platelet dysfunction*

---

† For a more specific care plan with nursing interventions/rationales and outcomes for clinical situations, such as medical diagnoses (e.g., chronic renal disease, acute kidney failure), surgical procedures (e.g., nephrectomy), treatments/procedures (e.g., hemodialysis, peritoneal dialysis), and 70 other clinical situations, refer to Carpenito-Moyet, L. J. (2009). *Nursing Care Plans and Documentation* (5th ed.). Philadelphia, PA: Lippincott, Williams & Wilkins.

Goals/Interventions

Refer to http://thePoint.lww.com/CarpenitoHB14e for goal and interventions for *Risk for Complications of Renal Insufficiency*

Refer to Section 1 for goals and interventions for specific related nursing diagnoses.

IMPAIRED URINARY ELIMINATION

Impaired Urinary Elimination

Maturational Enuresis

Functional Urinary Incontinence

Reflex Urinary Incontinence

Stress Urinary Incontinence

Continuous Urinary Incontinence

Urge Urinary Incontinence

Risk for Urge Urinary Incontinence

Overflow Urinary Incontinence

NANDA-I Definition

Dysfunction in urinary elimination

Defining Characteristics

Major (Must Be Present, One or More)

Reports or experiences a urinary elimination problem, such as:

Urgency*   Nocturia*
Dribbling   Incontinence*
Frequency*   Dysuria*
Bladder distention   Enuresis
Hesitancy*   Retention*
Large residual urine volumes

Related Factors

Pathophysiologic

Related to incompetent bladder outlet secondary to:
Congenital urinary tract anomalies

Related to decreased bladder capacity or irritation to bladder secondary to:
Infection*   Carcinoma
Glucosuria   Urethritis
Trauma

Related to diminished bladder cues or impaired ability to recognize bladder cues secondary to:
Cord injury/tumor/infection   Tabes dorsalis
Diabetic neuropathy   Demyelinating diseases
Brain injury/tumor/infection   Parkinsonism
Alcoholic neuropathy   Multiple sclerosis
Cerebrovascular accident   Alpha adrenergic agents

*Related to sensory motor impairment**

*Related to multiple causality**

*Related to anatomic obstruction**

Treatment Related

Related to effects of surgery on bladder sphincter secondary to:
Postprostatectomy   Extensive pelvic dissection

Related to diagnostic instrumentation

Related to decreased muscle tone secondary to:
General or spinal anesthesia   Epinephrine
Drug therapy (iatrogenic)   Diuretics
  Antihistamines   Anticholinergics
  Immunosuppressant therapy   Tranquilizers

Sedatives   After use of indwelling
Muscle relaxants   catheters

Situational (Personal, Environmental)

Related to weak pelvic floor muscles secondary to:
Obesity   Aging
Childbirth   Recent substantial weight loss

Related to inability to communicate needs

Related to bladder outlet obstruction secondary to:
Fecal impaction   Chronic constipation

Related to decreased bladder muscle tone secondary to:
Dehydration

Related to decreased attention to bladder cues secondary to:
Depression   Intentional suppression
Delirium   (self-induced deconditioning)
                                   Confusion

Related to environmental barriers to bathroom secondary to:
Distant toilets   Bed too high
Poor lighting   Side rails
Unfamiliar surroundings

Related to inability to access bathroom on time secondary to:
Caffeine/alcohol use   Impaired mobility

Maturational

Child
Related to small bladder capacity

Related to lack of motivation

 Author's Note

Impaired Urinary Elimination is too broad a diagnosis for effective clinical use; however, it is clinically useful until additional data can be collected. With more data the nurse can use a more specific diagnosis, such as *Stress Urinary Incontinence*, whenever possible. When the etiologic or contributing factors for incontinence have not been identified, the nurse could write a temporary diagnosis of *Impaired Urinary Elimination* related to unknown etiology, as evidenced by incontinence.

The nurse performs a focus assessment to determine whether the incontinence is transient, in response to an acute condition (e.g., infection, medication side effects), or established in response to various chronic neural or genitourinary conditions (Miller, 2009). In addition, the nurse should differentiate the type of incontinence: functional, reflex, stress, or urge.

Goal

The person will be continent (specify during day, night, 24 hours) as evidenced by the following indicators:

- Be able to identify the cause of incontinence.
- Provide rationale for treatments.

Interventions

Determine If There Is Acute Cause of Problem

- Infection (e.g., urinary tract, sexually transmitted disease, gonorrhea)
- Renal disease
- Renal calculi
- Medication effects
- Anesthesia effects

Refer to a Urologist If Acute Cause Is Determined

Assess to Determine Type If Incontinence Is the Problem

- History of continence
- Onset and duration (day, night, just certain times)
- Factors that increase incidence:
  - Coughing
  - Laughing
  - Standing
  - Turning in bed
  - Delay in getting to bathroom
  - When excited
  - Leaving bathroom
  - Running
- Perception of need to void: present, absent, diminished
- Ability to delay urination after urge
- Relief after voiding:
  - Complete
  - Continued desire to void after bladder is emptied

Refer to Specific Type of Incontinence Using Data from Assessment

Maturational Enuresis**

Definition

State in which a child experiences involuntary voiding during sleep that is not pathophysiologic in origin

Defining Characteristics

Reports or demonstrates episodes of involuntary voiding during sleep

Related Factors

Situational (Personal, Environmental)

Related to stressors (school, siblings)

Related to inattention to bladder cues

Related to unfamiliar surroundings

Maturational

Child

Related to small bladder capacity

Related to lack of motivation

Related to attention-seeking behavior

 Author's Note

Enuresis can result from physiologic or maturational factors. Certain etiologies, such as strictures, urinary tract infection, constipation, nocturnal epilepsy, and diabetes, should be ruled out when enuresis is present. These situations do not represent nursing diagnoses.

When enuresis results from small bladder capacity, failure to perceive cues because of deep sleep, inattention to bladder cues, or is associated with a maturational issue (e.g., new sibling, school pressures), the nursing diagnosis *Maturational Enuresis* is appropriate. Psychological problems usually are not the cause of enuresis but may result from lack of understanding or insensitivity to the problem. Interventions that punish or shame the child must be avoided.

** This diagnosis is not presently on the NANDA-I list but has been included for clarity and usefulness.

Urinary Continence, Knowledge: Enuresis, Family Functioning

Goal

The child will remain dry during the sleep cycle, as evidenced by the following indicator:

* The child and family will be able to list factors that decrease enuresis.

Urinary Incontinence Care: Enuresis, Urinary Habit Training, Anticipatory Guidance, Family Support

Interventions

Ascertain That Physiologic Causes of Enuresis Have Been Ruled Out

* Examples include infections, meatal stenosis, fistulas, pinworms, epispadias, ectopic ureter, and minor neurologic dysfunction (hyperactivity, cognitive delay).

Determine Contributing Factors

Refer to Related Factors.

Promote a Positive Parent–Child Relationship

* Explain to the parents and the child the physiologic development of bladder control.
* Offer reassurance to child that other children wet the bed at night and that he or she is not bad or sinful. Explain that there is a high rate of remission.

Reduce Contributing Factors, If Possible

Small Bladder Capacity
* After child drinks fluids, encourage him or her to postpone voiding to help stretch the bladder.

Sound Sleeper
* Have child void before retiring.
* Restrict fluids at bedtime.
* If child is awakened later (about 11 PM) to void, attempt to awaken child fully for positive reinforcement.

Too Busy to Sense a Full Bladder (If Daytime *Wetting Occurs*)

- Teach child awareness of sensations that occur when it is time to void.
- Teach child the ability to control urination (have him or her start and stop the stream; have him or her "hold" the urine during the day, even if for only a short time).
- Bladder retraining can help control dysfunctional voiding.
- Have child keep a record of how he or she is doing; emphasize dry days or nights (e.g., stars on a calendar).
- If child wets, have him or her explain or write down (if feasible) why he or she thinks it happened.
- With school age children, assess if the child is using the bathroom at school. Do they get sufficient bathroom breaks? Can a reminder device be used (vibrating watch)?

Initiate Health Teaching and Referrals, as Indicated

- For children with enuresis:
  - Teach child and parents the facts about enuresis.
  - Teach family techniques to control the adverse effects of enuresis (e.g., plastic mattress covers, use of sleeping bag [machine washable] when staying overnight away from home).
  - Explain that the child cannot control bed-wetting but that bed-wetting can be controlled with intervention (Morison, 1998).
  - Children who believe that they can be helped have the best chance of success (Morison, 1998).
- Without implying punishment, involve the child in bed changing for nocturnal enuresis (Ball & Bindler, 2008).
- Explain how the nocturnal enuresis alarm works.

Functional Urinary Incontinence

NANDA-I Definition

State in which a usually continent client experiences incontinence because of a difficulty or inability to reach the toilet in time

Defining Characteristics

Major (Must Be Present)

Incontinence before or during an attempt to reach the toilet

Related Factors

Pathophysiologic

Related to diminished bladder cues and impaired ability to recognize bladder cues secondary to:

Brain injury/tumor/infection   Demyelinating diseases
Alcoholic neuropathy   Progressive dementia
Cerebrovascular accident   Multiple sclerosis
Parkinsonism

Treatment Related

Related to decreased bladder tone secondary to:

Antihistamines   Anticholinergics
Immunosuppressant therapy   Tranquilizers
Epinephrine   Sedatives
Diuretics   Muscle relaxants

Situational (Personal, Environmental)

Related to impaired mobility

Related to decreased attention to bladder cues
Depression
Intentional suppression (self-induced deconditioning)
Confusion

Related to environmental barriers to using bathroom
Distant toilets/seat height   Side rails
Bed too high   Unfamiliar surroundings
Poor lighting   Clothing

Maturational

Older Adult

Related to motor and sensory losses

 NOC

Tissue Integrity, Urinary Continence, Urinary Elimination

Goal

The client will report no or decreased episodes of incontinence, as evidenced by the following indicators:

- Remove or minimize environmental barriers at home.
- Use proper adaptive equipment to assist with voiding, transfers, and dressing.
- Describe causative factors for incontinence.

NIC

Perineal Care, Urinary Incontinence Care, Prompted Voiding, Urinary Habit Training, Urinary Elimination Management, Teaching: Procedure/Treatment

Interventions

Assess Causative or Contributing Factors

Obstacles to Toilet

- Poor lighting, slippery floor, misplaced furniture and rugs, inadequate footwear, toilet too far, bed too high, side rails up
- Inadequate toilet (too small for walkers, wheelchair, seat too low/high, no grab bars)
- Inadequate signal system for requesting help
- Lack of privacy

Sensory/Cognitive Deficits

- Visual deficits (blindness, field cuts, poor depth perception)
- Cognitive deficits as a result of aging, trauma, stroke, tumor, infection

Motor/Mobility Deficits

- Limited upper and/or lower extremity movement/strength (inability to remove clothing)
- Barriers to ambulation (e.g., vertigo, fatigue, altered gait, hypertension)

Reduce or Eliminate Contributing Factors, If Possible

Environmental Barriers

- Assess path to bathroom for obstacles, lighting, and distance.
- Assess adequacy of toilet height and need for grab bars.
- Assess adequacy of room size.
- Assess if client can remove clothing easily.
- Provide a commode between bathroom and bed, if necessary.

Sensory/Cognitive Deficits

- For a client with diminished vision:
  - Ensure adequate lighting.
  - Encourage client to wear prescribed corrective lens.
  - Provide clear, safe pathway to bathroom.
  - Keep call bell easily accessible.
  - If bedpan or urinal is used, make sure it is within easy reach in the same location at all times.
  - Assess client for safety in bathroom.
  - Assess client's ability to provide self-hygiene.
- For a client with cognitive deficits:
  - Offer toileting reminders every 2 hours, after meals, and before bedtime.
  - Establish appropriate means to communicate need to void.
  - Answer call bell immediately.
  - Encourage wearing of ordinary clothes.
  - Provide a normal environment for elimination (use bathroom, if possible).
  - Allow for privacy while maintaining safety.
  - Allow sufficient time for task.
  - Reorient client to where he or she is and what task he or she is doing.
  - Be consistent in your approach to client.
  - Give simple step-by-step instructions; use verbal and nonverbal cues.
  - Give positive reinforcement for success.
  - Assess client for safety in bathroom.
  - Assess need for adaptive devices on clothing to make dressing and undressing easier.
  - Assess client's ability to provide self-hygiene.

Provide for Factors That Promote Continence

Maintain Optimal Hydration

- Increase fluid intake to 2000 to 3000 milliliters/day, unless contraindicated.
- Teach older adults not to depend on thirst sensations but to drink liquids even when not thirsty.
- Space fluids every 2 hours.
- Decrease fluid intake after 7 PM; provide only minimal fluids during the night.
- Avoid large amounts of tomato and orange juice.
- Avoid bladder irritants such as alcohol, caffeine, and aspartame (Smeltzer, Bare, Hinkle, & Cheever, 2010).
- Encourage intake of cranberry juice.

Maintain Adequate Nutrition to Ensure Bowel Elimination at Least Once Every 3 Days
- Promote micturition.

Promote Personal Integrity and Provide Motivation to Increase Bladder Control
- Encourage client to share feelings about incontinence and determine its effect on his or her social patterns.
- Convey that incontinence can be cured or at least controlled to maintain dignity.
- Use protective pads or garments only after conscientious reconditioning efforts have been completely unsuccessful after 6 weeks.
- Work to achieve daytime continence before expecting night-time continence.
  - Encourage socialization.
  - Discourage the use of bedpans.
  - Encourage and assist client to groom self.
  - If hospitalized, provide opportunities to eat meals outside bedroom (day room, lounge).
  - If fear or embarrassment is preventing socialization, instruct client to use sanitary pads or briefs temporarily until control is established.
  - Change clothes as soon as possible when wet to avoid indirectly sanctioning wetness.
  - Advise the oral use of chlorophyll tablets to deodorize urine and feces.
  - Refer to *Social Isolation* and *Ineffective Coping* for additional interventions, if indicated.

Promote Skin Integrity
- Identify clients at risk for development of pressure ulcers.
- Avoid harsh soaps and alcohol products.
- Keep moisture away from the skin.
- Refer to *Risk for Impaired Skin Integrity* for additional information.

Teach Prevention of Urinary Tract Infections

- Encourage regular, complete emptying of the bladder.
- Ensure adequate fluid intake.
- Keep urine acidic; avoid citrus juices, dark colas, coffee, tea, and alcohol, which act as irritants (Smeltzer, Bare, Hinkle, & Cheever, 2010).
- Monitor urine pH.
- Teach client to recognize abnormal changes in urine properties.
  - Increased mucus and sediment
  - Blood in urine (hematuria)

- Change in color (from normal straw colored) or odor
- Teach client to monitor for signs and symptoms of infection:
  - Elevated temperature, chills, and shaking
  - Changes in urine properties
  - Suprapubic pain
  - Painful urination
  - Urgency
  - Frequent small voids or frequent small incontinences
  - Increased spasticity in individuals with spinal cord injuries
  - Increased urine pH
  - Nausea/vomiting
  - Lower back, flank pain, or both

Explain Age-Related Effects on Bladder Function and That Urgency and Nocturia Do Not Necessarily Lead to Incontinence

Initiate Health Teaching Referral, When Indicated

- Refer to visiting nurse (occupational therapy department) for assessment of bathroom facilities at home.

✴ Geriatric Interventions

- Emphasize that incontinence is not an inevitable age-related event.
- Explain not to restrict fluid intake because of fear of incontinence.
- Explain not to rely on thirst as a signal to drink fluids.
- Teach the need to have easy access to bathroom at night. If needed, consider commode chair or urinal.

Reflex Urinary Incontinence

NANDA-I Definition

Involuntary loss of urine at somewhat predictable intervals when a specific bladder volume is reached

Defining Characteristics

Major (Must Be Present)*

Inability to voluntarily inhibit voiding or imitate voiding
Incomplete emptying with lesion above pontine micturition
   center

Incomplete emptying with lesion above sacral micturition
Predictable pattern of voiding
Sensation of urgency without voluntary inhibition of bladder
   contraction
Sensations associated with full bladder (e.g., sweating, restless-
   ness, abdominal discomfort)
No sensation of bladder fullness, urge to void or voiding

Related Factors

Pathophysiologic

*Related to impaired conduction of impulses above the reflex arc level
secondary to:*
Cord injury/tumor/infection

Related to post operative dribbling and incontinence secondary to:
Transurethral resection of the prostate
Prostate surgery

NOC

See *Functional Urinary Incontinence*.

Goal

The client will report a state of dryness that meets personal satisfaction, as evidenced by the following indicators:

• Have a residual urine volume of less than 50 milliliters.
• Use triggering mechanisms to initiate reflex voiding.

NIC

See also *Functional Urinary Incontinence*, Pelvic Muscle Exercises, Weight Management

Interventions

Assess for Causative and Contributing Conditions

• Refer to Related Factors.
• Explain rationale for treatment(s).

**Develop a Bladder Retraining or Reconditioning Program
(See Interventions Under Continuous Incontinence)**

Teach Techniques to Stimulate Reflex Voiding

• Cutaneous triggering mechanisms
• Repeated deep, sharp suprapubic tapping (most effective)

- Instruct client to:
  - Place self in a half-sitting position.
  - Tap directly at bladder wall at a rate of seven or eight times for 5 seconds (35 to 40 single blows).
  - Use only one hand.
  - Shift site of stimulation over bladder to find most successful site.
  - Continue stimulation until a good stream starts.
  - Wait approximately 1 minute; repeat stimulation until bladder is empty.
  - One or two series of stimulations without response signifies that nothing more will be expelled.
- If the preceding measures are ineffective, instruct client to perform each of the following for 2 to 3 minutes, waiting 1 minute between attempts:
  - Stroking glans penis
  - Lightly punching abdomen above inguinal ligaments
  - Stroking inner thigh
- Encourage client to void or trigger at least every 3 hours.
- Indicate on intake and output sheet which mechanism was used to induce voiding.
- People with abdominal muscle control should use the Valsalva maneuver during triggered voiding.
- Teach client that if he or she increases fluid intake, he or she also needs to increase the frequency of triggering to prevent overdistention.
- Schedule intermittent catheterization program (see *Continuous Incontinence*).

Initiate Health Teaching, as Indicated

Arrange an At-Home Assessment by a Home Health Nurse

- Teach bladder reconditioning program (see *Continuous Incontinence*).
- Teach intermittent catheterization (see *Continuous Incontinence*).
- Teach prevention of urinary tract infections (see *Continuous Incontinence*).
- If client is at high risk for dysreflexia, refer to *Dysreflexia*.

Stress Urinary Incontinence

NANDA-I Definition

Sudden leakage of urine with activities that increase intra-abdominal pressure

Defining Characteristics*

Observed or reported involuntary leakage of small amounts
   of urine:
   In the absence of detrusor contraction
   In the absence of an overactive bladder
   On exertion
   With coughing, laughing, sneezing, or all of these

Related Factors

Pathophysiologic

Related to incompetent bladder outlet secondary to:
Congenital urinary tract anomalies

Related to degenerative changes in pelvic muscles* and structural supports secondary to:
Estrogen deficiency

Related to intrinsic urethral sphincter*

Situational (Personal, Environmental)

Related to high intra-abdominal pressure* and weak pelvic muscles* secondary to:

Obesity	Poor personal hygiene
Sex	Smoking
Pregnancy	

Related to weak pelvic muscles and structural supports secondary to:

Recent substantial weight loss	Childbirth

Maturational

Older Adult
Related to loss of muscle tone

NOC

Refer to *Functional Urinary Incontinence*.

Goal

The client will report a reduction or elimination of stress incontinence, as evidenced by the following indicators:

• Be able to explain the cause of incontinence and rationale for
  treatments.

See also *Functional Incontinence*, Pelvic Muscle Exercise, Weight Management

Interventions

Determine Contributing Factors

Explain the Effect of Incompetent Floor Muscles on Continence

Teach Pelvic Muscle Exercises (Dougherty, 1998)

Teach How to Self-Assess Whether Exercises Are Being Done Correctly

- Stand with one foot elevated on a stool, insert finger in vagina, and feel the strength of the contraction. Evaluate the strength of the contraction on a scale of 0 to 5 (Sampselle & DeLancey, 1998):
  - 0 = No palpable contraction
  - 1 = Very weak, barely felt
  - 2 = Weak but clearly felt
  - 3 = Good but not maintained when moderate finger pressure is applied
  - 4 = Good but not maintained when intense finger pressure is applied
  - 5 = Maximum strength with strong resistance
- Use a mirror to observe whether the clitoris has downward movement and the anus tightens with contraction.
- Consult an incontinence specialist for use of vaginal weights for pelvic floor strengthening.

Provide Instructions for Pelvic Muscle Exercises

- Teach the client ways to strengthen the pelvic floor muscle.
- Tightening muscles as if you were trying to stop urination; this includes tightening the rectal muscles (Wilkinson & Van Leuven, 2007).
- Hold the contractions for 5 to 10 seconds and release. Relax between contractions taking care to keep contraction and relaxation times equal. If you contract for 10 seconds, relax for 10 seconds before next contraction (Wilkinson & Van Leuven, 2007).
- Perform 40 to 60 contractions divided into two to four sessions each time. These should be spread out through the day and incorporate different positions (sitting, standing, and lying; Wilkinson & Van Leuven, 2007).

- A good way to help clients remember to do exercises is to incorporate them into daily routine, such as stopping at a traffic light or washing dishes (Wilkinson & Van Leuven, 2007).
- Use the urine stop test to measure the effectiveness of a contraction by the time it takes to stop voiding. Advise not to perform the urine stop test more than once a day.

Initiate Health Teaching for People Who Continue to Remain Incontinent After Attempts at Bladder Reconditioning or Muscle Retraining

- Promote personal integrity (see *Continuous Incontinence*).
- Promote skin integrity (see *Continuous Incontinence*).
- Schedule intermittent catheterization program, if appropriate (see *Continuous Incontinence*).

Maternal Interventions

- For increased abdominal pressure during pregnancy:
  - Teach client to avoid prolonged standing.
  - Teach client the benefit of frequent voiding (at least every 2 hours).
  - Teach pelvic muscle exercises after delivery.

Continuous Urinary Incontinence**

Definition

State in which a client experiences continuous, unpredictable loss of urine* without distention or awareness of bladder fullness

Defining Characteristics

Constant flow of urine at unpredictable times without uninhibited bladder contractions/spasm or distention
Lack of bladder filling or perineal filling
Nocturia
Unawareness of incontinence
Incontinence refractory to other treatments

** This diagnosis is not presently on the NANDA-I list but has been included for clarity and usefulness.

Related Factors

Refer to *Impaired Urinary Elimination*.

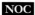

Refer to *Functional Urinary Incontinence*.

Goal

The client will be continent (specify during day, night, 24 hours), as evidenced by the following indicators:

- Identify the cause of incontinence and rationale for treatments.
- Identify daily goal for fluid intake.

NIC

See also *Functional Incontinence*, Environmental Management, Urinary Catheterization, Teaching: Procedure/Treatment, Tube Care: Urinary, Urinary Bladder Training

Interventions

Develop a Bladder Retraining or Reconditioning Program, Which Should Include Communication, Assessment of Voiding Pattern, Scheduled Fluid Intake, and Scheduled Voiding Times

Promote Communication Among All Staff Members and Among Individual, Family, and Staff

- Provide all staff with sufficient knowledge concerning the program planned.
- Assess staff's response to program.

Assess the Client's Potential for Participation in a Bladder-Retraining Program

- Cognition
- Desire to change behavior
- Ability to cooperate
- Willingness to participate

Provide Rationale for Plan and Acquire Client's Informed Consent

Encourage Client to Continue Program by Providing Accurate Information Concerning Reasons for Success or Failure

Assess Voiding Pattern

- Monitor and record:
  - Intake and output
  - Time and amount of fluid intake

- Type of fluid
- Amount of incontinence; measure if possible or estimate amount as small, moderate, or large
- Amount of void, whether it was voluntary or involuntary
- Presence of sensation of need to void
- Amount of retention (amount of urine left in the bladder after an unsuccessful attempt at manual triggering or voiding)
- Amount of residual (amount of urine left in the bladder after either a voluntary or manual triggered voiding; also called a *postvoid residual*)
- Amount of triggered urine (urine expelled after manual triggering [e.g., tapping, Credé's method])
- Identify certain activities that precede voiding (e.g., restlessness, yelling, exercise).
- Record in appropriate column.

Schedule Fluid Intake and Voiding Times

- Provide fluid intake of 2000 milliliters each day unless contraindicated.
- Discourage fluids after 7 PM.
- Provide caregiver education.
- Initially, bladder emptying is done at least every 2 hours and at least twice during the night; goal is 2- to 4-hour intervals.
- If the client is incontinent before scheduled voids, shorten the time between voids.
- If the client has a postvoid residual greater than 100 to 150 milliliters, schedule intermittent catheterization.

Reduce Incontinence-Related Irritant Dermatitis (Scardillo et al., 1999)

- Decrease the alkalizing effect of urine on the skin:
  - Use a no-rinse perineal cleanser.
  - Avoid fragrances, alcohol, and alkaline agents (found in many commercial soaps).
  - Apply moisturizer immediately after bathing, when pores are open.
  - Select a moisturizer that is occlusive (white petroleum, lanolin, emollients).
- Decrease injury with washing.
  - Do not try to remove all of the ointment with cleansing.
  - Gently wash skin, using little soap.
  - Dry skin gently by patting, not rubbing.
  - Use a moisture barrier product (e.g., Curity Moisture Barrier Cream; No Sting Barrier Film).

Schedule Intermittent Catheterization Program (ICP), if Indicated

- Monitor intake and output.
- Fluid intake should be at least 2000 milliliters/day.
- Use sterile catheterization technique in the hospital, clean technique at home.
- Desired catheter volumes are less than 500 milliliters.
- Increase or decrease the interval between catheterizations to obtain the desired catheter volumes.
- Usual catheterization times are every 4 to 6 hours.
- Urine volumes may increase at night; thus, it may be necessary to catheterize more frequently at night.
- Encourage the client to attempt to void before scheduled catheterization time.
- Initially obtain postvoid residuals at least every 6 hours.
- Terminate ICP when the bladder is consistently emptied voluntarily or by triggering with less than 50 milliliters residual urine after each void.

Teach ICP to Client and Family for Long-Term Management of Bladder

- Explain the reasons for the catheterization program.
- Explain the relation of fluid intake and the frequency of catheterization.
- Explain the importance of emptying the bladder at the prescribed time, regardless of circumstances, because of the hazards of an overdistended bladder (e.g., circulation contributes to infection, and stasis of urine contributes to bacterial growth).

Teach the Client About the Bladder Reconditioning Program

- Explain rationale and treatments.
- Explain the schedule of fluid intake, voiding attempts, manual triggering, and catheterization to control incontinence.
- Teach client and family the importance of positive reinforcement and adherence to program for best results.
- Refer to community nurses for assistance in bladder reconditioning if indicated.

Initiate Health Teaching

- If appropriate, teach intermittent catheterization.
- Instruct in prevention of urinary tract infection.
- For people living in the community, initiate a referral to the visiting nurse for follow-up and/or regular changes of an indwelling catheter.

Urge Urinary Incontinence

NANDA-I Definition

Involuntary passage of urine occurring soon after a strong sense of urgency to void

Defining Characteristics*

Observed or reported inability to reach toilet in time to avoid urine loss
Reports urinary urgency
Reports involuntary loss of urine with bladder contractions or bladder spasms

Related Factors

Pathophysiologic

Related to decreased bladder capacity secondary to:

Infection
Cerebrovascular accident
Trauma
Demyelinating diseases
Urethritis
Diabetic neuropathy
Neurogenic disorders or injury/tumor/infection injury
Alcoholic neuropathy
Brain Parkinsonism

Treatment Related

Related to decreased bladder capacity secondary to:
Abdominal surgery
After use of indwelling catheters

Situational (Personal, Environmental)

Related to irritation of bladder stretch receptors secondary to:
Alcohol
Caffeine
Excess fluid intake

Related to decreased bladder capacity secondary to:
Frequent voiding

Maturational

Child
Related to small bladder capacity

Older Adult
Related to decreased bladder capacity

NOC

Refer to *Functional Urinary Incontinence*

Goal

The client will report no or decreased episodes of incontinence (specify), as evidenced by the following indicators:

- Explain causes of incontinence.
- Describe bladder irritants.

NIC

Refer to *Functional Urinary Incontinence*

Interventions

Assess for Causative or Contributing Factors

Refer to Related Factors.

Assess Pattern of Voiding/Incontinence and Fluid Intake

- Maintain optimal hydration (see *Continuous Incontinence*).
- Assess voiding pattern (see *Continuous Incontinence*).

Reduce or Eliminate Causative and Contributing Factors, When Possible

Bladder Irritants
- Infection/inflammation
  - Refer to physician for diagnosis and treatment.
  - Initiate bladder reconditioning program (see *Continuous Incontinence*).
  - Explain the relation between incontinence and intake of alcohol, caffeine, and colas (irritants).
  - Explain the risk of insufficient fluid intake and its relation to infection and concentrated urine.

Diminished Bladder Capacity
- Determine time between urge to void and need to void (record how long client can delay urination).
- For a client with difficulty prolonging waiting time, communicate to personnel the need to respond rapidly to his or her request for assistance for toileting (note on care plan).

- Teach client to increase waiting time by increasing bladder capacity.
  - Determine volume of each void.
  - Ask client to "hold off" urinating as long as possible.
  - Give positive reinforcement.
  - Discourage frequent voiding that is the result of habit, not need.
  - Develop bladder reconditioning program (see *Continuous Incontinence*).

Overdistended Bladder

- Explain that diuretics are given to help reduce the water in the body; they work by acting on the kidneys to increase the flow of urine.
- Explain that in diabetes mellitus, insulin deficiency causes high levels of blood sugar. The high level of blood glucose pulls fluid from body tissues, causing osmotic diuresis and increased urination (polyuria).
- Explain that because of the increased urine flow, regular voiding is needed to prevent overdistention of the bladder.
- Assess voiding pattern (see *Continuous Incontinence*).
- Check postvoid residual; if greater than 100 milliliters, include intermittent catheterization in bladder reconditioning program.
- Initiate bladder reconditioning program (see *Continuous Incontinence*).

Uninhibited Bladder Contractions

- Assess voiding pattern (see *Continuous Incontinence*).
- Establish method to communicate urge to void (document on care plan).
- Communicate to personnel the need to respond rapidly to a request to void.
- Establish a planned-voiding pattern.
  - Provide an opportunity to void on awakening; after meals, physical exercise, bathing, and drinking coffee or tea; and before going to sleep.
  - Begin by offering use of bedpan, commode, or toilet every half hour initially, and gradually lengthen the time to at least every 2 hours.
  - If client has incontinent episode, reduce the time between scheduled voidings.
  - Document behavior/activity that occurs with void or incontinence (see *Continuous Incontinence*).
- Encourage client to try to "hold" urine until time to void, if possible.

- Consult primary care professional for pharmacologic interventions.
- Refer to *Continuous Incontinence* for additional information on developing a bladder reconditioning program.

Initiate Health Teaching

- Instruct client about prevention of urinary tract infections (refer to *Functional Incontinence*).

Risk for Urge Urinary Incontinence

NANDA-I Definition

At risk for involuntary passage of urine occurring soon after a strong sense of urgency to void

Risk Factors

Refer to Related Factors in *Urge Urinary Incontinence*.

 NOC

Refer to *Functional Urinary Incontinence*.

Goal

The person will report continued continence comfort as evidenced by the following indicators:

- Explain causes of incontinence.
- Explain strategies to maintain continence.

 NIC

Refer to *Functional Urinary Incontinence*.

Interventions

Refer to *Urge Urinary Incontinence*.

Overflow Urinary Incontinence**

NANDA-I Definition

Involuntary loss of urine associated with overdistention of the bladder

Defining Characteristics*

Bladder distention High residual volume observed after void
Observed or reported involuntary leakage of small volumes of
    urine
Nocturia

Related Factors

Pathophysiologic

Related to sphincter blockage secondary to:
Strictures   Prostatic enlargement
Ureterocele   Perineal swelling
Bladder neck contractures   Severe pelvic prolapse

Related to impaired afferent pathways or inadequacy secondary to:
Cord injury/tumor/infection   Multiple sclerosis
Brain injury/tumor/infection   Diabetic neuropathy
Cerebrovascular accident   Alcoholic neuropathy
Demyelinating diseases   Tabes dorsalis

Treatment Related

Related to bladder outlet obstruction or impaired afferent pathways
secondary to drug therapy (iatrogenic)*
Antihistamines   Decongestants*
Theophylline   Anticholinergics*
Epinephrine   Calcium channel blockers*
Isoproterenol

Situational (Personal, Environmental)

Related to bladder outlet obstruction secondary to:
Fecal impaction*

** Previously called *Urinary Retention.*

Related to detrusor hypocontractility secondary to:*
Deconditioned voiding
Association with stress or discomfort

NOC

Refer to *Functional Urinary Incontinence*

Goal

The client will achieve a state of dryness that meets personal satisfaction, as evidenced by the following indicators:

- Empty the bladder using Créde's or Valsalva maneuver with a residual urine of less than 50 milliliters if indicated.
- Void voluntarily.

NIC

See also *Functional Urinary Incontinence*, Overflow Retention Care, Urinary Bladder Training

Interventions

Refer to Related Factors.

Explain Rationale for Treatment

Develop a Bladder Retraining or Reconditioning Program
(*See Continuous Incontinence*)

Instruct About Methods to Empty Bladder

- Assist to a sitting position.
- Teach abdominal strain and Valsalva maneuver; instruct client to:
  - Lean forward on thighs.
  - Contract abdominal muscles, if possible, and strain or "bear down"; hold breath while straining (Valsalva maneuver).
  - Hold strain or breath until urine flow stops; wait 1 minute, and strain again as long as possible.
  - Continue until no more urine is expelled.
- Teach Credé's maneuver; instruct client to:
  - Place hands flat (or place fist) just below umbilical area.
  - Place one hand on top of the other.
  - Press firmly down and in toward the pelvic arch.
  - Repeat six or seven times until no more urine can be expelled.
  - Wait a few minutes and repeat to ensure complete emptying.

Indicate on the Intake and Output Record Which Technique Was Used to Induce Voiding

Obtain Postvoid Residuals After Attempts at Emptying Bladder; If Residual Urine Volumes Are Greater Than 100 Milliliters, Schedule Intermittent Catheterization Program (See Continuous Incontinence)

Initiate Health Teaching

- Teach bladder reconditioning program (refer to *Continuous Incontinence*).
- Teach intermittent catheterization (refer to *Continuous Incontinence*).
- Instruct client about prevention of urinary tract infections (refer to *Continuous Incontinence*).

RISK FOR VASCULAR TRAUMA

NANDA-I Definition

At risk for damage to a vein and its surrounding tissues related to the presence of a catheter and/or infused solutions

Risk Factors*

Treatment Related

Catheter type**
Catheter width**
Impaired ability to visualize the insertion site
Inadequate catheter fixation**
Infusion rate**

Insertions site**
Length of insertion time
Nature of solution (e.g., concentration, chemical irritant, temperature, pH)

🐾 Author's Note

This NANDA-I diagnosis represents a risk for all clients with intravenous catheters. Procedure manuals on the clinical unit should contain the correct placement, fixation, and monitoring of all intravenous sites. Nurses needing these guidelines should refer to the procedure manual. Practicing nurses do not need to have this diagnosis on the care plan.

** May indicate poor clinical practice.

Students should refer to their fundamentals of nursing text for specific techniques to start, secure, and monitor intravenous therapy. Consult with your faculty to determine if this should be written on your assigned client's care plan.

Clinically, certain intravenous medications (e.g., chemotherapy, vesicant medications) are extremely toxic and therefore require specific interventions to prevent occurrence and tissue necrosis. Interventions and goals for preventing and responding to extravasation of the intravenous vesicant medications will be outlined for this diagnosis. These interventions are usually also found in a procedure manual.

RISK FOR OTHER-DIRECTED VIOLENCE

Definition

At risk for behaviors in which an individual demonstrates that he or she can be physically, emotionally, and/or sexually harmful to others (NANDA-I)

State in which a client has been, or is at risk to be, assaultive toward others or the environment**

RISK FACTORS

Presence of Risk Factors (see Related Factors).

Related Factors

Pathophysiologic

Related to history of aggressive acts and perception of environment as threatening secondary to:

or

Related to history of aggressive acts and delusional thinking secondary to:

or

Related to history of aggressive acts and manic excitement secondary to:

or

** This statement added by Lynda Juall Carpenito for clarity and usefulness.

Related to history of aggressive acts and inability to verbalize feelings secondary to:

or

Related to history of aggressive acts and psychic overload secondary to:

Temporal lobe epilepsy	Hormonal imbalance
Head injury	Viral encephalopathy
Progressive central nervous system deterioration (brain tumor)	Mental retardation Minimal brain dysfunction

Related to toxic response to alcohol or drugs

Related to organic brain syndrome

Treatment Related

Related to toxic reaction to medication

Situational (Personal, Environmental)

Related to history of overt aggressive acts

Related to increase in stressors within a short period

Related to acute agitation

Related to suspiciousness

Related to persecutory delusions

Related to verbal threats of physical assault

Related to low frustration tolerance

Related to poor impulse control

Related to fear of the unknown

Related to response to catastrophic event

Related to response to dysfunctional family throughout developmental stages

Related to dysfunctional communication patterns

Related to drug or alcohol abuse

 Author's Note

The diagnosis *Risk for Other-Directed Violence* describes a client who has been assaultive or, because of certain factors (e.g., toxic response to alcohol or drugs, hallucinations or delusions, brain dysfunction), is at high risk for assaulting others. In such a situation, the nursing focus is on decreasing violent episodes and protecting the client and others.

The nurse should not use this diagnosis to address underlying problems such as anxiety or poor self-esteem, but instead should refer to the diagnoses *Anxiety*, *Ineffective Coping*, or both to focus on the sources of the violence (spouse, child, older adult). When domestic violence is present or suspected, the nurse should explore the diagnosis *Disabled Family Coping*. A client at risk for suicide would warrant the diagnosis *Risk for Suicide*.

NOC

Abuse Cessation, Abusive Behavior Self-Restraint, Aggression Self-Control, Impulse Self-Control

Goal

The client will refrain from abusive behaviors (in all forms) toward others, as evidenced by the following indicators (Varcarolis, 2011):

- Seeks assistance when emotions are escalating.
- Refrains from threatening, loud language toward others.
- Responds to external controls when at high risk for loss of control.
- Identifies factors contributing to abusive behaviors.
- Identifies calming strategies.
- Uses appropriate methods to express anger.

NIC

Abuse Protection Support, Anger Control Assistance, Environmental Management: Violence Prevention, Impulse Control Training, Crisis Intervention, Seclusion, Physical Restraint

Interventions

The nursing interventions for *Risk for Other-Directed Violence* apply to any client who is potentially violent, regardless of related factors.

Promote Interactions That Increase the Client's Sense of Trust

- Acknowledge the client's feelings (e.g., "You are having a rough time").
  - Be genuine and empathetic.
  - Tell the client that you will help him or her to control behavior and not do anything destructive.
  - Be direct and frank ("I can see you are angry").
  - Be consistent and firm.

- Set limits when the client poses a risk to others. Refer to *Anxiety* for further interventions for setting limits.
- Offer choices and options. At times, it is necessary to give in to some demands to avoid a power struggle.
- Encourage the client to express anger and hostility verbally instead of "acting out."
- Maintain client's personal space:
  - Do not touch the client.
  - Avoid feelings of physical entrapment of individual or staff.
- Be aware of your own feelings and reactions.
  - Do not take verbal abuse personally.
  - Remain calm if you are becoming upset; leave the situation to others, if possible.
  - After a threatening situation, discuss your feelings with other staff.
- Observe for cues of increasing anger (Boyd, 2005).
  - Reports of numbness, nausea, and vertigo
  - Choking sensation, chills, and prickly sensations
  - Increased muscle tone, clenched fists, set jaw, and eyebrows lower and drawn together
  - Lips pressed together to form a thin line
  - Flushing or paleness
  - "Goose bumps"
  - Twitching
  - Sweating

Initiate Immediate Management of the High-Risk Client

- Allow the client with acute agitation a space that is five times greater than that for a client who is in control. Do not touch the client unless you have a trusting relationship.
- Avoid physical entrapment of individual or staff.
- Convey empathy by acknowledging the client's feelings. Let the client know you will not let him or her lose control. Remind the client of previous successes with self-control.
- Do not approach a violent client alone. Often, the presence of three or four staff members is enough to reassure the client that you will not let him or her lose control. Use a positive tone; do not demand or cajole.
- Give the client control by offering alternatives (e.g., walking, talking).
- Set limits on actions, not feelings. Use concise, easily understood statements.
- Maintain eye contact, but do not stare. Stand at a friendly angle (45 degrees); keep an open posture if the client is standing, and sit when the client sits.
- Do not make promises you cannot keep.

- Avoid using "always" and "never."
- When interpersonal and pharmacologic interventions fail to control the angry, aggressive client, physical interventions (restraints, seclusion) are the final resort. Always follow hospital protocols (Varcarolis, 2011).

Establish an Environment That Reduces Agitation (Farrell et al., 1998)

- Decrease noise level.
- Give short, concise explanations.
- Control the number of persons present at one time.
- Provide a single or semiprivate room.
- Allow the client to arrange personal possessions.
- Be aware that darkness can increase disorientation and enhance suspiciousness.
- Decrease situations in which the client is frustrated.
- Provide music if the client is receptive.

Assist the Client to Maintain Control Over His or Her Behavior

- Establish the expectation that the client can control behavior, and continue to reinforce the expectation. Explain exactly which behavior is inappropriate and why.
- Give three options: two offer a choice, whereas the third is the consequence of violent behavior.
- Allow time for the client to make a choice.
- Provide positive feedback when the client is able to exercise restraint.
- Enforce consequences when indicated.
- Reassure the client that you will provide control if he or she cannot. ("I am concerned about you. I will get [more staff, medications] to keep you from doing anything impulsive.")
- Set firm, clear limits when a client presents a danger to self or others. ("Put the chair down.")
- Call the client by name in a calm, quiet, respectful manner.
- Avoid threats; refer to yourself, not policies, rules, or supervisors.
- Allow appropriate verbal expressions of anger. Give positive feedback.
- Set limits on verbal abuse. Do not take insults personally. Support others (clients, staff) who may be targets of abuse.
- Do not give attention to the client who is being verbally abusive. Tell the client what you are doing and why.
- Assist with external controls, as necessary.
  - Maintain observation every 15 to 30 minutes.
  - Remove items that the client could use as weapons (e.g., glass, sharp objects).

- Assess the client's ability to tolerate off-unit procedures.
- If the client is acutely agitated, be cautious with items such as hot coffee.

Plan for Unpredictable Violence

- Monitor for cues to potential aggression (Alvarey, 1998).

Verbal
- Morose silence
- Loud, demanding remarks
- Illogical responses
- Negative response to requests
- Demeaning remarks
- Overt hostility
- Threats
- Sarcasm
- Mistrust

Nonverbal Facial Expression
- Tense jaw
- Staring
- Clenched teeth
- Dilated pupils
- Lip biting
- Pulsing carotid

Nonverbal Body Language
- Hand twisting objects
- Stony withdrawal
- Aggression
- Confrontational stance
- Fist clenching, unclenching (slamming doors)
- Pounding, kicking
- Pacing
- Ensure availability of staff before potential violent behavior (never try to assist the client alone when physical restraint is necessary).
- Determine who will be in charge of directing personnel to intervene in violent behavior if it occurs.
- Ensure protection for self (door nearby for withdrawal, pillow to protect face).

Use Seclusion and/or Restraint, If Indicated

- Remove client from situation if environment is contributing to aggressive behavior, using the least amount of control needed (e.g., ask others to leave, and take client to quiet room).
- Reinforce that you are going to help the client control him or herself.

- Repeatedly tell the client what is going to happen before external control begins.
- Ensure that sufficient personnel (five) are present.
- Protect client from injuring self or others through use of restraints or seclusion.**
- When using seclusion, institutional policy provides specifics. The following are general measures:
  - Observe the client at least every 15 minutes.
  - Search the client before secluding to remove harmful objects.
  - Check seclusion room to see that safety is maintained.
  - Offer fluids and food periodically (in nonbreakable containers).
  - When approaching a client to be secluded, have sufficient staff present.
  - Explain concisely what is going to happen ("You will be placed in a room by yourself until you can better control your behavior"); give the client a chance to cooperate.
  - Assist with toileting and personal hygiene (assess the client's ability to be out of seclusion; a urinal or commode may need to be used).
  - If the client is taken out of seclusion, someone must be present continually.
  - Maintain verbal interaction during seclusion (provides information necessary to assess the client's degree of control).
  - When the client is allowed out of seclusion, a staff member needs to be in constant attendance to determine whether the client can handle additional stimulation.
- When using restraint, institutional policy provides specifics. The following are general measures:
  - A client in a four-point or two-point restraint must be in seclusion or with one-on-one nursing care for protection. Seclusion guidelines should be followed.
  - Restraints must be loosened every hour (one limb at a time).
  - Waist restraints must allow enough arm movement to enable eating/smoking and self-protection against falling.
  - Restraints should be padded.
  - Restraints never should be attached to side rails, but rather to the bed frame.
- Provide an opportunity to clarify the rationale for seclusion and to discuss the client's reactions after the seclusion period is over.

** May require a primary care professional's order.

Convene a Group Discussion After a Violent Episode in an Inpatient Unit

- Include all those who witnessed the episode (client, staff).
- Include client(s) exhibiting the violent behavior, if possible.
- Discuss what happened, the consequences, and the feelings of the community.

Assist the Client in Developing Alternative Coping Strategies When the Crisis Has Passed and Learning Can Occur

- Explore what precipitates the client's loss of control ("What was happening before you felt like hitting her?").
- Assist the client to recall the physical symptoms associated with anger.
- Teach to use deep breaths and relaxation breathing.
- Help the client to evaluate where in the chain of events change was possible.
  - Use role playing to practice communication techniques.
  - Discuss how issues of control interfere with communication.
  - Help the client recognize negative thinking patterns associated with low self-esteem.
- Help the client to practice negotiation skills with family and people in authority.
- Encourage increased recreational activities.
- Use group therapy to decrease sense of aloneness and increase communication skills.
- Instruct about or refer for assertiveness training.
- Instruct about or refer for negotiation skills development.

⚜ Pediatric Interventions

- Discuss with parents the methods of disciplining the child: Are they realistic? Appropriate? Effective?

To Manage Disruptive Behavior In Children (Varcarolis, 2011):

- Use a preset gesture or signal to remind child/adolescent to use self-control
- Move closer to child, put arm around child gently.
- Redirect attention to another activity.
- Use humor or kidding.
- Remove child from situation.
- Initiate therapeutic holding.
- Use promises and reward carefully.
- Use threats and punishment carefully.
- Discuss the risks of firearms in the home. Explore the storage of firearms and protective devices (e.g., lockboxes, trigger locks).

- Explore various sources of media violence (e.g., television, video games, music, movies).
- Explain strategies to prevent adverse effects of media (e.g., violence, commercials (Hockenberry, Wilson, 2007; Willis & Strasburger, 1998).
  - Watch television and videos with children: Limit to 2 hours or less a day.
  - If possible, avoid programs that emphasize violence.
  - Creatively illustrate when violent acts are punished.
  - Explore alternatives to violence (e.g., "What could the man have done besides shooting?")
  - When selecting programs, consider:
    - Are good characters violent?
    - Is the violence justified?
    - Are there negative consequences of violence?
  - Consider the child's age when selecting television programs and movies.
- Discuss programs and commercial content with child to emphasize (Davis, 1989):
  - You are smarter than what you see on TV
  - TV world is not real
  - Somebody is making money trying to sell you something
  - TV shows that some people are more important than others
- Engage the child and peers in a nonthreatening manner to discuss age-related violence (e.g., hitting, bullying, throwing objects, date rape).
- Role play high-risk situations, such as:
  - Finding a gun in a friend's house
  - Bullying a victim
  - Refusing sexual advances

RISK FOR SELF-DIRECTED VIOLENCE

NANDA-I Definition

At risk for behaviors in which an individual demonstrates that he or she can be physically, emotionally, and/or sexually harmful to self

Risk Factors*

Age 15 to 19
Age 45 or older
Engagement in autoerotic sexual acts

Author's Note

The remaining risk factors are risk factors for suicide (e.g., suicidal ideation or history of multiple suicide attempts). *Risk for Self-Directed Violence* should be replaced with *Risk for Suicide*. Refer to this diagnosis for additional content.

WANDERING

NANDA-I Definition

Meandering, aimless, or repetitive locomotion that exposes the individual to harm; frequently incongruent with boundaries

Defining Characteristics*

Continuous movement from place to place
Getting lost
Fretful locomotion
Frequent movement from place to place
Haphazard locomotion
Hyperactivity
Inability to locate significant landmarks in a familiar setting
Locomotion into unauthorized or private spaces
Locomotion resulting in unintended leaving of a premise
Long periods of locomotion without an apparent destination
Periods of locomotion interspersed with periods of non-
    locomotion (e.g., sitting, standing, sleeping)
Persistent locomotion in search of something
Pacing
Trespassing
Scanning behaviors
Searching behaviors
Locomotion that cannot be easily dissuaded
Shadowing a caregiver's locomotion

Related Factors

Pathophysiologic

*Related to impaired cerebral function** secondary to:*
Cerebrovascular accident

** This related factor must be present. Another related factor can also be
   present concurrently.

Mental retardation
Alzheimer's dementia or other dementia

Related to physiologic state or needs (e.g., hunger, thirst, pain, urination, constipation)*

Situational (Personal, Environmental)

Related to emotional state (e.g., frustration, anxiety, boredom, depression, or agitation)*

Related to overstimulating*/understimulating environment

Related to separation from familiar environment* (e.g., people, objects)

Maturational

Older Adult
Related to faulty judgments secondary to:
Medications (e.g., sedation,* hyperactivity)

 Author's Note

This approved NANDA-I diagnosis is more useful than *Risk for Injury*, which was previously used. *Risk for Injury* focuses on strategies to protect a client from injury. *Wandering* directs interventions to protect the client from injury in addition to addressing the reasons for the wandering behavior, if possible.

NOC

Risk Control, Elopement Propensity Risk, Safe Wandering, Family Functioning

Goal

The client will not elope or get lost, as evidenced by the following indicators for client and family:

- Ambulate safely.
- Caretakers will identify factors that contribute to wandering behaviors.
- Caretakers will anticipate wandering behaviors.

NIC

Surveillance: Safety, Environmental Management: Safety, Referral, Risk Identification, Security Enhancement

Interventions

Assess for Contributing Factors

- Anxiety
- Confusion
- Frustration
- Boredom
- Agitation
- Separation from familiar people and places
- Faulty judgments
- Physiologic urge (hunger, thirst, pain, urination, constipation)

Reduce or Eliminate Contributing Factors, If Possible

Anxiety/Agitation
Refer to *Anxiety* for interventions.

Unfamiliar Environment
- Select a familiar picture to exhibit on the client's door.
- Redirect the client if he or she is lost.
- Provide a safe route for walking.
- Encourage activities that involve exercise (e.g., sweeping, raking).
- Create nature scenes in the hallways (Cohen-Mansfield, 1998).
- Mark exit door with big signs.
- Place horizontal stripes on the exit door or use a cloth panel across the width of the door.

Physiologic Urges
- Anticipate need for toileting with a schedule.
- Schedule times for fluids and food.
- Evaluate for any pain.

Promote a Safe Environment

- Install locks on doors and windows.
- Install electronic devices with buzzers on doors and property boundaries.
- Use pressure-sensitive alarms (doormats, bed sensor, chair sensor).
- Provide regular opportunities for the client to walk with a companion or in a safe area.

Notify Others (Neighbors, Police, Others in Residence, Staff, Community Resources) About the Client's Wandering Behaviors

- Explain the use of electronic devices.
- Instruct others to notify the provider if they see the client wandering.
- Supply others with a recent photograph and current identification information (age, height, weight, hair color, description of clothes, identifying characteristics) of the client.
- Contact the local Alzheimer's association for safety programs.

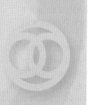

Section 2

Health Promotion/ Wellness Nursing Diagnoses

This section organizes all the health promotion/ wellness nursing diagnoses for individuals. *Readiness for Enhanced Self-Health Management* is a broad nursing diagnosis that can be useful if a specific wellness diagnosis does not address the targeted health topic. Some of the diagnoses included in this section represent unhealthy lifestyles. They have been included with a health promotion focus, e.g., Stress Overload, Sedentary Lifestyle, Risk-Prone Health Behavior.

Wellness nursing diagnoses are "a clinical judgment about an individual, group, or community in transition from a specific level of wellness to a higher level of wellness" (NANDA, 2007). A valid wellness nursing diagnosis has two requirements: (1) the client has a desire for increased wellness in a particular area and (2) the client is currently functioning effectively in a particular area.

Wellness nursing diagnoses are one-part statements with no related factors. The goals established by the client or group will direct their actions to enhance their health.

There is still confusion about the clinical usefulness of this type of diagnosis. The author believes that some of these diagnoses can be strengthened and are clinically useful, such as *Readiness for Enhanced Parenting* or *Readiness for Enhanced Community Coping*; whereas others, such as *Readiness for Enhanced Power, Readiness for Enhanced Urinary Elimination*, and other similar diagnoses, are questionable relative to clinical usefulness. Under each diagnosis, Author's Notes will elaborate on the clinical usefulness of the diagnosis.

Clinically, data that represent strengths can be important for nurses to know. These strengths can assist the nurse in selecting interventions to reduce or prevent a problem in another health pattern. If nurses want to designate strength, it should be documented as strength on the assessment form or care plan. If the client desires assistance in promoting a higher level of function, *Readiness for Enhanced (specify)* would be useful in certain settings, such as schools, community centers, and assisted living facilities. Interested clinicians can use these health-promotion/wellness nursing diagnoses and are invited to share their work with NANDA as well as the author.

Health Promotion/Wellness Assessment[†]

Subjective Data

Health Perception–Health Management Pattern

Ask the client to place one check next to the category in which they usually practice; place two checks for those they practice daily (Breslow, 2004):

- Three meals a day at regular times and no snacking
- Breakfast every day
- Moderate exercise two or three times a week
- 7 to 8 hours of sleep, not more or less
- No smoking
- Moderate weight
- No alcohol or in moderation

What Is the Client's/Family's Perception of Their Overall Health?

- What personal practices maintain their health?
- What sources does the client or family access to maintain or improve their healthy lifestyle?
- How could the client be healthier?

Nutrition–Metabolic Pattern

- What is the client's body mass index?
- Typical daily fluid intake
- Supplements (vitamins, types of snacks)
- Daily intake of whole grain or enriched breads, cereals, rice, or pasta.
- Three servings of fruit/fruit juice daily
- Unlimited raw or 5 to 8 servings of cooked non starch vegetables daily
- Skim or low-fat dairy products
- Meats and poultry trimmed of fat and skin
- No fried foods/snacks
- No or limited (fewer than two) sugar drinks (e.g., soda, ice tea, juices)
- Do you see a relationship among stress and tension, emotional upsets, and your eating habits?

Elimination Pattern

- Bowel elimination pattern? (Describe.)
  - Frequency (every 2–3 days), character (soft, bulky)
- Urinary elimination patter? (Describe.)
  - Character (amber, yellow, straw-colored)

[†] Carpenito-Moyet, 2007; Edelman & Mandle, 2010; Gordon, 2003.

Activity–Exercise Pattern
- Exercise pattern? (Type, frequency)
- Leisure activities? (Frequency)
- Energy level? (High, moderate, adequate, low)
- Are there barriers to exercising?
- What are five things that you do to play?
- What things do you do that make you feel good?

Sleep–Rest Pattern
- Satisfied and rested?
- Average hours of sleep per night
- Relaxation periods? (How often, how long)

Cognitive–Perceptual Pattern
- Satisfied with:
  - Decision making?
  - Memory?
  - Ability to learn?
- Describe briefly your educational background.

Self-Perception–Self-Concept Pattern
- Describe how you feel about:
  - Yourself
  - Your body? Changes?
- Do you have trouble expressing anger, sadness, happiness, love, and/or sexuality?
- What are your major strengths or personal qualities?
- What are your weaknesses or negative aspects?
- In your life right now, what is your most meaningful activity?
- How many more years do you expect to live, and how do you think you will die?
- How do you imagine your future?
- What would you like to accomplish in your future? Are there changes you need to make to accomplish this?

List the Most Important Events, Crises, Transitions, and/or Changes (Positive or Negative) in Your Life
- Take time to reflect on how they affected you. Place an asterisk in front of one or two that were especially important.

Roles–Relationships Pattern
- Satisfied with job? Need a change?
- Satisfied with role responsibilities?
- Describe your relationship with your family/partner.
- Describe your friendships (close, casual).
- List the most important people in your life right now and why they are important.

Sexuality–Reproductive Pattern
• Is sex an important aspect of your life?
• Are you currently in a sexual relationship?
• What would you want to change about your current sexual relationship?

Coping–Stress Tolerance Pattern
• List the most regular sources of stress in your life. How could you make them less stressful?
• How do you usually respond to stressful situations (get angry, withdraw, take it out on others, get sick, drink, eat)?
• What situations make you feel calm or relaxed?
• What situations make you feel anxious or upset? What can you do to make yourself feel better?

Values–Beliefs Pattern
• Write 10 things you most value in life.
• Would you describe yourself as a religious or spiritual person?
• How do your beliefs help you?

READINESS FOR ENHANCED BREASTFEEDING

NANDA-I Definition

A pattern of proficiency and satisfaction of the mother–infant dyad that is sufficient to support the breastfeeding process and can be strengthened

Defining Characteristics

Major (Must Be Present)

Mother's ability to position infant at breast to promote a successful latch-on response
Infant content after feeding
Regular and sustained suckling/swallowing at the breast
Infant weight patterns appropriate for age
Effective mother–infant communication patterns* (infant cues, maternal interpretation and response)

Minor (May Be Present)

Signs or symptoms of oxytocin release are present* (let-down or milk ejection reflex)

Adequate infant elimination patterns for age*
Eagerness of infant to nurse*
Maternal verbalization of satisfaction with breastfeeding

NOC
Knowledge: Breastfeeding

Goal

The mother will report an increase in confidence and satisfaction with breastfeeding, as evidenced by the following indicator:

• Identify two new strategies (specify) to enhance breastfeeding.

Interventions

Refer to the Internet for sites for resources and information on breastfeeding.
    Refer to *Ineffective Breastfeeding* for interventions to enhance breastfeeding.

READINESS FOR ENHANCED CHILDBEARING PROCESS

NANDA-I Definition

A pattern of preparing for and maintaining a healthy pregnancy, childbirth process, and care of the newborn that is sufficient for ensuring well-being and can be strengthened

Defining Characteristics*

During Pregnancy

Reports appropriate prenatal lifestyle (e.g., nutrition, elimination, sleep, body movement, exercise, personal hygiene)
Reports appropriate physical preparations
Reports managing unpleasant symptoms in pregnancy
Demonstrates respect for unborn baby

Reports a realistic birth plan
Prepares and seeks necessary newborn care items
Seeks necessary knowledge (e.g., of labor and delivery,
    newborn care)
Reports availability of support systems
Has regular prenatal health visits

During Labor and Delivery

Reports lifestyle (e.g., diet, elimination, sleep, body movement,
    personal hygiene) that is appropriate for the stage of labor
Responds appropriately to the onset of labor
Is proactive during labor and delivery
Uses relaxation techniques appropriate for the stage of labor
Demonstrates attachment behavior to the newborn baby
Uses support systems appropriately

After Birth

Demonstrates appropriate baby feeding techniques
Demonstrates appropriate breast care
Demonstrates attachment behavior to the baby
Demonstrates basic baby care techniques
Provides safe environment for the baby
Reports appropriate postpartum lifestyle (e.g., diet, elimination,
    sleep, body movement, exercise, personal hygiene)
Utilizes support system appropriately

 Author's Note

This NANDA-I nursing diagnosis represents the comprehensive care
that is needed to promote the following: healthy pregnancy, childbirth
and the postpartum process, enhanced relationships (mother, father,
infant, and siblings), and optimal care of the newborn. This care is beyond
the scope possible in this text. Refer to a text about maternal-child
health for the specific interventions for this diagnosis.

READINESS FOR ENHANCED COMFORT

NANDA-I Definition

A pattern of ease, relief, and transcendence in physical, psychospiritual, environmental, and/or social dimensions that is sufficient
for well-being and can be strengthened

Defining Characteristics*

Expresses desire to enhance comfort
Expresses desire to enhance feeling of contentment
Expresses desire to enhance relaxation
Expresses desire to enhance resolution of complaints

 Author's Note

This diagnosis is general and therefore does not direct specific interventions. It encompasses physical, psychological, spiritual, environmental, and social dimensions. It would be more clinically useful to focus on a particular dimension, such as *Readiness for Enhanced Spiritual Well-Being*.

READINESS FOR ENHANCED COMMUNICATION

NANDA-I Definition

A pattern of exchanging information and ideas with others that is sufficient for meeting one's needs and life's goals and can be strengthened

Defining Characteristics*

Able to speak and/or write a language
Expresses feelings
Expresses satisfaction with ability to share ideas with others
Expresses satisfaction with ability to share information with others
Expresses willingness to enhance communication
Forms phrases
Forms sentences
Forms words
Interprets nonverbal cures appropriately
Uses nonverbal cues appropriately

 Author's Note

This diagnosis represents a client with good communications skills. Interventions to enhance communication skills can be found in Section 1 in *Impaired Communication* and *Impaired Verbal Communication*.

READINESS FOR ENHANCED COPING

NANDA-I Definition

A pattern of cognitive and behavioral efforts to manage demands that are sufficient for well-being and can be strengthened

Defining Characteristics*

Acknowledges power
Aware of possible environmental changes
Defines stressors as manageable
Seeks knowledge of new strategies
Seeks social support
Uses a broad range of emotion-oriented strategies
Uses a broad range of problem-oriented strategies
Uses spiritual resources

Goal

The client will report increased satisfaction with coping with stressors, as evidenced by the following indicator:

• Identify two new strategies (specify) to enhance coping with stressors.

Interventions

If Anxiety Diminishes One's Effective Coping, Teach:

• Abdominal relaxation breathing
• Abdominal breathing while imagining a peaceful scene (e.g., ocean, woods, mountains)
• Imagine the feel of the warm sand on your feet, sun on your face, the sound of water.

Explain Reframing (Varcarolis, 2011)

• Reassess the situation; ask yourself:
  • What positive thing can come out of the situation?
  • What did I learn?
  • What would I do differently next time?

- What might be going on with my (boss, partner, sister friend) that would cause him or her to say or do that?
- Is she or he stressed out or having problems?

Acknowledge Stress-Reducing Tips for Living (Varcarolis, 2011)

- Exercise regularly, at least three times weekly
- Reduce caffeine intake
- Engage in meaningful, satisfying work
- Do not let work dominate your life
- Guard your personal freedom
- Choose your friends; associate with gentle people
- Live with and love whom you choose
- Structure your time as you see fit
- Set your own life goals
- Refer to the Internet for sites for resources and information about stress reduction techniques

READINESS FOR ENHANCED COMMUNITY COPING

Definition

A pattern of cognitive and behavioral efforts to manage demands that is sufficient for well-being and can be strengthened (NANDA-I)

A state in which a community's pattern for adaptation and problem solving is satisfactory for meeting the demands or needs of the community, but the community desires to improve management of current and future problems/stressors**

Defining Characteristics*

Acknowledges power
Aware of possible environmental changes
Defines stressors as manageable
Seeks knowledge of new strategies

Seek social support
Uses broad range of emotion-oriented strategies
Uses a broad range of problem-oriented strategies
Uses spiritual resources

** This definition has been added by the author for clarity and usefulness.

Author's Note

This diagnosis can be used to describe a community that wishes to improve an already effective pattern of coping. For a community to be assisted to a higher level of functioning, its basic needs for food, shelter, safety, a clean environment, and a supportive network must first be addressed. When these needs are met, programs can focus on higher functioning, such as wellness and self-actualization. Community programs can be designed after a community assessment and because of community requests. They can focus on enhancing health promotion with topics related to optimal nutrition, weight control, regular exercise programs, constructive stress management, social support, role responsibilities, and preparing for and coping with life events such as retirement, parenting, and pregnancy.

NOC

Community Competence, Community Health Status, Community Risk Control

Goal

The community (specify type of community, e.g., the town of Mullica Hill, the southeast neighborhood of South Tucson) will provide programs to improve (specify type of focus, e.g., nutrition), as evidenced by the following indicators:

- Identify health promotion needs as (specify: e.g., daily decrease in high-fat foods, increase in fruits and vegetables).
- Access resources needed (specify: e.g., local experts, nutritionist, college students).
- Develop programs (specify: health fair, school cafeteria, printed material) based on needs assessment.
- Implementation of policies for health (e.g., American Diabetes Association policy for healthy meals).

NIC

Program Development, Risk Identification, Community Health Development, Environmental Risk Protection

Interventions

Conduct Focus Groups to Discuss Programs to Assist Residents With Positive Coping With Developmental Tasks

- Arrange focus groups according to age, including diverse groups.

Plan Programs Targeted for a Specific Population

Adolescents (13 to 18 Years)
• Career planning
• Stress management

Young Adults (18 to 35 Years)
• Career selection
• Constructive relationships
• Balancing one's life
• Parenting issues

Middle Age (35 to 65 Years)
• Launching children
• Reciprocal relationships
• Aging parents
• Quality leisure time

Older Adults (65 Years and Older)
• Retirement issues
• Balancing one's life
• Anticipated losses
• Facts and myths of aging

All Ages
• Civic planning
• Meeting needs of all community members
• Crisis intervention
• Grieving
• Community involvement

Discuss Programs That Promote High-Level Wellness

• Optimal nutrition
• Weight control
• Exercise programs
• Socialization programs
• Effective problem solving
• Injury prevention
• Environmental quality

Define the Target Health Promotion Needs

• Analyze assessment of community.
• Prioritize the needs:
  • Organize the focus group responses
  • Probability of success
  • Cost:benefit ratio (e.g., resources available)
  • Potential for policy development

Select a Health Promotion Program

- Identify target population (e.g., entire community, older adults, adolescents).
- Delineate a timetable for the planning and implementation stages.

Meet With Community Groups (Health Centers, Faith-Based Groups, Government Agencies) to Review Findings of Focus Groups and to Discuss Collaborative Programming

Plan the Program

- Develop detailed program objectives and the evaluation framework to be used.
  - Content
  - Time needed
  - Ideal teaching method for targeting group
  - Teaching aids (e.g., large-print materials)
- Establish resources needed and sources.
  - Space
  - Transportation facilities
  - Optimal day of week
  - Optimal time of year
  - Supplies, audiovisual equipment
  - Financial (budgeted, donations)
- Market the program.
  - Media (e.g., newspaper, TV, radio)
  - Posters (food market, train station)
  - Flyers (distribute via school to home)
  - Word of mouth (religious organizations, community clubs, schools)
  - Guest speaker (community clubs, schools)

Provide Program and Evaluate Whether Desired Results (Objectives) Were Achieved

- Number of participants
- Negative feedback
- Objectives achieved
- Actual expenditures versus budgeted
- Statistics (e.g., bicycle accidents)
- Participant evaluations
- Adequate planning
- Revisions for future planning
- Shared responsibility
- Determine the strengths and limitations of the program and plan a new approach if indicated

READINESS FOR ENHANCED DECISION MAKING

NANDA-I Definition

A pattern of choosing a course of action that is sufficient for meeting short- and long-term health-related goals and can be strengthened

Defining Characteristics*

Expresses desire to enhance decision making
Expresses desire to enhance congruency of decisions with personal and/or sociocultural values and goals
Expresses desire to enhance risk–benefit analysis of decisions
Expresses desire to enhance understanding of choices and the meaning of the choices
Expresses desire to enhance use of reliable evidence for decisions

NOC
Decision-Making, Information Processing

Goal

The individual/group will report increased satisfaction with decision-making, as evidenced by the following indicator:

• Identify two new strategies (specify) to enhance decision making.

NIC
Decision-Making Support, Mutual Goal Setting

Interventions

Refer to Interventions for *Decisional Conflict*.
Refer to the Internet for sites for resources and information about decision making.

READINESS FOR ENHANCED FAMILY COPING

NANDA-I Definition

A pattern of management of adaptive tasks by primary person (family member, significant other, or close friend) involved with the client's health challenge that is sufficient for health and growth, in regard to self and in relation to the client, and can be strengthened

Defining Characteristics*

Significant person attempts to describe growth impact of crisis
Significant person moves in direction of enriching lifestyle
Significant person moves in direction of health promotion
Chooses experiences that optimize wellness*
Individual expresses interest in making contact with others who
    have experienced a similar situation

Related Factors

Refer to *Interrupted Family Processes*.

 Author's Note

This nursing diagnosis describes components found in *Interrupted Family Processes*. Until clinical research differentiates the category from the aforementioned categories, use *Interrupted Family Processes*, depending on the data presented.

READINESS FOR ENHANCED FAMILY PROCESSES

NANDA-I Definition

A pattern of family functioning that is sufficient to support the well-being of family members and can be strengthened

Defining Characteristics*

Expresses willingness to enhance family dynamics
Family functioning meets needs of family members
Activities support the safety and growth of family members
Communication is adequate
Relationships are generally positive; interdependent with
    community; family tasks are accomplished
Family roles are flexible and appropriate for developmental stages
Respect for family members is evident
Family adapts to change
Boundaries of family members are maintained
Energy level of family supports activities of daily living
Family resilience is evident
Balance exists between autonomy and cohesiveness

NOC

Family Environment: Internal

Goal

The family will expresses willingness to enhance family dynamics
and growth.

NIC

Family Involvement Promotion, Family Integrity Promotion

Interventions

**Discuss Elements That Influence Health Promotion in a Family
(Kaakinen et al., 2010)**

* Family culture
* Lifestyles patterns/role models
* Family nutrition
* Religion/spirituality
* Family processes
* Encourage the family to examine their patterns of communication
  (verbal, nonverbal) and family interactions (Kaakinen, 2010).
  * Are they effective?
  * Are all members involved in feeling sharing and decision
    making?
  * Is there positive, reinforcing interactions?
  * Are parent's role-modeling positive family processes?
* Convey that the family has the capacity to achieve a higher
  level of health and has the right to health information to make
  informed decisions.

- Elicit from family areas for growth and change. Assure the commitment of all family members (e.g., improved nutrition, exercising, family meals, group relaxation activities, family time).
- Determine one area for improvement and write a family self-care contract (Bomar, 2005; Kaakinen et al., 2010).
- Set a goal and time frame for initiating and frequency.
- Develop a plan.
- Assign responsibilities.
- Evaluate outcomes.
- Modify, renegotiate, or terminate.
- Direct family to seek resources independently (e.g., community resources, Web sites).
- Refer to *Interrupted Family Processes* for additional interventions for strengthening family functioning, promoting family integrity, mutual support, and positive functioning.

READINESS FOR ENHANCED FLUID BALANCE

NANDA-I Definition

A pattern of equilibrium between the fluid volume and the chemical composition of body fluids that is sufficient for meeting physical needs and can be strengthened

Defining Characteristics

Expresses willingness to enhance fluid balance
Stable weight
Moist mucous membranes
Food and fluid intake adequate for daily needs
Straw-colored urine with specific gravity within normal limits
Good tissue turgor
No excessive thirst
Urine output appropriate for intake
No evidence of edema or dehydration

 Author's Note

If a client has a pattern of equilibrium between fluid volume and the chemical composition of body fluids that is sufficient for meeting physical needs, how can this be strengthened? Would it be more useful to focus on education under the diagnosis *Risk for Deficient Fluid Volume*?

NOC

Fluid Balance, Hydration, Electrolyte Balance

Goal

The client will report increased satisfaction with fluid balance, as evidenced by the following indicator:

• Identify two new strategies (specify) to enhance fluid balance.

NIC

Fluid/Electrolyte Management

Interventions

Refer to Interventions for *Deficient Fluid Balance*.
Refer to the Internet for sites for resources and information about nutrition.

READINESS FOR ENHANCED HOPE

NANDA-I Definition

A pattern of expectations and desires for mobilizing energy on one's own behalf that is sufficient for well-being and can be strengthened

Defining Characteristics*

Expresses desire to enhance congruency of expectations with desires
Expresses desire to enhance ability to set achievable goals
Expresses desire to enhance problem solving to meet goals
Expresses desire to enhance belief in possibilities
Expresses desire to enhance spirituality and sense of meaning to life
Expresses desire to enhance interconnectedness with others
Expresses desire to enhance hope

NOC

Refer to *Hopelessness.*

Goal

The client will report increased hope, as evidenced by the following indicator:

• Identify two new strategies (specify) to enhance hope.

NIC

Refer to *Hopelessness*.
Refer to Internet sites for resources and information about hope.

Interventions

Refer to *Hopelessness* for interventions to promote hope.

READINESS FOR ENHANCED IMMUNIZATION STATUS

NANDA-I Definition

A pattern of conforming to local, national, and/or international standards of immunization to prevent infectious disease(s) that is sufficient to protect a person, family, or community and can be strengthened

Defining Characteristics*

Expresses desire to enhance immunization status
Expresses desire to enhance knowledge of immunization standards
Expresses desire to enhance behavior to prevent infectious disease
Expresses desire to enhance record-keeping of immunizations
Values immunizations as a health priority; expresses desire to
     enhance identification of possible problems associated with
     immunizations

 Author's Note

This diagnosis would apply to an individual or group that needs an immunization according to a national/international standard. All individuals qualify for immunization depending on their age or risk factors. The diagnosis *Risk for Altered Health Maintenance* could be use to describe client who needs immunizations and/or age-related screening such as mammograms. *Readiness for Enhanced Immunization* could be useful if the focus is on immunizations only.

Goal

The individual will verbalize acceptance of recommended immunizations, as evidenced by the following indicators:

• Can relate the benefits of the vaccine.
• Can indentify risks or side effects of vaccination.

Health-Promoting Behavior, Knowledge

Interventions

Determine if All Required Age-Related Immunizations Have Been Administered for Children

Explain the Rationale for Administration of Optional Vaccines (e.g., Risk Behaviors, Travel, Chronic Diseases)

Advise of the Risks of the Vaccine

- Hepatitis A
- Influenza
- Pneumococcal
- Human papillomavirus
- Zoster
- Typhoid
- Yellow fever
- Rabies

Access immunization schedules for children and adults (http:/www.cdc.gov/vaccines/recs).

- Hepatitis A is recommended for children aged 12 months or older and adults who live in areas with increased risks, travel to high-risk locations, or those who desire immunity.
- Pneumococcal vaccine (PCV7) is indicated for all children younger than 5 years old and should be completed with a single dose of PVC13. Adults 65 years of age or older should receive one dose. Children aged 6 to 18 years and adults with underlying medical conditions should receive a single dose of PVC13. Underlying conditions include chronic lung, liver, or cardiovascular diseases; diabetes mellitus; chronic alcoholism; smoking; asplenia; immunocompromised conditions; renal failure; cochlear implants; and central nervous system leaks. Administration of the vaccine can be repeated every 5 years.
- For detailed information about vaccine-related contraindications and precautions, visit the CDC Web site.

READINESS FOR ENHANCED ORGANIZED INFANT BEHAVIOR

NANDA-I Definition

A pattern of modulation of the physiologic and behavioral systems of functioning (i.e., autonomic, motor, state-organization, self-regulatory, and attention-interactional systems) in an infant that is sufficient for well-being and can be strengthened

Defining Characteristics[†]

Autonomic System

Regulated color and respiration

Reduced visceral signals (e.g., smooth)

Reduces tremors, twitches

Digestive functioning, feeding tolerance

Motor System

Smooth, well-modulated posture and tone
Synchronous smooth movements with:

Hand/foot clasping
Suck/suck searching
Grasping

Hand holding
Hand-to-mouth activity
Tucking

State System

Well-differentiated range of states
Clear, robust sleep states
Focused, shiny-eyed alertness with intent or animated facial expressions
Active self-quieting/consoling "ooh" face
Attentional smiling
Cooing

 Author's Note

This diagnosis describes an infant who is responding to the environment with stable and predictable autonomic, motor, and state cues. The focus of interventions is to promote continued stable development and to reduce excess environmental stimuli that may stress the infant. Because this is a wellness diagnosis, the use of related factors is not needed.
The nurse can write the diagnostic statement as *Readiness for Enhanced Organized Infant Behavior* as evidenced by ability to regulate autonomic, motor, and state systems to environmental stimuli.

NOC

Child Development: Specify Age, Sleep, Comfort Level

Goal

The infant will continue age-appropriate growth and development and not experience excessive environmental stimuli. The parent(s)

[†] Blackburn & Vandenberg, 1993

will demonstrate handling that promotes stability, as evidenced by the following indicators:

- Describe developmental needs of infant.
- Describe early signs of stress of exhaustion.
- Demonstrate:
  - Gentle, soothing touch
  - Melodic tone of voice, coos
  - Mutual gazing
  - Rhythmic movements
  - Acknowledgment of all baby's vocalizations
  - Recognition of soothing qualities of actions.

NIC

Developmental Care, Infant Care, Sleep Enhancement, Environmental Management: Comfort, Parent Education: Infant Attachment Promotion, Caregiver Support, Calming Technique

Interventions

Explain to Parents the Effects of Excess Environmental Stress on the Infant

Provide a List of Signs of Stress for Their Infant; Refer to *Disorganized Infant Behavior* for a List of Signs

Teach Parents to Terminate Stimulation if Infant Shows Signs of Stress

Model Developmental Interventions

- Offer only when the infant is alert (if possible, show parents examples of alert and not alert).
- Begin with one stimulus at a time (touch, voice).
- Provide intervention for a short time.
- Increase interventions according to infant's cues.
- Provide frequent, short interventions instead of infrequent, long-term ones.
- Stimulation (visual, auditory, vestibular, tactile, olfactory, gustatory)
- Periods of alertness
- Sleep requirements

Explain, Model, and Observe Parents Engaging in Developmental Interventions

Visual
- Eye contact
- Face-to-face experiences
- High-contrast colors, geometric shapes (e.g., black and white shapes on paper mobile); up to 4 weeks, simple mobiles of four dessert-size paper plates with stripes, four-square checkerboards,

a black dot, and a simple bull's eye, hung 10 to 13 inches from baby's eyes.

Auditory
- Use high-pitched vocalizations.
- Play classical music softly.
- Use a variety of voice inflections.
- Avoid loud talking.
- Call infant by name.
- Avoid monotone speech patterns.

Vestibular (Movement)
- Rock baby in chair.
- Place infant in sling and rock.
- Close infant's fist around a soft toy.
- Slowly change position during handling.
- Provide head support.

Tactile
- Use firm, gentle touch as initial approach.
- Use skin-to-skin contact in a warm room.
- Provide alternative textures (e.g., sheepskin, velvet, satin).
- Avoid stroking if responses are disorganized.

Olfactory
- Wear a light perfume.

Gustatory
- Allow non nutritive sucking (e.g., pacifier, hand in mouth).

Promote Adjustment and Stability in Caregiving Activities (Blackburn & Vandenberg, 1993; Merenstein & Gardner, 1998)

Waking
- Enter room slowly.
- Turn on light and open curtains slowly.
- Avoid walking baby if he or she is asleep.

Changing
- Keep room warm.
- Gently change position; contain limbs during movement.
- Stop changing if infant is irritable.

Feeding
- Time feedings with alert states.
- Hold infant close and, if needed, swaddle in a blanket.

Bathing
- Ventral openness may be stressful. Cover body parts not being bathed.
- Proceed slowly; allow for rest.
- Offer pacifier or hand to suck.

- Eliminate unnecessary noise.
- Use a soft, soothing voice.

Explain the Need to Reduce Environmental Stimuli When Taking the Infant Outside

- Shelter eyes from light.
- Swaddle the infant so his or her hands can reach the mouth. Protect from loud noises.

Praise Parent(s) for Interaction Patterns; Point Out Infant's Engaging Responses

Initiate Health Teaching and Referrals, as Needed

- Explain that developmental interventions will change with maturity. Refer to *Delayed Growth and Development* for specific age-related developmental needs.
- Provide parent(s) with resources for assistance at home (e.g., community resources).
- Refer to the Internet for sites for resources and information about preterm newborns.

READINESS FOR ENHANCED KNOWLEDGE (SPECIFY)

NANDA-I Definition

A pattern of cognitive information related to a specific topic, or its acquisition, that is sufficient for meeting health-related goals and can be strengthened

Defining Characteristics*

Expresses an interest in learning
Explains knowledge of the topic
Behaviors congruent with expressed knowledge
Describes previous experiences pertaining to the topic

Author's Note

Readiness for Enhanced Knowledge is broad. All nursing diagnoses—actual, risk, and wellness—seek to enhance knowledge. Once the specific area of enhanced knowledge is identified, refer to that specific diagnosis, for example, *Readiness for Enhanced Nutrition*, *Grieving*, *Risk for Ineffective Parenting*, *Deficient Health Behavior*, or *Ineffective Therapeutic Regimen*

Management. Readiness for Enhanced Knowledge is not needed because it lacks the reason for the desired or needed knowledge.

READINESS FOR ENHANCED NUTRITION

NANDA-I Definition

A pattern of nutrient intake that is sufficient for meeting metabolic needs and can be strengthened

Defining Characteristics*

Expresses willingness to enhance nutrition
Eats regularly
Consumes adequate food and fluid
Expresses knowledge of healthy food and fluid choices
Follows an appropriate standard for intake (e.g., MyPlate or
    American Diabetic Association guidelines)
Safe preparation and storage of food and fluids
Attitude toward eating and drinking is congruent with health goals

NOC
Nutritional Status, Teaching Nutrition

Goal

The client/group will report an increase in balanced nutrition, as evidenced by the following indicator:

• Identify two new strategies (specify) to enhance nutrition.

NIC
Nutrition Management, Nutrition Monitoring

Interventions

Refer to Internet sites for resources and information about nutrition:

• www.myplate.gov
• www.health.gov/dietaryguidelines

READINESS FOR ENHANCED PARENTING

NANDA-I Definition

A pattern of providing an environment for children or other dependent client(s)/person(s) that is sufficient to nurture growth and development and can be strengthened

Defining Characteristics*

Expresses willingness to enhance parenting
Children or other dependent client(s) express satisfaction with home environment
Emotional support of children or dependent client(s)/person(s)
Needs of children are met (e.g., physical and emotional) or needs of children/dependent client(s) are met
Exhibits realistic expectations of children/dependent person

⟳ Author's Note

Refer to *Interrupted Family Processes* for strategies to support effective family functioning and *Readiness for Enhanced Resiliency Resilience* for strategies to enhance parenting.

READINESS FOR ENHANCED POWER

NANDA-I Definition

A pattern of participating knowingly in change that is sufficient for well-being and can be strengthened

Defining Characteristics*

Expresses readiness to enhance awareness of possible changes to be made
Expresses readiness to enhance freedom to perform actions for change
Expresses readiness to enhance identification of choices that can be made for change
Expresses readiness to enhance involvement in creating change
Expresses readiness to enhance knowledge for participation in change

Expresses readiness to enhance participation in choices for daily
living and health
Expresses readiness to enhance power

NOC

Health Beliefs: Perceived Control, Participation: Health Care Decisions

Goal

The client/group will report increased power, as evidenced by the
following indicator:

• Identify two new strategies (specify) to enhance power.

NIC

Decision-Making Support, Self-Responsibility Facilitation, Teaching: Individual

Interventions

Refer to *Powerlessness* for strategies to increase power.

READINESS FOR ENHANCED RELATIONSHIP

NANDA-I Definition

A pattern of mutual partnership that is sufficient to provide each
other's needs and can be strengthened

Defining Characteristics*

Reports desire to enhance communication between partners
Reports satisfaction with sharing of information and ideas between
    partners
Reports satisfaction with fulfilling physical and emotional needs
    by one's partner
Demonstrates mutual respect between partners
Meets developmental goals appropriate for family life stage
Demonstrates well-balanced autonomy and collaboration between
    partners
Demonstrates mutual support in daily activities between partners;
    partners identify each other as a key person
Demonstrates understanding of partner's insufficiencies (physical,
    social)
Express satisfaction with complementary relation between partners

Goal

The client will report increased satisfaction with partnership, as evidenced by the following indicator:

• Identify two new strategies (specify) to enhance partnership.

Interventions

Teach to (Murray, Zentner, & Yakimo, 2009):

• Talk daily about feelings
• Elicit feelings of partner
• Explore "what if..." conversations

Vary Family Responsibilities, Schedule, Chores, and Roles

Engage Partner to Discuss Individual Problems and Validate Solutions or Ask for Partner's Opinion About the Problem

Establish a Support System That Can Help When Needed; Provide Such Support to Other Families or Individuals in Need

During Times of High Stress or Crises, Share Feelings of Guilt, Anger, or Helplessness

Engage in Activities Together as Partners, Family

Refer to the Internet for Sites and Resources for Coping with Difficult Family Situations (e.g., Death of Member, Ill Family Member)

READINESS FOR ENHANCED RELIGIOSITY

NANDA-I Definition

A pattern of reliance on religious beliefs and/or participation in rituals of a particular faith tradition that is sufficient for well-being and can be strengthened

Defining Characteristics

Expresses a desire to strengthen religious belief patterns.
Comfort or religion in the past

Questions harmful belief patterns
Rejects belief patterns that are harmful

Requests assistance expanding religious options

Requests assistance to increase participation in prescribed religious beliefs

Requests forgiveness

Requests reconciliation

Requests meeting with religious leaders/facilitators

Requests religious materials, experiences, or both

 Author's Note

This diagnosis represents a variety of foci. Request for forgiveness may be related to an actual nursing diagnosis such as *Grieving*, *Ineffective Individual Coping*, or *Compromised Family Coping*. Further assessment is needed for interventions. Refer to *Impaired Religiosity* in Section 1, for additional information.

READINESS FOR ENHANCED RESILIENCE

NANDA-I Definition

A pattern of positive responses to an adverse situation or crisis that is sufficient for optimizing human potential and can be strengthened

Defining Characteristics*

Access to resources

Demonstrates positive outlook

Effective use of conflict-management strategies

Enhances personal coping skills

Expresses desire to enhance resilience

Identifies available resources

Identifies support systems

Increases positive relationships with others

Involvement in activities

Makes progress toward goals

Presence of a crisis

Maintains safe environment

Sets goals

Takes responsibilities for actions

Uses effective communication skills

Verbalizes an enhanced sense of control

Verbalizes self control

Related Factors

Demographics that increase chance of maladjustment

Drug used

Gender

Inconsistent parenting

Low intelligence

Low maternal education
Large family size
Minority status
Parental mental illness
Poor impulse control
Poverty
Psychological disorders

Condition
Violence
Vulnerability factors that
    encompass indices that
    exacerbate the negative
    reflects of the risk

 Author's Note

This NANDA-I diagnosis focuses on the concept of resilience. Resilience is a strength that allows one to persevere and overcome difficulties. When faced with a crisis or problem, resilient people respond constructively with solutions or effective adaptation. Resilience is not a nursing diagnosis. It is an important and vital characteristic that can be nurtured and taught to children to assist them to cope with problematic life events.

The Defining Characteristics describe enhanced or effective coping. In contrast, the Related Factors are contributing factors for ineffective coping.

This author recommends:

- Using *Risk for Infective Coping* related to the Related Factors listed above to assist someone to prevent ineffective coping
- Using *Ineffective Coping* related to the above Related Factors if Defining Characteristics of *Ineffective Coping* exist. (Refer to Section 1 under *Ineffective Coping* for specific defining characteristics.)
- Referring to the interventions for promoting resiliency in children and adults (refer to Index under resiliency for specific pages).

READINESS FOR ENHANCED SELF-CARE

NANDA-I Definition

A pattern of performing activities for oneself that helps to meet health-related goals and can be strengthened

Defining Characteristics*

Expresses a desire to enhance independence in maintaining life
Expresses desire to enhance independence in maintaining health
Expresses desire to enhance knowledge of strategies of self-care
Expresses a desire to enhance responsibility for self-care
Expresses desire to enhance self-care

Author's Note

This diagnosis focuses more on improving self-care activities. Refer to *Self-Care Deficits* for interventions to improve self-care.

READINESS FOR ENHANCED SELF-CONCEPT

NANDA-I Definition

A pattern of perceptions or ideas about the self that is sufficient for well-being and can be strengthened

Defining Characteristics*

- Expresses willingness to enhance self-concept
- Expresses satisfaction with thoughts about self, sense of worthiness, role performance, body image, and personal identity
- Actions are congruent with expressed feelings and thoughts
- Expresses confidence in abilities
- Accepts strengths and limitations

 NOC

Quality of Life, Self-Esteem, Coping

Goal

The individual will report increased self-concept in (specify situation), as evidenced by the following indicator:

- Identify two new strategies (specify) to enhance self-concept.

NIC

Hope Instillation, Values Clarification, Coping Enhancement

Interventions

Refer to *Disturbed Self-Concept* for interventions to improve self-concept.

READINESS FOR ENHANCED SELF-HEALTH MANAGEMENT

NANDA-I Definition

A pattern of regulating and integrating into daily living a therapeutic regimen for the treatment of illness and its sequelae that is
sufficient for meeting health-related goals and can be strengthened

Defining Characteristics*

Expresses desire to manage the illness (e.g., treatment and
    prevention of sequelae)
Choices of daily living are appropriate for meeting goals
    (e.g., treatment, prevention)
Expresses little difficulty with prescribed regimens
Describes reduction of risk factors
No unexpected acceleration of illness symptoms

 Author's Note

This diagnosis can be used to focus on a personal or lifestyle change in a
specific area that is effective and can be enhanced to increase management
of an illness.

NOC

Adherence Behavior, Health Beliefs, Health Promoting Behaviors, Well-Being

Goal

The client will express a desire to move from wellness to a higher
level of wellness in management of a disease for condition (specify)
(e.g., nutrition, decision making), as evidenced by the following
indicators:

• Identify two new strategies (specify) to enhance management
  of a disease/condition

NIC

Health Education, Risk Identification, Values Classification, Behavior
Modification, Coping Enhancement, Knowledge: Health Resources

Interventions

The following interventions are appropriate for any health promotion/wellness nursing diagnosis that focuses on lifestyle changes and choices, for example, *Readiness for Enhanced Nutrition, Parenting, Sleep, Breastfeeding, Family Coping* and *Family Processes*. These areas of wellness and health promotion can be found readily in the self-help literature and on the Internet. Some of the interventions for the wellness nursing diagnoses, such as *Readiness for Enhanced Grieving, Readiness for Enhanced Coping*, or *Readiness for Enhanced Decision Making* can be found in Section 1, under the individual nursing diagnoses. For example, in *Decisional Conflict* there are interventions that can promote better decision making even for someone already making good decisions.

Complete Assessment of One or More or All Functional Health Patterns as the Individual Desires

Renew Data With Client or Group

- Does the client/group report good or excellent health?
- Does the client desire to learn a behavior to maximize health in a specific pattern?

Encourage the Client to Select Only One Wellness Focus at a Time (e.g., Exercise, Decrease Intake of Carbohydrates, Increase Intake of Water); Addressing Multiple Behavioral Changes at Once is Time Consuming, Which May Discourage the Change (Bodenheimer, MacGregor, & Shafiri, 2005).

Refer to Educational Resources About a Particular Focus (Print, Online); Examples of Generic Data-bases/Web sites Include:

- www.seekwellness.com/wellness/
- www.cdc.gov/—Centers for Disease Central and Prevention
- www.agingblueprint.org—focuses on aging well
- www.nhlbi.nih.gov—US Department of Health and Human Services
- www.ahrq.gov—US Preventive Services Task Force
- www.health.gov—various health topics
- www.nih.gov—National Institutes of Health
- www.fda.gov—Food and Drug Administration
- www.mbmi.org—Mind-Body Medical Institute
- www.ahha.org—American Holistic Health Association

Advise the Client to Contact the Nurse to Discuss the Outcome of Resource Review Via Telephone or E-Mail

Discuss the Strategies or Targeted Behavior Changes; Have the Client Record Realistic Goals and Time Frames That Are Highly Specific; Avoid Recommendations of "Exercise More" or "Eat Less"

- For example: Goal—I will reduce my daily intake of carbohydrates.
- Indicators—Reduce cookie intake from five to two each day.
- Change pasta to multigrain pasta.
- Reduce potato intake by 50% and replace with 50% root vegetables.

Ask the Client If You Can Contact Him or Her at Designated Intervals (Every Month, at 4 to 6 Months, at 1 Year); Call or E-Mail Client to Discuss Progress.

Advise the Client That This Process Can Be Repeated as They Desire in Other Functional Health Patterns

READINESS FOR ENHANCED SLEEP

NANDA-I Definition

A pattern of natural, periodic suspension of consciousness that provides adequate rest, sustains a desired lifestyle, and can be strengthened

Defining Characteristics*

Amount of sleep is congruent with developmental needs
Reports being rested after sleep
Expresses willingness to enhance sleep
Follows sleep routines that promote sleep habits
Uses medications to induce sleep on occasion

Goal

The individual will report satisfactory sleep pattern, as evidenced by the following indicator:

- Identify two new strategies (specify) to enhance sleep.

Interventions

Refer to *Disturbed Sleep Patterns* for strategies to promote sleep.

READINESS FOR ENHANCED SPIRITUAL WELL-BEING

NANDA-I Definition

A pattern of experiencing and integrating meaning and purpose in life through connectedness with self, others, art, music, literature, nature, and/or a power greater than oneself that is sufficient for well-being and can be strengthened.

Defining Characteristics[†]

Inner strength that nurtures:
   Sense of awareness
   Inner peace
   Sacred source
   Unifying force
   Trust relationships
Intangible motivation and commitment directed toward ultimate values of love, meaning, hope, beauty, and truth
Trusts relations with or in the transcendent that provide bases for meaning and hope in life's experiences and love in one's relationships
Has meaning and purpose to existence
Has connections with a power greater than self (e.g., reversance, prays, religious rituals)*
Has connections with art, music, literature, nature*

NOC
Hope, Spiritual Well-Being

Goal

The client will express enhanced spiritual harmony and wholeness, as evidenced by the following indicators:

• Maintain previous relationship with higher being.
• Continue spiritual practices not detrimental to health.

NIC
Spiritual Growth Facilitation, Spiritual Support, Hope

[†] Carson, 1999

Interventions

Refer to the Internet for resources and information about spiritual health.

READINESS FOR ENHANCED URINARY ELIMINATION

NANDA-I Definition

A pattern of urinary functions that is sufficient for meeting eliminatory needs and can be strengthened

Defining Characteristics*

Expresses willingness to enhance urinary elimination
Urine is straw colored with no odor
Specific gravity is within normal limits
Amount of output is within normal limits for age and other factors
Positions self for emptying of bladder
Fluid intake is adequate for daily needs

NOC

Fluid Balance, Hydration, Electrolyte Balance

Goal

The individual will report an increased balance in urinary elimination, as evidenced by the following indicator:

• Identify two new strategies (specify) to enhance urinary elimination.

NIC

Education: Fluid/Electrolyte

Interventions

• Refer to the Internet for resources and information about fluid balance:
  • www.health.gov/dietaryguidelines
  • www.seekwellness.com/wellness

Section 3

Diagnostic Clusters

This section presents medical conditions or clinical situations with associated nursing diagnoses and collaborative problems.

The following symbols are used in this section:

▲ This diagnosis was reported to be monitored for or managed frequently (75% to 100%).

Δ This diagnosis was reported to be monitored for or managed often (50% to 74%).

* This diagnosis was not included in the validation study.

† RC of (Risk for Complications of) is collaborative problems, not nursing diagnoses.

Part I
Medical Conditions

CARDIOVASCULAR/HEMATOLOGIC/ PERIPHERAL VASCULAR DISORDERS

Cardiac Conditions

Angina Pectoris

Collaborative Problems

Refer to *Heart Failure*.

Nursing Diagnoses**

- Anxiety related to chest pain secondary to effects of hypoxia
- Fear related to present status and unknown future
- Disturbed Sleep Pattern related to treatments and environment
- Risk for Constipation related to bed rest, change in lifestyle, and medications
- Activity Intolerance related to deconditioning secondary to fear of recurrent angina
- Risk for Disturbed Self-Concept related to perceived and/or actual role changes
- Risk for Impaired Home Maintenance related to angina or fear of angina
- Risk for Interrupted Family Processes related to impaired ability of person to assume role responsibilities
- Risk for Ineffective Sexuality Patterns related to fear of angina and altered self-concept

---

** List includes nursing diagnoses that may be associated with the medical diagnosis.

- Grieving related to actual or perceived losses secondary to cardiac condition
- Risk for Ineffective Self-Health Management related to insufficient knowledge of condition, home activities, diet, and medications

Heart Failure

Collaborative Problems

†∆ RC of Deep vein thrombosis
▲ RC of Hypoxia
∆ RC of Cardiogenic shock
* RC of Hepatic failure
* RC of Multiple organ failure
* RC of Hepatic insufficiency

Nursing Diagnoses

▲ Activity Intolerance related to insufficient oxygen for activities of daily living
∆ Imbalanced Nutrition: Less Than Body Requirements related to nausea; anorexia secondary to venous congestion of gastrointestinal tract and fatigue
∆ Ineffective Peripheral Tissue Perfusion related to venous congestion secondary to right-sided heart failure
▲ Anxiety related to breathlessness
* Fear related to progressive nature of condition
* Risk for Impaired Home Maintenance related to inability to perform activities of daily living secondary to breathlessness and fatigue
* (Specify) Self-Care Deficit related to dyspnea and fatigue
∆ Disturbed Sleep Pattern related to nocturnal dyspnea and inability to assume usual sleep position
▲ Risk for Excessive Fluid Volume: Edema related to decreased renal blood flow secondary to right-sided heart failure
∆ Powerlessness related to progressive nature of condition
∆ Risk for Ineffective Self-Health Management related to insufficient knowledge of low-salt diet, drug therapy (diuretic, digitalis), activity program, and signs and symptoms of complications

Endocarditis, Pericarditis
(Rheumatic, Infectious)

See also *Corticosteroid Therapy.* If child, see *Rheumatic Fever.*

Collaborative Problems

- RC of Congestive heart failure
- RC of Valvular stenosis
- RC of Cerebrovascular accident
- RC of Emboli (pulmonary, cerebral, renal, splenic, heart)
- RC of Cardiac tamponade

Nursing Diagnoses

- Activity Intolerance related to insufficient oxygen secondary to decreased cardiac output
- Risk for Ineffective Respiratory Function related to decreased respiratory depth secondary to pain
- Pain related to friction rub and inflammation process
- Risk for Ineffective Self-Health Management related to insufficient knowledge of etiology, prevention, antibiotic prophylaxis, and signs and symptoms of complications

Acute Coronary Syndrome
(Myocardial Infarction, Uncomplicated)

Collaborative Problems

- ▲ RC of Dysrhythmias
- ▲ RC of Cardiogenic shock
- ▲ RC of Thromboembolism
- • RC of Recurrent myocardial infarction

Nursing Diagnoses

- ▲ Anxiety related to acute pain secondary to cardiac tissue ischemia
- * Fear related to pain, present status, and unknown future
- * Disturbed Sleep Pattern related to treatments and environment
- • Risk for Constipation related to decreased peristalsis secondary to medication effects, decreased activity, and change in diet
- ▲ Activity Intolerance related to insufficient oxygen for activities of daily living secondary to cardiac tissue ischemia
- * Risk for Disturbed Self-Concept related to perceived or actual role changes
- • Risk for Impaired Home Maintenance related to angina or fear of angina

▲ Anxiety/Fear (individual, family) related to unfamiliar situation, unpredictable nature of condition, negative effect on lifestyle, possible sexual dysfunction

* Risk for Interrupted Family Processes related to impaired ability of ill person to assume role responsibilities

* Risk for Ineffective Sexuality Patterns related to fear of angina and altered self-concept

Δ Grieving related to actual or perceived losses secondary to cardiac condition

Δ Risk for Ineffective Self-Health Management related to insufficient knowledge of hospital routines, treatments, conditions, medications, diet, activity progression, signs and symptoms of complications, reduction of risks, follow-up care, community resources

Hematologic Conditions

Anemia

Collaborative Problems

- RC of Bleeding
- RC of Cardiac failure
- RC of Iron overload (repeated transfusion)

Nursing Diagnoses

- Activity Intolerance related to impaired oxygen transport secondary to diminished red blood cell count
- Risk for Infection related to decreased resistance secondary to tissue hypoxia and/or abnormal white blood cells (neutropenia, leukopenia)
- Risk for Injury: Bleeding tendencies related to thrombocytopenia and splenomegaly
- Risk for Impaired Oral Mucous Membrane related to gastrointestinal mucosal atrophy
- Risk for Ineffective Self-Health Management related to insufficient knowledge of condition, nutritional requirements, and drug therapy

Aplastic Anemia

Collaborative Problems

- RC of Fatal aplasia
- RC of Pancytopenia
- RC of Bleeding
- RC of Hypoxia
- RC of Sepsis

Nursing Diagnoses

- Activity Intolerance related to insufficient oxygen secondary to diminished red blood cell count
- Risk for Infection related to increased susceptibility secondary to leukopenia
- Risk for Impaired Oral Mucous Membrane related to tissue hypoxia and vulnerability
- Risk for Ineffective Self-Health Management related to insufficient knowledge of causes, prevention, and signs and symptoms of complications

Pernicious Anemia

See also *Anemia*.

Nursing Diagnoses

- Impaired Oral Mucous Membrane related to sore red tongue secondary to papillary atrophy and inflammatory changes
- Diarrhea/Constipation related to gastrointestinal mucosal atrophy
- Risk for Imbalanced Nutrition: Less Than Body Requirements related to anorexia secondary to sore mouth
- Risk for Ineffective Self-Health Management related to insufficient knowledge of chronicity of disease and vitamin B treatment

Disseminated Intravascular Coagulation (DIC)

See also underlying disorders (e.g., *Obstetric, Infections, Burns*), *Anticoagulant Therapy*.

Collaborative Problems

- RC of Bleeding
- RC of Renal failure
- RC of Microthrombi (renal, cardiac, pulmonary, cerebral, gastrointestinal)

Nursing Diagnoses

- Fear related to treatments, environment, and unpredictable outcome
- Interrupted Family Processes related to critical nature of the situation and uncertain prognosis
- Anxiety related to insufficient knowledge of causes and treatment

Polycythemia Vera**

Collaborative Problems

- RC of Thrombus formation
- RC of Bleeding
- RC of Hypertension
- RC of Congestive heart failure
- RC of Peptic ulcer
- RC of Gout

Nursing Diagnoses

- Imbalanced Nutrition: Less Than Body Requirements related to anorexia, nausea, and vasocongestion
- Activity Intolerance related to insufficient oxygen secondary to pulmonary congestion and tissue hypoxia
- Risk for Infection related to hypoxia secondary to vasocongestion
- Risk for Ineffective Self-Health Management related to insufficient knowledge of fluid requirements, exercise program, and signs and symptoms of complications

Peripheral Vascular Conditions

Deep Vein Thrombosis

See also *Anticoagulant Therapy*, if indicated.

Collaborative Problems

- ▲ RC of Pulmonary embolism
- ▲ RC of Chronic leg edema
- Δ RC of Chronic stasis ulcers

** This diagnosis was not included in the validation study.

Nursing Diagnoses

- Risk for Constipation related to decreased peristalsis secondary to immobility
- △ Risk for Ineffective Respiratory Function related to immobility
- △ Risk for Impaired Skin Integrity related to chronic ankle edema
- ▲ Acute Pain related to impaired circulation for ambulation
- △ Risk for Ineffective Self-Health Management related to insufficient knowledge of prevention of recurrence of deep vein thrombosis and signs and symptoms of complications

Hypertension

Collaborative Problems

- RC of Retinal hemorrhage
- RC of Cerebrovascular accident
- RC of Cerebral hemorrhage
- RC of Renal failure

Nursing Diagnoses

- Risk for Noncompliance related to negative side effects of prescribed therapy versus the belief that no treatment is needed without the presence of symptoms
- Risk for Ineffective Sexuality Patterns related to decreased libido or erectile dysfunction secondary to medication side effects
- Risk for Ineffective Self-Health Management related to insufficient knowledge of condition, diet restrictions, medications, risk factors, and follow-up care

Varicose Veins**

Collaborative Problems

- RC of Vascular rupture
- RC of Bleeding
- RC of Thrombosis

Nursing Diagnoses

- Chronic Pain related to engorgement of veins
- Risk for Ineffective Self-Health Management related to insufficient knowledge of condition, treatment options, and risk factors

---

** This diagnosis was not included in the validation study.

Peripheral Arterial Disease
(Atherosclerosis, Arteriosclerosis)

Collaborative Problems

- RC of Stroke (cerebrovascular accident)
- RC of Ischemic ulcers
- RC of Claudication
- RC of Acute arterial thrombosis
- RC of Hypertension

Nursing Diagnoses

- Risk for Impaired Tissue Integrity related to compromised circulation
- Chronic Pain related to muscle ischemia during prolonged activity
- Risk for Injury related to decreased sensation secondary to chronic atherosclerosis
- Risk for Infection related to compromised circulation
- Risk for Injury related to effects of orthostatic hypotension
- Activity Intolerance related to claudication
- Risk for Ineffective Self-Health Management related to insufficient knowledge of condition, management of claudication, risk factors, foot care, and treatment plan

Raynaud's Disease

Collaborative Problems

- RC of Acute arterial occlusion
- RC of Ischemic ulcers
- RC of Gangrene

Nursing Diagnoses

- Acute Pain related to ischemia secondary to acute vasospasm
- Risk for Impaired Tissue Integrity: Ischemic ulcers related to vasospasm
- Fear related to potential loss of work secondary to work-related aggravating factors
- Risk for Ineffective Self-Health Management related to insufficient knowledge of condition, risk factors, and self-care

Venous Stasis Ulcers
(Postphlebitis Syndrome)

Collaborative Problems

- ▲ RC of Cellulitis
- * RC of Thrombosis

Nursing Diagnoses

- * Ineffective Peripheral Tissue Perfusion related to dependent position of legs
- * Risk for Infection related to compromised circulation
- ▲ Chronic Pain related to ulcers and debridement treatments
- Δ Risk for Disturbed Body Image related to chronic open wounds and response of others to appearance
- Δ Risk for Ineffective Self-Health Management related to lack of knowledge of condition, prevention of complications, risk factors, and treatment

RESPIRATORY DISORDERS

Adult Respiratory Distress Syndrome

See also *Mechanical Ventilation* (under Part 7, *Diagnostic and Therapeutic Procedures*).

Collaborative Problems

- • RC of Electrolyte imbalances
- • RC of Hypoxemia

Nursing Diagnoses

- • Anxiety related to implications of condition and critical care setting
- • Powerlessness related to condition and treatments (ventilator, monitoring)

Chronic Obstructive Pulmonary Disease
(Emphysema, Bronchitis)

Collaborative Problems

- ▲ RC of Hypoxemia
- Δ RC of Right-sided heart failure

Nursing Diagnoses

▲ Ineffective Airway Clearance related to excessive and tenacious secretions

Δ Risk for Imbalanced Nutrition: Less Than Body Requirements related to anorexia secondary to dyspnea, halitosis, and fatigue

▲ Activity Intolerance related to insufficient oxygen for activities and fatigue

Impaired Verbal Communication related to dyspnea

▲ Anxiety related to breathlessness and fear of suffocation

Δ Powerlessness related to feeling of loss of control and lifestyle restrictions

Δ Disturbed Sleep Pattern related to cough, inability to assume recumbent position, and environmental stimuli

Δ Risk for Ineffective Self-Health Management related to insufficient knowledge of condition, treatments, prevention of infection, breathing exercises, risk factors, signs and symptoms of complications

Pleural Effusion

See also underlying disorders (*Heart Disease, Cirrhosis, Malignancy*).

Collaborative Problems

• RC of Respiratory failure
• RC of Pneumothorax (post-thoracentesis)
• RC of Hypoxemia
• RC of Hemothorax

Nursing Diagnoses

• Activity Intolerance related to insufficient oxygen for activities of daily living
• Risk for Imbalanced Nutrition: Less Than Body Requirements related to anorexia secondary to pressure on abdominal structures
• Impaired Comfort related to accumulation of fluid in pleural space
• (Specify) Self-Care Deficits related to fatigue and dyspnea

Pneumonia

Collaborative Problems

▲ RC of Respiratory insufficiency
Δ RC of Septic shock
Δ RC of Paralytic ileus

Nursing Diagnoses

- Risk for Hyperthermia related to infectious process
▲ Activity Intolerance related to insufficient oxygen for activities of daily living
Δ Risk for Impaired Oral Mucous Membrane related to mouth breathing, frequent expectoration, and decreased fluid intake secondary to malaise
* Risk for Deficient Fluid Volume related to increased insensible fluid loss secondary to fever and hyperventilation
Δ Risk for Imbalanced Nutrition: Less Than Body Requirements related to anorexia, dyspnea, and abdominal distention secondary to air swallowing
▲ Ineffective Airway Clearance related to pain, increased tracheobronchial secretions, and fatigue
* Risk for Infection Transmission related to communicable nature of the disease
* Impaired Comfort related to hyperthermia and malaise
* Risk for Impaired Skin Integrity related to prescribed bed rest
Δ Risk for Ineffective Self-Health Management related to lack of knowledge of condition, infection transmission, prevention of recurrence, diet, signs and symptoms of recurrence, and follow-up care

Pulmonary Embolism

See also *Anticoagulant Therapy*.

Collaborative Problem

- RC of Hypoxemia

Nursing Diagnoses

- Risk for Impaired Skin Integrity related to immobility and prescribed bed rest
- Risk for Ineffective Self-Health Management related to insufficient knowledge of anticoagulant therapy and signs and symptoms of complications

METABOLIC/ENDOCRINE DISORDERS

Addison's Disease

Collaborative Problems

- RC of Addisonian crisis (shock)
- RC of Electrolyte imbalances (sodium, potassium)
- RC of Hypoglycemia

Nursing Diagnoses

- Risk for Imbalanced Nutrition: Less Than Body Requirements related to anorexia and nausea
- Risk for Deficient Fluid Volume related to excessive loss of sodium and water secondary to polyuria
- Diarrhea related to increased excretion of sodium and water
- Risk for Disturbed Self-Concept related to appearance changes secondary to increased skin pigmentation and decreased axillary and pubic hair (female)
- Risk for Injury related to postural hypotension secondary to fluid/electrolyte imbalances
- Risk for Ineffective Self-Health Management related to insufficient knowledge of disease, signs and symptoms of complications, risks for crisis (infection, diarrhea, decreased sodium intake, diaphoresis), overexertion, dietary management, identification (card, medallion), emergency kit, and pharmacologic management

Aldosteronism, Primary

Collaborative Problems

- RC of Hypokalemia
- RC of Alkalosis
- RC of Hypertension
- RC of Hypernatremia

Nursing Diagnoses

- Impaired Comfort related to excessive urine excretion and polydipsia
- Risk for Deficient Fluid Volume related to excessive urinary excretion
- Risk for Ineffective Self-Health Management related to insufficient knowledge of condition, surgical treatment, and effects of corticosteroid therapy

Cirrhosis

(Laënnec's Disease)

See also *Substance Abuse*, if indicated.

Collaborative Problems

- ▲ RC of Bleeding
- Δ RC of Hypokalemia
- Δ RC of Portal systemic encephalopathy
- * RC of Negative nitrogen balance
- ▲ RC of Medication toxicity (opiates, short-acting barbiturates, major tranquilizers)
- Δ RC of Renal insufficiency
- * RC of Anemia
- * RC of Esophageal varices

Nursing Diagnoses

- ▲ Pain related to liver enlargement and ascites
- Δ Diarrhea related to excessive secretion of fats in stool secondary to liver dysfunction
- * Risk for Injury related to decreased prothrombin production and synthesis of substances used in blood coagulation
- ▲ Imbalanced Nutrition: Less Than Body Requirements related to anorexia, impaired protein, fat, glucose metabolism, and impaired storage of vitamins (A, C, K, D, E)
- * Risk for Ineffective Respiratory Function related to pressure on diaphragm secondary to ascites
- * Risk for Disturbed Self-Concept related to appearance changes (jaundice, ascites)
- * Risk for Infection related to leukopenia secondary to enlarged, overactive spleen and hypoproteinemia
- Δ Impaired Comfort: Pruritus related to accumulation of bilirubin pigment and bile salts on skin
- ▲ Risk for Impaired Tissue Integrity related to edema and ascites secondary to portal hypertension
- Δ Risk for Ineffective Self-Health Management related to insufficient knowledge of pharmacologic contraindications, nutritional requirements, signs and symptoms of complications, and risks of alcohol ingestion

Cushing's Syndrome

Collaborative Problems

- • RC of Hypertension
- • RC of Congestive heart failure

- RC of Psychosis
- RC of Electrolyte imbalance (sodium, potassium)

Nursing Diagnoses

- Disturbed Self-Concept related to physical changes secondary to disease process (moon face, thinning of hair, truncal obesity, virilism)
- Risk for Infection related to excessive protein catabolism and depressed leukocytic phagocytosis secondary to hyperglycemia
- Risk for Injury: Fractures related to osteoporosis
- Risk for Impaired Skin Integrity related to loss of tissue, edema, and dryness
- Ineffective Sexuality Patterns related to loss of libido and cessation of menses (female) secondary to excessive adrenocorticotropic hormone production
- Risk for Ineffective Self-Health Management related to insufficient knowledge of disease and diet therapy (high protein, low cholesterol, low sodium)

Diabetes Mellitus

Collaborative Problems

Acute Complications
- ▲ RC of Ketoacidosis (DKA)
- Δ RC of Hyperosmolar hyperglycemic nonketotic coma (HHNC)
- ▲ RC of Hypoglycemia
- ▲ RC of Infections

Chronic Complications
- • Macrovascular
- ▲ RC of Cardiac artery disease
- ▲ RC of Peripheral vascular disease
- • Microvascular
- Δ RC of Retinopathy
- ▲ RC of Neuropathy
- Δ RC of Nephropathy

Nursing Diagnoses

- Δ Risk for Injury related to decreased tactile sensation, diminished visual acuity, and hypoglycemia
- Δ Fear (client, family) related to diagnosis of diabetes, potential complications of diabetes, insulin injection, negative effect on lifestyle
- Δ Risk for Ineffective Coping (client, family) related to chronic disease, complex self-care regimen, and uncertain future

▲ Imbalanced Nutrition: More Than Body Requirements related to intake in excess of activity expenditures, lack of knowledge, and ineffective coping

Δ Risk for Ineffective Sexuality Patterns (male) related to erectile problems secondary to peripheral neuropathy or psychological conflicts

Δ Risk for Ineffective Sexuality Patterns (female) related to frequent genitourinary problems and physical and psychological stressors of diabetes

Δ Powerlessness related to the future development of complications of diabetes (blindness, amputations, kidney failure, painful neuropathy)

* Risk for Loneliness related to visual impairment/blindness

Δ Risk for Noncompliance related to the complexity and chronicity of the prescribed regimen

Δ Risk for Ineffective Self-Health Management related to insufficient knowledge of condition, self-monitoring of blood glucose, medications, American Diabetes Association exchange diet, treatment of hypoglycemia, weight control, sick-day care, exercise program, foot care, signs and symptoms of complications, and community resources

Hepatitis (Viral)

Collaborative Problems

* RC of Hepatic failure
* RC of Coma
* RC of Subacute hepatic necrosis
* RC of Fulminant hepatitis
* RC of Portal systemic encephalopathy
Δ RC of Hypokalemia
Δ RC of Bleeding
Δ RC of Drug toxicity
Δ RC of Renal failure
Δ RC of Progressive liver degeneration

Nursing Diagnoses

* Fatigue related to reduced metabolism by liver
▲ Risk for Infection Transmission related to contagious nature of virus type A and type B
▲ Imbalanced Nutrition: Less Than Body Requirements related to anorexia, epigastric distress, and nausea
* Risk for Deficient Fluid Volume related to lack of desire to drink
Δ Impaired Comfort related to accumulation of bilirubin pigment and bile salts

*   Risk for Injury related to reduced prothrombin synthesis and reduced vitamin K absorption

Δ   Pain related to swelling of inflamed liver

*   Deficient Diversional Activity related to the monotony of confinement and isolation precautions

Δ   Risk for Ineffective Self-Health Management related to insufficient knowledge of condition, rest requirements, precautions to prevent transmission, nutritional requirements, and contraindications

Hyperthyroidism
(Thyrotoxicosis, Graves' Disease)

Collaborative Problems

- RC of Thyroid storm
- RC of Cardiac dysrhythmias

Nursing Diagnoses

- Imbalanced Nutrition: Less Than Body Requirements related to intake less than metabolic needs secondary to excessive metabolic rate
- Activity Intolerance related to fatigue and exhaustion secondary to excessive metabolic rate
- Diarrhea related to increased peristalsis secondary to excessive metabolic rate
- Impaired Comfort related to heat intolerance and profuse diaphoresis
- Risk for Impaired Corneal Tissue Integrity related to inability to close eyelids secondary to exophthalmos
- Risk for Injury related to tremors
- Risk for Hyperthermia related to lack of metabolic compensatory mechanism secondary to hyperthyroidism
- Risk for Ineffective Self-Health Management related to insufficient knowledge of condition, treatment regimen, pharmacologic therapy, eye care, dietary management, and signs and symptoms of complications

Hypothyroidism
(Myxedema)

Collaborative Problems

- RC of Atherosclerotic heart disease
- RC of Normochromic, normocytic anemia
- RC of Acute organic psychosis

- RC of Myxedemic coma
- RC of Metabolic
- RC of Hematologic

Nursing Diagnoses

- Imbalanced Nutrition: More Than Body Requirements related to intake greater than metabolic needs secondary to slowed metabolic rate
- Activity Intolerance related to insufficient oxygen secondary to slowed metabolic rate
- Constipation related to decreased peristaltic action secondary to decreased metabolic rate and decreased physical activity
- Impaired Skin Integrity related to edema and dryness secondary to decreased metabolic rate and infiltration of fluid into interstitial tissues
- Impaired Comfort related to cold intolerance secondary to decreased metabolic rate
- Risk for Impaired Social Interaction related to listlessness and depression
- Risk for Ineffective Self-Health Management related to insufficient knowledge of condition, treatment regimen, dietary management, signs and symptoms of complications, pharmacologic therapy, and contraindications

Obesity

Nursing Diagnoses

- Ineffective Coping related to increased food consumption secondary to response to external stressors
- Chronic Low Self-Esteem related to feelings of self-degradation and the response of others to the condition
- Risk-Prone Health Behavior related to multiple factors resulting in imbalance between caloric intake and energy expenditure

Pancreatitis

Collaborative Problems

Δ   RC of Hypovolemia/Shock
*   RC of Hemotologic
*   RC of Acute Respiratory Distress Syndrome
Δ   RC of Hypercalcemia
▲   RC of Hyperglycemia
*   RC of Sepsis
*   RC of Acute renal failure

Nursing Diagnoses

▲ Acute Pain related to nasogastric suction, distention of pancreatic capsule, and local peritonitis

* Risk for Deficient Fluid Volume related to decreased intake secondary to nausea and vomiting

▲ Imbalanced Nutrition: Less Than Body Requirements related to vomiting, anorexia, and impaired digestion secondary to decreased pancreatic enzymes

Δ Diarrhea related to excessive excretion of fats in stools secondary to insufficient pancreatic enzymes

Δ Ineffective Denial related to inability to accept the consequences of one's alcohol abuse or dependency

Δ Risk for Ineffective Self-Health Management related to insufficient knowledge of disease process, treatments, contraindications, dietary management, and follow-up care

GASTROINTESTINAL DISORDERS

Esophageal Disorders
(Esophagitis, Hiatal Hernia)

Collaborative Problems

• RC of Bleeding
• RC of Gastric ulcers

Nursing Diagnoses

• Risk for Imbalanced Nutrition: Less Than Body Requirements related to anorexia, heartburn, and dysphagia
• Impaired Comfort: Heartburn related to regurgitation and eructation
• Risk for Ineffective Self-Health Management related to insufficient knowledge of condition, dietary management, hazards of alcohol and tobacco, positioning after meals, pharmacologic therapy, and weight reduction (if indicated)

Gastroenterocolitis/Enterocolitis

Collaborative Problem

• RC of Fluid/Electrolyte imbalances

Nursing Diagnoses

- Risk for Deficient Fluid Volume related to vomiting and diarrhea
- Acute Pain related to abdominal cramping, diarrhea, and vomiting secondary to vascular dilatation and hyperperistalsis
- Risk for Ineffective Self-Health Management related to insufficient knowledge of condition, dietary restrictions, and signs and symptoms of complications

Hemorrhoids/Anal Fissure
(Nonsurgical)

Collaborative Problems

- RC of Bleeding
- RC of Bowel strangulation
- RC of Thrombosis

Nursing Diagnoses

- Acute Pain related to pressure on defecation
- Risk for Constipation related to fear of pain on defecation
- Risk for Ineffective Self-Health Management related to insufficient knowledge of condition, bowel routine, diet instructions, exercise program, and perianal care

Inflammatory Bowel Disease
(Crohn's Disease, Ulcerative Colitis)

Collaborative Problems

- ▲ RC of Gastrointestinal bleeding
- ▲ RC of Fluid/Electrolyte imbalances
- ▲ RC of Anemia
- ▲ RC of Intestinal obstruction
- Δ RC of Renal calculi
- Δ RC of Fistula/Fissure/Abscess

Nursing Diagnoses

- ▲ Chronic Pain related to intestinal inflammatory process
- ▲ Diarrhea related to intestinal inflammatory process
- * Constipation related to inadequate dietary intake of fiber
- * Risk for Impaired Skin Integrity (Perianal) related to diarrhea and chemical irritants
- Δ Risk for Ineffective Coping related to chronicity of condition and lack of definitive treatment

▲ Imbalanced Nutrition: Less Than Body Requirements related to dietary restrictions, nausea, diarrhea, and abdominal
cramping associated with eating or painful ulcers of the oral
mucous membrane

Δ Risk for Ineffective Self-Health Management related to
insufficient knowledge of condition, diagnostic tests, prognosis,
treatment, and signs and symptoms of complications

Peptic Ulcer Disease

Collaborative Problems

▲ RC of Bleeding
▲ RC of Perforation
Δ RC of Pyloric obstruction

Nursing Diagnoses

▲ Acute/Chronic Pain related to lesions secondary to increased
gastric secretions
▲ Constipation/Diarrhea related to effects of medications on
bowel function
Δ Risk for Ineffective Self-Health Management related to insufficient knowledge of disease process, contraindications, signs
and symptoms of complications, and treatment regimen

RENAL/URINARY TRACT DISORDERS

Acute Kidney Failure

Collaborative Problems

▲ RC of Fluid overload
▲ RC of Metabolic acidosis
▲ RC of Electrolyte imbalances
* RC of Hypertension
* RC of Pulmonary edema
* RC of Dysrthmias
* RC of Gastrointestinal Bleeding

Nursing Diagnoses

Δ Imbalanced Nutrition: Less Than Body Requirements related to anorexia, nausea, vomiting, loss of taste, loss of smell,
stomatitis, and unpalatable diet
▲ Risk for Infection related to invasive procedures

* Anxiety related to present status and unknown prognosis
* Risk for Ineffective Self-Health Management related to insufficient knowledge of condition, dietary restriction, daily recording, pharmacologic therapy, signs and symptoms of complications, follow-up visits, and community resources

Chronic Kidney Disease

See also *Peritoneal Dialysis* and *Hemodialysis*, if indicated.

Collaborative Problems

▲ RC of Fluid/Electrolyte imbalances
Δ RC of Gastrointestinal bleeding
* RC of Hyperparathyroidism
* RC of Pathologic fractures
* RC of Malnutrition
▲ RC of Anemia
▲ RC of Fluid overload
Δ RC of Hypoalbuminemia
Δ RC of Polyneuropathy
Δ RC of Congestive heart failure
* RC of Pulmonary edema
Δ RC of Metabolic acidosis
Δ RC of Pleural effusion
  RC of Pericarditis, cardiac tamponade

Nursing Diagnoses

▲ Imbalanced Nutrition: Less Than Body Requirements related to anorexia, nausea/vomiting, loss of taste/smell, stomatitis, and unpalatable diet
• Ineffective Sexuality Patterns related to decreased libido, impotence, amenorrhea, sterility, fatigue
* Disturbed Self-Concept related to effects of limitation on achievement of developmental tasks
* Risk for Caregiver Role Strain related to long-term care needs secondary to disability and treatment requirements
* Impaired Comfort related to (examples) fatigue, headaches, fluid retention, anemia
* Fatigue related to insufficient oxygenation secondary to anemia
Δ Impaired Comfort: Pruritus related to calcium phosphate or urate crystals on skin
▲ Risk for Infection related to invasive procedures
Δ Powerlessness related to progressively disabling nature of illness
▲ Risk for Ineffective Self-Health Management related to insufficient knowledge of condition, dietary restriction, daily recording, pharmacologic therapy, signs and symptoms of complications, follow-up visits, and community resources

Neurogenic Bladder

Collaborative Problems

- RC of Renal calculi
- RC of Autonomic dysreflexia

Nursing Diagnoses

- Risk for Impaired Skin Integrity related to constant irritation from urine
- Risk for Infection related to retention of urine or introduction of urinary catheter
- Risk for Loneliness related to embarrassment from wetting self in front of others and fear of odor from urine
- Overflow Urinary Incontinence related to chronically overfilled bladder with loss of sensation of bladder distention *or*
- Reflex Urinary Incontinence related to absence of sensation to void and loss of ability to inhibit bladder contraction *or*
- Urge Urinary Incontinence related to disruption of the inhibitory efferent impulses secondary to brain or spinal cord dysfunction
- Risk for Dysreflexia related to reflex stimulation of sympathetic nervous system secondary to loss of autonomic control
- Risk for Ineffective Self-Health Management related to insufficient knowledge of etiology of incontinence, management, bladder retraining programs, signs and symptoms of complications, and community resources

Urinary Tract Infections
(Cystitis, Pyelonephritis, Glomerulonephritis)

See also *Acute Kidney Failure.*

Nursing Diagnoses

- Chronic Pain related to inflammation and tissue trauma
- Impaired Comfort related to inflammation and infection
- Risk for Imbalanced Nutrition: Less Than Body Requirements related to anorexia secondary to malaise
- Risk for Ineffective Coping related to the chronicity of the condition
- Risk for Ineffective Self-Health Management related to insufficient knowledge of prevention of recurrence (adequate fluid intake, frequent voiding, hygiene measures [post-toileting], and voiding after sexual activity), signs and symptoms of recurrence, and pharmacologic therapy

Urolithiasis
(Renal Calculi)

Collaborative Problems

Δ RC of Pyelonephritis
▲ RC of Renal insufficiency

Nursing Diagnoses

▲ Acute Pain related to inflammation secondary to irritation of calculi and smooth muscle spasms
* Diarrhea related to renointestinal reflexes
Δ Risk for Ineffective Self-Health Management related to insufficient knowledge of prevention of recurrence, dietary restrictions, and fluid requirements

---

NEUROLOGIC DISORDERS

Brain Tumor

Because this disorder can cause alterations varying from minimal to profound, the following possible nursing diagnoses reflect individuals with varying degrees of involvement.

See also *Surgery (General, Cranial); Cancer.*

Collaborative Problems

• RC of Increased intracranial pressure
• RC of Paralysis
• RC of Hyperthermia
• RC of Motor losses
• RC of Sensory losses
• RC of Cognitive losses

Nursing Diagnoses

• Risk for Injury related to gait disorders, vertigo, or visual disturbances, secondary to compression/displacement of brain tissue
• Anxiety related to implications of condition and uncertain future
• (Specify) Self-Care Deficit related to inability to perform/ difficulty in performing activities of daily living secondary to sensory–motor impairments
• Imbalanced Nutrition: Less Than Body Requirements related to dysphagia and fatigue

- Grieving related to actual/perceived loss of function and uncertain future
- Impaired Physical Mobility related to sensory–motor impairment
- Acute Pain related to compression/displacement of brain tissue and increased intracranial pressure
- Interrupted Family Processes related to the nature of the condition, role disturbances, and uncertain future
- Disturbed Self-Concept related to interruption in achieving/failure to achieve developmental tasks (childhood, adolescence, young adulthood, middle age)
- Risk for Deficient Fluid Volume related to vomiting secondary to increased intracranial pressure
- Risk for Injury related to impaired/uncontrolled sensory–motor function

Cerebrovascular Accident

Because this disorder can cause alterations varying from minimal to profound, the following possible nursing diagnoses reflect individuals with varying degrees of involvement.

Collaborative Problems

▲ RC of Increased intracranial pressure
▲ RC of Pneumonia
▲ RC of Atelectasis

Nursing Diagnoses

* Disturbed Sensory Perception: (specify) related to hypoxia and compression or displacement of brain tissue
▲ Impaired Physical Mobility related to decreased motor function of (specify) secondary to damage to upper motor neurons
▲ Impaired Communication related to dysarthria or aphasia
▲ Risk for Injury related to visual field, motor, or perception deficits
* Activity Intolerance related to deconditioning secondary to fatigue and weakness
* Disuse Syndrome
Δ Continuous Incontinence related to loss of bladder tone, loss of sphincter control, or inability to perceive bladder cues
▲ (Specify) Self-Care Deficit related to impaired physical mobility or confusion
Δ Impaired Swallowing related to muscle paralysis or paresis secondary to damage to upper motor neurons
Δ Grieving (Family, Individual) related to loss of function and inability to meet role responsibilities

△ Risk for Impaired Social Interaction related to difficulty communicating and embarrassment regarding disabilities

△ Risk for Deficient Fluid Volume related to dysphagia, difficulty in obtaining fluids secondary to weakness or motor deficits

△ Risk for Impaired Home Maintenance related to altered ability to maintain self at home secondary to sensory/motor/cognitive deficits and lack of knowledge by caregivers of home care, reality orientation, bowel/bladder program, skin care, signs and symptoms of complications, and community resources

▲ Functional Incontinence related to inability or difficulty in reaching toilet secondary to decreased mobility or motivation

△ Unilateral Neglect related to (specify site) secondary to right hemispheric brain damage

* Risk for Caregiver Role Strain related to complex care requirements secondary to (specify sensory or motor deficits)

△ Risk for Disturbed Self-Concept related to effects of prolonged debilitating condition on achieving developmental tasks and lifestyle

* Risk for Ineffective Self-Health Management related to insufficient knowledge of condition, pharmacologic therapy, self-care activities of daily living, home care, speech therapy, exercise program, community resources, self-help groups, and signs and symptoms of complications

* Wandering related to impaired cerebral function secondary to cerebrovascular accident

Nervous System Disorders
(Degenerative, Demyelinating, Inflammatory, Myasthenia Gravis, Multiple Sclerosis, Muscular Dystrophy, Parkinson's Disease, Guillain–Barré Syndrome, Amyotrophic Lateral Sclerosis)

Because the responses associated with these disorders can range from minimal to profound, the following possible diagnoses reflect individuals with varying degrees of involvement.

Collaborative Problems

* RC of Renal failure
* RC of Pneumonia
* RC of Atelectasis
* RC of Acute respiratory dysfunction
* RC of Autonomic nervous system dysfunction
* RC of Peripheral nervous system dysfunction
* RC of Decreased cardiac output

Nursing Diagnoses

- Risk for Disturbed Self-Concept related to the effects of prolonged debilitating condition on lifestyle and on achieving developmental tasks
- Risk for Injury related to visual disturbances, unsteady gait, sensory losses, weakness, or uncontrolled movements
- Impaired Verbal Communication related to dysarthria secondary to ataxia of muscles of speech
- Risk for Imbalanced Nutrition: Less Than Body Requirements related to dysphagia/chewing difficulties secondary to cranial nerve impairment
- Activity Intolerance related to fatigue and difficulty in performing activities of daily living
- Disuse Syndrome
- Impaired Physical Mobility related to effects of muscle rigidity, tremors, and slowness of movement on activities of daily living
- Impaired Swallowing related to cerebellar lesions
- Fatigue related to extremity weakness, spasticity, fear of injury, and stressors
- Overflow Urinary Incontinence related to sensory/motor deficits
- Chronic Sorrow (Client, Family) related to nature of disease and uncertain prognosis
- Ineffective Sexuality Patterns (female) related to loss of libido, fatigue, and decreased perineal sensation
- Interrupted Family Processes related to nature of disorder, role disturbances, and uncertain future
- Risk for Deficient Diversional Activity related to inability to perform usual job-related/recreational activities
- Risk for Loneliness related to mobility difficulties and associated embarrassment
- Impaired Home Maintenance related to inability to care for/difficulty in caring for self/home secondary to disability or unavailable or inadequate caregiver
- Parental Role Conflict related to disruptions secondary to disability
- Caregiver Role Strain related to continuous, multiple care needs
- (Specify) Self-Care Deficits related to (examples) headaches, muscular spasms, joint pain, fatigue, paresis/paralysis
- Powerlessness related to the unpredictable nature of the condition (e.g., remissions/exacerbations)
- (Specify) Urinary Incontinence: related to poor sphincter control and spastic bladder
- Ineffective Airway Clearance related to impaired ability to cough
- Risk for Ineffective Self-Health Management related to insufficient knowledge of condition, treatments, prevention of infection, stress management, aggravating factors, signs and symptoms of complications, and community resources

Presenile Dementia
(Alzheimer's Disease, Huntington's Disease)

See also *Nervous System Disorders.*

Nursing Diagnoses

- Risk for Injury related to lack of awareness of environmental hazards
- Chronic Confusion related to inability to evaluate reality secondary to cerebral neuron degeneration Impaired Physical Mobility related to gait instability
- Risk for Interrupted Family Processes related to effects of condition on relationships, role responsibilities, and finances
- Impaired Home Maintenance related to inability to care for/ difficulty in caring for self/home or inadequate or unavailable caregiver
- Unilateral Neglect related to (specify site) secondary to neurologic pathology
- (Specify) Self-Care Deficit related to (specify)
- Decisional Conflict related to placement of person in a care facility
- Caregiver Role Strain related to multiple care needs and insufficient resources
- Wandering related to impaired cerebral function secondary to Alzheimer's dementia

Seizure Disorders
(Epilepsy)

If the client is a child, see also *Developmental Problems/Needs.*

Collaborative Problem

- RC of Staus epilepticus

Nursing Diagnoses

- * Risk for Injury related to uncontrolled tonic–clonic movements during seizure episode
- ▲ Risk for Ineffective Airway Clearance related to relaxation of tongue and gag reflexes secondary to disruption in muscle innervation
- Risk for Loneliness related to fear of embarrassment secondary to having a seizure in public
- * Risk for Delayed Growth and Development related to interruption in achieving/failure to achieve developmental tasks (adolescence, young adulthood, middle age)

*   Risk for Impaired Oral Mucous Membrane related to effects of drug therapy on oral tissue

*   Fear related to unpredictable nature of seizures and embarrassment

Δ   Risk for Ineffective Self-Health Management related to insufficient knowledge of condition, medication, activity, care during seizures, environmental hazards, and community resources

Spinal Cord Injury[†]

Collaborative Problems

Δ   RC of Electrolyte imbalances
*   RC of Spinal shock
*   RC of Neurogenic shock
▲   RC of Respiratory complications
Δ   RC of Paralytic ileus
Δ   RC of Gastrointestinal bleeding
▲   RC of Thrombophlebitis
Δ   RC of Fracture/Dislocation
Δ   RC of Cardiovascular insufficiency
▲   RC of Hypoxemia
▲   RC of Urinary retention
*   RC of Pyelonephriris
Δ   RC of Renal insufficiency

Nursing Diagnoses

▲   Self-Care Deficit related to sensory/motor deficits secondary to level of spinal cord injury

*   Impaired Verbal Communication related to impaired ability to speak secondary to tracheostomy

*   Fear related to possible abandonment by others, changes in role responsibilities, effects of injury on lifestyle, multiple tests and procedures, or separation from support systems

Δ   Interrupted Family Processes related to adjustment requirements, role disturbances, and uncertain future

*   Risk for Aspiration related to inability to cough secondary to level of injury

Δ   Risk for Impaired Home Maintenance related to insufficient knowledge of the effects of altered skin, bowel, bladder, respiratory, thermoregulation, and sexual function and their management, signs and symptoms of complications, follow-up care, and community resources

▲   Anxiety related to perceived effects of injury on lifestyle and unknown future

▲ Chronic Sorrow related to loss of body function and its effects on lifestyle

Δ Risk for Loneliness (individual/family) related to disability or requirements for the caregiver(s)

Δ Risk for Caregiver Role Strain related to continuous, multiple care needs, inadequate resources, and coping mechanisms

* Risk for Disturbed Self-Concept related to effects of disability on achieving developmental tasks and lifestyle

* Risk for Deficient Fluid Volume related to difficulty obtaining liquids

* Risk for Imbalanced Nutrition: More Than Body Requirements related to imbalance of intake versus activity expenditures

* Risk for Imbalanced Nutrition: Less Than Body Requirements related to anorexia and increased metabolic requirements

* Risk for Deficient Diversional Activity related to effects of limitations on ability to participate in recreational activities
  • Reflex Urinary Incontinence or Overflow Urinary Incontinence
  • Related to bladder atony secondary to sensory–motor deficits

* Disuse Syndrome

* Risk for Injury related to impaired ability to control movements and sensory–motor deficits

* Risk for Infection related to urinary stasis, repeated catheterizations, and invasive procedures (skeletal tongs, tracheostomy, venous lines, surgical sites)

Δ Risk for Ineffective Sexuality Patterns related to physiologic, sensory, and psychological effects of disability on sexuality or function

Δ Bowel Incontinence (Reflex) related to lack of voluntary sphincter control secondary to spinal cord injury at the 11th thoracic vertebra (T_{11})

Δ Bowel Incontinence (Areflexia) related to lack of voluntary sphincter control secondary to spinal cord injury involving sacral reflex arc (S_2-S_4)

Δ Risk for Dysreflexia related to reflex stimulation of sympathetic nervous system secondary to loss of autonomic control

* Risk for Ineffective Self-Health Management related to insufficient knowledge of condition, treatment regimen, rehabilitation, and assistance devices

Unconscious Individual

See also *Mechanical Ventilation*, if indicated.

Collaborative Problems

* RC of Respiratory insufficiency
▲ RC of Pneumonia

▲ RC of Atelectasis
▲ RC of Fluid/Electrolyte imbalances
* RC of Negative nitrogen balance
* RC of Bladder distention
* RC of Seizures
* RC of Stress ulcers
* RC of Increased intracranial pressure
Δ RC of Sepsis
▲ RC of Thrombophlebitis
* RC of Renal calculi
Δ RC of Urinary tract infection

Nursing Diagnoses

* Risk for Infection related to immobility and invasive devices (tracheostomy, Foley catheter, venous lines)
* Risk for Impaired Corneal Tissue Integrity related to corneal drying secondary to open eyes and lower tear production
* Family Anxiety/Fear related to present state of individual and uncertain prognosis
• Risk for Impaired Oral Mucous Membrane related to inability to perform own mouth care and pooling of secretions
▲ Continuous Incontinence related to unconscious state
Δ Disuse Syndrome
Δ Powerlessness (family) related to feelings of loss of control and restrictions on lifestyle
▲ Risk for Ineffective Airway Clearance related to stasis of secretions secondary to inadequate cough and decreased mobility

SENSORY DISORDERS

Ophthalmic Disorders
(Cataracts, Detached Retina, Glaucoma, Inflammations)

See also *Cataract Extractions; Scleral Buckle/Vitrectomy.*

Collaborative Problem

• RC of Increased intraocular pressure

Nursing Diagnoses

• Risk for Injury related to visual limitations
• Acute Pain related to (examples) inflammation (lid, lacrimal structures, conjunctiva, uveal tract, retina, cornea, sclera), infection, increased intraocular pressure, ocular tumors

- Risk for Noncompliance related to negative side effects of prescribed therapy versus the belief that no treatment is needed without the presence of symptoms
- Risk for Loneliness related to fear of injury or embarrassment outside home environment
- Risk for Impaired Home Maintenance related to impaired ability to perform activities of daily living secondary to impaired vision
- (Specify) Self-Care Deficit related to impaired vision
- Anxiety related to actual or possible vision loss and perceived impact of chronic illness on lifestyle
- Risk for Disturbed Self-Concept related to effects of visual limitations
- Risk for Ineffective Self-Health Management related to insufficient knowledge of condition, eye care, medications, safety measures, activity restrictions, and follow-up care

Otic Disorders
(Infections, Mastoiditis, Trauma)

Nursing Diagnoses

- Risk for Injury related to disturbances of balance and impaired ability to detect environmental hazards
- Impaired Verbal Communication related to difficulty understanding others secondary to impaired hearing
- Risk for Impaired Social Interaction related to difficulty in participating in conversations
- Risk for Loneliness related to the lack of contact with others secondary to fear and embarrassment of hearing losses
- Acute Pain related to inflammation, infection, tinnitus, or vertigo
- Fear related to actual or possible loss of hearing
- Risk for Ineffective Self-Health Management related to insufficient knowledge of condition, medications, prevention of recurrence, hazards (swimming, air travel, showers), signs and symptoms of complications, and hearing aids

INTEGUMENTARY DISORDERS

Dermatologic Disorders
(Dermatitis, Psoriasis, Eczema)

Nursing Diagnoses

- Impaired Skin Integrity related to lesions and inflammatory response
- Impaired Comfort related to dermal eruptions and pruritus

- Risk for Impaired Social Interaction related to fear of embarrassment and negative reactions of others
- Risk for Disturbed Self-Concept related to appearance and response of others
- Risk for Ineffective Self-Health Management related to insufficient knowledge of condition, topical agents, and contraindications

Pressure Ulcers[†]

Collaborative Problem

Δ RC of Sepsis

Nursing Diagnoses

▲ Risk for Infection related to exposure of ulcer base to fecal/urinary drainage
▲ Impaired Tissue Integrity related to mechanical destruction of tissue secondary to pressure, shear, and friction
*   Impaired Home Maintenance related to complexity of care or unavailable caregiver
▲ Imbalanced Nutrition: Less Than Body Requirements related to anorexia secondary to (specify)
▲ Impaired Physical Mobility related to imposed restrictions, deconditioned status, loss of motor control, or altered mental status
*   Excess Fluid Volume: Edema related to (specify)
*   Continuous Incontinence related to (specify)
Δ Risk for Ineffective Self-Health Management related to insufficient knowledge of etiology, prevention, treatment, and home care

Skin Infections
(Impetigo, Herpes Zoster, Fungal Infections)

Collaborative Problems

- RC of Postherpetic neuralgia
- RC of Keratitis
- RC of Uveitis
- RC of Corneal ulceration
- RC of Blindness

Nursing Diagnoses

- Impaired Skin Integrity related to lesions and pruritus
- Impaired Comfort related to dermal eruptions and pruritus

- Risk for Infection Transmission related to contagious nature of the organism
- Risk for Ineffective Self-Health Management related to insufficient knowledge of condition (causes, course), prevention, treatment, and skin care

Thermal Injuries
(Burns, Severe Hypothermia)

Acute Period
Collaborative Problems

- ▲ RC of Hypovolemia/Shock
- * RC of Fluid overload
- * RC of Anemia
- Δ RC of Negative nitrogen balance
- ▲ RC of Electrolyte imbalance
- Δ RC of Metabolic acidosis
- ▲ RC of Respiratory Insufficiency
- ▲ RC of Sepsis
- * RC of Emboli
- ▲ RC of Graft rejection/infection
- * RC of Hypothermia
- Δ RC of Curling's ulcer
- Δ RC of Paralytic ileus
- * RC of Stress diabetes
- * RC of Pneumonia
- Δ RC of Renal insufficiency
- * RC of Compartment syndrome

Nursing Diagnoses

- ▲ Risk for Infection related to loss of protective layer secondary to thermal injury
- ▲ Imbalanced Nutrition: Less Than Body Requirements related to increased caloric requirement secondary to thermal injury and inability to ingest sufficient quantities to meet increased requirements
- * Impaired Physical Mobility related to acute pain secondary to thermal injury and treatments
- Δ (Specify) Self-Care Deficit related to impaired range-of-motion ability secondary to pain
- * Fear related to painful procedures and possibility of death
- * Risk for Loneliness related to infection control measures and separation from family and support systems

* Disuse Syndrome
* Disturbed Sleep Pattern related to position restrictions, pain, and treatment interruptions
* Risk for Disturbed Sensory Perception related to (examples) excessive environmental stimuli, stress, imposed immobility, sleep deprivation, protective isolation
▲ Grieving (family, individual) related to actual or perceived impact of injury on life, appearance, relationships, lifestyle
▲ Anxiety related to sudden injury, treatments, uncertainty of outcome, and pain
* Anxiety related to pain secondary to thermal injury treatments and immobility
▲ Acute Pain related to thermal injury treatments and immobility

Postacute Period

If individual is a child, see also *Developmental Problems/Needs.*

Collaborative Problem

• RC of Same as in acute period

Nursing Diagnoses

Δ Deficient Diversional Activity related to monotony of confinement
* Risk for Loneliness related to embarrassment and response of others to injury
* Powerlessness related to inability to control situation
Δ Risk for Disturbed Self-Concept related to effects of thermal injury on achieving developmental tasks (child, adolescent, adult)
* Fear related to uncertain future and effects of injury on life-style, relationships, occupation
* Impaired Home Maintenance related to long-term requirements of treatments
Δ Risk for Ineffective Self-Health Management related to insufficient knowledge of exercise program, wound care, nutritional requirements, pain management, signs and symptoms of complications, and burn prevention and follow-up care

MUSCULOSKELETAL/CONNECTIVE TISSUE DISORDERS

Fractured Jaw

Collaborative Problem

• RC of Dislocation

Nursing Diagnoses

• Risk for Aspiration related to inadequate cough secondary to pain and fixative devices
• Impaired Oral Mucous Membrane related to difficulty in performing oral hygiene secondary to fixation devices
• Impaired Verbal Communication related to fixation devices
• Acute Pain related to tissue trauma and fixation device
• Risk for Imbalanced Nutrition: Less Than Body Requirements related to inability to ingest solid food secondary to fixation devices
• Risk for Ineffective Self-Health Management related to insufficient knowledge of mouth care, nutritional requirements, signs and symptoms of infection, and procedure for emergency wire cutting (e.g., vomiting)

Fractures

See also *Casts*.

Collaborative Problems

▲ RC of Neurovascular compromise
▲ RC of Fat embolism
▲ RC of Bleeding/Hematoma formation
* RC of Osteomyelitis
* RC of Compartment syndrome
* RC of Contracture
▲ RC of Thromboemboli

Nursing Diagnoses

* Acute Pain related to tissue trauma and immobility
▲ Impaired Physical Mobility related to tissue trauma secondary to fracture
* Disuse Syndrome
• Risk for Infection related to invasive fixation devices

▲ (Specify) Self-Care Deficit related to limitation of movement secondary to fracture
* Deficient Diversional Activity related to boredom of confinement secondary to immobilization devices
* Risk for Impaired Home Maintenance related to (examples) fixation device, impaired physical mobility, unavailable support system
* Interrupted Family Processes related to difficulty of ill person in assuming role responsibilities secondary to limited motion
Δ Risk for Ineffective Self-Health Management related to insufficient knowledge of condition, signs and symptoms of complications, activity restrictions

Low Back Pain

Collaborative Problem

• RC of Herniated nucleus pulposus

Nursing Diagnoses

• Pain related to (examples) acute lumbosacral strain, weak muscles, osteoarthritis of spine, unstable lumbosacral ligaments, spinal stenosis, intervertebral disk problem
• Impaired Physical Mobility related to decreased mobility and flexibility secondary to muscle spasm
• Risk for Ineffective Coping related to effects of chronic pain on lifestyle
• Risk for Interrupted Family Processes related to impaired ability to meet role responsibilities (financial, home, social)
• Risk for Ineffective Self-Health Management related to insufficient knowledge of condition, exercise program, noninvasive pain relief methods (relaxation, imagery), proper posture and body mechanics, and risk factors (smoking, inactivity, overweight)

Osteoporosis

Collaborative Problems

• RC of Fractures
• RC of Kyphosis
• RC of Paralytic ileus

Nursing Diagnoses

• Acute/Chronic Pain related to muscle spasm and fractures
• Ineffective Self-Health Management related to insufficient daily physical activity

- Imbalanced Nutrition: Less Than Body Requirements related to inadequate dietary intake of calcium, protein, and vitamin D
- Impaired Physical Mobility related to limited range of motion secondary to skeletal changes
- Fear related to unpredictable nature of condition
- Risk for Ineffective Self-Health Management related to insufficient knowledge of condition, risk factors, nutritional therapy, and prevention

Inflammatory Joint Disease

Collaborative Problems

- RC of Septic arthritis
- RC of Sjogren's syndrome
- RC of Neuropathy
- RC of Anemia, leukopenia
- RC of Avascular necrosis
- RC of Cardiopulmonary effects
- RC of Diabetes mellitus
- RC of Septic shock

Nursing Diagnoses

- Chronic Pain related to local and systemic inflammatory lesions
- (Specify) Self-Care Deficit related to loss of motion, muscle weakness, pain, stiffness, or fatigue
- Powerlessness related to physical and psychological changes imposed by the disease
- Ineffective Coping related to the stress imposed by unpredictable exacerbations
- (Specify) Self-Care Deficit related to limitations secondary to disease process
- Fatigue related to effects of chronic inflammatory process
- Risk for Impaired Oral Mucous Membrane related to effects of medications or Sjögren's syndrome
- Impaired Home Maintenance related to impaired ability to perform household responsibilities secondary to limited mobility and pain
- Disturbed Sleep Pattern related to pain or secondary to fibrositis
- Impaired Physical Mobility related to pain and limited joint motion
- Ineffective Sexuality Patterns related to pain, fatigue, difficulty in assuming positions, and lack of adequate lubrication (female) secondary to disease process
- Risk for Loneliness related to ambulation difficulties and fatigue

- Interrupted Family Processes related to difficulty/inability of ill person to assume role responsibilities secondary to fatigue and limited motion
- Risk for Ineffective Self-Health Management related to insufficient knowledge of condition, pharmacologic therapy, home care, stress management, and quackery

INFECTIOUS/IMMUNODEFICIENT DISORDERS

Lupus Erythematosus
(Systemic)

See also *Rheumatic Diseases; Corticosteroid Therapy.*

Collaborative Problems

- RC of Sepsis
- RC of Polymyositis, Serositis, Pericarditis, Pleuritis
- RC of Vasculitis
- RC of Hematologic abnormalities
- RC of Raynaud's disease
- RC of Neuropsychiatric disorders

Nursing Diagnoses

- Powerlessness related to unpredictable course of disease
- Ineffective Coping related to unpredictable course and altered appearance
- Risk for Loneliness related to embarrassment and the response of others to appearance
- Risk for Disturbed Self-Concept related to inability to achieve developmental tasks secondary to disabling condition and changes in appearance
- Risk for Injury related to increased dermal vulnerability secondary to disease process
- Fatigue related to decreased mobility and effects of chronic inflammation
- Risk for Ineffective Self-Health Management related to insufficient knowledge of condition, rest versus activity requirements, pharmacologic therapy, signs and symptoms of complications, risk factors, and community resources

Meningitis/Encephalitis

Collaborative Problems

- RC of Fluid/Electrolyte imbalances
- RC of Cerebral edema
- RC of Adrenal damage
- RC of Circulatory collapse
- RC of Bleeding
- RC of Seizures
- RC of Sepsis
- RC of Alkalosis
- RC of Increased intracranial pressure

Nursing Diagnoses

- Risk for Infection Transmission related to contagious nature of organism
- Acute Pain related to headache, fever, neck pain secondary to meningeal irritation
- Activity Intolerance related to fatigue and malaise secondary to infection
- Risk for Impaired Skin Integrity related to immobility, dehydration, and diaphoresis
- Risk for Impaired Oral Mucous Membrane related to dehydration and impaired ability to perform mouth care
- Risk for Imbalanced Nutrition: Less Than Body Requirements related to anorexia, fatigue, nausea, and vomiting
- Risk for Ineffective Respiratory Function related to immobility and pain
- Risk for Injury related to restlessness and disorientation secondary to meningeal irritation
- Interrupted Family Processes related to critical nature of situation and uncertain prognosis
- Anxiety related to treatments, environment, and risk of death
- Risk for Ineffective Self-Health Management related to insufficient knowledge of condition, treatments, pharmacologic therapy, rest/activity balance, signs and symptoms of complications, follow-up care, and prevention of recurrence

Sexually Transmitted Infections/Diseases

Nursing Diagnoses

- Risk for Infection Transmission related to lack of knowledge of the contagious nature of the disease and reports of high-risk behaviors

- Anxiety related to nature of the condition and its implications for lifestyle with genital herpes/warts diagnosis
- Grieving related to loss of trust in partner secondary to infidelity
- Acute Pain related to inflammatory process
- Risk for Loneliness related to fear of transmitting disease to others, e.g., genital herpes, HIV
- Risk for Ineffective Self-Health Management related to insufficient knowledge of condition, modes of transmission, consequences of repeated infections, and prevention of recurrences

Acquired Immunodeficiency Syndrome (AIDS) (Adult)

See also *End-Stage Cancer.*

Collaborative Problems

▲ RC of Opportunistic infections
▲ RC of Myelosuppression
▲ RC of Sepsis
* RC of Neuropathy
* RC of Peripheral Nephropathy

Nursing Diagnoses

* Chronic Pain related to headache, fever secondary to inflammation of cerebral tissue
▲ Fatigue related to effects of disease, stress, chronic infections, and nutritional deficiency
* Risk for Impaired Skin Integrity related to perineal and anal tissue excoriation secondary to diarrhea and chronic genital candidal or herpes lesions
* Imbalanced Nutrition: Less Than Body Requirements related to chronic diarrhea, gastrointestinal malabsorption, fatigue, anorexia, or oral/esophageal lesions
▲ Risk for Infection Transmission related to contagious nature of blood and body secretions
Δ Risk for Loneliness related to fear of rejection or actual rejection of others secondary to fear
* Hopelessness related to nature of the condition and poor prognosis
Δ Powerlessness related to unpredictable nature of condition
▲ Interrupted Family Processes related to the nature of the AIDS condition, role disturbance, and uncertain future
Δ Anxiety related to perceived effects of illness on lifestyle and unknown future

△ Chronic Sorrow related to loss of body function and its effects on lifestyle

▲ Risk for Infection related to increased susceptibility secondary to compromised immune system

▲ Risk for Impaired Oral Mucous Membrane related to compromised immune system

△ Risk for Caregiver Role Strain related to multiple needs of ill person and chronicity

△ Risk for Ineffective Self-Health Management related to insufficient knowledge of condition, medications, home care, infection control, and community resources

NEOPLASTIC DISORDERS

Cancer

Cancer: Initial Diagnosis
See also specific types.

Nursing Diagnoses

▲ Anxiety related to unfamiliar hospital environment, uncertainty about outcomes, feelings of helplessness and hopelessness, and insufficient knowledge about cancer and treatment

▲ Grieving related to potential loss of body function and the perceived losses associated with cancer on lifestyle

* Powerlessness related to uncertainty about prognosis and outcome of cancer treatment

▲ Interrupted Family Processes related to fears associated with recent cancer diagnosis, disruptions associated with treatments, financial problems, and uncertain future

△ Decisional Conflict related to treatment modality choices

△ Risk for Disturbed Self-Concept related to changes in lifestyle, role responsibilities, and appearance

△ Risk for Loneliness related to fear of rejection or actual rejection secondary to fear

△ Risk for Spiritual Distress related to conflicts centering on the meaning of life, cancer, spiritual beliefs, and death

* Risk for Ineffective Self-Health Management related to insufficient knowledge of cancer, cancer treatment options, diagnostic tests, effects of treatment, treatment plan, and support services

(Cancer: General)
(Applies to Malignancies in Varied Sites and Stages)
Nursing Diagnoses

- Impaired Oral Mucous Membranes related to (examples) disease process, therapy, radiation, chemotherapy, inadequate oral hygiene, and altered nutritional/hydration status
- Risk for Ineffective Sexuality Patterns related to (examples) fear, grieving, changes in body image, anatomic changes, pain, fatigue (treatments, disease), or change in role responsibilities
- Acute/Chronic Pain related to disease process and treatments
- Diarrhea related to (examples) disease process, chemotherapy, radiation, and medications
- Constipation related to (examples) disease process, chemotherapy, radiation therapy, immobility, dietary intake, and medications
- Disturbed Self-Concept related to (examples) anatomic changes, role disturbances, uncertain future, disruption of lifestyle
- (Specify) Self-Care Deficit related to fatigue, pain, or depression
- Risk for Infection related to altered immune system
- Imbalanced Nutrition: Less Than Body Requirements related to anorexia, fatigue, nausea, and vomiting secondary to disease process and treatments
- Risk for Injury related to disorientation, weakness, sensory/perceptual deterioration, or skeletal/muscle deterioration
- Disuse Syndrome
- Risk for Deficient Fluid Volume related to (examples) altered ability/desire to obtain fluids, weakness, vomiting, diarrhea, depression, and fatigue
- Risk for Impaired Home Maintenance related to (examples) lack of knowledge, lack of resources (support system, equipment, finances), motor deficits, sensory deficits, cognitive deficits, and emotional deficits
- Risk for Impaired Social Interaction related to fear of rejection or actual rejection of others after diagnosis
- Powerlessness related to inability to control situation
- Interrupted Family Processes related to (examples) stress of diagnosis/treatments, role disturbances, and uncertain future
- Grieving (Family, Individual) related to actual, perceived, or anticipated losses associated with diagnosis
- Risk for Ineffective Self-Health Management related to insufficient knowledge of disease, misconceptions, treatments, home care, and support agencies

Cancer: End Stage
See also specific types.

Collaborative Problems

- RC of Hypercalcemia
- RC of Intracerebral metastasis
- RC of Malignant effusions
- RC of Opioid toxicity
- RC of Pathologic fractures
- RC of Spinal cord compression
- RC of Superior vena cava syndrome
- RC of Negative nitrogen imbalance
- RC of Myelosuppression
- RC of Bowel Obstruction
- RC of Hepatoxicity
- RC of Increased Intracranial pressure
- RC of Cardiotoxicity

Nursing Diagnoses

- See also *Cancer (General)*.
- Imbalanced Nutrition: Less Than Body Requirements related to decreased oral intake, increased metabolic demands of tumor, and altered lipid metabolism
- Impaired Comfort related to pruritus secondary to dry skin and biliary obstruction
- Ineffective Airway Clearance related to inability to cough up secretions secondary to weakness, increased viscosity, and pain
- Impaired Physical Mobility related to pain, sedation, weakness, fatigue, and edema
- (Specify) Self-Care Deficit related to fatigue, weakness, sedation, pain, or decreased sensory/perceptual capacity
- Activity Intolerance related to hypoxia, fatigue, malnutrition, and decreased mobility
- Grieving related to terminal illness, impending death, functional losses, and withdrawal of, or from, others
- Hopelessness related to overwhelming functional losses or impending death
- Disturbed Self-Concept related to dependence on others to meet basic needs and decrease in functional ability
- Powerlessness related to change from curative status to palliative status
- Caregiver Role Strain related to multiple care needs and concern about ability to manage home care
- Risk for Spiritual Distress related to fear of death, overwhelming grief, belief system conflicts, and unresolved conflicts
- Death Anxiety related to effects of disease process

- Risk for Impaired Home Maintenance related to insufficient knowledge of home care, pain management, signs and symptoms of complications, and community resources available

Colorectal Cancer

See also *Cancer (General)*.

Nursing Diagnoses

- Risk for Ineffective Sexuality Patterns (male) related to inability to have or sustain an erection secondary to surgical procedure on perineal structures
- Risk for Ineffective Self-Health Management related to insufficient knowledge of ostomy care, supplies, dietary management, signs and symptoms of complications, and community services

Part 2

Surgical Procedures

General Surgery

Preoperative Period

Nursing Diagnoses

- Fear related to surgical experience, loss of control, and unpredictable outcome
- Anxiety related to preoperative procedures (surgical permit, diagnostic studies, Foley catheter, diet and fluid restrictions, medications, skin preparation, waiting area for family) and postoperative procedures (disposition [recovery room, intensive care unit], medications for pain, coughing/turning/leg exercises, tube/drain placement, nothing by mouth [NPO]/diet restrictions, bed rest)

Postoperative Period

Collaborative Problems

- RC of Urinary retention
- RC of Bleeding
- RC of Hypovolemia/Shock
- RC of Pneumonia
- RC of Peritonitis
- RC of Thrombophlebitis
- RC of Paralytic ileus
- RC of Evisceration/Dehiscence

Nursing Diagnoses

- Risk for Infection related to site for bacterial invasion
- Risk for Ineffective Respiratory Function related to postanesthesia state, postoperative immobility, and pain
- Acute Pain related to incision, flatus, and immobility

- Risk for Constipation related to decreased peristalsis secondary to the effects of anesthesia, immobility, and pain medication
- Risk for Imbalanced Nutrition: Less Than Body Requirements related to increased protein/vitamin requirements for wound healing and decreased intake secondary to pain, nausea, vomiting, and diet restrictions
- Risk for Ineffective Self-Health Management related to insufficient knowledge of home care, incisional care, signs and symptoms of complications, activity restriction, and follow-up care

Amputation
(Lower Extremity)

Preoperative Period
See also *Surgery (General)*.

Nursing Diagnoses

▲ Anxiety related to insufficient knowledge of postoperative routines, postoperative sensations, and crutch-walking techniques

Postoperative Period
Collaborative Problems

▲ RC of Edema of stump
▲ RC of Bleeding
▲ RC of Hematoma site
* RC of Delayed wound healing

Nursing Diagnoses

* Disuse Syndrome
▲ Grieving related to loss of limb and its effects on lifestyle
▲ Acute/Chronic Pain related to phantom limb sensations secondary to peripheral nerve stimulation or abnormal impulses to CNS
▲ Risk for Injury related to altered gait and hazards of assistive devices
Δ Risk for Impaired Home Maintenance related to architectural barriers
Δ Risk for Disturbed Body Image related to perceived negative effects of amputation and response of others to appearance
▲ Risk for Injury related to contracture formation secondary to impaired movement and pain

Δ Risk for Ineffective Self-Health Management related to insufficient knowledge of activities of daily living adaptations, stump care, prosthesis care, gait training, and follow-up care

Aneurysm Resection
(Abdominal Aortic)

See also *Surgery (General)*.

Preoperative Period
Collaborative Problems

▲ RC of Rupture of aneurysm

Postoperative Period
Collaborative Problems

▲ RC of Distal vessel thrombosis or emboli
▲ RC of Kidney failure
Δ RC of Mesenteric ischemia/thrombosis
Δ RC of Spinal cord ischemia

Nursing Diagnoses

▲ Risk for Infection related to location of surgical incision
* Risk for Ineffective Sexuality Patterns (male) related to possible loss of ejaculate and erections secondary to surgery
Δ Risk for Ineffective Self-Health Management related to insufficient knowledge of home care, activity restrictions, signs and symptoms of complications, and follow-up care

Anorectal Surgery

See also *Surgery (General)*.

Preoperative Period
See *Hemorrhoids/Anal Fissure*.

Postoperative Period
Collaborative Problems

• RC of Bleeding
• RC of Urinary retention

Nursing Diagnoses

- Risk for Constipation related to fear of pain
- Risk for Infection related to surgical incision and fecal contamination
- Risk for Ineffective Self-Health Management related to insufficient knowledge of wound care, prevention of recurrence, nutritional requirements (diet, fluid), exercise program, and signs and symptoms of complications

Arterial Bypass Graf of Lower Extremity
(Aortic, Iliac, Femoral, Popliteal)

See also *Surgery (General)*; *Anticoagulant Therapy*.

Postoperative Period
Collaborative Problems

- ▲ RC of Thrombosis of graft
- Δ RC of Compartment syndrome
  RC of Lymphocele
- ▲ RC of Disruption of anastomosis

Nursing Diagnoses

- ▲ Risk for Infection related to location of surgical incision
- ▲ Acute Pain related to increased tissue perfusion to previous ischemic tissue
- Δ Risk for Impaired Tissue Integrity related to immobility and vulnerability of heels
- Δ Risk for Ineffective Self-Health Management related to insufficient knowledge of wound care, signs and symptoms of complications, activity restrictions, and follow-up care

Arthroscopy, Arthrotomy, Meniscectomy, Bunionectomy

See also *Surgery (General)*.

Postoperative Period
Collaborative Problems

- RC of Hematoma formation
- RC of Neurovascular impairments
- RC of Bleeding
- RC of Effusion

Nursing Diagnoses

- Risk for Ineffective Self-Health Management related to insufficient knowledge of home care, incision care, activity restrictions, signs of complications, and follow-up care

Breast Surgery
(Lumpectomy, Mastectomy)

See also *Cancer (General); Surgery (General)*.

Preoperative Period

▲ Anxiety/Fear related to perceived effects of breast surgery and cancer on (immediate concerns of pain, edema and postdischarge concerns regarding relationships, work and prognosis

Postoperative Period

Collaborative Problems

▲ RC of Neurovascular compromise

Nursing Diagnoses

- ▲ Risk for Impaired Physical Mobility (shoulder, arm) related to lymphedema, nerve/muscle damage, and pain
- ▲ Risk for Injury related to compromised lymph, motor, and sensory function in affected arm
- ▲ Grieving related to loss of breast and change in appearance
- ▲ Risk for Ineffective Self-Health Management related to insufficient knowledge of wound care, exercises, breast prosthesis, signs and symptoms of complications, hand/arm precautions, community resources, and follow-up care

Carotid Endarterectomy

See also *Surgery (General)*.

Preoperative Period

Nursing Diagnoses

Δ Anxiety related to anticipated surgery and unfamiliarity with preoperative and postoperative routines and postoperative sensations

Postoperative Period

Collaborative Problems

▲ RC of Thrombosis
▲ RC of Hypotension
▲ RC of Hypertension
▲ RC of Bleeding
▲ RC of Cerebral infarction
▲ RC of Cranial nerve impairment
▲ RC of Facial nerve impairment
▲ RC of Hypoglossal nerve impairment
▲ RC of Glossopharyngeal nerve impairment
Δ RC of Vagus nerve impairment
Δ RC of Local nerve impairment (peri-incisional numbness of skin)
▲ RC of Respiratory obstruction

Nursing Diagnoses

Δ Risk for Injury related to syncope secondary to vascular insufficiency
Δ Risk for Ineffective Self-Health Management related to insufficient knowledge of home care, signs and symptoms of complications, risk factors, activity restrictions, and follow-up care

Cataract Extraction

Postoperative Period

Collaborative Problem

▲ RC of Bleeding

Nursing Diagnoses

Δ Acute Pain related to surgical procedure
▲ Risk for Infection related to increased susceptibility secondary to surgical interruption of eye surface
▲ Risk for Injury related to visual limitations, presence in unfamiliar environment, limited mobility, and postoperative presence of eye patch
Δ Risk for Loneliness related to decreased socialization and altered visual acuity and fear of falling
Δ Risk for Impaired Home Maintenance related to inability to perform activities of daily living secondary to activity restrictions and visual limitations

▲ Risk for Ineffective Self-Health Management related to insufficient knowledge of activities permitted and restricted, medications, complications, and follow-up care

Cesarean Section

See *Surgery (General); Postpartum Period.*

Cholecystectomy

See also *Surgery (General).*

Postoperative Period

Collaborative Problem

• RC of Peritonitis

Nursing Diagnoses

• Risk for Ineffective Respiratory Function related to high abdominal incision and splinting secondary to pain
• Risk for Impaired Oral Mucous Membrane related to NPO state and mouth breathing secondary to nasogastric intubation

Colostomy

See also *Surgery (General).*

Postoperative Period

Collaborative Problems

▲ RC of Peristomal ulceration/herniation
▲ RC of Stomal necrosis, retraction, prolapse, stenosis, obstruction

Nursing Diagnoses

Δ Grieving related to implications of cancer diagnosis
▲ Risk for Disturbed Self-Concept related to effects of ostomy on body image and lifestyle
Δ Risk for Ineffective Sexuality Patterns related to perceived negative impact of ostomy on sexual functioning and attractiveness

- Risk for Sexual Dysfunction related to physiologic impotence secondary to damaged sympathetic nerves (male) or inadequate vaginal lubrication (female)
Δ Risk for Loneliness related to decreased socialization and anxiety about possible odor and leakage from appliance
▲ Risk for Ineffective Self-Health Management related to insufficient knowledge of stoma pouching procedure, colostomy irrigation, peristomal skin care, perineal wound care, and incorporation of ostomy care into activities of daily living

Corneal Transplant
(Penetrating Keratoplasty)

See also *Surgery (General)*.

Postoperative Period
Collaborative Problems

* RC of Endophthalmitis
▲ RC of Increased intraocular pressure
* RC of Epithelial defects
* RC of Graft failure

Nursing Diagnoses

Δ Risk for Infection related to nonintact ocular tissue
▲ Acute Pain related to surgical procedure
▲ Risk for Ineffective Self-Health Management related to insufficient knowledge of eye care, resumption of activities, medications/medication administration, signs and symptoms of complications, and long-term follow-up care

Coronary Artery Bypass Grafting (CABG)

See also *Surgery (General)*.

Postoperative Period
Collaborative Problems

▲ RC of Cardiovascular insufficiency
▲ RC of Respiratory insufficiency
▲ RC of Renal insufficiency
* RC of Hyperthermia
* RC of Postcardiotomy delirium

Nursing Diagnoses

▲ Acute Pain related to surgical incisions, chest tubes, and immobility secondary to lengthy surgery
Impaired Physical Mobility related to surgical incisions, chest tubes, and fatigue

Δ Fear related to transfer from intensive environment of the critical care unit and potential for complications Impaired Verbal Communication related to endotracheal tube (temporary)

Δ Interrupted Family Processes related to disruption of family life, fear of outcome (death, disability), and stressful environment (intensive care unit)

Δ Risk for Disturbed Self-Concept related to the symbolic meaning of the heart and changes in lifestyle

Δ Risk for Ineffective Self-Health Management related to insufficient knowledge of incisional care, pain management (angina, incisions), signs and symptoms of complications, condition, pharmacologic care, risk factors, restrictions, stress management techniques, and follow-up care

Cranial Surgery

See also *Surgery (General); Brain Tumor* for preoperative and postoperative care.

Postoperative Period

Collaborative Problems

▲ RC of Increased intracranial pressure
▲ RC of Cerebral/Cerebellar dysfunction
* RC of Hypoxemia
▲ RC of Seizures
▲ RC of Brain hemorrhage, hematomas, hygroma
▲ RC of Cranial nerve dysfunctions
* RC of Cardiac dysrhythmias
▲ RC of Fluid/Electrolyte imbalances
Δ RC of Meningitis/Encephalitis
▲ RC of Sensory–motor losses
▲ RC of Hypothermia/Hyperthermia
Δ RC of Antidiuretic hormone secretion disorders
▲ RC of Cerebrospinal fluid leaks
▲ RC of Hygromas
* RC of Brain shifts/Herniations
* RC of Hydrocephalus
* RC of Gastrointestinal bleeding

Nursing Diagnoses

▲ Acute Pain related to compression/displacement of brain tissue and increased intracranial pressure

△ Risk for Impaired Corneal Tissue Integrity related to inadequate lubrication secondary to tissue edema

△ Risk for Ineffective Self-Health Management related to insufficient knowledge of wound care, signs and symptoms of complications, restrictions, and follow-up care

Dilatation and Curettage

See also *Surgery (General)—Preoperative and Postoperative.*

Postoperative Period

Collaborative Problem

• RC of Bleeding

Nursing Diagnoses

• Risk for Ineffective Self-Health Management related to insufficient knowledge of condition, home care, signs and symptoms of complications, and activity restrictions

Enucleation

Postoperative Period

Collaborative Problems

▲ RC of Bleeding
• RC of Abscess

Nursing Diagnoses

△ Risk for Injury related to visual limitations and presence in unfamiliar environment

△ Grieving related to loss of eye and its effects on lifestyle

△ Risk for Disturbed Self-Concept related to effects of change in appearance on lifestyle

△ Risk for Loneliness related to changes in body image and altered vision

△ Risk for Impaired Home Maintenance related to inability to perform activities of daily living secondary to change in visual abilities

△ Risk for Ineffective Self-Health Management related to insufficient knowledge of activities permitted, self-care activities, medications, complications, and plans for follow-up care

Fractured Hip and Femur

See also *Surgery (General)*.

Postoperative Period
Collaborative Problems

▲ RC of Hypovolemia/Shock
▲ RC of Pulmonary embolism
▲ RC of Sepsis
▲ RC of Fat emboli
▲ RC of Compartment syndrome
△ RC of Peroneal nerve palsy
▲ RC of Displacement of hip joint
▲ RC of Venous stasis/Thrombosis
• RC of Avascular necrosis of femoral head

Nursing Diagnoses

▲ (Specify) Self-Care Deficit related to prescribed activity restriction
▲ Disuse syndrome
△ Fear related to anticipated postoperative dependence
△ Risk for Disturbed Sensory Perceptions related to unfamiliar environment, pain, and immobility
△ Risk for Ineffective Self-Health Management related to insufficient knowledge of activity restrictions, assistive devices, home care, follow-up care, and supportive services

Hysterectomy
(Vaginal, Abdominal)

See also *Surgery (General)*.

Postoperative Period
Collaborative Problems

▲ RC of Vaginal bleeding
* RC of Urinary retention (postcatheter removal)
* RC of Fistula formation
▲ RC of Deep vein thrombosis

▲ RC of Trauma (ureter, bladder, rectum)
* RC of Neurological deficits secondary to epidural therapy

Nursing Diagnoses

* Risk for Infection related to surgical intervention and presence of urinary catheter
▲ Risk for Disturbed Self-Concept related to significance of loss
* Grieving related to loss of body part and childbearing ability
Δ Risk for Ineffective Self-Health Management related to insufficient knowledge of perineal/incisional care, signs of complications, activity restrictions, loss of menses, hormone therapy, and follow-up care

Ileostomy

Postoperative Period

Collaborative Problems

▲ RC of Peristomal ulceration/herniation
▲ RC of Stomal necrosis, retraction, prolapse, stenosis, obstruction
▲ RC of Fluid and electrolyte imbalances
* RC of Ileanal Kock pouchitis
* RC of Failed nipple valve (Kock Pouch)
* RC of Ileal reservoir pouchitis (Kock Pouch)
* RC of Cholelithiasis
* RC of Urinary calculi

Nursing Diagnoses

▲ Risk for Disturbed Self-Concept related to effects of ostomy on body image
Δ Risk for Ineffective Sexuality Patterns related to perceived negative impact of ostomy on sexual functioning and attractiveness
Δ Risk for Loneliness related to decreased socialization and anxiety about possible odor and leakage from appliance
Δ Risk for Ineffective Self-Health Management related to insufficient knowledge of stoma pouching procedure, peristomal skin care, perineal wound care, and incorporation of ostomy care into activities of daily living
Δ Risk for Ineffective Self-Health Management related to insufficient knowledge of care of ileoanal reservoir
Δ Risk for Ineffective Self-Health Management related to insufficient knowledge of intermittent intubation of Kock continent ileostomy

Laminectomy

See also *Surgery (General)*.

Postoperative Period

Collaborative Problems

- ▲ RC of Neurosensory impairments
- * RC of Bowel/Bladder dysfunction
- ▲ RC of Paralytic ileus
- * RC of Cord edema
- * RC of Skeletal misalignment
- Δ RC of Cerebrospinal fistula
- * RC of Hematoma
- ▲ RC of Urinary retention

Nursing Diagnoses

- * Risk for Injury related to vertigo secondary to postural hypotension
- ▲ Acute Pain related to muscle spasms (back, thigh) secondary to surgical trauma
- * (Specify) Self-Care Deficit related to activity restrictions
- ▲ Risk for Ineffective Self-Health Management related to insufficient knowledge of home care, brace care, activity restrictions, and exercise program

Radical Neck Dissection
(Laryngectomy)

See also *Surgery (General); Cancer (General); Tracheostomy*.

Postoperative Period

Collaborative Problems

- * RC of Hypoxemia
- ▲ RC of Flap rejection
- ▲ RC of Bleeding
- ▲ RC of Carotid artery rupture
- * RC of Cranial nerve injury
- * RC of Infection

Nursing Diagnoses

- ▲ Risk for Impaired Physical Mobility: Shoulder, head related to removal of muscles, nerves, flap graft reconstruction, and surgical trauma

▲ Risk for Disturbed Self-Concept related to change in appearance
▲ Risk for Ineffective Self-Health Management related to insufficient knowledge of wound care, signs and symptoms of complications, exercises, and follow-up care

Ophthalmic Surgery

See also *Surgery (General)*.

Postoperative Period
Collaborative Problems

△ RC of Wound dehiscence/evisceration
△ RC of Increased intraocular pressure
△ RC of Retinal detachment
* RC of Dislocation of lens implant
* RC of Choroidal hemorrhage
* RC of Endophthalmitis
* RC of Hyphema
* RC of Hypopyon
△ RC of Blindness

Nursing Diagnoses

△ Risk for Infection related to increased susceptibility secondary to surgical trauma
▲ Risk for Injury related to visual limitations, presence in unfamiliar environment, and presence of postoperative eye patches Feeding, Bathing Self-Care Deficit related to activity restrictions, visual impairment, or presence of eye patch(es)
▲ Risk for Disturbed Sensory Perceptions related to insufficient input secondary to impaired vision or presence of unilateral/bilateral eye patches
▲ Risk for Ineffective Self-Health Management related to insufficient knowledge of activities permitted and restricted, medications, complications, and follow-up care

Otic Surgery
(Stapedectomy, Tympanoplasty, Myringotomy, Tympanic Mastoidectomy)

See also *Surgery (General)*.

Postoperative Period

Collaborative Problems

- RC of Bleeding
- RC of Facial paralysis
- RC of Infection
- RC of Impaired hearing/deafness

Nursing Diagnoses

- Impaired Communication related to decreased hearing
- Risk for Loneliness related to embarrassment of not being able to hear in a social setting
- Risk for Injury related to vertigo
- Risk for Ineffective Self-Health Management related to insufficient knowledge of signs and symptoms of complications (facial nerve injury, vertigo, tinnitus, gait disturbances, and ear discharge), ear care, contraindications, and follow-up care

Nephrectomy

See also *Surgery (General)*.

Collaborative Problems

- ▲ RC of Hypovolemia/Shock
- ▲ RC of Paralytic ileus
- ▲ RC of Renal insufficiency
- Δ RC of Pyelonephritis
- Δ RC of Ureteral stent dislodgement
- Δ RC of Pneumothorax secondary to thoracic approach

Nursing Diagnoses

- Δ Impaired Physical Mobility related to distention of renal capsule and incision
- ▲ Risk for Ineffective Respiratory Function related to pain on breathing and coughing secondary to location of incision
- ▲ Risk for Ineffective Self-Health Management related to insufficient knowledge of hydration requirements, nephrostomy care, and signs and symptoms of complications

Renal Transplant

See also *Corticosteroid Therapy; Surgery (General)*.

Collaborative Problems

▲ RC of Hemodynamic instability
▲ RC of Hypervolemia/Hypovolemia
▲ RC of Hypertension/Hypotension
▲ RC of Renal insufficiency (donor kidney). Examples:
* Ischemic damage before implantation
* Hematoma
* Rupture of anastomosis
* Bleeding at anastomosis
* Renal vein thrombosis
* Renal artery stenosis
* Blockage of ureter (kinks, clots)
* Kinking of ureter, renal artery
▲ RC of Rejection of donor tissue
▲ RC of Excessive immunosuppression
▲ RC of Electrolyte imbalances (potassium, phosphate)
▲ RC of Deep vein thrombosis
▲ RC of Sepsis

Nursing Diagnoses

▲ Risk for Infection related to altered immune system secondary to medications
▲ Risk for Impaired Oral Mucous Membrane related to increased susceptibility to infection secondary to immunosuppression
△ Risk for Disturbed Self-Concept related to transplant experience and potential for rejection
▲ Fear related to possibility of rejection and death
▲ Risk for Noncompliance related to complexity of treatment regimen (diet, medications, record-keeping, weight, blood pressure, urine testing) and euphoria (post-transplant)
▲ Risk for Ineffective Self-Health Management related to insufficient knowledge of prevention of infection, activity progression, dietary management, daily recording (intake, output, weights, urine testing, blood pressure, temperature), pharmacologic therapy, daily urine testing (protein), signs and symptoms of rejection/infection, avoidance of pregnancy, follow-up care, and community resources

Thoracic Surgery

See also *Surgery (General)*; *Mechanical Ventilation*.

Postoperative Period

Collaborative Problems

* * RC of Atelectasis
* * RC of Pneumonia
* ▲ RC of Respiratory insufficiency
* ▲ RC of Pneumothorax, hemothorax
* Δ RC of Bleeding
* ▲ RC of Pulmonary embolism
* ▲ RC of Subcutaneous emphysema
* Δ RC of Mediastinal shift
* ▲ RC of Acute pulmonary edema
* Δ RC of Thrombophlebitis

Nursing Diagnoses

* ▲ Acute Pain related to surgical incision, chest tube sites, and immobility secondary to lengthy surgery
* ▲ Ineffective Airway Clearance related to increased secretions and diminished cough secondary to pain and fatigue
* • Activity Intolerance related to reduction in exercise capacity secondary to loss of alveolar ventilation
* ▲ Impaired Physical Mobility related to restricted arm and shoulder movement secondary to pain and muscle dissection and imposed position restrictions
* • Grieving related to loss of body part and its perceived effects on lifestyle
* * Risk for Ineffective Self-Health Management related to insufficient knowledge of condition, pain management, shoulder/arm exercises, incisional care, breathing exercises, splinting, prevention of infection, nutritional needs, rest versus activity, respiratory toilet, and follow-up care

Tonsillectomy

See also *Surgery (General)*.

Collaborative Problems

* • RC of Airway obstruction
* • RC of Aspiration
* • RC of Bleeding

Nursing Diagnoses

* • Risk for Deficient Fluid Volume related to decreased fluid intake secondary to pain on swallowing

- Risk for Imbalanced Nutrition: Less Than Body Requirements related to decreased intake secondary to pain on swallowing
- Risk for Ineffective Self-Health Management related to insufficient knowledge of rest requirements, nutritional needs, signs and symptoms of complications, pain management, positioning, and activity restrictions

Total Joint Replacement
(Hip, Knee, or Shoulder Replacement)

See also *Surgery (General)*.

Postoperative Period
Collaborative Problems

▲ RC of Fat emboli
* RC of Bleeding/Hematoma formation
▲ RC of Dislocation/Subluxation of joint
* RC of Stress fractures
▲ RC of Neurovascular compromise
* RC of Synovial herniation
▲ RC of Thromboemboli
▲ RC of Sepsis

Nursing Diagnoses

▲ Risk for Impaired Skin Integrity related to immobility and incision
* Activity Intolerance related to fatigue, pain, and impaired gait
* Impaired Home Maintenance related to postoperative flexion restrictions
▲ Risk for Constipation related to activity restriction
▲ Risk for Injury related to altered gait and assistive devices
Δ Risk for Ineffective Self-Health Management related to insufficient knowledge of activity restrictions, use of supportive devices, rehabilitative program, follow-up care, apparel restrictions, signs of complications, supportive services, and prevention of infection

Transurethral Resection
(Prostate [Benign Hypertrophy or Cancer], Bladder Tumor)

See also *Surgery (General)*.

Postoperative Period

Collaborative Problems

- RC of Oliguria/Anuria
- RC of Bleeding
- RC of Perforated bladder (intraoperative)
- RC of Hyponatremia
- RC of Sepsis
- RC of Occlusion of drainage devices
- RC of Prostatectomy
- RC of Clot formation

Nursing Diagnoses

- Acute Pain related to bladder spasms, clot retention, or back and leg pain
- Risk for Ineffective Self-Health Management related to insufficient knowledge of fluid requirements, activity restrictions, catheter care, urinary control, follow-up, and signs and symptoms of complications

Urostomy

See also *Surgery (General)*.

Postoperative Period

Collaborative Problems

- Δ RC of Internal urine leakage
- ▲ RC of Urinary tract infection
- ▲ RC of Peristomal ulceration/herniation
- ▲ RC of Stomal necrosis, retraction, prolapse, stenosis, obstruction

Nursing Diagnoses

- Δ Risk for Disturbed Self-Concept related to effects of ostomy on body image
  Risk for Ineffective Sexuality Patterns related to perceived negative impact of ostomy on sexual functioning and attractiveness
- * Risk for Ineffective Sexuality Patterns related to erectile dysfunction (male) or inadequate vaginal lubrication (female)
- Δ Risk for Loneliness related to anxiety about possible odor and leakage from appliance

▲ Risk for Ineffective Self-Health Management related to insufficient knowledge of stoma pouching procedure, colostomy irrigation, peristomal skin care, perineal wound care, incorporation of ostomy care into activities of daily living

Δ Risk for Ineffective Self-Health Management related to insufficient knowledge of intermittent self-catheterization of Kock continent urostomy

Radical Vulvectomy

See also *Surgery (General); Anticoagulant Therapy.*

Postoperative Period

Collaborative Problems

▲ RC of Hypovolemia/Shock
▲ RC of Urinary retention
▲ RC of Sepsis
Δ RC of Pulmonary embolism
▲ RC of Thrombophlebitis

Nursing Diagnoses

▲ Acute Pain related to effects of surgery and immobility
▲ Grieving related to loss of body function and its effects on lifestyle
Δ Risk for Ineffective Sexuality Patterns related to negative impact of surgery on sexual functioning and attractiveness
Δ Risk for Ineffective Self-Health Management related to insufficient knowledge of home care, wound care, self-catheterization, and follow-up care

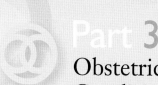

Part 3
Obstetric/Gynecologic Conditions

PRENATAL PERIOD (GENERAL)

Nursing Diagnoses

- Nausea related to elevated estrogen levels, decreased blood sugar, or decreased gastric motility and pressure on cardiac sphincter from enlarged uterus
- Constipation related to decreased gastric motility and pressure of uterus on lower colon
- Activity Intolerance related to fatigue and dyspnea secondary to pressure of enlarging uterus on diaphragm and increased blood volume
- Risk for Impaired Oral Mucous Membranes related to hyperemic gums secondary to estrogen and progesterone levels
- Risk for Injury related to syncope/hypotension secondary to peripheral venous pooling secondary to peripheral venous pooling
- Risk for Ineffective Self-Health Management related to insufficient knowledge of (examples) effects of pregnancy on body systems (cardiovascular, integumentary, gastrointestinal, urinary, pulmonary, musculoskeletal), psychosocial domain, sexuality/sexual function, family unit (spouse, children), fetal growth and development, nutritional requirements, hazards of smoking, excessive alcohol intake, drug abuse, excessive caffeine intake, excessive weight gain, signs and symptoms of complications (vaginal bleeding, cramping, gestational diabetes, excessive edema, preeclampsia), preparation for childbirth (classes, printed references)

Abortion, Induced

Preprocedure Period

Nursing Diagnosis

- Anxiety related to significance of decision, procedure, and post procedure care

Postprocedure Period

Collaborative Problems

- RC of Bleeding
- RC of Infection

Nursing Diagnoses

- Risk for Ineffective Coping related to unresolved emotional responses (guilt) to societal, moral, religious, and familial opposition
- Risk for Interrupted Family Processes related to effects of procedure on relationships (disagreement about decisions, previous conflicts [personal, marital], or adolescent identity problems)
- Risk for Ineffective Self-Care Management related to insufficient knowledge of self-care (hygiene, breast care), nutritional needs, expected bleeding, cramping, signs and symptoms of complications, resumption of sexual activity, contraception, sex education as indicated, comfort measures, expected emotional responses, follow-up appointment, and community resources

Extrauterine Pregnancy
(Ectopic Pregnancy)

Collaborative Problems

- RC of Bleeding
- RC of Shock
- RC of Sepsis
- RC of Acute pain

Nursing Diagnoses

- Grieving related to loss of fetus
- Fear related to possibility of not being able to have successful pregnancies

Hyperemesis Gravidarum

Collaborative Problems

- RC of Negative nitrogen balance

Nursing Diagnoses

- Risk for Imbalanced Nutrition: Less Than Body Requirements related to loss of nutrients and fluid secondary to vomiting
- Risk for Deficient Fluid Volume related to prolonged vomiting
- Self-Health Management related to insufficient knowledge of condition, signs and symptoms to monitor for, home management strategies and when to access medical care.

Gestational Hypertension

See also *Prenatal Period; Postpartum Period; RC of Nonassuring Fetal Status.*

Collaborative Problems

- RC of Malignant hypertension
- RC of Seizures
- RC of Proteinuria
- RC of Visual disturbances
- RC of Coma
- RC of Renal failure
- RC of Cerebral edema
- RC of Fetal compromise

Nursing Diagnoses

- Fear related to the effects of condition on self, pregnancy, and infant
- Risk for Injury related to vertigo, visual disturbances, or seizures
- Risk for Ineffective Self-Health Management related to insufficient knowledge of dietary restrictions, signs and symptoms of complications, conservation of energy, pharmacologic therapy, comfort measures for headaches and backaches and when to access medical care

Pregnant Adolescent

See also *General Prenatal, Intrapartum Period,* and *Postpartum Period.*

Prenatal

Collaborative Problem

- RC of Gestational hypertension

Nursing Diagnoses

- Interrupted Family Processes related to stressors associated with adolescent pregnancy and future implications for family
- Risk for Imbalanced Nutrition: Less Than Body Requirements related to maternal growth needs and lower nutritional stores secondary to adolescence
- Disturbed Self-Concept related to pregnancy-associated body changes and conflict with adolescent and parenting roles
- Risk for Loneliness related to negative response of peer group to pregnancy
- Risk for Infection related to insufficient knowledge of prevention of urinary tract infection and increased vulnerability secondary to effects of pregnancy on renal and ureteral anatomy

Postpartum

Nursing Diagnoses

- Risk for Impaired Parenting related to conflicting developmental tasks of adolescence and parenthood
- Decisional Conflict related to caregiver of infant, adoption options, or living arrangements

Uterine Bleeding During Pregnancy
(Placenta Previa, Abruptio Placentae, Uterine Rupture, Nonmalignant Lesions, Hydatidiform Mole)

See also *Postpartum Period.*

Collaborative Problems

- RC of Hypovolemia/Shock
- RC of Disseminated intravascular coagulation
- RC of Renal failure
- RC of Nonassuring fetal status
- RC of Sepsis

Nursing Diagnoses

- Fear related to effects of bleeding on pregnancy and infant
- Impaired Physical Mobility related to increased bleeding in response to activity
- Grieving related to anticipated possible loss of pregnancy and loss of expected child
- Fear related to possibility of subsequent future complications of pregnancy

INTRAPARTUM PERIOD (GENERAL)

Collaborative Problems

- RC of Hemorrhage (placenta previa, abruptio placentae)
- RC of Nonassuring fetal status
- RC of Hypertension
- RC of Uterine rupture

Nursing Diagnoses

- Acute Pain related to uterine contractions during labor
- Fear related to unpredictability of uterine contractions and possibility of having an impaired baby
- Anxiety related to insufficient knowledge of relaxation/breathing exercises, positioning and procedures (preparations [bowel, skin], frequent assessments, anesthesia [regional, inhalation])

POSTPARTUM PERIOD

General Postpartum Period

Collaborative Problems

- RC of Hemorrhage
- RC of Uterine atony
- RC of Retained placental fragments
- RC of Lacerations
- RC of Hematomas
- RC of Urinary retention

Nursing Diagnoses

- Risk for Infection related to bacterial invasion secondary to trauma during labor, delivery, and episiotomy
- Risk for Ineffective Breastfeeding related to inexperience or pain secondary to engorged breasts
- Acute Pain related to trauma to perineum during labor and delivery, hemorrhoids, engorged breasts, and involution of uterus
- Risk for Constipation related to decreased intestinal peristalsis (post delivery) and decreased activity
- Risk for Impaired Parenting related to (examples) inexperience, feelings of incompetence, powerlessness, unwanted child, disappointment with child, or lack of role models
- Stress Incontinence related to tissue trauma during delivery
- Risk for Situational Low Self-Esteem related to changes that persist after delivery (skin, weight, lifestyle)
- Risk for Ineffective Self-Health Management related to insufficient knowledge of postpartum routines, hygiene (breast, perineum), exercises, sexual counseling (contraception), nutritional requirements (infant, maternal), infant care, stresses of parenthood, adaptation of father, sibling, parent–infant bonding, postpartum emotional responses, sleep/rest requirements, household management, community resources, management of discomforts (breast, perineum), and signs and symptoms of complications

MISCARRIAGE, SPONTANEOUS

Nursing Diagnoses

- Fear related to possibility of subsequent miscarriages
- Grieving related to loss of pregnancy

MASTITIS (LACTATIONAL)

Collaborative Problem

• RC of Abscess

Nursing Diagnoses

• Acute Pain related to inflammation of breast tissue
• Risk for Ineffective Breastfeeding related to interruption secondary to inflammation
• Risk for Ineffective Self-Health Management related to insufficient knowledge of need for breast support, breast hygiene, breastfeeding restrictions, and signs and symptoms of abscess formation

FETAL/NEWBORN DEATH

Nursing Diagnoses

• Interrupted Family Processes related to emotional trauma of loss on each family member
• Grieving related to loss of infant
• Fear related to the possibility of future fetal deaths

CONCOMITANT MEDICAL CONDITIONS (CARDIAC DISEASE [PRENATAL, POSTPARTUM], DIABETES [PRENATAL, POSTPARTUM])

Cardiac Disease

See also *Cardiac Disorders; Prenatal Period; Postpartum Period.*

Collaborative Problems

• RC of Congestive heart failure
• RC of Gestational hypertension (preeclampsia, eclampsia)
• RC of Nonassuring fetal status

Nursing Diagnoses

• Fear related to effects of condition on self, pregnancy, and infant
• Activity Intolerance related to increased metabolic requirements (pregnancy) in presence of compromised cardiac function
• Impaired Home Maintenance related to impaired ability to perform role responsibilities during and after pregnancy

- Risk for Interrupted Family Processes related to disruption of activity restrictions and fears of effects on lifestyle
- Risk for Ineffective Self-Health Management related to insufficient knowledge of dietary requirements, prevention of infection, conservation of energy, signs and symptoms of complications, and community resources

DIABETES (PRENATAL)

See also *Prenatal Period; Diabetes Mellitus; Postpartum Period.*

Collaborative Problems

- RC of Hypoglycemia/Hyperglycemia
- RC of Hydramnios
- RC of Acidosis
- RC of Gestational hypertension

Nursing Diagnoses

- Risk for Impaired Skin Integrity related to excessive skin stretching secondary to hydramnios
- Risk for Infection related to susceptibility to monilial infection
- Acute Pain related to cerebral edema or hyperirritability
- Risk for Ineffective Self-Health Management related to insufficient knowledge of effects of pregnancy on diabetes, effects of diabetes on pregnancy, nutritional requirements, insulin requirements, signs and symptoms of complications, and need for frequent blood/urine samples

DIABETES (POSTPARTUM)

See also *Postpartum Period (General).*

Collaborative Problems

- RC of Hypoglycemia
- RC of Hyperglycemia
- RC of Hemorrhage (secondary to uterine atony from excessive amniotic fluid)
- RC of Gestational hypertension

Nursing Diagnoses

- Anxiety related to separation from infant secondary to the special care needs of infant
- Risk for Infection of perineal area related to depleted host defenses and depressed leukocytic phagocytosis secondary to hyperglycemia

- Risk for Ineffective Self-Health Management related to insufficient knowledge of risks of future pregnancies, birth control methods, types contraindicated, and special care requirements for infant

ENDOMETRIOSIS

Collaborative Problems

- RC of Hypermenorrhea
- RC of Polymenorrhea

Nursing Diagnoses

- Chronic Pain related to response of displaced endometrial tissue (abdominal, peritoneal) to cyclic ovarian hormonal stimulation
- Ineffective Sexuality Patterns related to painful intercourse or infertility
- Anxiety related to unpredictable nature of disease
- Risk for Ineffective Self-Health Management related to insufficient knowledge of condition, myths, pharmacologic therapy, and potential for pregnancy

PELVIC INFLAMMATORY DISEASE

Collaborative Problems

- RC of Septicemia
- RC of Abscess formation
- RC of Pneumonia
- RC of Pulmonary embolism

Nursing Diagnoses

- Acute Pain related to malaise, increased temperature secondary to infectious process
- Risk for Deficient Fluid Volume related to inadequate intake, fatigue, pain, and fluid losses secondary to elevated temperature
- Chronic Pain related to inflammatory process
- Risk for Ineffective Coping: Depression related to chronicity of condition and lack of definitive diagnosis/treatment
- Risk for Ineffective Self-Health Management related to insufficient knowledge of condition, nutritional requirements, signs and symptoms of complications, prevention of sexually transmitted diseases, and sleep/rest requirements

Part 4

Neonatal Conditions

Neonate, Normal

Collaborative Problems

- RC of Hypothermia
- RC of Hypoglycemia
- RC of Hyperbilirubinemia
- RC of Bradycardia

Nursing Diagnoses

- Risk for Infection related to vulnerability of infant, lack of normal flora, environmental hazards, and open wound (umbilical cord, circumcision)
- Risk for Ineffective Airway Clearance related to oropharynx secretions
- Risk for Impaired Skin Integrity related to susceptibility to nosocomial infection and lack of normal skin flora
- Ineffective Thermoregulation related to newborn extrauterine transition
- Risk for Ineffective Infant's Health Management related to insufficient knowledge of (specify) (see *Postpartum Period*)

Neonate, Premature

See also *Family of High-Risk Neonate.*

Collaborative Problems

- RC of Cold stress
- RC of Apnea
- RC of Bradycardia
- RC of Hypoglycemia
- RC of Acidosis
- RC of Hypocalcemia
- RC of Sepsis

- RC of Seizures
- RC of Pneumonia
- RC of Hyperbilirubinemia

Nursing Diagnoses

- Risk for Constipation related to decreased intestinal motility and immobility
- Risk for Aspiration related to immobility and increased secretions
- Risk for Infection related to vulnerability of infant, lack of normal flora, environmental hazards, and open wounds (umbilical cord, circumcision)
- Risk for Impaired Skin Integrity related to susceptibility to nosocomial infection (lack of normal skin flora)
- Ineffective Thermoregulation related to newborn transition to extrauterine environment
- Ineffective Infant Feeding Pattern related to lethargy secondary to prematurity
- Risk for Sudden Infant Death Syndrome related to increased vulnerability secondary to prematurity

Neonate, Postmature, Small for Gestational Age (SGA), Large for Gestational Age (LGA)

Collaborative Problems

- RC of Asphyxia at birth
- RC of Meconium aspiration
- RC of Hypoglycemia
- RC of Polycythemia (SGA)
- RC of Edema (generalized, cerebral)
- RC of CNS depression
- RC of Renal tubular necrosis
- RC of Impaired intestinal absorption
- RC of Birth injuries (shoulder) (LGA)

Nursing Diagnoses

- Risk for Impaired Skin Integrity related to absence of protective vernix and prolonged exposure to amniotic fluid (LGA)
- Ineffective Infant Feeding Pattern related to lethargy
- Risk for Infection Transmission related to contagious nature of organism
- Risk for Injury related to uncontrolled tonic–clonic movements

Neonate with Meningomyelocele

See also *Normal Neonate; Family of High-Risk Neonate.*

Collaborative Problems

- RC of Hydrocephalus
- RC of Neurovascular insufficiency (below lesion)

Nursing Diagnoses

- Risk for Trauma related to vulnerability of meningomyelocele
- Overflow Incontinence related to effects of spinal cord injury on bladder function
- Risk for Impaired Skin Integrity related to inability to move lower extremities

Neonate with Congenital Heart Disease (Preoperative)

See also *Normal Neonate; Family of High-Risk Neonate.*

Collaborative Problems

- RC of Congestive heart failure
- RC of Dysrhythmias
- RC of Decreased cardiac output

Nursing Diagnoses

- Risk for Ineffective Infant Feeding Pattern related to difficulty breathing and fatigue

Neonate of a Mother With Diabetes

See also *Neonate, Normal; Family of High-Risk Neonate.*

Collaborative Problems

- RC of Hypoglycemia
- RC of Hypocalcemia
- RC of Polycythemia
- RC of Hyperbilirubinemia
- RC of Sepsis
- RC of Acidosis
- RC of Hyaline membrane disease
- RC of Respiratory distress syndrome
- RC of Venous thrombosis

Nursing Diagnoses

- Risk for Deficient Fluid Volume related to increased urinary excretion and osmotic diuresis

High-Risk Neonate

See also *Family of High-Risk Neonate*.

Collaborative Problems

- RC of Hypoxemia
- RC of Shock
- RC of Respiratory distress
- RC of Seizures
- RC of Hypotension
- RC of Septicemia

Nursing Diagnoses

- Disorganized Infant Behavior related to immature CNS and excess stimulation
- Risk for Infection related to vulnerability of infant, lack of normal flora, environmental hazards, open wounds (umbilical cord, circumcision), and invasive lines
- Ineffective Infant Feeding Pattern related to (specify)
- Risk for Ineffective Respiratory Function related to increased oropharyngeal secretions
- Risk for Impaired Skin Integrity related to susceptibility to nosocomial infection secondary to lack of normal skin flora
- Ineffective Thermoregulation related to newborn transition to extrauterine environment

Family of High-Risk Neonate

Nursing Diagnoses

- Chronic Sorrow related to realization of present or future loss for family and child
- Interrupted Family Processes related to effect of extended hospitalization on family (role responsibilities, finances)
- Anxiety related to unpredictable prognosis
- Risk for Impaired Parenting related to inadequate bonding secondary to parent–child separation or failure to accept impaired child

Hyperbilirubinemia
(Rh Incompatibility, ABO Incompatibility)

See also *Family of High-Risk Neonate; Neonate, Normal*.

Collaborative Problems

- RC of Anemia
- RC of Jaundice
- RC of Kernicterus
- RC of Hepatosplenomegaly
- RC of Hydrops fetalis (cardiac failure, hypoxia, anasarca, and pericardial, pleural, and peritoneal effusions)
- RC of Renal failure (phototherapy complications, hyperthermia/hypothermia, dehydration, priapism, "bronze baby" syndrome)

Nursing Diagnoses

- Risk for Impaired Corneal Tissue Integrity related to exposure to phototherapy light and continuous wearing of eye pads
- Risk for Impaired Skin Integrity related to diarrhea, urinary excretion of bilirubin, and exposure to phototherapy light

Neonate of Narcotic-Addicted Mother

See also *Family of High-Risk Neonate; Neonate, Normal; Substance Abuse by Mother.*

Collaborative Problems

- RC of Hyperirritability/Seizures
- RC of Withdrawal
- RC of Hypocalcemia
- RC of Hypoglycemia
- RC of Sepsis
- RC of Dehydration
- RC of Electrolyte imbalances

Nursing Diagnoses

- Risk for Impaired Skin Integrity related to generalized diaphoresis and marked rigidity
- Diarrhea related to increased peristalsis secondary to hyperirritability
- Disturbed Sleep Pattern related to hyperirritability
- Risk for Injury related to frantic sucking of fists
- Risk for Injury related to uncontrolled tremors or tonic–clonic movements
- Disturbed Sensory Perceptions related to hypersensitivity to environmental stimuli
- Ineffective Infant Feeding Pattern related to lethargy
- Risk for Sudden Infant Death Syndrome related to increased vulnerability secondary to maternal drug use

Respiratory Distress Syndrome

See also *High-Risk Neonate; Mechanical Ventilation.*

Collaborative Problems

- RC of Hypoxemia
- RC of Atelectasis
- RC of Acidosis
- RC of Sepsis
- RC of Hyperthermia

Nursing Diagnoses

- Activity Intolerance related to insufficient oxygenation of tissues secondary to impaired respirations
- Risk for Infection related to vulnerability of infant, lack of normal flora, environmental hazards (personnel, other newborns, parents), and open wounds (umbilical cord, circumcision)
- Risk for Impaired Skin Integrity related to susceptibility to nosocomial infection and lack of normal skin flora

Sepsis

See also *Neonate, Normal; Family of High-Risk Neonate; High-Risk Neonate.*

Collaborative Problems

- RC of Anemia
- RC of Respiratory distress
- RC of Hypothermia/Hyperthermia
- RC of Hypotension
- RC of Edema
- RC of Seizures
- RC of Hepatosplenomegaly
- RC of Hemorrhage
- RC of Jaundice
- RC of Meningitis
- RC of Pyarthrosis

Nursing Diagnoses

- Risk for Impaired Skin Integrity related to edema and immobility
- Diarrhea related to intestinal irritation secondary to infecting organism
- Risk for Injury related to uncontrolled tonic–clonic movements and hematopoietic insufficiency

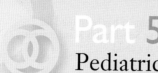

Part 5
Pediatric/Adolescent Disorders

Developmental Problems/Needs Related to Chronic Illness
(Permanent Disability, Multiple Handicaps, Developmental Disability [Mental/Physical], Life-Threatening Illness)

Nursing Diagnoses**

- Chronic Sorrow (parental) related to anticipated losses secondary to condition

Diabetes mellitus	Neoplastic disorders
Anorexia nervosa (psychiatric disorders)	Fractures
	Congestive heart failure
Spinal cord injury	Pneumonia
Head trauma	

- Interrupted Family Processes related to adjustment requirements for situation: (examples) time, energy (emotional, physical), financial, and physical care
- Risk for Impaired Home Maintenance related to inadequate resources, housing, or impaired caregiver(s)
- Risk for Parental Role Conflict related to separations secondary to frequent hospitalizations
- Risk for Loneliness (child/family) related to decreased socialization due to the disability and the requirements of the caregiver(s)
- Risk for Impaired Parenting related to abuse, rejection, overprotection secondary to inadequate resources or coping mechanisms
- Decisional Conflict related to illness, health care interventions, and parent–child separation
- (Specify) Self-Care Deficit related to illness limitations or hospitalization
- Risk for Delayed Growth and Development related to impaired ability to achieve developmental tasks
- Caregiver Role Strain related to multiple ongoing care needs secondary to restrictions imposed by disease, disability, or treatments

---

** For additional pediatric medical diagnoses, see the adult diagnoses and Developmental Problems/Needs.

- Ineffective Child's Health Management has been used for clinical usefulness since Ineffective Self-Health Management does not apply when the patient is a child

Anxiety/School Phobia

Nursing Diagnoses

- Anxiety related to altered self-esteem, change in environment, fear of separation, and negative responses (peers, family)
- Ineffective Coping related to inadequate problem-solving skills and denial of problem
- Disturbed Self-Esteem related to negative peer responses, perceived mental deficits, and unrealistic expectations in performance

Acquired Immunodeficiency Syndrome (Child)

See also *Acquired Immunodeficiency Syndrome (Adult)*; *Developmental Problems/Needs Related to Chronic Illness*.

Nursing Diagnoses

- Risk for Infection Transmission related to exposure to stool and other secretions during diaper changes or failure of child to follow handwashing procedure after toileting
- Imbalanced Nutrition: Less Than Body Requirements related to lactose intolerance, need for double the usual recommended daily allowance, anorexia secondary to oral lesions, and malaise
- Delayed Growth and Development related to decreased muscle tone secondary to encephalopathy
- Interrupted Family Processes related to the impact of the child's condition on role responsibilities, siblings, and finances and negative responses of relatives, friends, and community
- Risk for Ineffective Child's Health Management related to insufficient knowledge of modes of transmission, risks of live virus vaccines, avoidance of infections, school attendance, and community resources

Asthma

See also *Developmental Problems/Needs*.

Collaborative Problems

- RC of Hypoxemia
- RC of Corticosteroid therapy
- RC of Respiratory acidosis

Nursing Diagnoses

* Ineffective Airway Clearance related to bronchospasm and increased pulmonary secretions
* Fear related to breathlessness and recurrences
* Risk for Ineffective Child's Health Management related to insufficient knowledge of condition, environmental hazards (smoking, allergens, weather), prevention of infection, breathing/relaxation exercises, signs and symptoms of complications, pharmacologic therapy, fluid requirements, behavioral modification, and daily diary recording of peak flows

Attention Deficit Disorder

Collaborative Problems

* RC of Adverse effects of CNS stimulants

Nursing Diagnoses

* Activity Intolerance related to delayed physical, emotional, or mental capacity and fatigue
* Ineffective Coping related to fatigue and delayed development
* Delayed Growth and Development related to delayed maturation secondary to genetic, physical, and mental disability
* Risk for Injury related to motor deficits and hyperactivity
* Disturbed Self-Esteem related to lack of success in school and negative peer interactions
* Impaired Social Interaction related to delayed social development and poor peer acceptance

Celiac Disease

See also *Developmental Problems/Needs.*

Collaborative Problems

* RC of Severe malnutrition/dehydration
* RC of Anemia
* RC of Altered blood coagulation
* RC of Osteoporosis
* RC of Electrolyte imbalances
* RC of Metabolic acidosis
* RC of Shock
* RC of Delayed growth

Nursing Diagnoses

- Risk for Imbalanced Nutrition: Less Than Body Requirements related to malabsorption, dietary restrictions, and anorexia
- Diarrhea related to decreased absorption in small intestines secondary to damaged villi resulting from toxins from undigested gliadin
- Risk for Deficient Fluid Volume related to fluid loss in diarrhea
- Risk for Ineffective Child's Health Management related to insufficient knowledge of dietary management, restrictions, and requirements

Cerebral Palsy**

See also *Developmental Problems/Needs.*

Collaborative Problems

- RC of Contractures
- RC of Seizures
- RC of Respiratory infections

Nursing Diagnoses

- Risk for Injury related to inability to control movements
- Risk for Imbalanced Nutrition: Less Than Body Requirements related to sucking difficulties (infant) and dysphagia
- (Specify) Self-Care Deficit related to sensory–motor impairments
- Impaired Verbal Communication related to impaired ability to speak words related to facial muscle involvement
- Risk for Deficient Fluid Volume related to difficulty obtaining or swallowing liquids
- Risk for Deficient Diversional Activity related to effects of limitations on ability to participate in recreational activities
- Risk for Ineffective Child's Health Management related to insufficient knowledge of disease, pharmacologic regimen, activity program, education, community services, and orthopedic appliances

Child Abuse
(Battered Child Syndrome, Child Neglect)

See also *Fractures, Burns; Failure to Thrive.*

** Because disabilities associated with cerebral palsy can be varied (hemiparesis, quadriparesis, diplegia, monoplegia, triplegia, paraplegia), the nurse will have to specify clearly the child's limitations in the diagnostic statements.

Collaborative Problems

- RC of Failure to thrive
- RC of Malnutrition

Nursing Diagnoses

- Disabled Family Coping related to presence of factors that contribute to child abuse: (examples) lack of or unavailability of extended family, economic problems (inflation, unemployment); lack of role model as a child, high-risk children (unwanted, of undesired gender or appearance, physically or mentally handicapped, hyperactive, terminally ill); and high-risk parents (single, adolescent, emotionally disturbed, alcoholic, drug addicted, or physically ill)
- Ineffective Coping (child abuser) related to (examples) history of abuse by own parents and lack of warmth and affection from them, social isolation (few friends or outlets for tensions), marked lack of self-esteem with low tolerance for criticism, emotional immaturity and dependency, distrust of others, inability to admit need for help, high expectations for/of child (perceiving child as a source of emotional gratification), and unrealistic desire for child to give pleasure
- Ineffective Coping (nonabusing parent) related to passive and compliant response to abuse
- Fear related to possibility of placement in a shelter or foster home
- Parental Fear related to responses of others, possible loss of child, and criminal prosecution
- Risk for Imbalanced Nutrition: Less Than Body Requirements related to inadequate intake secondary to lack of knowledge or neglect
- Impaired Parenting related to insufficient knowledge of parenting skills (discipline, expectations), constructive stress management, signs and symptoms of abuse, high-risk groups, child protection laws, and community services

Cleft Lip and Palate

See also *Developmental Problems/Needs; Surgery (General)*.

Preoperative Period

Nursing Diagnoses

- Risk for Imbalanced Nutrition: Less Than Body Requirements related to impaired sucking secondary to cleft lip

Postoperative Period

Collaborative Problems

- RC of Respiratory distress
- RC of Failure to thrive (organic)

Nursing Diagnoses

- Impaired Physical Mobility related to restricted activity secondary to use of restraints
- Risk for Ineffective Infant Feeding Pattern related to impaired muscle development and impaired sucking.
- Risk for Ineffective Infant's Health Management related to insufficient knowledge of condition, feeding and suctioning techniques, surgical site care, risks for otitis media (dental/oral problems), and referral to speech therapist

Communicable Diseases

See also *Developmental Problems/Needs.*

Nursing Diagnoses

- Acute Pain related to pruritus, fatigue, malaise, sore throat, and elevated temperature
- Risk for Infection Transmission related to contagious agents
- Risk for Deficient Fluid Volume related to increased fluid loss secondary to elevated temperature or insufficient oral intake secondary to malaise
- Risk for Imbalanced Nutrition: Less Than Body Requirements related to anorexia and sore throat or pain on chewing (mumps)
- Risk for Ineffective Airway Clearance related to increased mucus production (whooping cough)
- Risk for Ineffective Child's Health Management related to insufficient knowledge of condition, transmission, prevention, immunizations, and skin care

Congenital Heart Disease

See also *Developmental Problems/Needs Related to Chronic Illness.*

Collaborative Problems

- RC of Congestive heart failure
- RC of Pneumonia
- RC of Hypoxemia
- RC of Cerebral thrombosis
- RC of Digoxin toxicity

Nursing Diagnoses

- Activity Intolerance related to insufficient oxygenation secondary to heart defects
- Risk for Imbalanced Nutrition: Less Than Body Requirements related to inadequate sucking, fatigue, and dyspnea
- Risk for Ineffective Child's Health Management related to insufficient knowledge of condition, prevention of infection, signs and symptoms of complications, digoxin therapy, nutrition requirements, and community services

Convulsive Disorders

See also *Developmental Problems/Needs; Mental Disabilities*, if indicated.

Collaborative Problems

- RC of Respiratory arrest

Nursing Diagnoses

- Risk for Injury related to uncontrolled movements of seizure activity
- Anxiety related to embarrassment and fear of seizure episodes
- Risk for Ineffective Coping related to restrictions, parental overprotection, and parental indulgence
- Risk for Ineffective Child's Health Management related to insufficient knowledge of condition/cause, pharmacologic therapy, treatment during seizures, and environmental hazards (water, driving, heights)

Craniocerebral Trauma

Collaborative Problems

- RC of Increased intracranial pressure
- RC of Hemorrhage
- RC of Tentorial herniation
- RC of Cranial nerve dysfunction

Nursing Diagnoses

- Acute Pain related to compression/displacement of cerebral tissue
- Risk for Injury related to uncontrolled tonic–clonic movements during seizure episode or somnolence
- Risk for Ineffective Child's Health Management related to insufficient knowledge of condition, signs and symptoms of complications, post-traumatic syndrome, activity restrictions, and follow-up care

Cystic Fibrosis

See also *Developmental Problems/Needs.*

Collaborative Problems

- RC of Bronchopneumonia, atelectasis
- RC of Paralytic ileus

Nursing Diagnoses

- Ineffective Airway Clearance related to mucopurulent secretions
- Risk for Imbalanced Nutrition: Less Than Body Requirements related to need for increased calories and protein secondary to impaired intestinal absorption, loss of fat and fat-soluble vitamins in stools
- Constipation/Diarrhea related to excessive or insufficient pancreatic enzyme replacement
- Activity Intolerance related to impaired oxygen transport secondary to mucopurulent secretions
- Risk for Ineffective Child's Health Management related to insufficient knowledge of condition (genetic transmission), risk of infection, pharmacologic therapy (side effects, ototoxicity, renal toxicity), equipment, nutritional therapy, salt replacement requirements, breathing exercises, postural drainage, exercise program, and community resources (Cystic Fibrosis Foundation)

Down Syndrome

See also *Developmental Problems/Needs; Mental Disabilities,* if indicated.

Nursing Diagnoses

- Risk for Ineffective Respiratory Function related to decreased respiratory expansion secondary to decreased muscle tone, inadequate mucus drainage, and mouth breathing
- Risk for Impaired Skin Integrity related to rough, dry skin surface and flaccid extremities
- Risk for Constipation related to decreased gastric motility
- Risk for Imbalanced Nutrition: More Than Body Requirements related to increased caloric consumption secondary to boredom in the presence of limited physical activity and decreased metabolic rate
- (Specify) Self-Care Deficit related to physical limitations
- Ineffective Infant Feeding Pattern related to neurologic impairment
- Risk for Ineffective Child's Health Management related to insufficient knowledge of condition, home care, education, and community services

Dysmenorrhea

Nursing Diagnosis

- Acute Pain related to insufficient knowledge of comfort measures, menstrual physiology, and nutritional management.

Failure to Thrive (Nonorganic)

See also *Developmental Problems/Needs*.

Collaborative Problems

- RC of Metabolic dysfunction
- RC of Dehydration

Nursing Diagnoses

- Imbalanced Nutrition: Less Than Body Requirements related to inadequate intake secondary to lack of emotional and sensory stimulation or lack of knowledge of caregiver
- Disturbed Sensory Perceptions related to history of insufficient sensory input from primary caregiver
- Insomnia related to anxiety and apprehension secondary to parental deprivation
- Impaired Parenting related to (examples) insufficient knowledge of parenting skills, impaired caregiver, impaired child, lack of support system, lack of role model, relationship problems, unrealistic expectations for child, unmet psychological needs
- Impaired Home Maintenance related to difficulty of caregiver with maintaining a safe home environment
- Risk for Ineffective Infant's Health Management related to insufficient knowledge of growth and development requirements, feeding guidelines, risk for child abuse, parenting skills, and community agencies

Glomerular Disorders
(Glomerulonephritis: Acute, Chronic; Nephrotic Syndrome: Congenital, Secondary, Idiopathic)

See also *Developmental Problems/Needs; Corticosteroid Therapy*.

Collaborative Problems

- RC of Anasarca (generalized edema)
- RC of Hypertension
- RC of Azotemia
- RC of Sepsis

818 SECTION 3 • Diagnostic Clusters

- RC of Malnutrition
- RC of Ascites
- RC of Pleural effusion
- RC of Hypoalbuminemia

Nursing Diagnoses

- Risk for Infection related to increased susceptibility during edematous phase and lowered resistance secondary to corticosteroid therapy
- Risk for Impaired Skin Integrity related to (examples) immobility, lowered resistance, edema, or frequent application of collection bags
- Imbalanced Nutrition: Less Than Body Requirements related to dietary restrictions, anorexia secondary to fatigue, malaise, and pressure on abdominal structures (edema)
- Fatigue related to circulatory toxins, fluid and electrolyte imbalances
- Deficient Diversional Activity related to hospitalization and impaired ability to perform usual activities
- Risk for Ineffective Child's Health Management related to insufficient knowledge of condition, etiology, course, treatments, signs and symptoms of complications, pharmacologic therapy, nutritional/fluid requirements, prevention of infection, home care, follow-up care, and community services

Hemophilia

See also *Developmental Problems/Needs.*

Collaborative Problem

- RC of Hemorrhage

Nursing Diagnoses

- Acute/Chronic Pain related to joint swelling and limitations secondary to hemarthrosis
- Risk for Impaired Physical Mobility related to joint swelling and limitations secondary to hemarthrosis
- Risk for Impaired Oral Mucous Membranes related to trauma from coarse food and insufficient dental hygiene
- Risk for Ineffective Child's Health Management related to insufficient knowledge of condition, contraindications (e.g., aspirin), genetic transmission, environmental hazards, and emergency treatment to control bleeding

Hydrocephalus

See also *Developmental Problems/Needs Related to Chronic Illness.*

Collaborative Problems

- RC of Increased intracranial pressure
- RC of Sepsis (post shunt procedure)

Nursing Diagnoses

- Risk for Impaired Skin Integrity related to impaired ability to move head secondary to size
- Risk for Injury related to inability to support large head and strain on neck
- Risk for Imbalanced Nutrition: Less Than Body Requirements related to vomiting secondary to cerebral compression and irritability
- Risk for Ineffective Child's Health Management related to insufficient knowledge of condition, home care, signs and symptoms of infection, increased intracranial pressure, and emergency treatment of shunt

Infectious Mononucleosis
(Adolescent)

Collaborative Problems

- RC of Splenetic dysfunction, enlargement
- RC of Hepatic dysfunction

Nursing Diagnoses

- Activity Intolerance related to fatigue secondary to infectious process
- Acute Pain related to sore throat, malaise, and headaches
- Risk for Imbalanced Nutrition: Less Than Body Requirements related to sore throat and malaise
- Risk for Infection Transmission related to contagious condition
- Risk for Ineffective Self-Health Management related to insufficient knowledge of condition, communicable nature, diet therapy, risks of alcohol ingestion (with hepatic dysfunction), signs and symptoms of complications (hepatic, splenic, neurologic, hematologic), and activity restrictions

Legg–Calvé–Perthes Disease

See also *Developmental Problems/Needs.*

Collaborative Problem

- RC of Permanently deformed femoral head

Nursing Diagnoses

- Acute/Chronic Pain related to joint dysfunction
- Risk for Impaired Skin Integrity related to immobilization devices (casts, braces)
- (Specify) Self-Care Deficit related to pain and immobilization devices
- Risk for Ineffective Self-Health Management related to insufficient knowledge of disease, weight-bearing restrictions, application/maintenance of devices, and pain management at home

Leukemia

See also *Chemotherapy; Radiation Therapy; Cancer (General); Developmental Problems/Needs.*

Collaborative Problems

- RC of Hepatosplenomegaly
- RC of Increased intracranial edema
- RC of Metastasis (brain, lungs, kidneys, gastrointestinal tract, spleen, liver)
- RC of Hypermetabolism
- RC of Hemorrhage
- RC of Dehydration
- RC of Myelosuppression
- RC of Lymphadenopathy
- RC of CNS involvement
- RC of Electrolyte imbalance

Nursing Diagnoses

- Risk for Infection related to increased susceptibility secondary to leukemic process and side effects of chemotherapy
- Risk for Loneliness related to effects of disease and treatments on appearance and embarrassment
- Risk for Injury related to bleeding tendencies secondary to leukemic process and side effects of chemotherapy
- Powerlessness related to inability to control situation
- Risk for Delayed Growth and Development related to impaired ability to achieve developmental tasks secondary to limitations of disease and treatments
- Risk for Ineffective Child's Health Management related to insufficient knowledge of disease process, treatment, signs and symptoms of complications, reduction of risk factors, and community resources

Meningitis (Bacterial)

See also *Developmental Problems/Needs*.

Collaborative Problems

- RC of Peripheral circulatory collapse
- RC of Disseminated intravascular coagulation
- RC of Increased intracranial pressure/hydrocephalus
- RC of Visual/Auditory nerve palsies
- RC of Paresis (hemiparesis, quadriparesis)
- RC of Subdural effusions
- RC of Respiratory distress
- RC of Seizures
- RC of Fluid/Electrolyte imbalances

Nursing Diagnoses

- Risk for Injury related to seizure activity secondary to infectious process
- Acute Pain related to nuchal rigidity, muscle aches, immobility, and increased sensitivity to external stimuli secondary to infectious process
- Impaired Physical Mobility related to intravenous infusion, nuchal rigidity, and restraining devices
- Risk for Impaired Skin Integrity related to immobility
- Risk for Ineffective Child's Health Management related to insufficient knowledge of condition, antibiotic therapy, and diagnostic procedures

Meningomyelocele

See also *Developmental Problems/Needs*.

Collaborative Problems

- RC of Hydrocephalus/Shunt infections
- RC of Increased intracranial pressure
- RC of Urinary tract infections

Nursing Diagnoses

- Reflex Incontinence related to sensory–motor dysfunction
- Risk for Infection related to vulnerability of meningomyelocele sac
- Risk for Impaired Skin Integrity related to sensory–motor impairments and orthopedic appliances
- (Specify) Self-Care Deficit related to sensory–motor impairments
- Impaired Physical Mobility related to lower limb impairments

- Parental Grieving related to birth of infant with defects
- Risk for Ineffective Child's Health Management related to insufficient knowledge of condition, home care, orthopedic appliances, self-catheterization, activity program, and community services

Mental Disabilities

See also *Developmental Problems/Needs.*

Nursing Diagnoses

- (Specify) Self-Care Deficit related to sensory–motor deficits
- Impaired Communication related to impaired receptive skills or impaired expressive skills
- Risk for Loneliness (family, child) related to fear and embarrassment of child's behavior/appearance
- Risk for Ineffective Child's Health Management related to insufficient knowledge of condition, child's potential, home care, and community services

Muscular Dystrophy

See also *Developmental Problems/Needs.*

Collaborative Problems

- RC of Seizures
- RC of Respiratory infections
- RC of Metabolic failure

Nursing Diagnoses

- Risk for Injury related to inability to control movements
- Risk for Imbalanced Nutrition: Less Than Body Requirements related to sucking difficulties (infant) and dysphagia
- Ineffective Infant Feeding Pattern related to muscle weakness and impaired coordination
- (Specify) Self-Care Deficit related to sensory–motor impairments
- Impaired Verbal Communication related to impaired ability to speak secondary to facial muscle involvement
- Risk for Impaired Physical Mobility related to muscle weakness
- Risk for Imbalanced Nutrition: More Than Body Requirements related to increased caloric consumption in presence of decreased metabolic needs secondary to limited physical activity
- Chronic Sorrow (parental) related to progressive, terminal nature of disease
- Impaired Swallowing related to sensory–motor deficits
- Risk for Hopelessness related to progressive nature of disease

- Risk for Deficient Diversional Activity related to effects of limitations on ability to participate in recreational activities
- Risk for Ineffective Child's Health Management related to insufficient knowledge of disease, pharmacologic regimen, activity program, education, and community services

Obesity

See also *Developmental Problems/Needs.*

Nursing Diagnoses

- Ineffective Coping related to increased food consumption in response to stressors
- Ineffective Self-Health Management related to the need for exercise program, nutrition counseling, and behavioral modification
- Disturbed Self-Concept related to feelings of self-degradation and response of others (peers, family, others) to obesity
- Interrupted Family Processes related to responses to and effects of weight loss therapy on parent–child relationship
- Risk for Impaired Social Interaction related to inability to initiate and maintain relationships secondary to feelings of embarrassment and negative responses of others
- Risk for Ineffective Self-Health Management related to insufficient knowledge of condition, etiology, course, risks, therapies available, destructive versus constructive eating patterns, and self-help groups

Osteomyelitis

See also *Developmental Problems/Needs.*

Collaborative Problems

- RC of Infective emboli
- RC of Side effects of antibiotic therapy (hematologic, renal, hepatic)

Nursing Diagnoses

- Acute Pain related to swelling, hyperthermia, and infectious process of bone
- Deficient Diversional Activity related to impaired mobility and long-term hospitalization
- Risk for Imbalanced Nutrition: Less Than Body Requirements related to anorexia secondary to infectious process
- Risk for Constipation related to immobility
- Risk for Impaired Skin Integrity related to mechanical irritation of cast/splint
- Risk for Injury: Pathologic Fractures related to disease process

- Risk for Ineffective Child's Health Management related to insufficient knowledge of condition, wound care, activity restrictions, signs and symptoms of complications, pharmacologic therapy, and follow-up care

Parasitic Disorders

See also *Developmental Problems/Needs*.

Nursing Diagnoses

- Risk for Imbalanced Nutrition: Less Than Body Requirements related to anorexia, nausea, vomiting, and deprivation of host nutrients by parasites
- Impaired Skin Integrity related to pruritus secondary to emergence of parasites (pinworms) onto perianal skin, lytic necrosis, and tissue digestion
- Diarrhea related to parasitic irritation to intestinal mucosa
- Acute Pain related to parasitic invasion of small intestines
- Risk for Infection Transmission related to contagious nature of parasites
- Risk for Ineffective Child's Health Management related to insufficient knowledge of condition, mode of transmission, and prevention of reinfection

Pediculosis

Nursing Diagnoses

- Risk for Infection related to lesions
- Impaired Comfort: Pruritus related to lesions
- Risk for Infection Transmission related to insufficient knowledge of modes of transmission, treatment, and prevention
- Risk for Ineffective Child's Health Management related to insufficient resources, low prioritization of problem, or repeated infections

Poisoning

See also *Dialysis*, if indicated; *Unconscious Individual*.

Collaborative Problems

- RC of Respiratory alkalosis
- RC of Metabolic acidosis
- RC of Hemorrhage

- RC of Fluid/Electrolyte imbalances
- RC of Burns (acid/alkaline)
- RC of Aspiration
- RC of Blindness

Nursing Diagnoses

- Acute Pain related to heat production secondary to poisoning (e.g., salicylate)
- Fear related to invasive nature of treatments (gastric lavage, dialysis)
- Anxiety (parental) related to uncertainty of situation and feelings of guilt
- Risk for Poisoning related to insufficient knowledge of home treatment of accidental poisoning, and poison prevention (storage, teaching, poisonous plants, locks)

Respiratory Tract Infection (Lower)

See also *Developmental Problems/Needs; Adult Pneumonia.*

Collaborative Problems

- RC of Hyperthermia
- RC of Respiratory insufficiency
- RC of Septic shock
- RC of Paralytic ileus

Nursing Diagnoses

- Acute Pain related to hyperthermia, malaise, and respiratory distress
- Risk for Imbalanced Nutrition: Less Than Body Requirements related to anorexia secondary to dyspnea and malaise
- Anxiety related to breathlessness and apprehension
- Risk for Deficient Fluid Volume related to insufficient intake secondary to dyspnea and malaise
- Risk for Ineffective Self-Health Management related to insufficient knowledge of condition, prevention of recurrence, and treatment

Rheumatic Fever

See also *Developmental Problems/Needs.*

Collaborative Problem

- RC of Endocarditis

Nursing Diagnoses

- Deficient Diversional Activity related to prescribed bed rest
- Imbalanced Nutrition: Less Than Body Requirements related to anorexia and malaise
- Acute Pain related to arthralgia
- Risk for Injury related to choreic movements
- Risk for Ineffective Child's Health Management related to insufficient knowledge of condition, signs and symptoms of complications, long-term antibiotic therapy, prevention of recurrence, and risk factors (e.g., surgery, dental)

Rheumatoid Arthritis
(Juvenile)

See also *Developmental Problems/Needs; Corticosteroid Therapy.*

Collaborative Problems

- RC of Pericarditis
- RC of Ocular Infections

Nursing Diagnoses

- Impaired Physical Mobility related to pain and restricted joint movement
- Acute Pain related to swollen, inflamed joints and restricted movement
- Fatigue related to chronic inflammatory process
- Risk for Ineffective Child's Health Management related to insufficient knowledge of condition, pharmacologic therapy, exercise program, rest versus activity, myths, and community resources

Reye's Syndrome

See also *Unconscious Individual*, if indicated.

Collaborative Problems

- RC of Renal failure
- RC of Increased intracranial pressure
- RC of Fluid/Electrolyte imbalances
- RC of Hepatic failure
- RC of Shock
- RC of Seizures
- RC of Coma
- RC of Respiratory distress
- RC of Diabetes insipidus

Nursing Diagnoses

- Parental Anxiety related to diagnosis and uncertain prognosis
- Risk for Injury related to uncontrolled tonic–clonic movements
- Risk for Infection related to invasive monitoring procedures
- Acute Pain related to hyperpyrexia and malaise secondary to disease process
- Fear related to separation from family, sensory bombardment (intensive care, treatments), and unfamiliar experiences
- Interrupted Family Processes related to critical nature of syndrome, hospitalization of child, and separation of family members
- Grieving related to actual, anticipated, or possible death of child
- Risk for Impaired Skin Integrity related to immobility
- Risk for Ineffective Child's Health Management related to insufficient knowledge of condition, treatment, and complications

Scoliosis

See also *Developmental Problems/Needs.*

Nursing Diagnoses

- Impaired Physical Mobility related to restricted movement secondary to braces
- Risk for Impaired Skin Integrity related to mechanical irritation of brace
- Risk for Noncompliance related to chronicity and complexity of treatment regimen
- Risk for Falls related to restricted range of motion
- Risk for Ineffective Child's Health Management related to insufficient knowledge of condition, treatment, exercises, environmental hazards, care of appliances, follow-up care, and community services

Sickle Cell Anemia

See also *Developmental Problems/Needs.*

Collaborative Problems

- RC of Sickling crisis of transfusion therapy
- RC of Thrombosis and infarction
- RC of Cholelithiasis

Nursing Diagnoses

- Ineffective Peripheral Tissue Perfusion related to viscous blood and occlusion of microcirculation
- Acute Pain related to viscous blood and tissue hypoxia

- (Specify) Self-Care Deficit related to pain and immobility of exacerbations
- Risk for Ineffective Child's Health Management related to insufficient knowledge of hazards, signs and symptoms of complications, fluid requirements, and hereditary factors

Tonsillitis

See also *Tonsillectomy*, if indicated.

Collaborative Problems

- RC of Otitis media
- RC of Rheumatic fever (β-hemolytic streptococci)

Nursing Diagnoses

- Risk for Deficient Fluid Volume related to inadequate fluid intake secondary to pain
- Risk for Ineffective Child's Health Management related to insufficient knowledge of condition, treatments, nutritional/fluid requirements, and signs and symptoms of complications

Wilms' Tumor

See also *Developmental Problems/Needs; Nephrectomy; Cancer (General)*.

Collaborative Problems

- RC of Metastases to liver, lung, bone, brain
- RC of Sepsis
- RC of Tumor rupture

Nursing Diagnoses

- Anxiety related to (examples) age-related concerns (separation, strangers, pain), response of others to visible signs (alopecia), and uncertain future
- Parental Anxiety related to (examples) unknown prognosis, painful procedures, treatments (chemotherapy), and feelings of inadequacy
- Grieving related to actual, anticipated, or possible death of child Spiritual Distress related to nature of disease and its possible disturbances in belief systems
- Risk for Ineffective Child's Health Management related to insufficient knowledge of condition, prognosis, treatments (side effects), home care, nutritional requirements, follow-up care, and community services

Part 6
Mental Health Disorders

Affective Disorders
(Depression)

Nursing Diagnoses

- Dressing/Grooming Self-Care Deficit related to decreased interest in body, inability to make decisions, and feelings of worthlessness
- Ineffective Coping related to internal conflicts (guilt, low self-esteem) or feelings of rejection
- Risk for Loneliness related to inability to initiate activities to reduce isolation secondary to low energy levels
- Complicated Grieving related to unresolved grief, prolonged denial, and repression
- Chronic Low Self-Esteem related to feelings of worthlessness and failure secondary to (specify)
- Compromised Family Coping related to marital discord and role conflicts secondary to effects of chronic depression
- Powerlessness related to unrealistic negative beliefs about self-worth or abilities
- Disturbed Thought Processes related to negative cognitive set (overgeneralizing, polarized thinking, selected abstraction, arbitrary inference)
- Ineffective Sexuality Patterns related to decreased sex drive, loss of interest and pleasure
- Deficient Diversional Activity related to a loss of interest or pleasure in usual activities and low energy levels
- Impaired Home Maintenance related to inability to make decisions or concentrate
- Risk for Self-Harm related to feelings of hopelessness and loneliness
- Insomnia related to difficulty falling asleep or early morning awakening secondary to emotional stress
- Constipation related to sedentary lifestyle, insufficient exercise, or inadequate diet

- Risk for Imbalanced Nutrition: More Than Body Requirements related to increased intake versus decreased activity expenditures secondary to boredom and frustration
- Risk for Imbalanced Nutrition: Less Than Body Requirements related to anorexia secondary to emotional stress
- Risk for Ineffective Self-Health Management related to insufficient knowledge of condition, behavior modification, therapy options (pharmacologic, electroshock), and community resources

Alcoholism

Collaborative Problems

- RC of Delirium tremens
- RC of Autonomic hyperactivity
- RC of Seizures
- RC of Alcoholic hallucinosis
- RC of Hypertension
- RC of Hypoglycemia

Nursing Diagnoses

- Imbalanced Nutrition: Less Than Body Requirements related to anorexia
- Risk for Deficient Fluid Volume related to abnormal fluid loss secondary to vomiting and diarrhea
- Risk for Injury related to disorientation, tremors, or impaired judgment
- Risk for Violence related to chemical withdrawal with impulsive behavior, disorientation, tremors, or impaired judgment
- Disturbed Sleep Pattern related to irritability, tremors, and nightmares
- Anxiety related to loss of control, memory losses, and fear of withdrawal
- Ineffective Coping related to inability to manage stressors constructively without drugs/alcohol
- Impaired Social Interaction related to alcoholic problematic behavior with emotional immaturity, irritability, high anxiety, impulsive behavior, or aggressive responses
- Ineffective Sexuality Patterns related to impotence/loss of libido secondary to altered self-concept and substance abuse
- Ineffective Family Coping related to disruption in marital dyad and inconsistent limit setting
- Disabled Family Coping related to the destructive effects of alcoholic family member on family functioning and each family member
- Risk for Ineffective Self-Health Management related to insufficient knowledge of condition, treatments available, high-risk situations, and community resources

Anorexia Nervosa

Collaborative Problems

- RC of Anemia
- RC of Hypotension
- RC of Dysrhythmias
- RC of Amenorrhea

Nursing Diagnoses

- Imbalanced Nutrition: Less Than Body Requirements related to exercise in excess of caloric intake, refusal to eat, self-induced vomiting following eating, or laxative abuse
- Disturbed Self-Concept related to inaccurate perception of self as obese
- Risk for Deficient Fluid Volume related to vomiting and excessive weight loss
- Activity Intolerance related to fatigue secondary to malnutrition
- Ineffective Coping related to self-induced vomiting, denial of hunger, and insufficient food intake secondary to feelings of loss of control and inaccurate perceptions of body states
- Compromised Family Coping related to marital discord and its effect on family members
- Constipation related to insufficient food and fluid intake
- Impaired Social Interaction related to inability to form relationships with others or fear of trusting relationships with others
- Fear related to implications of a maturing body and dissatisfaction with relationships with others

Anxiety and Adjustment Disorders
(Phobias, Anxiety States, Traumatic Stress Disorders, Adjustment Reactions)

See also *Substance Abuse Disorders*, if indicated.

Nursing Diagnoses

- Impaired Social Interaction related to effects of behavior and actions on forming and maintaining relationships
- Anxiety related to irrational thoughts or guilt
- Ineffective Coping related to inadequate psychological resources to adapt to a traumatic event
- Disturbed Sleep Pattern related to recurrent nightmares
- Ineffective Coping related to altered ability to manage stressors constructively secondary to (examples) physical illness, marital discord, business crisis, natural disasters, or developmental crisis

- Risk for Ineffective Self-Health Management related to insufficient knowledge of condition, pharmacologic therapy, and legal system regarding violence

Bipolar Disorder
(Mania)

Nursing Diagnoses

- Defensive Coping related to unrealistic expectations secondary to exaggerated sense of self-importance and abilities
- Impaired Social Interaction related to alienation from others secondary to overt hostility, overconfidence, or manipulation of others
- Risk for Other Directed Violence related to impaired reality testing, impaired judgment, or compromised ability to control behavior
- Disturbed Sleep Pattern related to hyperactivity
- Disturbed Thought Processes related to biochemical disturbances
- Risk for Deficient Fluid Volume related to altered sodium excretion secondary to lithium therapy
- Noncompliance related to feelings of no longer requiring medication
- Risk for Ineffective Self-Health Management related to insufficient knowledge of condition, pharmacologic therapy, and follow-up care

Childhood Behavioral Disorders
(Attention Deficit Disorders, Learning Disabilities)

Nursing Diagnoses

- Impaired Social Interaction related to inattention, impulsivity, or hyperactivity
- Chronic Sorrow (parental) related to anticipated losses secondary to condition
- Interrupted Family Processes related to adjustment requirements for situation: (examples) time, energy, money, physical care, and prognosis
- Risk for Other-Directed Violence related to history of aggressive acts and (specify)
- Risk for Impaired Home Maintenance related to inadequate resources, inadequate housing, or impaired caregivers
- Risk for Loneliness (child, family) related to disability and requirements for caregivers
- Risk for Impaired Parenting related to inadequate resources or inadequate coping mechanisms
- Disturbed Self-Concept related to effects of limitations on achievement of developmental tasks

Obsessive–Compulsive Disorder

Nursing Diagnoses

- (Specify) Self-Care Deficit related to ritualistic obsessions interfering with performance of activities of daily living
- Noncompliance related to poor concentration and poor impulse control secondary to obsessive thought patterns
- Risk for Loneliness related to fear of vulnerability associated with need for closeness and embarrassment about ritualistic behavior
- Anxiety related to the perceived threat of actual or anticipated events

Paranoid Disorders

Nursing Diagnoses

- Impaired Social Interaction related to feelings of mistrust and suspicion of others
- Ineffective Denial related to unrealistic expectations secondary to inability to accept own feelings and responsibility for actions
- Risk for Imbalanced Nutrition: Less Than Body Requirements related to reluctance to eat secondary to fear of poisoning
- Impaired Thought Processes related to unknown etiology (e.g., repressed fears, drug use, abuse)
- Risk for Loneliness related to fear and mistrust of situations and others

Personality Disorders

Examples: Schizoid, Histrionic, Antisocial, Passive-Aggressive, Borderline, Paranoid, Narcissistic, Schizotypal, Avoidant, Dependent, Compulsive

Nursing Diagnoses

- Ineffective Coping related to biochemical changes with faulty thinking secondary (specify mental disorder)
- Ineffective Coping related to biochemical changes with poor impulse control and low frustration level
- Impaired Social Interaction related to unrealistic expectations of relationships and impaired ability to maintain enduring attachments
- Ineffective Coping related to resistance (procrastination, stubbornness, intentional inefficiency) in responses to responsibilities (role, social)

Schizophrenic Disorders

Nursing Diagnoses

- Risk for Other-Directed Violence related to responding to delusional thoughts or hallucinations
- Risk for Self-Mutilation related to responding to delusional thoughts or hallucinations
- Impaired Verbal Communication related to incoherent/illogical speech pattern and side effects of medications
- Impaired Social Interaction related to biochemical disturbances with preoccupation with egocentric and illogical ideas and extreme suspiciousness
- Impaired Home Maintenance related to impaired judgment, inability to self-initiate activity, and loss of skills over long course of illness

Somatoform Disorders
(Somatization, Hypochondriasis, Conversion Reactions)

See also *Affective Disorders*, if indicated.

Nursing Diagnoses

- Impaired Social Interaction related to effects of multiple somatic complaints and complaining on relationships
- Ineffective Coping related to unrealistic fear of having a disease despite reassurance to contrary
- Risk for Disabled Family Coping related to chronicity of illness
- Noncompliance related to impaired judgments and thought disturbances
- Dressing Self-Care Deficit related to loss of skills and lack of interest in body and appearance
- Deficient Diversional Activity related to apathy, inability to initiate goal-directed activities, and loss of skills
- Disturbed Self-Concept related to feelings of worthlessness and lack of ego boundaries
- Risk for Ineffective Self-Health Management related to insufficient knowledge of condition, pharmacologic therapy, tardive dyskinesia, occupational skills, and follow-up care

Part 7
Diagnostic and Therapeutic Procedures

Angioplasty
(Percutaneous, Transluminal, Coronary, Peripheral)

Preprocedure Period

Nursing Diagnoses

• Anxiety/Fear (individual, family) related to health status, angioplasty procedure, routines, outcome, and possible need for cardiac surgery

Postprocedure Period

Collaborative Problems

▲ RC of Dysrhythmias
▲ RC of Acute coronary occlusion (clot, spasm, collapse)
▲ RC of Myocardial infarction
▲ RC of Arterial dissection or rupture
▲ RC of Hemorrhage/Hematoma at angioplasty site
* RC of Paresthesia distal to site
* RC of Arterial thrombosis
* RC of Embolization (peripheral)

Nursing Diagnoses

▲ Impaired Physical Mobility related to prescribed bed rest and restricted movement of involved extremity
▲ Risk for Ineffective Self-Health Management related to insufficient knowledge of care of insertion site, discharge activities, diet, medications, signs and symptoms of complications, exercises, and follow-up care

Anticoagulant Therapy

Collaborative Problem

▲ RC of Hemorrhage

Nursing Diagnoses

Δ Risk for Ineffective Self-Health Management related to insufficient knowledge of administration schedule, identification card/band, contraindications, dietary precautions and signs and symptoms of bleeding

Cardiac Catheterization

Postprocedure Period

Collaborative Problems

▲ RC of Systemic (allergic reaction)
▲ RC of Cardiac (dysrhythmias, myocardial infarction, pulmonary edema)
* RC of CVA
▲ RC of Circulatory (hematoma formation or hemorrhage at entry site, hypovolemia, thromboembolic phenomenon)

Nursing Diagnoses

* Impaired Comfort related to tissue trauma and prescribed postprocedure immobilization
Δ Risk for Ineffective Self-Health Management related to insufficient knowledge of site care, signs and symptoms of complications, and follow-up care

Casts

Collaborative Problems

▲ RC of Compartment syndrome
▲ RC of Infection/Sepsis

Nursing Diagnoses

* Risk for Injury related to hazards of crutch-walking and impaired mobility secondary to cast
▲ Risk for Impaired Skin Integrity related to pressure of cast on skin surface
▲ (Specify) Self-Care Deficit related to limitation of movement secondary to cast
* Risk for Ineffective Respiratory Function related to imposed immobility or restricted respiratory movement secondary to cast (body)
* Deficient Diversional Activity related to boredom and inability to perform usual recreational activities

▲ Risk for Ineffective Self-Health Management related to insufficient knowledge of cast care, signs and symptoms of complications, use of assistive devices, and hazards

Chemotherapy

See also *Cancer (General)*.

Collaborative Problems

* * RC of Necrosis/Phlebitis at intravenous site
* * RC of Thrombocytopenia
* * RC of Anemia
* * RC of Leukopenia
* Δ RC of Peripheral nerve toxicosis
* ▲ RC of Anaphylactic reaction
* Δ RC of CNS toxicity
* Δ RC of Congestive heart failure
* ▲ RC of Electrolyte imbalance
* ▲ RC of Extravasation of vesicant drugs
* Δ RC of Hemorrhagic cystitis
* ▲ RC of Myelosuppression
* ▲ RC of Renal insufficiency/calculi

Nursing Diagnoses

* * Risk for Deficient Fluid Volume related to gastrointestinal fluid losses secondary to vomiting
* * Risk for Infection related to altered immune system secondary to effects of cytotoxic agents or disease process
* * Risk for Interrupted Family Processes related to interruptions imposed by treatment and schedule on patterns of living
* * Risk for Ineffective Sexuality Patterns related to amenorrhea and sterility (temporary/permanent) secondary to effects of chemotherapy on testes/ovaries
* * Risk for Injury related to bleeding tendencies
* ▲ Anxiety related to prescribed chemotherapy, insufficient knowledge of chemotherapy, and self-care measures
* ▲ Fatigue related to effects of anemia, malnutrition, persistent vomiting, and sleep pattern disturbance
* Δ Risk for Constipation related to autonomic nerve dysfunction secondary to vinca alkaloid administration and inactivity
* ▲ Diarrhea related to intestinal cell damage, inflammation, and increased intestinal motility
* ▲ Acute Pain related to gastrointestinal cell damage, stimulation of vomiting center, fear, and anxiety

▲ Risk for Impaired Skin Integrity related to persistent diarrhea, malnutrition, prolonged sedation, and fatigue
▲ Imbalanced Nutrition: Less Than Body Requirements related to anorexia, taste changes, persistent nausea/vomiting, and increased metabolic rate
▲ Impaired Oral Mucous Membrane related to dryness and epithelial cell damage secondary to chemotherapy
Δ Disturbed Self-Concept related to change in lifestyle, role, alopecia, and weight loss or gain

Corticosteroid Therapy

Collaborative Problems

Δ RC of Peptic ulcer
* RC of Pseudotumor cerebri
▲ RC of Steroid-induced diabetes
Δ RC of Osteoporosis
Δ RC of Hypertension
Δ RC of Hypokalemia

Nursing Diagnoses

▲ Risk for Excess Fluid Volume related to sodium and water retention
▲ Risk for Infection related to immunosuppression secondary to corticosteroid therapy
Δ Risk for Imbalanced Nutrition: More Than Body Requirements related to increased appetite
Δ Risk for Disturbed Body Image related to appearance changes (e.g., abnormal fat distribution, increased production of androgens)
Δ Risk for Ineffective Self-Health Management related to insufficient knowledge of administration schedule, adverse reactions, signs and symptoms of complications, hazards of adrenal insufficiency, and potential causes of adrenal insufficiency

Electroconvulsive Therapy (ECT)

Postprocedure Period

Collaborative Problems

• RC of Hypertension
• RC of Dysrhythmias

Nursing Diagnoses

- Risk for Injury related to uncontrolled tonic–clonic movements and disorientation, confusion post-treatment
- Acute Pain related to headaches, muscle aches, nausea secondary to seizure activity and tissue trauma
- Risk for Aspiration related to post-ECT somnolence
- Anxiety related to memory losses and disorientation secondary to effects of ECT on cerebral function

Electronic Fetal Monitoring (Internal)

See also *Intrapartum Period (General)*.

Postinsertion

Collaborative Problems

- RC of Fetal scalp laceration
- RC of Perforated uterus

Nursing Diagnoses

- Impaired Physical Mobility related to restrictions secondary to monitor cords

Enteral Nutrition

Collaborative Problems

- ▲ RC of Hypoglycemia/Hyperglycemia
- ▲ RC of Hypervolemia
- Δ RC of Hypertonic dehydration
- ▲ RC of Electrolyte and trace mineral imbalances
- Δ RC of Mucosal erosion

Nursing Diagnoses

- ▲ Risk for Infection related to gastrostomy incision and enzymatic action of gastric juices on skin
- ▲ Impaired Comfort related to cramping, distention, nausea, vomiting related to type of formula, administration rate, temperature, or route
- ▲ Diarrhea related to adverse response to formula, rate, or temperature

▲ Risk for Aspiration related to position of tube and of individual
Δ Risk for Ineffective Self-Health Management related to insufficient knowledge of nutritional indications/requirements,
   home care, and signs and symptoms of complications

External Arteriovenous Shunting

Collaborative Problems

▲ RC of Thrombosis
▲ RC of Bleeding

Nursing Diagnoses

▲ Risk for Ineffective Self-Health Management related to insufficient knowledge of catheter care, precautions, emergency
   measures, prevention of infection, and activity limitations

Hemodialysis

See also *Chronic Kidney Failure.*

Collaborative Problems

* RC of Anaphylaxis/Allergies
▲ RC of Fluid imbalances
▲ RC of Electrolyte imbalance (potassium, sodium)
▲ RC of Dialysis disequilibrium syndrome
Δ RC of Transfusion reaction
▲ RC of Hemorrhage
* RC of Disruption of vascular access
Δ RC of Dialysate leakage
▲ RC of Clotting
* RC of Hemolysis
▲ RC of Hypertension/Hypotension
▲ RC of Dialysis disequilibrium syndrome
▲ RC of Air embolism
▲ RC of Sepsis
Δ RC of Pyrogen reaction

Nursing Diagnoses

* Risk for Injury to (vascular) access site related to vulnerability
* Risk for Infection related to direct access to bloodstream
   secondary to vascular access
▲ Powerlessness related to need for treatments to live despite
   effects on lifestyle

▲ Interrupted Family Processes related to the interruptions of role responsibilities caused by the treatment schedule

▲ Risk for Infection Transmission related to frequent contacts with blood and high risk for hepatitis B

* Risk for Ineffective Self-Health Management related to insufficient knowledge of rationale of treatment, care of site, precautions, emergency treatments (disconnected, bleeding, clotting), pretreatment instructions, and daily assessments (bruit, blood pressure, weight)

Hemodynamic Monitoring

See also *Medical Conditions* for the specific medical diagnosis.

Collaborative Problems

* RC of Sepsis
▲ RC of Hemorrhage
* RC of Bleeding
* RC of Vasospasm
* RC of Tissue ischemia/hypoxia
▲ RC of Thrombosis/Thrombophlebitis
▲ RC of Pulmonary embolism, air embolism
▲ RC of Arterial spasm

Nursing Diagnoses

▲ Risk for Infection related to invasive lines
Δ Impaired Physical Mobility related to position restrictions secondary to hemodynamic monitoring
Δ Anxiety related to impending procedure, loss of control, and unpredictable outcome
* Risk for Ineffective Self-Health Management related to insufficient knowledge of purpose, procedure, and associated care

Hickman Catheter

Collaborative Problems

• RC of Air embolism
• RC of Bleeding
• RC of Thrombosis

Nursing Diagnoses

• Risk for Infection related to direct access to bloodstream
• Risk for Impaired Home Maintenance related to lack of knowledge of catheter management

Long-Term Venous Catheter

Collaborative Problems

- △ RC of Pneumothorax
- ▲ RC of Hemorrhage
- △ RC of Embolism/Thrombosis
- ▲ RC of Sepsis

Nursing Diagnoses

- ▲ Anxiety related to upcoming insertion of catheter and insufficient knowledge of procedure
- ▲ Risk for Infection related to catheter's direct access to bloodstream
- △ Risk for Ineffective Self-Health Management related to insufficient knowledge of home care, signs and symptoms of complications, and community resources

Mechanical Ventilation

See also *Tracheostomy*.

Collaborative Problems

- * RC of Tracheal necrosis
- △ RC of Gastrointestinal bleeding
- * RC of Tension pneumothorax
- △ RC of Oxygen toxicity
- ▲ RC of Respiratory insufficiency
- ▲ RC of Atelectasis
- * RC of Ventilation acquired pneumonia (VAP)
- ▲ RC of Decreased cardiac output

Nursing Diagnoses

- ▲ Impaired Verbal Communication related to effects of intubation on ability to speak
- △ Disuse Syndrome
- ▲ Risk for Infection related to disruption of skin layer secondary to tracheostomy
- * Interrupted Family Processes related to critical nature of situation and uncertain prognosis
- △ Fear related to the nature of the situation, uncertain prognosis of ventilator dependence, or weaning
- * Risk for Disturbed Sensory Perceptions related to excessive environmental stimuli and decreased input of meaningful stimuli secondary to treatment and critical care unit

▲ Risk for Ineffective Airway Clearance related to increased secretions secondary to tracheostomy, obstruction of inner cannula, or displacement of tracheostomy tube

▲ Powerlessness related to dependency on respirator, inability to talk, and loss of mobility

▲ Risk for Dysfunctional Ventilatory Weaning Response related to unsatisfactory weaning attempts, respiratory muscle fatigue secondary to mechanical ventilation, increased work of breathing, supine position, protein–calorie malnutrition, inactivity, and/or fatigue

* Risk for Disturbed Self-Concept related to mechanical ventilation, dependence on achieving developmental tasks, and lifestyle changes

Pacemaker Insertion

Postprocedure Period

Collaborative Problems

▲ RC of Cardiac dysfunction
▲ RC of Pacemaker malfunction
Δ RC of Rejection of unit
Δ RC of Necrosis near pulse generator site
* RC of Hemorrhage (site, rupture of vessel)

Nursing Diagnoses

* Acute Pain related to insertion site and prescribed postprocedure immobilization

Δ Impaired Physical Mobility related to incisional site pain, activity restrictions, and fear of lead displacements

* Risk for Infection related to operative site

Δ Risk for Ineffective Self-Health Management related to insufficient knowledge of activity restrictions, precautions, signs and symptoms of complications, electromagnetic interference (microwave ovens, arc welding equipment, gasoline engines, electric motors, antitheft devices, power transmitters), pacemaker function (daily pulse taking, signs of impending battery failure), activity restrictions, and follow-up care

Peritoneal Dialysis

Collaborative Problems

* RC of Fluid imbalances
Δ RC of Electrolyte imbalances

Δ RC of Hemorrhage
* RC of Sepsis
▲ RC of Bowel/Bladder perforation
▲ RC of Hyperglycemia
* RC of Peritonitis
▲ RC of Inflow/Outflow problems
▲ RC of Uremia

Nursing Diagnoses

▲ Risk for Infection related to access to peritoneal cavity, catheter exit site, and use of high-dextrose concentration in dialysis solution
* Risk for Injury to catheter site related to vulnerability
Δ Risk for Ineffective Breathing Pattern related to immobility, pressure, and pain
Δ Impaired Comfort related to catheter insertion, instillation of dialysis solution, outflow, suction, and chemical irritation of peritoneum
Δ Imbalanced Nutrition: Less Than Body Requirements related to anorexia
* Risk for Excessive Fluid Volume related to fluid retention secondary to catheter problems (kinks, blockages) or position
Δ Risk for Interrupted Family Processes related to the effects of interruptions of the treatment schedule on role responsibilities
Δ Powerlessness related to chronic illness and the need for continuous treatment
* Impaired Home Maintenance related to insufficient knowledge of treatment procedure
Δ Risk for Ineffective Self-Health Management related to insufficient knowledge of rationale for treatment, medications, home dialysis procedure, signs and symptoms of complications, community resources, and follow-up care

Radiation Therapy
(External)

Postprocedure Period

Collaborative Problems

* RC of Cerebral edema, Increased intracranial pressure (site dependent)
Δ RC of Myelosuppression
* RC of Mucositis, esophagitis, pneumonitis
Δ RC of Fluid/Electrolyte imbalances
Δ RC of Inflammation

* RC of Pleural effusion (site specific)
* RC of Myelitis, parotitis

Nursing Diagnoses

▲ Anxiety related to prescribed radiation therapy and insufficient knowledge of treatments and self-care measures

Δ Acute Pain related to stimulation of the vomiting center and damage to the gastrointestinal mucosal cells secondary to radiation

▲ Fatigue related to systemic effects of radiation therapy

• Acute Pain related to damage to sebaceous and sweat glands secondary to radiation

Δ Risk for Impaired Oral Mucous Membrane related to dry mouth or inadequate oral hygiene

▲ Impaired Skin Integrity related to effects of radiation on epithelial and basal cells and effects of diarrhea on perineal area

▲ Imbalanced Nutrition: Less Than Body Requirements related to decreased oral intake, reduced salivation, mouth discomfort, dysphagia, nausea/vomiting, and increased metabolic rate

Δ Disturbed Self-Concept related to alopecia, skin changes, weight loss, sterility, and changes in role, relationships, and lifestyle

Δ Grieving related to changes in lifestyle, role, finances, functional capacity, body image, and health losses

Δ Interrupted Family Processes related to imposed changes in family roles, relationships, and responsibilities

* Diarrhea related to increased peristalsis secondary to irradiation of abdomen/lower back

* Risk for Infection related to moist skin reaction

* Activity Intolerance related to fatigue secondary to treatments or transportation

* Risk for Ineffective Self-Health Management related to insufficient knowledge of skin care and signs of complications

Total Parenteral Nutrition
(Hyperalimentation Therapy)

Collaborative Problems

▲ RC of Sepsis
▲ RC of Hyperglycemia
Δ RC of Air embolism
* RC of Sepsis
* RC of Perforation
Δ RC of Pneumothorax, hydrothorax, hemothorax

Nursing Diagnoses

Δ Risk for Infection related to catheter's direct access to bloodstream

* Risk for Impaired Skin Integrity related to continuous skin surface irritation secondary to catheter and adhesive

* Risk for Impaired Oral Mucous Membrane related to inability to ingest food/fluid

Δ Risk for Ineffective Self-Health Management related to insufficient knowledge of home care, signs and symptoms of complications, catheter care, and follow-up care (laboratory studies)

Tracheostomy

Postoperative Period

Collaborative Problems

▲ RC of Hypoxemia

▲ RC of Hemorrhage

▲ RC of Tracheal edema

Nursing Diagnoses

▲ Risk for Ineffective Airway Clearance related to increased secretions secondary to tracheostomy, obstruction of inner cannula, or displacement of tracheostomy tube

▲ Risk for Infection related to excessive pooling of secretions and bypassing of upper respiratory defenses

▲ Impaired Verbal Communication related to inability to produce speech secondary to tracheostomy

* Risk for Ineffective Sexuality Patterns related to change in appearance, fear of rejection

▲ Risk for Ineffective Self-Health Management related to insufficient knowledge of tracheostomy care, precautions, signs and symptoms of complications, emergency care, and follow-up care

Bibliography

Ackley, B. J., Ladwig, G. B., Swan, B. A., & Tucker, S. J. (2008). *Evidence-based nursing care guidelines: Medical-surgical interventions.* St. Louis: Mosby Elsevier.

Acute Pain Management Guideline Panel. (1992). *Acute pain management in infants, children, and adolescents: Operative and medical procedures.* Quick Reference Guide for Clinicians. AHCPR Pub. No. 92-0020. Rockville, MD: Agency for Health Care Policy and Research, Public Health Service, U.S. Department of Health and Human Services.

Addams, S., & Clough, J. A. (1998). Modalities for mobilization. In A. B. Mahler, S. Salmond, & T. Pellino (Eds.), *Orthopedic nursing.* Philadelphia: W. B. Saunders.

Agency for Health Care Policy and Research [AHCPR] Panel for the Prediction and Prevention of Pressure Ulcers in Adults. (1992, May). *Pressure ulcers in adults: Prediction and prevention.* Clinical Practice Guidelines Number 3, AHCPR, Bulletin No. 92–0047. Rockville, MD: Agency for Health Care Policy & Research, Public Health Services, U.S. Department of Health and Human Services.

Alfaro-LeFevre, R. (2010). *Applying nursing process: A tool for critical thinking* (7th ed.). Philadelphia: Lippincott Williams & Wilkins.

Algase, D. L. (1999). Wandering: A dementia-compromised behavior. *Journal of Gerontological Nursing, 25*(9), 10–16.

Allender, J. A., Rector, C., & Warner, K. (2010). *Community health nursing: Promoting and protecting the public* (7th ed.). Philadelphia: Lippincott.

American Academy of Pediatrics. (2000). Task force on infant sleep position and Sudden Infant Death Syndrome: Changing concepts of Sudden Infant Death Syndrome; implications for infants sleeping environment and sleep position. *Pediatrics, 105*(3), 650–656.

American Academy of Pediatrics (AAP) Committee on Fetus and Newborn, American Academy of Pediatrics Section on Surgery, Canadian Paediatric Society Fetus and Newborn Committee, Batton, D. G., Barrington, K. J., & Wallman, C. (2006). Prevention and management of pain in the neonate: An update. *Pediatrics, 118*(5), 2231–2241.

American Association of Critical Care Nurses (AACN) from AACN Ethics Work Group. (2004). *The 4 A's to rise above moral distress.* Aliso Viejo, CA: Author.

American Association of Retired Persons. (2009). AARP statement to the 53rd session of the United Nations Commission on the Status of Women. Retrieved from http://www.un.org/womenwatch/daw/csw/53sess.htm

American Nurse's Association. (2003). *Nursing's Social Policy statement* (2nd ed.). Silver Spring, MD: Author.

American Nurse's Association. (2010). Just culture. Retrieved from www.justculture.org/Downloads/ANA_Just_Culture.pdf

American Psychiatric Association. (2000). *Diagnostic and statistical manual of mental disorders* (4th ed., text revision). Washington, DC: Author.

American Psychiatric Association. (2004). *DSM IV-TR: Diagnostic and statistical manual of mental disorders* (5th ed., text revision). Washington, DC: Author.

Anderson, J. E. (2000). Co-sleeping: Can we ever put the issue to rest? *Contemporary Pediatrics, 17*(6), 98–102, 109–110, 113–114.

Anetzberger, G. J. (1987). *The etiology of elder abuse by adult offspring.* Springfield, IL: Charles C. Thomas.

Arizona baby steps to breastfeeding success. (2010). Retrieved from http://www.azdhs.gov/phs/bnp/gobreastmilk/BFAzBabySteps.htm

Askin, D., & Wilson, D. (2007). The high risk newborn and family. In M. J. Hockenberry & D. Wilson (Eds.), *Wong's nursing care of infants and children* (8th ed.). St. Louis: Mosby Elsevier.

Asthma and Allergy Foundation of America. (2011). Reducing allergens in the home: A room-by-room guide. Retrieved from msdh.ms.gov/msdhsite/_static/resources/2111.pdf

Ball, J., & Bindler, R. (2008). *Pediatric nursing: Caring for children* (4th ed.). Upper Saddle River, NJ: Pearson Prentice Hall.

Bamberger, J. D., Unick, J., Klein, P., Fraser, M., Chesney, M., & Katz, M. H. (2000). Helping the urban poor stay on antiretroviral HIV drug therapy. *American Journal of Public Health, 90*(5), 699–701.

Bandura, A. (1982). Self-efficacy mechanism in human agency. *American Psychology, 37*(3), 122–147.

Banks, J. B. (2002). Childhood discipline: Challenges for clinicians and parents. *American Family Physician, 66*(8), 1447–1452.

Barnhouse, A. (1987). Development of the nursing diagnosis of translocation syndrome with critical care patients. Unpublished master's thesis. Kent, OH: Kent State University.

Beckstrand, R. L., Callsiter, L. C., & Kirchhoff, K. T. (2006). Providing a "Good Death": Critical care nurse's suggestions for improving end-of-life care. *American Journal of Critical Care, 15*(1), 38–45.

Bengtsson-Tops, A., Saveman, B. I., & Tops, D. (2009). Staff experience and understanding of working with abused women suffering from mental illness. *Health and Social Care in the Community, 17*(5), 459–465. doi:10.1111/j.1365-2524.2009.00843.x

Bennett, C. (2003). Urgent urological management of the paraplegic/quadriplegic patient. *Urologic Nursing, 23*(6), 436–437.

Bennett, R. (2000). Acute gastrointestinal and associated conditions. In R. Barker, J. Burton, & P. Zieve (Eds.), *Principles of ambulatory medicine.* Baltimore: Williams & Wilkins.

Bergstrom, N., Allman, R., Alvarez, O., Bennett, M., Carlson, C., Frantz, R., . . . Yarkony, G. (1994). *Treatment of pressure ulcers.* Clinical practice guideline (No. 15). Rockville, MD: Agency for Health Care Policy and Research, AHCPR Publication No. 95-0652.

Bhardwaj, A., Mirski, M. A., & Ulatowski, J. A. (2004). *Handbook of neurocritical care.* Totowa, NJ: Humana Press.

Blackburn, S. (1993). Assessment and management of neuralgic dysfunction. In C. Kenner, A. Brueggemeyer, & L. Gunderson (Eds.), *Comprehensive neonatal nursing.* Philadelphia: W. B. Saunders.

Blackburn, S., & Vandenberg, K. (1993). Assessment and management of neonatal neurobehavioral development. In C. Kenner, A. Brueggemeyer, & L. Gunderson (Eds.), *Comprehensive neonatal nursing.* Philadelphia: W. B. Saunders.

Bodenheimer, T., MacGregor, K., & Shafiri, C. (2005). *Helping patients manage their chronic conditions.* California Healthcare Foundation. Retrieved from http://www.chcf.

org/topics/chronicdisease/index.cfm?itemID=111768

Botolfsen, P., Helbostad, J. L., Moe-Nilssen, R., & Wall, J. C. (2008). Reliability and concurrent validity of the Expanded Timed Up-and-Go test in older people with impaired mobility. *Physiotherapy Research International, 13*(2), 94–106.

Boyd, M. A. (2005). *Psychiatric nursing: Contemporary practice.* Philadelphia: Lippincott Williams & Wilkins.

Bozzette, M. (1993). Observations of pain behavior in the NICU: An exploratory study. *Journal of Perinatal and Neonatal Nursing, 7*(1), 76–87.

Breslin, E. H. (1992). Dyspnea-limited response in chronic obstructive pulmonary disease: Reduced unsupported arm activities. *Rehabilitation Nursing, 17*(1), 12–20.

Bridges, E. J., & Dukes, M. S. (2005). Cardiovascular aspects of septic shock: Pathophysiology, monitoring, and treatment. *Critical Care Nurse, 25*(2), 14–42.

Brothers, B. M., and Anderson, B. L. (2009) Hopelessness as a predictor of depressive symptoms for breast cancer patients coping with recurrence. *Psycho-Oncology, 18,* 267–275. DOI: 10.1002/pon.1394

Bulechek, G., Butcher, H., & Dochterman, J. M. (2008). *Nursing interventions classification (NIC)* (5th ed.). St. Louis: Mosby.

Burgess, A. W. (1995). Rape-trauma syndrome: A nursing diagnosis. *Occupational Health Nursing, 33*(8), 405–410.

Burke, M. L., Hainsworth, M. A., Eakes, G. G., & Lindgren, C. L. (1992). Current knowledge and research on chronic sorrow: A foundation for inquiry. *Death Studies, 16*(3), 231–245.

Burkhart, L., & Solari-Twadell, A. (2001). Spirituality and religiousness: Differentiating the diagnoses through a review of the nursing literature. *International Journal of Nursing Terminologies and Classifications, 12*(2), 44–54.

Burnside, I., & Haight, B. (1994). Reminiscence and life review: Therapeutic interventions for older people. *Nurse Practitioner, 19*(4), 55–60.

Camp-Sorrell, D. (2007). Chemotherapy: Toxicity management. In C. Yarbro, M. H. Frogge, M. Goodman, & S. Groenwald (Eds.), *Career nursing* (6th ed.). Boston: Jones and Bartlett.

Carpenito, L. J. (2013). *Nursing diagnosis: Application to clinical practice* (14th ed.). Philadelphia: Lippincott Williams & Wilkins.

Carpenito-Moyet, L. J. (2007). *Understanding the nursing process: Concept mappping and care planning for students.* Philadelphia: Lippincott Williams & Wilkins.

Carscadden, J. S. (1993). *On the cutting edge: A guide for working with people who self injure* (pp. 29–34). London, Ontario: London Psychiatric Hospital.

Carson, V. B. (1989). *Spiritual dimensions of nursing practice.* Philadelphia: W. B. Saunders.

Carson, V. B. (1999). *Mental health nursing: The nurse-patient journey* (2nd ed.). Philadelphia: W. B. Saunders.

Carson V. M., & Smith-DiJulio, K. (2006). Sexual assault. In E. Varcarolis, V. M. Carson, & N. C. Shoemaker (Eds.), *Foundations of psychiatric-mental health nursing* (5th ed.). Philadelphia: W. B. Saunders.

Cassells, J. M., & Redman, B. K. (1989). Preparing students to be moral agents in clinical nursing practice. *Nursing Clinics of North America, 24,* 463–473.

Centers for Disease Control and Prevention. (2000). Youth risk behavior surveillance. *Morbidity and Mortality Weekly Report, 49*(5), 1–94.

Centers for Disease Control and Prevention. (2003). Male batterers. Retrieved from www.cdc.gov/ncipc/factsheet/malebat.htm

Centers for Disease Control and Prevention. (2004). Retrieved from http://www.bt.cdc.gov/ncidod/dhap/gl_isolation_ptII.htm/

Centers for Disease Control and Prevention. (2008). HIV Transmission Rates in US. Retrieved February 25, 2009 from www.cdc.gov/hiv/topics/surveillance/resources/fact-sheets/transmission.htm

Chan, L. (1998). Effectiveness of a music therapy intervention on relaxation and anxiety for patients receiving ventilation assistance. *Heart and Lung, 27*(3), 169–176.

Christophersen, E. R. (1992). Discipline. *Pediatric Clinics of North America, 39*, 395–411.

Cohen-Mansfield, J. (1998). The effects of an enhanced environment on nursing home residents who pace. *Gerontologist, 38*(2), 199–208.

Cohen-Mansfield, J., & Werner, P. (1998). Determinants of the effectiveness of one to one social interactions for treating verbally disruptive behaviors. *Journal of Mental Health and Aging, 4*(3), 323–324.

Comfort, M., Sockloff, A., Loverro, J., & Kaltenbach, K. (2003). Multiple predictors of substance-abusing women's treatments and life outcomes: A prospective longitudinal study. *Addictive Behaviors, 28*(2), 199–224.

Cooley, M. E., Yeomans, A. C., & Cobb, S. C. (1986). Sexual and reproductive issues for women with Hodgkin's disease. II. Application of PLISSIT model. *Cancer Nursing, 9*, 248–255.

Cowen, P. S. (1999). Child neglect: Injuries of omission. *Pediatric Nursing, 25*(4), 401–418.

Cutcliffe, J. R. (2004). The inspiration of hope in bereavement counseling. *Issues in Mental Health Nursing, 25*(2), 165–190.

Davis, A. J. (1989). Clinical nurses' ethical decision making in situations of informed consent. *Advanced Nursing Science, 11*(3), 63–69.

DeFabio, D. C. (2000). Fluid and nutrient maintenance before,

during, and after exercise. *Journal of Sports Chiropractic and Rehabilitation, 14*(2), 21–24, 42–43.

DeJong, N. W., Patiwael, J. A., de Groot, H., Burdorf, A., & Gerth van Wijk, R. (2011). Natural rubber latex allergy among healthcare workers: Significant reduction of sensitization and clinical relevant latex allergy after introduction of powder-free latex gloves. *Journal of Allergy and Clinical Immunology, 127*(2), AB70.

Deloian, B. J., & Berry, A. (2009). Developmental management in pediatric primary care. In C. E. Burns, A. M. Dunn, M. A. Brady, N. B. Starr, & C. G. Blosser (Eds.), *Pediatric Primary Care* (pp. 53–70). St. Louis: Saunders Elsevier.

Denison, B. (2004). Touch the pain away. *Holistic Nursing Practice, 18*(3), 142–151.

Dennis, H. (1984). Remotivation therapy groups. In I. M. Burnside (Ed.), *Working with the elderly group: Process and techniques* (2nd ed.). Monterey, CA: Jones & Bartlett.

Dennis, K. (2004). Weight management in women. *Nursing Clinics of North America, 39*(14), 231–241.

Dougherty, M. (1998). Current status of research on pelvic muscles strengthening techniques. *Journal of Wound, Ostomy, and Continence, 25*(3), 75–83.

Dudek, S. (2009). *Nutrition essentials for nursing practice* (6th ed.). Philadelphia: Lippincott Williams & Wilkins.

Dunst, C. J., Trivette, C. M., Davis, M., & Cornwell, J. (1988). Enabling and empowering families of children with health impairments. *Children's Health Care, 17*, 71–81.

Dunwoody, C., Krenziscbek, D., Pasero, C., Rathmell, J., & Polomano, R. (2008). Assessment, physiological monitoring, and consequences of inadequately treated pain. *Pain Management Nursing, 9*(1), S11–S21.

Dzurec, L. C. (2000). Fatigue and relatedness experiences

of inordinately tired women: Fourth quarter. *Journal of Nursing Scholarship*, *32*(4), 339–345.

Eakes, G. (1995). Chronic sorrow: The lived experience of parents of chronically mentally ill individuals. *Archives of Psychiatric Nursing*, *9*(2), 77–84.

Eckert, R. M. (2001). Understanding anticipatory nausea. *Continuing Education*, *28*(10), 1553–1560.

Edelman, C. H., & Mandle, C. (2010). *Health promotion throughout the life span* (7th ed.). St. Louis: Mosby–Year Book.

Edgerly, E. S., & Donovick, P. J. (1998). Neuropsychological correlates of wandering in persons with Alzheimer's disease. *American Journal of Alzheimer's Disease*, *13*(6), 317–329.

Emick-Herring, B., & Wood, P. (1990). A team approach to neurologically based swallowing disorders. *Rehabilitation Nursing*, *15*, 126–132.

Essen, J., & Blegen, M. (1991). Social isolation. In M. Maas, K. Backwater, & N. Hardy (Eds.), *Nursing diagnoses and interventions for the elderly*. Redwood City, CA: Addison-Wesley Nursing.

Evans, L. K., Strumpf, N. E., & Williams, C. C. (1992). Limiting use of physical restraints: A prerequisite for independent functioning. In E. Calkins, A. Ford, & P. Katz (Eds.), *The practice of geriatrics* (2nd ed.). Philadelphia: W. B. Saunders.

Farrell, S., Harmon, R., & Hastings, S. (1998). Nursing management of acute psychotic episodes. *Nursing Clinics of North America*, *33*(1), 187–200.

Feinstein, N., Torgerson, K. L., & Atterbury, J. (Eds.). (2003). *Fetal heart monitoring principles and practices* (3rd ed.). Dubuque, IA: Kendall-Hunt.

Fetterman, L. G., & Lemburg, L. (2004). A silent killer—Often preventable. *American Journal of Critical Care*, *13*(5), 431–436.

Field, T., Peck, M., Hernandez Reif, M., Krugman, S., Burman, I., &

Ozment-Schenck, L. (2000). Postburn itching, pain, and psychological symptoms are reduced with massage therapy. *Journal of Burn Care Rehabilitation*, *21*(3), 189–193.

Finkelman, A. W. (2000). Self-management for psychiatric patient at home. *Home Care Provider*, *5*(6), 95–101.

Flandermyer, A. A. (1993). The drug exposed neonate. In C. Kenner, A. Brueggemeyer, & L. Gunderson (Eds.), *Comprehensive neonatal nursing*. Philadelphia: W. B. Saunders.

Fleitas, J. (2000). When Jack fell down. . . . Jill came tumbling after. Siblings in the web of illness and disability. *MCN: American Journal of Maternal-Child Nursing*, *25*(5), 267–273.

Fuhrman, M. P. (1999). Diarrhea and tube feeding. *Nutritional Clinical Practice*, *14*(2), 83–84.

Fulmer, T., & Paveza, G. (1998). Neglect in the elderly. *Nursing Clinics of North America*, *33*(3), 457–466.

Gage, J., Everett, K., & Bullock, L. (2006). Integrative review of parenting in nursing research. *Journal of Nursing Scholarship*, *38*(1), 56–62.

Gallup Poll. (2009). Honesty and ethics poll finds congress' image tarnished. Retrieved from www.gallup/poll124625/honesty-ethics-poll

Gardner, D. L., & Campbell, B. (1991). Assessing postpartum fatigue. *Maternal-Child Nursing Journal*, *16*(5), 264–266.

Geisman, L. K. (1989). Advances in weaning from mechanical ventilation. *Critical Care Nursing Clinics of North America*, *1*(4), 697–705.

Giger, J., & Davidhizar, R. (2008). *Transcultural nursing*. St. Louis: Mosby-Year Book.

Gilbert, E. S. (2007). *Manual of high risk pregnancy and delivery* (4th ed.). St. Louis: Mosby.

Gordon, M. (1982). Historical perspective: The National Group for Classification of Nursing Diagnoses. In M. J. Kim & D. A. Moritz (Eds.), *Classification of nursing diagnoses: Proceedings of the fourth national conference.* New York: McGraw-Hill.

Gordon, M. (1994). *Nursing diagnosis: Process and application.* St. Louis: Mosby-Year Book.

Grainger, R. (1990). Anxiety interrupters. *American Journal of Nursing, 90*(2), 14–15.

Gray, J. (1995). *Mars and Venus in the bedroom: A guide to lasting romance and passion.* New York: Harper Collins.

Grealish, L., Lomasney, A., & Whiteman, B. (2000). Foot massage. A nursing intervention to modify the distressing symptoms of pain and nausea in patients hospitalized with cancer. *Cancer Nursing, 23,* 237–243.

Grober, M. (Ed.). (1984). *Dysphagia.* Oxford, UK: Butterworth-Heinemann.

Hagen, B. (2001). Nursing home placement. *Journal of Gerontological Nursing, 27*(2), 44–53.

Hagan, J. F., Shaw, J. S., & Duncan, P. M. (Eds.). (2008). *Bright futures: Guidelines for health supervision of infants, children, and adolescents* (3rd ed.). Elk Grove Village, IL: American Academy of Pediatrics.

Hale, T. W. (2010). *Medications and mother's milk* (14th ed.). Amarillo, TX: Hale Publications.

Hall, G. R. (1991). Altered thought processes: Dementia. In M. Maas, K. Buckwalter, & M. Hardy (Eds.), *Nursing diagnoses and interventions for the elderly.* Menlo Park, CA: Addison-Wesley Nursing.

Hall, G. R. (1994). Caring for people with Alzheimer's disease using the conceptual model of progressively lowered stress threshold in the clinical setting. *Nursing Clinics of North America, 29,* 129–141.

Hall, G. R., & Buckwalter, K. C. (1987). Progressively lowered stress threshold: A conceptual model for care of adults with

Alzheimer's disease. *Archives of Psychiatric Nursing, 1,* 399–406.

Hammell, K. W., Miller, W. C., Forwell, S. J., & Jacobsen, B. A. (2009). Fatigue and spinal cord injury: A qualitative analysis. *Spinal Cord, 47,* 44–49. doi: 10.1038/sc2008.68

Harkulich, J., & Brugler, C. (1988). Nursing diagnosis—translocation syndrome: Expert validation study. Partial funding granted by the Peg Schiltz Fund, Delta Xi Chapter, Sigma Theta Tau International. Indianapolis, IN: Sigma Theta Tau International.

Hatton, C. L., & McBride, S. (1984). *Suicide: Assessment and intervention.* Norwalk, CT: Appleton-Century-Crofts.

Heinrich, L. (1987). Care of the female rape victim. *Nurse Practitioner, 12*(11), 9.

Herman-Staab, B. (1994). Screening, management and appropriate referral for pediatric behavior problems. *Nurse Practitioner, 19*(7), 40–49.

Herth, K. (1993). Hope in the family caregiver of terminally ill people. *Journal of Advanced Nursing, 18,* 538–547.

Hickey, J. (2006). *The clinical practice of neurological and neurosurgical nursing* (5th ed.). Philadelphia: Lippincott Williams & Wilkins.

Hiltunen, E. (1987). Diagnostic content validity of the nursing diagnosis: Decisional conflict. In A. M. McLane (Ed.). *Classification of nursing diagnoses: Proceedings of the seventh conference.* St. Louis: Mosby.

Hinds, P., Martin, J., & Vogel, R. (1987). Nursing strategies to influence adolescent hopefulness during oncologic illness. *Journal of the Association of Pediatric Oncology Nurses, 4*(1/2), 14–23.

Hockenberry, M. J. (2011). Family influences on child health promotion. In M. J. Hockenberry & D. Wilson (Eds.), *Wong's nursing care of infants and children* (pp. 46–67). St. Louis, MO: Elsevier Mosby.

Hockenberry, M. J., & Wilson, D. (2009). *Wong's essentials of pediatric nursing* (6th ed.). St. Louis: Mosby.

Hockenberry, M. J., & Wilson, D., (2007). *Wong's nursing care of infants and children* (8th ed.). Elsevier.

Holditch-Davis, D., & Blackburn, S. (2007). Neurobehavioral development. In C. Kenner & J. W. Lott (Eds.), *Comprehensive neonatal care: an interdisciplinary approach* (4th ed., pp. 448–479). St. Louis: Saunders Elsevier.

Holmstrom, L., & Burgess, A. W. (1975). Development of diagnostic categories: Sexual traumas. *American Journal of Nursing, 75,* 1288–1291.

Hooyman, N. R. & Kramer, B. J. (2006). *Living through loss: Interventions across the life span.* New York: Columbia University Press.

Iezzoni, L. F., O'Day, B., Keleen, M. A., & Harker, H. (2004). Improving patient care: Communicating about health care: Observations from persons who are deaf or hard of hearing. *Annals of Internal Medicine, 140*(5), 356–362.

Institute for Healthcare Improvement. (2008). Implement the ventilator bundle: Elevation of the head of the bed. Retrieved from www.ihi.org/IHI/Topics/ CriticalCare/IntensiveCare/ Changes/IndividualChanges/ Elevationoftheheadofthebed.htm

Janssen, J., & Giberson, D. (1988). Remotivation therapy. *Journal of Gerontological Nursing, 14*(6), 31–34.

Jennings, P. (1997). The aging spirit. Faith and hope—therapeutic tools for case managers. *Aging Today, 18*(2), 17.

Jenny, J. (1987). Knowledge deficit: Not a nursing diagnosis. *Image: Journal of Nursing Scholarship, 19*(4), 184–185.

Jenny, J., & Logan, J. (1991). Interventions for the nursing diagnosis Dysfunctional Ventilatory Weaning Response: A qualitative study. In R. M. Carroll-Johnson (Ed.), *Classification of nursing diagnoses.* Philadelphia: J. B. Lippincott.

Johnson, B. S. (1995). *Child, adolescent and family psychiatric nursing.* Philadelphia: J. B. Lippincott.

Johnson-Crowley, N. (1993). Systematic assessment and home follow-up. In C. Kenner, A. Brueggemeyer, & L. Gunderson (Eds.), *Comprehensive neonatal nursing.* Philadelphia: W. B. Saunders.

Jones, P. E., & Jakob, D. F. (1984). Anxiety revisited from a practice perspective. In M. J. Kim, G. K. McFarland, & A. M. McLane (Eds.), *Classification of nursing diagnoses: Proceedings of the fifth national conference.* St. Louis: C. V. Mosby.

Kaakinen, J. R., Gedaly-Duff, V., Hanson, S. M. H., & Padgett, D. (2010). *Family health care nursing: Theory, practice, and research* (4th ed.). Philadelphia: F. A. Davis.

Kavchak-Keyes, M. A. (2000). Autonomic hyperreflexia. *Rehabilitation Nursing, 25*(1), 31–35.

Keegan, L. (2000). Protocols for practice: Applying research at the bedside. Alternative and complementary modalities for managing stress and anxiety. *Critical Care Nurse, 20*(3), 93–96.

Kendrick, K. D., & Robinson, S. (2000). Spirituality: Its relevance and purpose for clinical nursing in the new millennium. *Journal of Clinical Nursing, 9*(5), 701–705.

Kimball, M. J., & Williams-Burgess, C. (1995). Failure to thrive: The silent epidemic of the elderly. *Archives of Psychiatric Nursing, 9*(2), 99–105.

Kono, A., Kai, I., Sakato, C., & Rubenstein, L. (2004). Frequency of going outdoors: A predictor of functional and psychosocial change among ambulatory frail elders living at home. *Journals of Gerontology Series A: Biological Sciences and Medical Sciences, 59*(3), 275–280.

Kovalesky, A. (2004). Women with substance abuse concerns. *Nursing Clinics of North America, 39*(1), 205–217.

Krieger, D. (1987). *The therapeutic touch: How to use your hands to help or to heal.* Englewood Cliffs, NJ: Prentice-Hall.

Landis, C., & Moc, K. (2004). Sleep and menopause. *Nursing Clinics of North America, 39*(1), 97–115.

Larson, C. E. (2000). Evidence-based practice. Safety and efficacy of oral rehydration therapy for treatment of diarrhea and gastro-enteritis in pediatrics. *Pediatric Nursing, 26*(2), 177–179.

LaSala, C. A., & Bjarnason, D. (2010). Creating workplace environments that support moral courage. *The Online Journal of Issues in Nursing, 15*(3), 1–11. Retrieved from http://www.nursingworld.org/OJIN

Ledray, L. E. (2001). Evidence collection and care of the sexually assault survivor: SANE-SART response. Retrieved from www.vaw.umn.edu/ documents/commissioned/2forensicvidence.htlm

Leuner, J., Coler, M., & Norris, J. (1994). Self-esteem. In M. Rantz & P. LeMone (Eds.), *Classification of nursing diagnosis: Proceedings of the eleventh conference.* Glendale, CA: CINAHL.

Levin, R. F., Krainovitch, B. C., Bahrenburg, E., & Mitchell, C. A. (1989). Diagnostic content validity of nursing diagnoses. *Image: Journal of Nursing Scholarship, 21*(1), 40–44.

Lindeman, M., Hokanson, J., & Batek, J. (1994). The alcoholic family. *Nursing Diagnosis, 5*(2), 65–73.

Lindgren, C. L., Burke, M. L., Hainsworth, M. A., & Eakes, G. G. (1992). Chronic sorrow: A lifespan concept. *Scholarly Inquiry for Nursing Practice, 24*(6), 27–42.

Logan, J., & Jenny, J. (1990). Deriving a new nursing diagnosis through qualitative research: Dysfunctional ventilatory weaning response. *Nursing Diagnosis, 1*(1), 37–43.

Logan, J., & Jenny, J. (1991). Interventions for the nursing diagnosis Dysfunctional Ventilatory Weaning Response: A qualitative study. In R. M. Carroll-Johnson (Ed.), *Classification of nursing diagnoses: Proceedings of the ninth conference* (pp. 141–147). Philadelphia: J. B. Lippincott.

Lugina, H. I., Christensson, K., Massawe, S., Nystrom, L., & Lindmark, G. (2001). Change in maternal concerns during the 6 weeks postpartum period: A study of primaparous mothers in Dar es Salaam, Tanzania. *Journal of Midwifery and Women's Health, 46*(4), 248–257.

Lusardi P., Jodka, P., Stambovsky, M., Stadnicki, B., Babb, B., Plouffe, D., . . . Montonye, M. (2011). The going home initiative: Getting critical care patients home with hospice. *Critical Care Nurse, 31*(5), 46–57.

Lutz, K. F., Anderson, L. S., Riesch, S. K., Pridham, K. A., & Becker, P. T. (2009). Furthering the understanding of parent-child relationships: a nursing scholarship review series. Part 2: grasping the early parenting experience-the insider view. *Journal of the Society of Pediatric Nurses, 14*, 262–284.

Lyon, B. A. (2002). Cognitive self-care skills: A model for managing stressful lifestyles. *Nursing Clinics of North America, 37*(2), 285–294.

Macauley, M., Pettersen, L., Fader, M., Brooks, R., & Cottenden, R. (2004). A multicenter evaluation of absorbent products for children with incontinence and disabilities. *Journal of WOCN, 31*(4), 235–244.

Maddox, T. (2002). Adverse reactions to contrast material: Recognition, prevention, and treatment. *American Family Physician, Oct 1; 66*(7), 1229–1234.

Magnan, M. A. (1987). *Activity intolerance: Toward a nursing theory of activity.* Paper presented at the Fifth Annual Symposium of the Michigan Nursing Diagnosis Association, Detroit.

Maher, A. B., Salmond, S. W., & Pellino, T. (1998). *Orthopedic nursing* (2nd ed.). Philadelphia: W. B. Saunders.

Maier-Lorentz, M. M. (2000). Effective nursing interventions for the management of Alzheimer's disease. *Journal of Neuroscience Nursing, 32*(3), 153–157.

Maklebust, J. (2005). Choosing the right support surface. *Advances in Skin and Wound Care, 18*(3), 158–161.

Maklebust, J., & Sieggreen, M. Y. (1996). Attacking on all fronts. How to conquer pressure ulcers. *Nursing, 26*(12), 34–39.

Maresca, T. (1986). Assessment and management of acute diarrheal illness in adults. *Nurse Practitioner, 11*(11), 15–16.

Maroni, J. (1989). Impaired social interactions. In G. McFarland, & E. McFarlane (Eds.), *Nursing diagnosis and interventions.* St. Louis: C. V. Mosby.

May, J. (1996). Fathers: The forgotten parent. *Pediatric Nursing, 22*(3), 243–271.

May, K. A., & Mahlmeister, L. R. (1994). *Maternal and neonatal nursing: Family-centered care* (3rd ed.). Philadelphia: J. B. Lippincott.

May, R. (1977). *The meaning of anxiety.* New York: W. W. Norton.

Maynard, C. K. (2004). Assess and manage somatization. *Holistic Nursing Practice, 18*(2), 54–60.

Mayo Clinic Staff. (2011). Allergy-proof your house. Retrieved from http://www.mayoclinic.com/health/allergy/HQ01514

McFarland, G., & Wasli, E. (2000). Manipulation in nursing diagnosis and process. In B. S. Johnson (Ed.), *Psychiatric-mental health nursing* (5th ed.; p. 147). Philadelphia: J. B. Lippincott.

McFarland, G., Wasli, E., & Gerety, E. (1996). *Nursing diagnoses and process in psychiatric mental health nursing* (5th ed.). Philadelphia: J. B. Lippincott.

McLane, A., & McShane, R. (1986). Empirical validation of defining characteristics of constipation: A study of bowel elimination practices of healthy adults. In M. E. Hurley (Ed.), *Classification of nursing diagnoses: Proceedings of the sixth conference* (pp. 448–455). St. Louis: Mosby.

McMillan, J., DeAngelis, C., Feigin, R., & Warshaw, J. (1999). *Oski's pediatrics: Principles and practice.* Philadelphia: Lippincott Williams & Wilkins.

Meehan, T. G. (1991). Therapeutic touch. In G. Bulechek & J. McCloskey (Eds.), *Nursing interventions: Essential nursing treatments.* Philadelphia: W. B. Saunders.

Melnyk, B., Feinstein, N., Moldenhouer, Z., & Small, L. (2001). Coping of parents of children who are chronically ill. *Pediatric Nursing, 27*(6), 548–558.

Merenstein, G. B., & Gardner, S. L. (1998). *Handbook of neonatal intensive care* (4th ed.). St. Louis: Mosby-Year Book.

Miller, C. (2009). *Nursing for wellness in older adults* (5th ed.). Philadelphia: Lippincott Williams & Wilkins.

Mina, C. (1985). A program for helping grieving parents. *Maternal-Child Nursing Journal, 10,* 118–121.

Mohr, W. K. (2009). *Psychiatric-mental health nursing: Adaptation and growth* (6th ed.). Philadelphia: Lippincott Williams & Wilkins.

Monsen, R. B. (1999). Mothers' experiences of living worried when parenting children with spina bifida. *Journal of Pediatric Nursing, 14*(3), 157–163.

Moorhead, S., Johnson, M., Maas, M., & Swanson, E. (2008). *Nursing outcomes classification (NOC).* St. Louis: Mosby.

Morison, M. (1998). Family attitudes to bed-wetting and their influence on treatment. *Professional Nurse, 13*(5), 321–325.

Morton, P., Fontaine, D., Hudak, C., & Gallo, B. (2005). *Critical care nursing* (8th ed.). Philadelphia: Lippincott Williams & Wilkins.

Movaffaghi, Z., Hasanpoor, M., Farsi, M., Hooshmand, P., & Abrishami, F. (2006). Effects of therapeutic touch on blood hemoglobim and hematocrit. *Journal of Holistic Nursing, 24*(1), 41–48.

Murray, J. S. (2000). A concept analysis of social support as experienced by siblings of children with cancer. *Journal of Pediatric Nursing, 15*(5), 313–322.

Murray, R. B., Zentner, J. P., & Yakimo, R. (2009). *Health promotion strategies through the life span* (8th ed.). Upper Saddle River, NJ: Pear-Prentice Hall.

NANDA International. (2007). *NANDA nursing diagnosis: Definitions and classifications.* Philadelphia: Author.

NANDA International. (2012). *Nursing diagnoses: Definitions and classification 2012–2014.* Ames, IA: Wiley-Blackwell.

National Comprehensive Cancer Network. (2008). *Oral mucositis is often underrecognized and undertreated.* Retrieved from www.nccn.org/professionals/meetings/13thannual/highlights

National Safety Council. (2000). *Injury facts.* Itaska, IL: National Safety Council.

Newman, J., & Pittman, T. (2006). *The ultimate breastfeeding book of answers* (3rd ed.). New York: Three Rivers Press.

Nicoll, L. H. (2002). Heat in motion: Evaluating and managing temperature. *Nursing, 32*(5), s1–s12.

Norris, J., & Kunes-Connell, M. (1987). Self-esteem disturbance: A clinical validation study. In A. McLane (Ed.), *Classification of nursing diagnoses: Proceedings of the seventh NANDA national conference.* St. Louis: Mosby.

Northington, L. (2000). Chronic sorrow in caregivers of school age children with sickle cell disease: A grounded theory approach. *Issues in Comprehensive Pediatric Nursing, 23*(3), 141–154.

O'Brien, M. E. (2010). *Spirituality in nursing: Standing on holy ground* (4th ed.). Boston: Jones and Bartlett.

Owen, M., & Grier, M. (1987). *Infection risk assessment guide.* Orange, CA: Unpublished.

Palmer, B. (2006, March 4). *Breastfeeding and frenulums.* Paper presented at the Bay Area Lactation Associates Conference, Berkley, CA.

Pasero. C., & McCaffery, M. (2011). *Pain assessment and pharmaceutical management,* New York: Mosby.

Pearlin, L., Mullan, J., Semple, S., & Skaff, M. (1990). Caregiving and the stress process: An overview of concepts and their measures. *The Gerontologist, 30,* 583–594.

Pfeffer, C. R. (1981). Development issues among children of separation and divorce. In I. R. Stuart & L. E. Abt (Eds.), *Children of separation and divorce: Management and treatment.* New York: Van Nostrand Reinhold.

Pillitteri, A. (2010). *Maternal and child health nursing* (6th ed.). Philadelphia: Lippincott Williams & Wilkins.

Polomeno, V. (1999). Sex and babies: Pregnant couples' postnatal sexual concerns. *Journal of Perinatal Education, 8*(4), 9–18.

Porth, C. M. (2011). *Essentials of pathophysiology: Concepts of altered health states* (3rd ed.). Philadelphia: Lippincott Williams & Wilkins.

Puchalski, C. M., & Ferrell, B. (2010). *Making health care whole: Integrating spirituality into patient care.* West Conshohocken, PA: Templeton Press.

Puterbough, C. (1991). Hypothermia related to exposure and surgical interventions. *Today's OR Nurse, 13*(7), 32–33.

Quinn, C. (1994). The four A's of restraint reduction: Attention, assessment, anticipation, avoidance. *Orthopaedic Nursing, 13*(2), 11–19.

Rantz, M. (1991). Diversional activity deficit. In M. Maas, K. Buckwalter, & M. Hardy (Eds.), *Nursing diagnoses and interventions for the elderly.*

Redwood City, CA: Addison-Wesley Nursing.

Rasin, J. (1990). Confusion. *Nursing Clinics of North America, 25,* 909–918.

Rateau, M. R. (2000). Confusion and aggression in restrained elderly persons undergoing hip repair surgery. *Applied Nursing Research, 13*(1), 50–54.

Reeder, S., Martin, L., & Koniak-Griffin, D. (1997). *Maternity nursing* (18th ed.). Philadelphia: Lippincott-Raven.

Regalado, M., Sareen, H., Inkelas, M., Wissow, L., & Halfon, N. (2004). Parents' discipline of young children: Results from the National Survey of Early Childhood Health. *Pediatrics, 113*(5), 1952–1958.

Reichel, S. M. (1958). Shearing force as a factor in decubitus ulcers in paraplegics. *Journal of the American Medical Association, 166*(7), 762–763.

Rhoten, D. (1982). Fatigue and the postsurgical patient. In C. Norris (Ed.), *Concept clarification in nursing.* Rockville, MD: Aspen Systems.

Robbins, J. B., & Pozniak, M. A. (2010). Contrast media tutorial. Retrieved from https:// www.radiology.wisc.edu/ fileShelf/contrastCorner/ files/ ContrastAgentsTutorial.pdf

Roberts, B. L. (2001). Managing delirium in adult intensive care patients. *Critical Care Nurse, 21*(1), 48–55.

Rothrock, J. C. (2003). *Alexander's care of the patient in surgery* (12th ed.). St. Louis: Mosby.

Sampselle, C., & DeLancey, J. (1998). Anatomy of female continence. *Journal of Wound, Ostomy and Continence Nursing, 25*(3), 63–74.

Santrock, J. (2004). *Life-Span Development* (9th ed.). Boston: McGraw-Hill.

Scardillo, J., & Aronovitch, S. A. (1999). Successfully managing incontinence-related irritant dermatitis across the lifespan. *Ostomy Wound Management, 45*(4), 36–44.

Schoenfelder, D. P. (2000). A fall prevention program for elderly individuals. *Journal of Gerontological Nursing, 26*(3), 43–45.

Shields, C. (1992). Family interaction and caregivers of Alzheimer's disease patients: Correlates of depression. *Family Process, 31*(3), 19–32.

Shrago, L., & Bocar, D. (1990). The infant's contribution to breastfeeding. *Journal of Obstetric, Gynecologic, and Neonatal Nursing, 19*(3), 209–211.

Shua-Haim, J., Sabo, M., & Ross, J. (1999). Constipation in the elderly: A practical approach. *Clinical Geriatrics, 7*(12), 91–99.

Siddiqi, N. (2011). Contrast medium reactions. *Medscape.* Retrieved from http://emedicine.medscape. com/article/422855-overview

Simpson, K. R., & Creehan, P. A. (2007). *AWHONN's perinatal nursing* (3rd ed.). Philadelphia: Lippincott Williams & Wilkins.

Singh, J., & Daftary, A. (2008). Iodinated contrast media and their adverse reactions. *Journal of Nuclear Medicine Technology, 36*(2), 69–74.

Smeltzer, S., Bare, B., Hinkle, J., & Cheever, K. (2010). *Brunner & Suddarth's textbook of medical-surgical nursing* (12th ed.). Philadelphia: Lippincott Williams & Wilkins.

Smith, L. (1999). Family-centered decision-making: A model for parent participation. *Journal of Neonatal Nursing, 5*(6), 31–33.

Soholt, D. (1990). *A life experience: Making a health care treatment decision.* Unpublished master's thesis. Brookings, SD: South Dakota State University.

Somani, B. K. (2009). Autonomic dysreflexia: A medical emergency with spinal cord injury. *International Journal of Clinical Practice, 63*(3), 350–352. doi: 10.1111/j.1742-1241.2008.01844.x

Stang, I., & Mittelmark, M. B. (2008). Learning as an empowerment process in breast cancer self-help groups. *Journal of Clinical Nursing, 18*(14), 2049–2057.

Stanley, M., & Beare, P. G. (2000). *Gerontological nursing*. Philadelphia: F. A. Davis.

Starling, B. P., & Martin, A. C. (1990). Adult survivors of parental alcoholism: Implications for primary care. *Nursing Practice, 15*(7), 16–24.

Stephenson, N. L., Weinrich, S. P., & Tavakoli, A. S. (2000). The effects of foot reflexology on anxiety and pain in patients with breast and lung cancer. *Oncology Nursing Forum, 27*, 67–72.

Stuart, G. W., & Sundeen, S. (2002). *Principles and practice of psychiatric nursing* (6th ed.). St. Louis: Mosby-Year Book.

Swadener-Culpepper, L. (2010). Continuous lateral rotation therapy. *Critical Care Nurse, 30*(2), S5–S7. Retrieved from Medline Database.

Swift, C., Calcutawalla, S., & Elliot, R. (2007). Nursing attitudes towards recording of religious and spiritual data. *British Journal of Nursing, 16*(20), 1279–1282.

Taylor, E. J. (2000). Spiritual and ethical end-of-life concerns. In C. H. Yarbro, M. H. Frogge, M. Goodman, & S. L. Groenwald. *Cancer nursing: Principles and practice* (5th ed.). Boston: Jones and Bartlett.

Taylor, S. E., Klein, L. C., Lewis, B., & Petal, C. (2000). Biobehavioral responses to stress in females: Tend and befriend, not fight-or-flight. *Psychology Review, 107*(3), 411–429.

Taylor-Loughran, A., O'Brien, M., LaChapelle, R., & Rangel, S. (1989). Defining characteristics of the nursing diagnoses fear and anxiety: A validation study. *Applied Nursing Research, 2*, 178–186.

Teel, C. S. (1991). Chronic sorrow: Analysis of the concept. *Journal of Advanced Nursing, 16*(11), 1311–1319.

Thomas, K. A. (1989). How the NICU environment sounds to a preterm infant. *MCN: American Journal of Maternal Child Nursing, 14*(4), 249–251.

Thomas, S. P. (1998). Assessing and intervening with anger disorders. *Nursing Clinics of North America, 33*(1), 121–134.

Thorns, A., & Edmonds, P. (2000). The management of pruritus in palliative care patients. *European Journal of Palliative Care, 7*(1), 9–12.

Townsend, M. C. (1994). *Nursing diagnosis in psychiatric nursing* (3rd ed.). Philadelphia: F. A. Davis.

Tusaie, K., & Dyer, J. (2004). Resilience: A historical review of the construct. *Holistic Nursing Practice, 18*(1), 3–8.

Vandenberg, K. (1990). The management of oral nippling in the sick neonate, the disorganized feeder. *Neonatal Network, 9*(1), 9–16.

VandenBerg, K. (2007). State systems development in high-risk newborns in the neonatal intensive care unit: Identification and management of sleep, alertness, and crying. *Journal Perinatal & Neonatal Nursing, 21*(2), 130–139.

Vanezis, M., & McGee, A. (1999). Mediating factors in the grieving process of the suddenly bereaved. *British Journal of Nursing, 8*(14), 932–937.

Varcarolis, E. M. (2011) *Manual of psychiatric nursing care plans* (4th ed.). St. Louis: Saunders.

Varcarolis, E. M., Carson, V. B., & Shoemaker, N. C. (2010). *Foundations of psychiatric mental health nursing* (6th ed.). Philadelphia: W. B. Saunders.

Vickers, J. L., & Carlisle, C. (2000). Choices and control: Parental experiences in pediatric terminal home care. *Journal of Pediatric Oncology Nursing, 17*(1), 12–21.

Vincent, K. G. (1985). The validation of a nursing diagnosis. *Nursing Clinics of North America, 20*(4), 631–639.

Voith, A. M., Frank, A. M., & Pigg, J. S. (1987). Validations of fatigue as a nursing diagnosis. In A. McLane (Ed.), *Classification of nursing diagnoses: Proceedings of the seventh national conference* (p. 280). St. Louis: Mosby.

Walker, M. (2006). *Breastfeeding management for the clinician: Using the evidence.* Sudbury, WA: Jones & Bartlett.

Walsh, K. & Kowanko, I. (2002). Nurses' and patients' perceptions of dignity. *International Journal of Nursing Practice, 8*(3), 143–151.

Weeks, S. K., Hubbartt, E., & Michaels, T. K. (2000). Keys to bowel success. *Rehabilitation Nursing, 25*(2), 66–80.

Whitley, G. (1994). Concept analysis in nursing diagnosis research. In R. Carroll-Johnson & M. Paquette (Eds.), *Classification of nursing diagnosis: Proceedings of the tenth conference.* Philadelphia: J. B. Lippincott.

Wilkinson, J., & Van Leuven, K. (2007). *Fundamentals of nursing: Theory, concepts & applications.* Philadelphia: F. A. Davis.

Williams, A. M. (2000). Distress and hardiness: a comparison of African-American and white caregivers. *Journal of National Black Nurses' Association. 11*(1), 21–26.

Willis, D., & Porche, D. (2004). Male battering of intimate partners: Theoretical underpinnings, intervention approaches, and implications. *Nursing Clinics of North America, 39*(2), 271–282.

Willis, E., & Strasburger, V. (1998). Media violence. *Pediatric Clinics of North America, 45*(2), 319–331.

Winslow, B., & Carter, P. (1999). Patterns of burden in wives who care for husbands with dementia. *Nursing Clinics of North America, 34*(2), 275–287.

Woods, S. L., & Ehrat, K. S. (2009). *The art of EKG interpretation: A elf-instructional text* (7th ed.). Dubuque, Iowa: Kendall-Hunt.

Worden, W. (2002). *Grief counseling and grief therapy* (3rd ed.). New York: Springer.

Wound Ostomy Continence Nursing (WOCN). (2003). *Guideline for prevention and management of pressure ulcers.* Glenview, IL: WOCN.

Wright, L. M. (2004). *Spirituality, suffering, and illness: Ideas for healing.* Philadelphia: F.A. Davis Co.

Wysocki, T., & Wayne, W. (1992). Childhood diabetes and the family. *Practical Diabetology, 11*(20), 29–32.

Yakimo, R. (2006), Perspectives on psychiatric consultation liaison nursing. *Perspectives in Psychiatric Care, 42,* 59–62.

Yarbro, C. H., Wujcik, D., & Gobel, B. (2011). *Cancer nursing: Principles and practice* (7th ed.). Boston: Jones and Bartlett.

Yokom, C. J. (1984). The differentiation of fear and anxiety. In M. J. Kim, G. K. McFarland, & A. M. McLane (Eds.), *Classification of nursing diagnoses: Proceedings of the fifth national conference.* St. Louis: C. V. Mosby.

Young, M. G. (2001). Providing care for the caregiver. *Patient Care for the Nurse Practitioner, 2,* 36–47.

Zerwich, J. (1992). Laying the groundwork for family self-help: Locating families, building trust and building strength. *Public Health Nursing, 9*(1), 15–21.

Zuzelo, P. R. (2007). Exploring the moral distress of registered nurses. *Nursing Ethics, 14*(3), 344–359.

Index

Page numbers followed by *t* or *b* indicate tables and boxes, respectively. Nursing diagnoses are in **bold**.